Chronic Pain: Assessment, Diagnosis and Treatment

Chronic Pain: Assessment, Diagnosis and Treatment

Editor: Pam Kellner

FOSTER ACADEMICS

www.fosteracademics.com

www.fosteracademics.com

FOSTER ACADEMICS

Cataloging-in-Publication Data

Chronic pain : assessment, diagnosis and treatment / edited by Pam Kellner.
p. cm.
Includes bibliographical references and index.
ISBN 978-1-63242-477-8
1. Chronic pain. 2. Chronic pain--Diagnosis. 3. Chronic pain--Treatment. 4. Pain--Physiological aspects.
5. Pain medicine. I. Kellner, Pam.
RB127 .C47 2017
616.047 2--dc23

Foster Academics,
118-35 Queens Blvd., Suite 400,
Forest Hills, NY 11375, USA

ISBN 978-1-63242-477-8 (Hardback)

Printed and bound in China.

Contents

Preface

The world is advancing at a fast pace like never before. Therefore, the need is to keep up with the latest developments. This book was an idea that came to fruition when the specialists in the area realized the need to coordinate together and document essential themes in the subject. That's when I was requested to be the editor. Editing this book has been an honour as it brings together diverse authors researching on different streams of the field. The book collates essential materials contributed by veterans in the area which can be utilized by students and researchers alike.

Pain and pain management is defined as the science of treating and diagnosing chronic pain. This book on chronic pain explores topics related to intense pain, its treatment and recurrent musculoskeletal pain. Some of the most popular treatments for chronic pain include physical therapy, international procedures, etc. The objective of this book is to give a general view of the different areas of chronic pain such as its diagnosis and treatment. It brings forth some of the most innovative concepts and elucidates the unexplored aspects of chronic pain. With state-of-the-art inputs by acclaimed experts of this field, this book targets students and professionals.

Each chapter is a sole-standing publication that reflects each author's interpretation. Thus, the book displays a multi-facetted picture of our current understanding of applications and diverse aspects of the field. I would like to thank the contributors of this book and my family for their endless support.

Editor

Antiplatelet Effect of Catechol Is Related to Inhibition of Cyclooxygenase, Reactive Oxygen Species, ERK/p38 Signaling and Thromboxane A_2 Production

Mei-Chi Chang[1]ⓢ, Hsiao-Hua Chang[2]ⓢ, Tong-Mei Wang[2], Chiu-Po Chan[3]ⓢ, Bor-Ru Lin[4], Sin-Yuet Yeung[3], Chien-Yang Yeh[2], Ru-Hsiu Cheng[1], Jiiang-Huei Jeng[2]*

1 Biomedical Science Team, Chang Gung University of Science and Technology, Taoyuan,Taiwan, **2** Laboratory of Pharmacology & Toxicology, Graduate Institute of Clinical Dentistry and Department of Dentistry, National Taiwan University Hospital and National Taiwan University Medical College, Taipei, Taiwan, **3** Department of Dentistry, Chang Gung Memorial Hospital and Chang Gung University, Taipei, Taiwan, **4** Department of Diagnotherapeutics, National Taiwan University Hospital, Taipei, Taiwan

Abstract

Catechol (benzenediol) is present in plant-derived products, such as vegetables, fruits, coffee, tea, wine, areca nut and cigarette smoke. Because platelet dysfunction is a risk factor of cardiovascular diseases, including stroke, atherosclerosis and myocardial infarction, the purpose of this study was to evaluate the anti-platelet and anti-inflammatory effect of catechol and its mechanisms. The effects of catechol on cyclooxygenase (COX) activity, arachidonic acid (AA)-induced aggregation, thromboxane B_2 (TXB_2) production, lactate dehydrogenase (LDH) release, reactive oxygen species (ROS) production and extracellular signal-regulated kinase (ERK)/p38 phosphorylation were determined in rabbit platelets. In addition, its effect on IL-1β-induced prostaglandin E_2 (PGE_2) production by fibroblasts was determined. The *ex vivo* effect of catechol on platelet aggregation was also measured. Catechol (5-25 μM) suppressed AA-induced platelet aggregation and inhibited TXB_2 production at concentrations of 0.5–5 μM; however, it showed little cytotoxicity and did not alter U46619-induced platelet aggregation. Catechol (10–50 μM) suppressed COX-1 activity by 29–44% and COX-2 activity by 29–50%. It also inhibited IL-1β-induced PGE_2 production, but not COX-2 expression of fibroblasts. Moreover, catechol (1–10 μM) attenuated AA-induced ROS production in platelets and phorbol myristate acetate (PMA)-induced ROS production in human polymorphonuclear leukocytes. Exposure of platelets to catechol decreased AA-induced ERK and p38 phosphorylation. Finally, intravenous administration of catechol (2.5–5 μmole/mouse) attenuated *ex vivo* AA-induced platelet aggregation. These results suggest that catechol exhibited anti-platelet and anti-inflammatory effects, which were mediated by inhibition of COX, ROS and TXA_2 production as well as ERK/p38 phosphorylation. The anti-platelet effect of catechol was confirmed by *ex vivo* analysis. Exposure to catechol may affect platelet function and thus cardiovascular health.

Editor: Xin-Yuan Guan, The University of Hong Kong, China

Funding: The authors would like to thank Miss HF Jeng for her technical assistance. This study is supported by grants from National Science Council (NSC102-2314-B-255-003-MY2, NSC102-2628-B-255-001-MY3, NSC101-2320-B-255-002, NSC-100-2314-B-002-094 and NSC-101-2320-B-255-002) and Chang Gung Memorial Hospital (CMRPF1C0011, CMRPF1C0012, NMRPF3C0091, NMRPF3C0061). The funders had no role in study design, data collection and analysis, decision to publish, or preparation of the manuscript.

Competing Interests: The authors have declared that no competing interests exist.

* Email: jhjeng@ntu.edu.tw

ⓢ These authors contributed equally to this work.

Introduction

Various benzenediols (e.g., catechol, resorcinol, hydroquinone [HQ]) are present in many plant-derived products, including vegetables, areca nut, fruits, grains, coffee, tea, beer, and wine [1–3]. Many catechol (i.e., pyrocatechol) derivatives have been suggested to have therapeutic potential. Phenol and catechol (1,2-benzenediol) are two major metabolites identified in the urine of workers occupationally exposed to benzene. In addition, catechol and HQ (e.g., 1,4-benzenediol) levels in peripheral blood may be a marker of exposure to benzene or cigarette smoke [4]. However, the effect of catechol on human health remains to be investigated.

Catechol scavenges diphenylpicrylhydrazyl radicals and reactive oxygen species (ROS) [5]. The structure of catechin and hydroxychavicol may be responsible for its ROS scavenging and anti-platelet activities [6]. However, Lee and Lin [7] found that catechol, pyrogallol and 1,2,4-benzenetriol may gerenate ROS and exhibit mutagenicity. In addition, catechol and HQ may antagonize transforming growth factor-β (TGF-β)-induced elimination of transformed cells suggesting a co-carcinogenic effect [8].

In many countries, cardiovascular diseases, such as atherosclerosis, stroke and myocardial infarction, are responsible for a great proportion of human morbidity and mortality [9]. Platelets play important roles in thrombosis and hemostasis through platelet adhesion, activation and aggregation; their aggregation may be

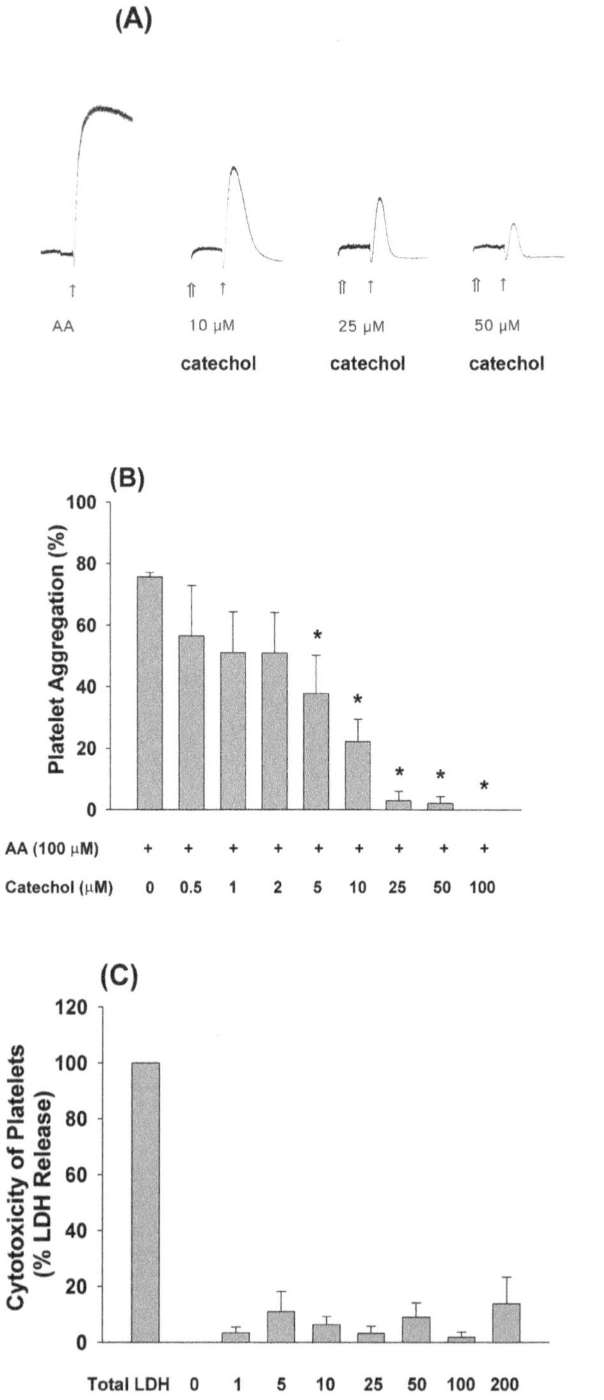

Figure 1. Inhibition of AA-induced platelet aggregation by different concentrations of catechol. (A) One representative picture of AA-induced platelet aggregation and its inhibition by catechol was shown. (B) Quantitative analysis of AA (100 μM)-induced platelet aggregation and its inhibition by catechol (0.5–100 μM). Results were expressed as % of platelet aggregation (n = 5–8). (C) Cytotoxicity of catechol to platelets. Results were expressed as % of LDH release (n = 3). ↑ indicates the addition of AA, and ⇑ indicates the addition of catechol. *indicates significant difference when compared with AA-treated group (P<0.05).

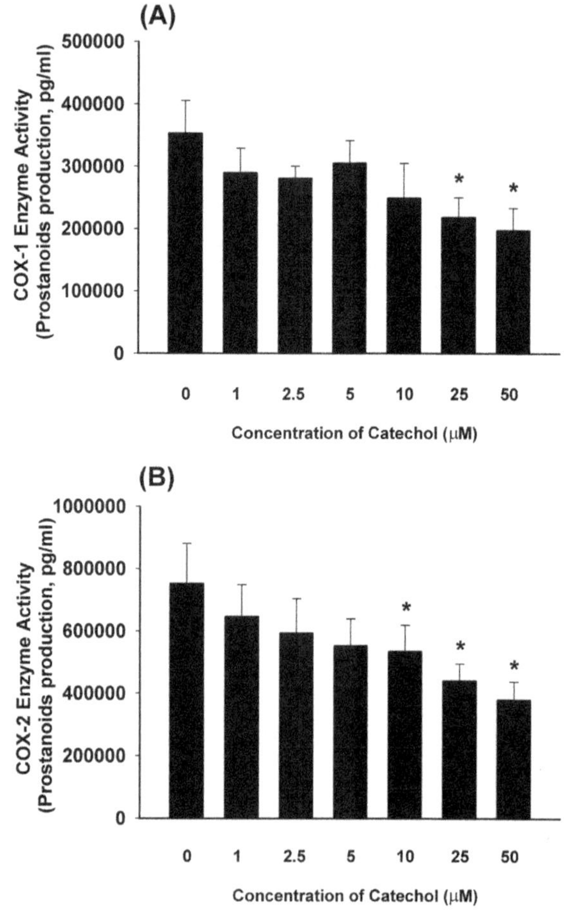

Figure 2. Effect of different concentrations of catechol on the (A) COX-1 enzyme activity (n = 6), and (B) COX-2 enzyme activity (n = 6). Results were expressed as COX-1 and COX-2 enzyme activity as indicated by PGE_2 production (pg/mL). *indicated statistically significant difference when compared with solvent (DMSO) control group (0) (p<0.05).

initiated by various agonists, including adenosine diphosphate (ADP), thrombin, collagen, and prostaglandin endoperoxides. In addition, secretion of the contents of intracellular granules may accompany platelet aggregation, which may further recruit additional platelets to induce full aggregation and subsequent gross thrombus formation. Aberrant platelet activation may directly or indirectly induce blood clot formation, thrombosis and sustained vascular wall inflammation, resulting in cardiovascular diseases (e.g. atherosclerosis and cardiovascular attack) [10,11]. Although catechol has been shown to inhibit arachidonic acid (AA)-induced platelet aggregation [12,13], limited mechanistic information is available about its possible anti-platelet and anti-thrombotic effects or toxicity in cardiovascular cells.

Considering the frequency that humans are exposed catechol (pyrocatechol) along with its potential pharmacological or toxicological effects, the anti-platelet and anti-inflammatory effects of catechol and related signaling mechanisms (e.g., cyclooxygenase [COX] inhibition, thromboxane, ROS, ERK/p38 phosphorylation, etc.) were assessed in this study to determine its effects on cardiovascular health.

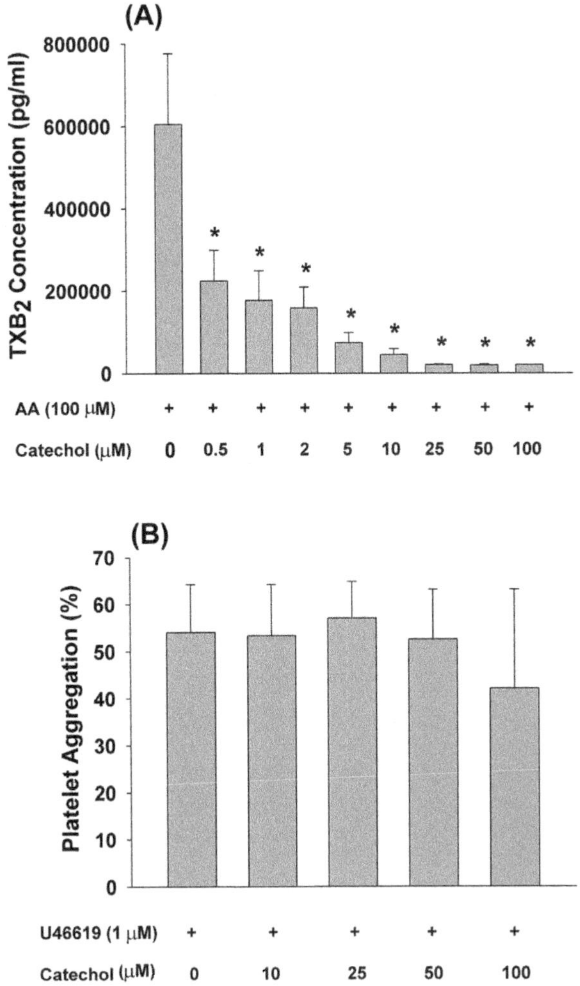

Figure 3. Effect of catechol on AA-induced TXB_2 production in platelets, (A). Results were expressed as TXB_2 production (n = 5). *denotes statistically significant difference when compared with the group that treated by solvent (DMSO) plus AA, (B) Effect of catechol (10–100 μM) on U46619 (1 μM)-induced platelet aggregation (n = 3).

Materials and Methods

Materials

Catechol (pyrocatechol), arachidonic acid (AA), U46619 (a thromboxane receptor agonist), 2′,7′-diacethyl-chlorofluorescein (DCFH-DA), lactate dehydrogenase (LDH) assay kits, superoxide dismutase (SOD), N-acetyl-L-cysteine (NAC) and sodium citrate were obtained from Sigma (St. Louis, MO, USA). Thromboxane B_2 (TXB_2) ELISA kits, prostaglandin E_2 (PGE_2) ELISA kits and a COX inhibitor screening assay were purchased from Cayman Chemical Company (Ann Arbor, MI, USA). Primary antibodies against COX-2, GAPDH (sc-32233) and phospho-extracellular signal-regulated protein kinase (p-ERK) (sc-7383) were purchased from Santa Cruz Biotechnology (Santa Cruz, CA, USA). The p-p38 antibody was obtained from Cell Signaling Technology (Beverly, MA, USA).

Platelet aggregation assay

Washed rabbit platelets were isolated from animals in the Animal Center of National Taiwan University Hospital as previously described [14–16] and were suspended in Tyrodes solution containing 1 mM calcium and 0.35% bovine serum albumin (BSA). Catechol (final concentration of 0.5–100 μM) was added to the platelets for 3 min after which AA (100 μM) or U46619 (1 μM, a TXA_2 receptor agonist) was added, and platelet aggregation was measured using the turbidimetric method described by Born and Cross [17] using an aggregometer (Model 600B, Payton Associates, ON, Canada). The percentage of aggregation inhibition was calculated as described by Teng et al. [18]. All animal studies were approved by the Ethics Committee of the Chang Gung University of Science and Technology and National Taiwan University Hospital.

Lactate dehydrogenase (LDH) activity assay

Following exposure of platelets to catechol (1–200 μM) for 9 min, LDH activity in the supernatant and total cell lysate was determined as an index of platelet damage using LDH activity assay kits [6,16]. The measurement was dependent on the spectrophotometric method as described by Wroblewski and La Due [19]. LDH generated by injured platelets was compared (in a percentage basis) with the total LDH activity of platelets dissolved in 0.1% Triton X-100 (v/v).

Thromboxane B_2 (TXB_2) assay

Platelets were preincubated with catechol (0.5–100 μM) for 3 min and then treated with or without AA (100 μM). EDTA (2 mM) and indomethacin (50 μM) were then added to the platelet suspension. After centrifugation at 14,000 rpm for 2 min, TXB_2 levels were measured with Cayman ELISA kits according to the manufacturer's instructions [6,15].

Effects of catechol on COX-1 and COX-2 enzyme activity

The direct effect of catechol on COX-1 and COX-2 enzymatic activities was measured using the COX inhibitor screening assay according to the manufacturer's instructions [6]. In brief, catechol (final 1–50 μM) was incubated with COX-1 or COX-2 in a reaction buffer for 10 min. Thereafter, AA was added as a substrate and incubated for an additional 2 min. This was followed by the addition of 0.1 N HCl and saturated stannous fluoride solution to stop the reaction. COX-1- or COX-2-mediated PGE_2 production was then measured using the Cayman ELISA kits.

Fluorimetric assay of ROS production in platelets and PMNs

Platelet ROS production was determined by measuring the platelet 2′,7′-dichlorofluorescein (DCF) fluorescence as described by Iuliano et al. [20] with slight modification. Briefly, washed platelets (5×10^8/mL) were preincubated with 10 μM 2′,7′-diacethyl- chlorofluorescein (DCFH-DA) at 37°C for 30 min. After centrifugation and washing, 200 μL of platelets (5×10^8/mL) were added to each well of a 96-well plate containing various concentrations of catechol (final concentrations of 1–50 μM). Then AA (final 100 μM), and the emitted DCF fluorescence was measured immediately by a Gemini XPS microplate spectrofluorometer (Molecular Devices Corporation, Sunnyvale, CA, USA) at an excitation of 485 nm and emission of 535 nm for 15 min. The fluorescence of DCF-labeled platelets without exposure to AA was used as a reference of basal level ROS production.

Human polymorphonuclear leukocytes (PMNs) were isolated as previousy described [16], by the approval of Ethics Committee, National Taiwan University Hospital. Briefly, heparinized blood was mixed with 3% dextran at a ratio of 1:1 (v/v) in a 50 mL conical tube and placed upright for 20–25 min at room

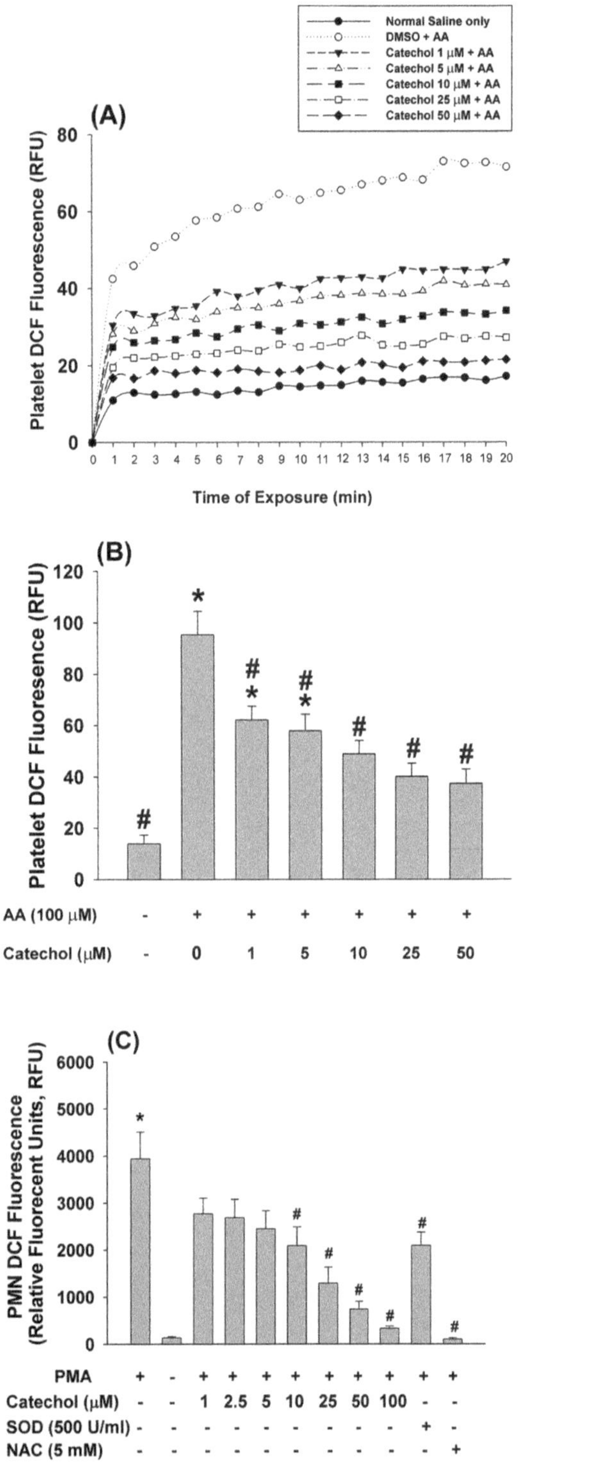

Figure 4. Effect of catechol on AA-induced ROS production in platelets, (A). The DCF fluorescence of platelets after exposure to AA with/without catechol was measured. One representative histogram of DCF fluorescence was shown. Results were expressed as relative fluorescent unit (RLU). (B) Quantitative DCF fluorescence of platelets after exposure to AA with/without pretreatment by solvent control (DMSO) or catechol. *denotes significant difference ($p<0.05$) when compared with normal saline treated group (NC). #denotes statistically significant difference when compared with solvent (DMSO)+AA group ($n=4$). (C) Catechol also prevented PMA-induced ROS production in isolated human PMN ($n=6$). *denotes significant difference ($p<0.05$) when compared with control group. #denotes statistically significant difference when compared with vehicle + PMA group

temperature. Then, 10 mL of Ficoll-Hypaque lymphocyte separation medium (LSM1077-PAA Labs, Pasching, Austria) was added, mixed and density-gradient centrifuged at 400×g for 40 min at 4°C. After hypotonic lysis of the erythrocytes, the isolated PMNs (final 4×10^6 cells/mL) were counted and resuspended in 1× Hanks' balanced salt solution (HBSS) containing 10 μM DCFH-DA for 40 min. Cells were washed with HBSS prior to the addition of phorbol myristate acetate (PMA, final 1 μM) with and without catechol (1–100 μM) pretreatment. The emitted DCF fluorescence was measured using a Gemini XPS microplate spectrofluorometer at an excitation of 485 nm and emission of 535 nm for 20 min. SOD and NAC was used to prevent PMA-induced ROS production by PMNs.

Effect of catechol on AA-induced ERK and p38 phosphorylation in platelets

The prepared platelets (1×10^9 platelets/mL) were resuspended in Tyrode's solution containing 1 mM $CaCl_2$ and 0.35% BSA, and 0.5 mL of the platelet suspension was placed into an aggregometer with constant stirring. Various amounts of catechol were added and preincubated for 3 min followed by addition of AA (100 μM) for 5 min. After addition of 0.5 mL of Laemmli sample buffer (75 mM Tris-HCl, 2% SDS, 15% glycerol, 3% 2-mercaptoethanol, pH 6.8) to terminate the reaction and for platelet lysis, cell lysates were boiled for 5 min, and 40 μL of cell lysates were subjected to 8% SDS-PAGE. After transfer to a PVDF membrane, blots were probed using anti-GAPDH, anti-p-ERK and anti-p-p38 antibodies as described previously [16]. For some western blot results, Image J software was used for quantitative analysis. The results were expressed as folds of control (as 1).

Ex vivo platelet aggregation of platelet-rich plasma (PRP)

After intravenous injection of catechol (0.5–5 μmole/mouse), blood was drawn from each mouse by heart puncture [21]. Whole blood containing anticoagulant (3.8% sodium citrate in 9:1 (v/v)) was placed in an Eppendorf tube and centrifuged at 60×g for 4 min to prepare PRP. AA-induced *ex vivo* platelet aggregability of PRP was measured with an aggregometer as previously described [6,16,21].

Effect of catechol on IL-1β-induced PGE2 production and COX-2 expression of dental pulp cells

PGE_2 level of dental pulp and its induction by IL-1β is crucial to the pathogenesis of pulpitis and pulpal pain [22,23]. To know the anti-inflammatory effect, we tested whether catechol may prevent IL-1β-induced COX-2 expression and PGE_2 production of pulp cells in this study. Human dental pulp cells were cultured as described previously [14]. For PGE_2 analysis, 1×10^5 pulp cells were inoculated onto 24-well culture plates. After 24 h, medium was changed, and catechol (50 and 100 μM) was added for a 30 min pretreatment followed by addition of IL-1β (5 ng/mL) for an additional 24 h. Culture medium was collected for PGE_2 analysis by ELISA. Viability of pulp cells was evaluated by MTT assay as previously [16], because pulp cells are attached to culture wells that is different from platelets floating in the buffer. For analysis of COX-2 expression, 1.5×10^6 pulp cells were inoculated onto 10-cm culture dishes. After 24 h, medium was changed, and catechol (50 and 100 μM) was added for a 30 min pretreatment, followed by addition of IL-1β (5 ng/mL) for an additional 24 h. Cell lysate of cultured pulp cells were prepared and subjected to western blotting as above (section 2.7.) except that anti-GAPDH and anti-COX-2 antibodies were used.

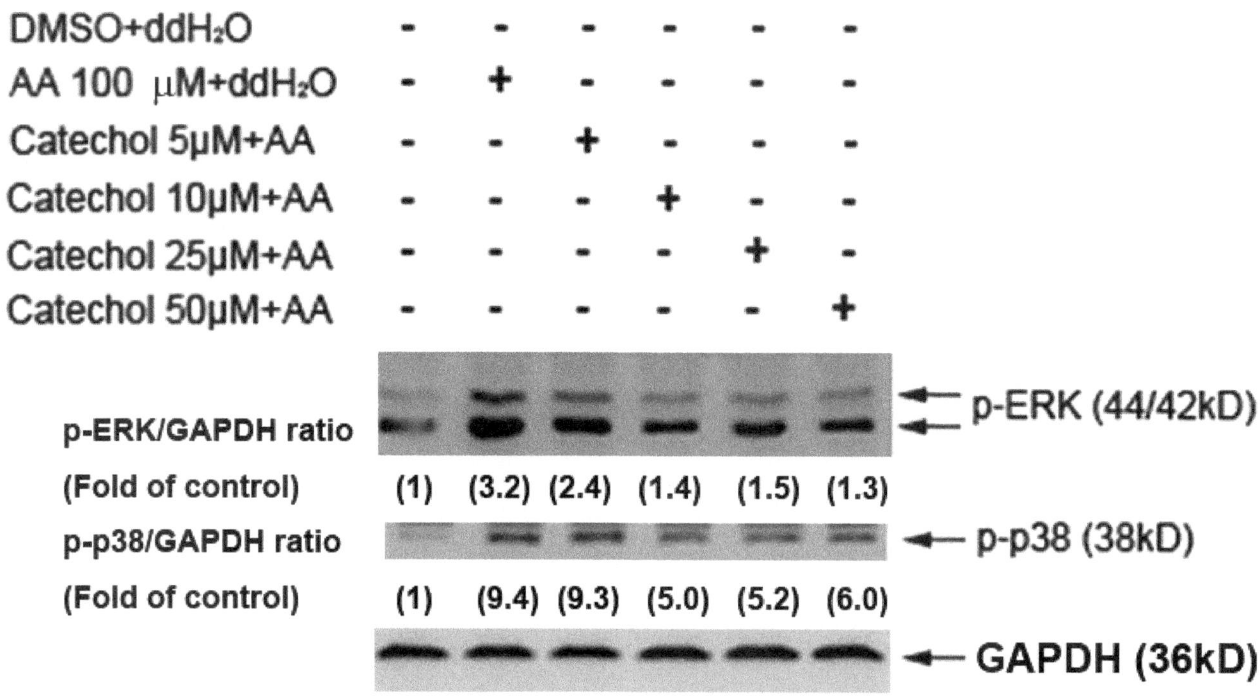

Figure 5. Effect of catechol on AA-induced p38 and ERK phosphrylation in platelets. One representative western blotting picture was shown. Expression of GAPDH was used as control. Quantitative results of p-ERK/GAPDH and p-p38/GAPDH ratio were measured by Image J analysis and expressed as fold of control (the value in parenthesis).

Statistical analysis

Three or more independent experiments were performed. Results were expressed as percentage of inhibition on AA-induced platelet aggregation and TXB_2 synthesis. One-way ANOVA and post-hoc Tukey test were used for statistical analysis.

Results

Effects of catechol on platelet aggregation

The effects of catechol on platelet aggregation were first analyzed. As shown in **Figure 1A**, catechol suppressed AA-induced platelet aggregation at concentrations ≥10 μM. Quantitative analysis revealed that 5, 10 and 25 μM catechol inhibited AA-induced platelet aggregation by 50%, 71% and 94%, respectively (***p*<0.05; Figure 1B**), and 100 μM catechol completely inhibited AA-induced platelet aggregation (***p*<0.05; Figure 1B**). However, it did not significantly induce platelet cytoxicity at concentrations of 1–200 μM as determined by LDH release (**Figure 1C**).

Inhibition of COX-1 and COX-2 activities by catechol

The anti-platelet effect of catechol can be partly explained by its inhibition of COX-1 activity. As shown in **Figure 2A**, catechol inhibited COX-1 activity by 29%, 38% and 44% at concentrations of 10, 25 and 50 μM, respectively (***p*<0.05**;). Accordingly, catechol also inhibited COX-2 enzymatic activity by 29%, 42% and 50% at concentrations of 10, 25 and 50 μM, respectively (***p*<0.05; Figure 2B**).

Effect of catechol on AA-induced platelet TXB_2 production and U46619-induced platelet aggregation

We next assessed the effects of catechol on AA-induced TXB_2 production by platelets. As shown in **Figure 3A**, catechol suppressed AA-induced TXB_2 production by 64% and 88% at concentrations of 0.5 and 5 μM, respectively (***p*<0.05**).

U46619 (1 μM), a TXA2 receptor agonist, can stimulate platelet aggregation. This effect was not significantly altered by catechol at concentrations ranging from 10–100 μM (**Figure 3B**).

Effects of catechol on AA-induced ROS production by platelets

Exposure of platelets to AA rapidly stimulated cellular ROS production as analyzed by an increase in DCF fluorescence. Pre-incubation with catechol attenuated AA-induced DCF fluorescence in platelets (**Figure 4A**). At concentrations of 1 and 10 μM, catechol effectively suppressed AA-induced ROS production by 35% and 49% (***p*<0.05; Figure 4B**). Moreover, the PMA-induced ROS production in isolated human PMNs as indicated by an increase in DCF fluorescence. This was inhibited by SOD (500 U/mL), N-acetyl-L-cysteine (NAC, 5 mM) as well as catechol (10–100 μM) (***p*<0.05; Figure 4C**).

Effects of catechol on AA-induced p38 and ERK phosphorylation in platelets

Mitogen-activated protein kinases (MAPKs), such as ERK and p38, are important for the regulation of platelet aggregation. To determine whether the anti-platelet effect of catechol is due to its attenuation of MAPK signaling, we incubated platelets in AA and found that it rapidly stimulated ERK and p38 phosphorylation (**Figure 5**). However, pre-incubation of platelets with catechol (5–50 μM) attenuated AA-induced ERK and p38 phosphorylation as analyzed by Western blot analysis. Quantitatively, AA stimulated ERK and p38 phosphorylation to 3.2–fold and 9.4–fold of control, respectively (**Figure 5**). Catechol (10–50 μM) decreased the AA-

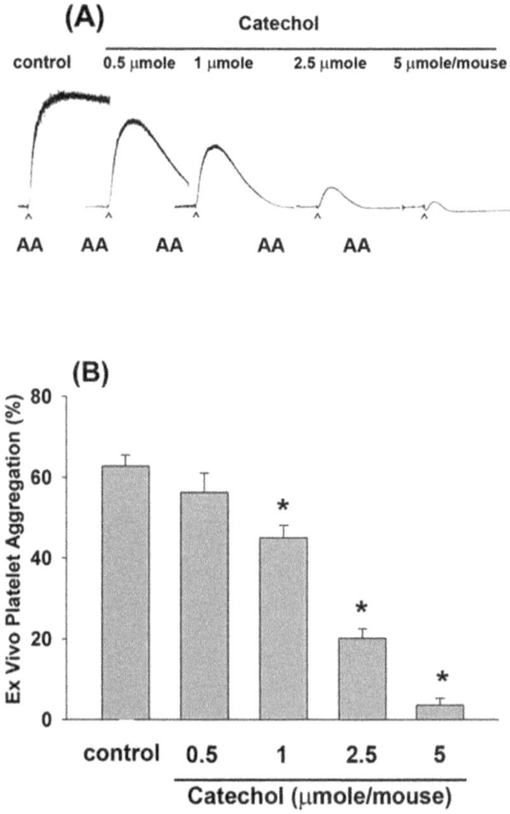

Figure 6. *Ex vivo* platelet aggregation by AA and its inhibition by administration of catechol. (A) Intravenous administration of catechol (0.5–5 μmole/mouse) inhibited the AA-induced platelet aggregation *ex vivo*. One representative picture of platelet aggregation was shown with more similar results. (B) Inhibition of AA-induced platelet aggregation *ex vivo* by intravenous administration of different amounts of catechol (0.5–5 μmole/mouse) into mice. (n = 7). *denotes significant difference when compared with solvent control group ($p < 0.05$).

induced p-ERK and p-p38 expression to 1.3–1.5 fold and 5.0–6.0 fold of control, respectively (**Figure 5**).

Effects of catechol on *ex vivo* platelet aggregation induced by AA

Intravenous administration of catechol suppressed AA-induced platelet aggregation *ex vivo* at concentrations higher than 1 μmole/mouse (**Figure 6A**). Specifically, 2.5 and 5 μmole catechol/mouse significantly inhibited *ex vivo* AA-induced platelet aggregation by 68% and 94%, respectively (***p*<0.05; Figure 6B**).

Effects of catechol on the growth, PGE2 production and COX-2 expression of dental pulp cells

Catechol inhibited COX-1 and COX-2 activities (**Figures 2A and 2B**). Because we have found that IL-1β stimulates COX-2 expression and PGE_2 production by pulp cells [23], we further analyzed whether catechol may have anti-inflammatory effect and could inhibit IL-1β-induced PGE_2 production of pulp cells. Exposure to 50 and 100 μM catechol with/without IL-1β showed little effect on pulp cell morphology as compared with control pulp cells (**Figure 7A**), and minimal cytotoxicity with 50 and 100 μM catechol was observed (**Figure 7B**). However, catechol (50 and 100 μM) almost completely inhibited the IL-1β-induced PGE_2 production by pulp cells (**Figure 7C**). Western blotting analysis further found that catechol (50 and 100 μM) by itself slightly stimulated COX-2 protein expression of pulp cells. In addition, pretreatment by catechol and co-incubation with IL-1β showed no marked stimulation and even enhanced the IL-1β-induced COX-2 expression (**Figure 7D**), suggesting a possible compensatory response.

Discussion

Catechol is present in a number of food products and cosmetic ingrediens. It can be rapily absorbed by oral, dermal and inhalaton of exposure. Skin application of catechol for 30 min results in absorption of 0.4% of applied dose through human skin and a 24-h application of 4% catechol results in 53% absorption from skin, where it can be metabolized to reactive benzoquinone metabolites or other toxic quinone species by myeloperoxidase [24,25]. It is also a metabolite of benzene and toluene [4]. In this study, catechol exhibits anti-platelet effects at low concentrations, suggesting its potential role in the prevention of cardiovascular diseases at low levels. Consistently, catechol, resorcinol (1,3-benzenediol) and hydroquinone have been previously shown to suppress AA-induced rabbit platelet aggregation although with varying levels of potency (about μM concentrations) [12]. Catechol also inhibits collagen-induced platelet aggregation at concentration of 100 μM, and a catechol group of phenolics has been suggested to responsible for its anti-platelet effect on collagen-induced platelet aggregation [13,26]. In the present study, catechol significantly inhibits AA-induced platelet aggregation even at concentrations higher than 5 μM, which is in general agreement with the results described by Kitagawa et al. [12]. It is well known that platelet dysfunction plays a critical role in the pathogenesis of cardiovascular diseases [9–11]; therefore, exposure to catechol or consumption of catechol-containing products at suitable amounts may potentially prevent cardiovascular diseases via its anti-platelet effect.

AA-induced platelet aggregation is mediated by COX-1 activation, TXA_2 production and subsequent activation of thromboxane receptors and the downstream signaling to induce full platelet aggregation. In this stdy, the anti-platelet effect of catechol may be partly due to its inhibition of COX-1 enzymatic activity given that platelets only express COX-1 and the binding and inhibition of catechol on COX and phospholipase A_2 (PLA_2) has been reported [27,28]. Consistently, catechol almost completely inhibited AA-induced platelet production of TXA_2, which interacts with platelet thromboxane receptor and induces full platelet aggregation. But catechol showed only partial inhibition on COX activity. This indicates that catechol possibly also affects other critical molecules such as ROS and PLA_2 as mentioned previously [28]. As a stable TXA_2 metabolite, TXB_2 was obviously inhibited by catechol in AA-stimulated platelets. Binding of TXA_2 to platelet TXA_2 receptors may further induce downstream signaling for platelet aggregation [29]. Platelet TXA_2 production is mediated mainly through metabolism of AA by COX-1 to produce TXA_2, that may bind and activate thromboxane receptor to induce further full platelet activation. The TXA_2 receptor agonist, U46619, was shown to stimulate marked platelet aggregation. However, catechol showed little inhibitory effect on U46619-induced platelet aggregation, suggesting that the anti-platelet effect of catechol is associated with COX-1 inhibition and that it cannot suppress platelet aggregation signaling downstream of thromboxane receptors.

The anti-platelet effect of catechol was not due to cytotoxicity as no obvious changes in platelet extracellular and intracellular LDH

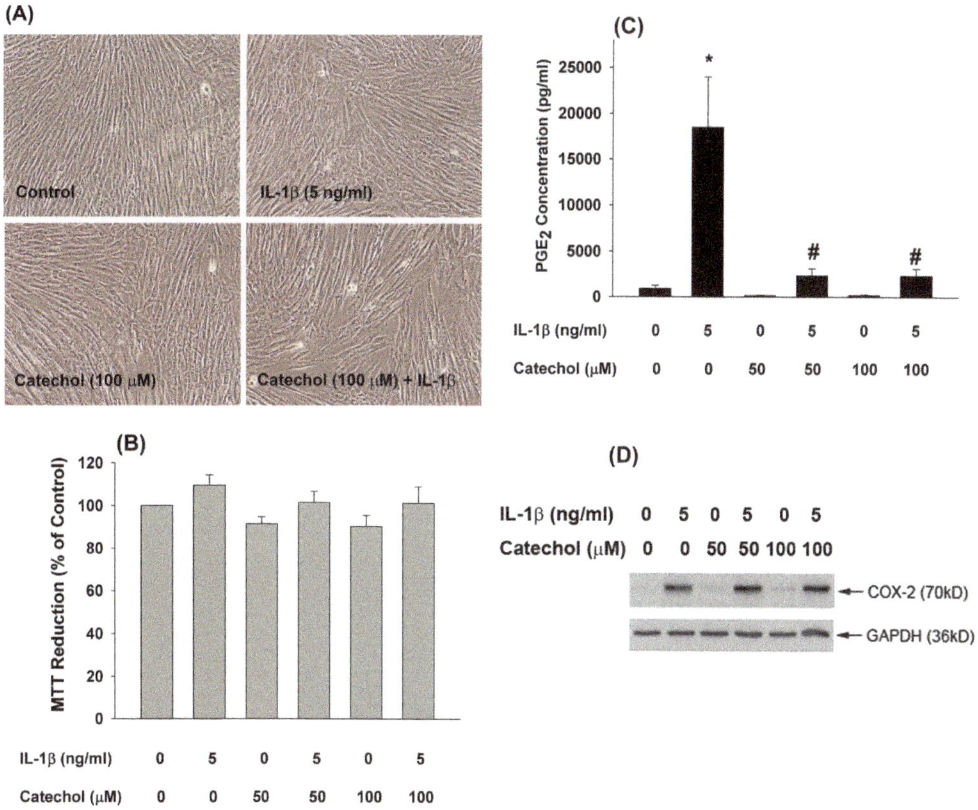

Figure 7. Catechol inhibited the IL-1β-induced PGE_2 production of pulp cells. Pulp cells were pretreated with catechol with/without further co-incubation by IL-1β for 24-hours. (A) morphology of control fibroblasts, pulp fibroblasts exposed to IL-1β for 24-hours, Pulp fibroblasts incubated with 0.1 mM catechol for 24-hours, and Pulp fibroblasts exposure to 0.1 mM catechol with IL-1β for 24-hours, (B) Viable cells were estimated by MTT assay. MTT reduction was shown as % of control (Mean ± SE) (n = 8). *denotes significant difference ($p<0.05$) when compared with solvent control group. (C) PGE_2 level in the cultured medium was measured and the PGE_2 concentration was shown as pg/ml (Mean ± SE) (n = 7). *denotes significant difference when compared with solvent control group; #denotes significant difference ($p<0.05$) when compared with IL-1β solely group. (D) COX-2 expression of pulp cells after exposure to IL-1β with/without pretreatment and co-incubation by catechol. One representative western blotting result was shown.

levels were noted after exposure to catechol. Catechol is not toxic to glioblastoma cells at concentrations below 0.2 mM [30]; however, it induces a 44% increase in esophageal cell death at 35 μM [4], suggesting that it exhibits differential cytotoxicity that is cell type-dependent.

ROS may regulate many physiological and pathological processes in the pulmonary and cardiovascular systems [31,32]. ROS and redox changes also critically modulate platelet function [20,33]. In this study, we found that AA stimulated ROS production in platelets, which was suppressed by catechol. Catechol further inhibited PMA-induced ROS production in PMNs, which is suggestive of a potential role as an anti-oxidant and anti-inflammatory mediator. Thus, the anti-platelet and anti-inflammatory effects of catechol are possibly related to its scavenging ROS or attenuation of ROS production in platelets. Consistently, the catechol group within the B-ring of flavonoids is responsible for their anti-oxidant effects toward PMA-induced oxidative burst [34] and 1,1-diphenyl-2-picrylhydrazyl free radicals [35]). However, at higher concentrations (150–600 μM), catechol is toxic to cultured Muller cells possibly via ROS production [36]. Therefore, more *in vitro* and *in vivo* studies are necessary to further clarify the beneficial and detrimental effects of catechol exposure.

ERK and p38 MAPKs play an important role in the regulation of platelet granule secretion, ATP release and platelet aggregation as well as the stimulation of myosin light chain to stimulate blood clot retraction [37,38]. Some anti-platelet agents, including caffeic acid phenethyl ester, simvastatin and davallialactone, suppress platelet activation via inhibition of p38 and ERK [38–40]. Inhibition of both ERK and p38 phosphorylation is required to suppress AA-induced platelet aggregation [41]. In this study, we found that catechol effectively prevented AA-induced ERK and p38 MAPK phosphorylation, which is crucial for platelet AA release and TXA_2 production [39]. At comparable concentrations, catechol obviously inhibited AA-induced platelet aggregation and TXA_2 production in the present study, suggesting that the inhibitory effect of catechol on platelet TXA_2 production is possibly mediated by blocking p38 and ERK signaling or other upstream signaling molecules such as phospholipase C (PLC), protein kinase C, glycoproein $\alpha II_b\beta_3$, proline-rich tyrosine kinase 2 [42–44], and that it may have therapeutic potential as an anti-platelet agent.

In the present study, intravenous administration of catechol to mice inhibited *ex vivo* platelet aggregation, indicating that catechol may have anti-platelet effects even in the presence of plasma. Because catechol inhibits both COX-1 and COX-2 activities, we further analyzed the effects of catechol on IL-1β-induced PGE_2

production of oral fibroblasts, especially given that it exhibits anti-microbial and anti-inflammatory activities by suppression of leukotriene B_4 production in rat peritoneal exudate cells [45]. Therefore, catechol may increase the PGE_2/leukotriene B_4 ratio in PMNs. These phenols also inhibit PGE_2 production in whole blood. Low concentrations of catechol stimulated PGE_2 formation in PMNs; however, a repression was noted at high concentrations [46]. Vascular wall inflammation is related to platelet activation and constitutes a major pathogenic event in atherosclerosis [10]. Stimulation of COX-2 expression and PGE_2 production is crucial for tissue inflammation, pain response and cardiovascular disease [23,47,48]. Dental pulp is a specialized connective tissue popularly suffered from inflammatory and pain response, where IL-1β and PGE_2 are involved [22]. Recently, we observed the stimulation of PGE_2 by IL-1β and possible activation of pulp cells via prostaglandin EP receptors, and suppression of IL-1β-induced PGE_2 production in pulpal fibroblasts by plant phenolic was noted [16,23]. In this study, catechol also attenuated the IL-1β-induced PGE_2 production, but no COX-2 expression of pulp cells. These results support the anti-inflammatory effect of catechol. The inhibition of IL-1β-induced PGE_2 production of pulp cells by catechol is possibly due to its direct interaction with COX-2 and inhibition of COX-2 enzyme activities, but not due to its suppression of COX-2 protein expression.

Conclusions

Catechol exhibits anti-platelet and anti-inflammatory effects. The anti-platelet effects of catechol are related to its inhibition of platelet COX activity, TXA_2 production, ROS production as well as ERK/p38 signaling. The anti-platelet effect of catechol was confirmed using an *ex vivo* study. Catechol further suppresses PMA-induced ROS production in PMNs, which is suggestive of possible anti-inflammatory properties. Catechol also exhibits anti-inflammatory effects via inhibition of COX-2 activity and IL-1β-induced prostaglandin production. Catechol showed little cytotoxicity at concentrations below 0.1 mM. Taken together, exposure to catechol or suitable consumption of catechol-containing food/nutritional supplements, such as marine algae tablets or plants, may be beneficial to cardiovascular health. Delineation of its full pharmacological potential requires further investigation.

Author Contributions

Conceived and designed the experiments: JHJ MCC CPC. Performed the experiments: MCC HHC CPC TMW BRL SYY. Analyzed the data: MCC HHC CYY RHC. Contributed reagents/materials/analysis tools: MCC. Contributed to the writing of the manuscript: MCC JHJ.

References

1. DeCaprio AP (1999) The toxicology of hydroquinone-relevance to occupational and environmental exposure. Crit Rev Toxicol 29: 283–330.
2. McGregor D (2007) Hydroquinone: an evaluation of the human risks from its carcinogenic and mutagenic properties. Crit Rev Toxicol 37: 887–914.
3. IARC (1985) Betel quid and areca nut chewing. Monographs on the evaluation of the carcinogenic risk of chemicals to humans. IARC Scientific Publications No 37, IARC, Lyon, pp. 141–202.
4. Myburg RB, Dutton MF, Chuturgoon AA (2002) Cytotoxicity of fumonisin B1, diethylnitrosamine and catechol on the SNO esophageal cancer cell line. Environ Health Perspect 110: 813–815.
5. Thavasi V, Bettens RP, Leong LP (2009) Temperature and solvent effects on radical scavenging ability of phenols. J Phys Chem A 113: 3068–3077.
6. Chang MC, Uang BJ, Tsai CY, Wu HL, Lin BR, et al. (2007) Hydroxychavicol, a novel betel leaf component, inhibits platelet aggregation by suppression of cyclooxygenase, thromboxane production and calcium mobilization. Br J Pharmacol 152: 73–92.
7. Lee SF, Lin JK (1994) Generation of hydrogen peroxide, superoxide anion and hydroxyl free radical from polyphenols and active benzene metabolites: Their possible role in mutagenesis. J Biomed Sci 1: 125–130.
8. Schaefer D, Jurgensmeier JM, Baur G (1995) Catechol interferes with TGF-beta-induced elimination of transformed cells by normal cells: implicatios for the survival of transformed cells during carcinogenesis. Int J Cancer 60: 520–526.
9. Alexandru N, Popov D, Georgescu A (2012) Platelet dysfunction in vascular pathologies and how can it be treated. Thromb Res 129: 116–126.
10. Tsoumani ME, Kalantzi KI, Goudevenos IA, Tselepis AD (2012) Platelet-mediated inflammation in cardiovascular disease. Potential role of platelets-endothelium interaction. Curr Vasc Pharmacol 10: 39–549.
11. Willoughby S, Holmes A, Losalzo J (2002). Platelets and cardiovascular disease. European Journal of Cardiovascular Nursing. 1:273–288.
12. Kitagawa S, Fujisawa H, Baba S, Kametani F (1991) Inhibitory effect of catechol derivatives on arachidonic acid-induced aggregation of rabbit platelets. Chem Pharm Bull 39: 1062–1064.
13. Ostertag LM, O'Kennedy N, Horgan GW, Kroon PA, Duthie GG, et al. (2011) In vitro antiplatelet effects of simple plant-derived phenolic compounds are only found at high, non-physiological concentrations. Mol Nutr Food Res 55: 1624–1636.
14. Chang MC, Chan CP, Ho YS, Lee JJ, Lin PS, et al. (2009) Signaling pathways for induction of platelet aggregation by SAS tongue cancer cells – a mechanism of hematogenous metastasis. J Oral Pathol Med 38: 434–440.
15. Jeng JH, Chen SY, Liao CH, Tung YY, Lin BR, et al. (2002). Modulation of platelet aggregation by areca nut and betel leaf ingredients: roles of reactive oxygen species and cyclooxygenase. Free Radic Biol Med 32: 860–871.
16. Chang MC, Chang HH, Chan CP, Chou HY, Chang BE, et al. (2012) Antiplatelet effect of phloroglucinol is related to inhibition of cyclooxygenase, reactive oxygen species, ERK/p38 signaling and thromboxane A(2) production. Toxicol Appl Pharmacol 263: 287–295.
17. Born GVR, Cross MJ (1963). The aggregation of blood platelets. J Physiol 168: 178–195.
18. Teng CM, Ko FN (1988) Comparison of the platelet aggregation induced by three thrombin-like enzymes of snake venoms and thrombin. Thromb Haemost 59: 304–309.
19. Wroblewski F, La Due JS (1955). Lactic dehydrogenase activity in blood. Proc Soc Exp Biol Med USA 90: 210–213.
20. Iuliano L, Pedersen JZ, Pratico D, Rotilio G, Violi F (1994). Role of hydroxyl radicals in the activation of human platelets. Eur J Biochem 221: 695–704.
21. Chang MC, Lin HK, Peng HC, Huang TF (1998) Antithrombotic effect of crotalin, a platelet membrane glycoprotein lb antagonist from venom of Crotalus atrox. Blood 91: 1582–1589.
22. Martinho FC, Chiesa WM, Leite FR, Cirelli JA, Gomes BP (2012) Correlation between clinical/radiographic features and inflammatory cytokine networks produced by macrophages stimulated with endodontic content. J Endod 38: 740–750.
23. Chang MC, Chen YJ, Tai TF, Tai MR, Li MY, et al. (2006) Cytokine-induced prostaglandin E2 production and cyclooxygenase-2 expression in dental pulp cells: downstream calcium signalling via activation of prostaglandin EP receptor. Int Endod J 39: 819–826.
24. Jung CT, Wickett RR, Desai PB, Bronaugh RL (2003) In vitro and in vivo percutaneous absorption of catechol. Food Chem Toxicol 41: 885–895.
25. Subrahmanyam VV, Kolachana P, Smith MT (1991) Metabolism of hydroquinone by human myeloperoxidase: mechanisms of stimulation by other phenolic compounds. Arch Biochem Biophys 286: 76–84.
26. Wright B, Tindall MJ, Lovegrove JA, Gibbins JM (2013) Investigating flavonoids as molecular templates for the design of small-molecule inhibitors of cell signaling. J Food Science 78: N1921–1928.
27. Laughton MJ, vans PJ, Moroney MA, Hoult J, Halliwell B (1991) Inhibition of mammalian 5-lipoxygenase and cyclooxygenase by flavonoids and phenolic dietary additives: relationship to antioxidant activity and to iron-reducing ability. Biochem Pharmacol 42: 1673–1681.
28. Dileep KV, Tintu I, Mandal PK, Karthe P, Haridas M, et al. (2012) Binding of PLA2 may contribute to the anti-inflammatory activity of catechol. Chem Biol drug Des 79: 143–147.
29. Lopez-Farre A, Sanchez de Miguel L, Monton M, Jimenez A, Lopez-Bloya A, et al. (2001) Angiotensin II AT(I) receptor antagonists and platelet activation. Nephrol Dial Transplant 16 Suppl 1: 45–49.
30. De Oliveira DM, Pitanga BP, Grangeiro MS, Lima RM, Costa MF, et al. (2010) Catechol cytotoxicity in vitro: induction of glioblastoma cell death by apoptosis. Hum Exp Toxicol 29: 199–212.
31. Al Ghouleh I, Khoo NK, Knaus UG, Griendling KK, Touyz RM, et al. (2011) Oxidase and peroxidase in cardiovascular and lung disease: new concept in reactive oxygen species signaling. Free Radic Biol Med 51: 1271–1288.
32. Zinkevich NS, Gutterman DD (2011) ROS-induced ROS release in vascular biology: redox-redox signaling. Am J Physiol Heart Circ Physiol 301: H647–H653.
33. Essex DW (2009) Redox control of platelet function. Antioxid Redox Signal 11: 1191–1225.

34. Ribeiro D, Freitas M, Tome SM, Silva AM, Porto G, et al. (2013) Modulation of human neutrophils' oxidative burst by flavonoids. Eur J Med Chem 67: 280–292.
35. De Martino L, Mencherini T, Mancini E, Aquino RP, De Almeida LF, et al. (2012) In vitro phytotoxicity and antioxidant activity of selected flavonoids. Int J Mol Sci 13: 5406–5419.
36. Mansoor S, Gupta N, Luczy-Bachman G, Limb GA, Kuppermann BD, et al. (2010) Protective effects of memantine and epicatechin on catechol-induced cytotoxicity to Muller cells in vitro. Toxicology 271: 107–114.
37. Flavaris P, Li Z, Zhang G, Zheng Y, Liu J, et al. (2009) Two distinct roles of mitogen-activated protein kinases in platelets and a novel Rac1-MAPK-dependent integrin outside-in retractile signaling pathway. Blood 113: 893–901.
38. Hsiao G, Lee JJ, Lin KH, Shen CH, Fong TH, et al. (2007) Characterization of a novel and potent collagen antagonist, caffeic acid phenethyl ester in human platelets: in vitro and in vivo studies. Cardiovasc Res 75: 782–792.
39. Lee YM, Chen WF, Chou DS, Jayakumar T, Hou SY, et al. (2010) Cyclic nucleotides and mitogen-activated protein kinases: regulation of simvastatin in platelet activation. J Biomed Sci 17: 45.
40. Kim SD, Lee IK, Lee WM, Cho JY, Park HJ, et al. (2008) The mechanism of antiplatelet activity of davallialactone: involvement of intracelluar calcium ions, extracellular signal-regulated kinase 2 and p38 mitogen-activated protein kinase. Eur J Pharmacol 584: 367–367.
41. McNicol A, Jackson EC (2003) Inhibition of the MEK/ERK pathway has no effect on agonist-induced aggregation of human platelets. Biochem Pharmacol 65: 1243–1250.
42. Lee YM, Chen WF, Chou DS, Jayakumar T, Hou SY, et al. (2010) Cyclic nucleotides and mitogen-activated protein kinases: regulation of simvastatin in platelet activation. J Biomed Sci 17: 45–54.
43. Yacoub D, Theoret JF, Villeneuve L, Abou-Saleh H, Mourad W, et al. (2006) Essential role of protein kinase Cδ in platele signaling, $\alpha_{IIb}\beta_3$ activation, and thromboxane A_2 release. J Biol Chem 281: 30024–30035.
44. Sun L, Feng S, Resendiz JC, Lu X, Durante W, et al. (2004) Role of the Pyk2-MAP kinase-cPLA2 signaling pathway in shear-dependent platelet aggregation. Ann Biomed Eng 32: 1193–1201.
45. Yamada K, Shoji K, Mori M, Ueyama T, Matsuo N, et al. (1999) Structure-activity relationship of polyphenols on inhibition of chemical mediator release from rat peritoneal exudate cells. In Vitro Cell Dev Biol Anim 35: 169–174.
46. Alanko J, Riutta A, Vapaatalo H (1995) Phenols inhibit prostaglandin E_2 synthesis in A23187-stimulated human whole blood and modify the ratio of arachidonic acid metabolites. Prostaglangins Leukot Essent Fatty Acids 52: 299–301.
47. Beck J, Garcia R, Heiss G, Vokonas PS, Offenbacher S (1996) Periodontal disease and cardiovascular disease. J Periodontol 67 (10 Suppl): 1123–1137.
48. Wang M, Song WL, Cheng Y, Fitzgerald GA (2008) Microsomal prostaglandin E synthase-1 inhibition in cardiovascular inflammatory disease. J Intern Med 263: 500–505.

2

Early Exposure to Volatile Anesthetics Impairs Long-Term Associative Learning and Recognition Memory

Bradley H. Lee[1], John Thomas Chan[1], Obhi Hazarika[1], Laszlo Vutskits[2], Jeffrey W. Sall[1]*

1 Department of Anesthesia and Perioperative Care, University of California San Francisco, San Francisco, California, Unites States of America, **2** Department of Anesthesiology, Pharmacology and Intensive Care, University Hospital of Geneva, Geneva, Switzerland

Abstract

Background: Anesthetic exposure early in life affects neural development and long-term cognitive function, but our understanding of the types of memory that are altered is incomplete. Specific cognitive tests in rodents that isolate different memory processes provide a useful approach for gaining insight into this issue.

Methods: Postnatal day 7 (P7) rats were exposed to either desflurane or isoflurane at 1 Minimum Alveolar Concentration for 4 h. Acute neuronal death was assessed 12 h later in the thalamus, CA1-3 regions of hippocampus, and dentate gyrus. In separate behavioral experiments, beginning at P48, subjects were evaluated in a series of object recognition tests relying on associative learning, as well as social recognition.

Results: Exposure to either anesthetic led to a significant increase in neuroapoptosis in each brain region. The extent of neuronal death did not differ between groups. Subjects were unaffected in simple tasks of novel object and object-location recognition. However, anesthetized animals from both groups were impaired in allocentric object-location memory and a more complex task requiring subjects to associate an object with its location and contextual setting. Isoflurane exposure led to additional impairment in object-context association and social memory.

Conclusion: Isoflurane and desflurane exposure during development result in deficits in tasks relying on associative learning and recognition memory. Isoflurane may potentially cause worse impairment than desflurane.

Editor: Yael Abreu-Villaça, Universidade do Estado do Rio de Janeiro, Brazil

Funding: Funding for the study was provided through National Institutes of Health Grant GM086511 to JWS, the University of California San Francisco Department of Anesthesia and Perioperative Care Hamilton Award to JWS, and by Swiss National Science Foundation Grant 31003A_130625 to LV. The funders had no role in study design, data collection and analysis, decision to publish, or preparation of the manuscript.

Competing Interests: The authors have declared that no competing interests exist.

* Email: sallj@anesthesia.ucsf.edu

Introduction

Every day, anesthetics are used around the world in newborns and infants who undergo medical procedures. There is growing concern that anesthetics can significantly alter the developing brain, and animal models have shown that exposure to anesthetics at an early age lead to neuronal death and long-term cognitive dysfunction [1–3]. Epidemiologic studies suggest that humans are also susceptible to long-term cognitive effects after anesthesia [4,5].

Our knowledge of cognitive effects in humans has been, until recently [6], limited to retrospective studies that typically assess global tests of learning and behavior [4,5,7,8]. For instance, most of these epidemiologic studies identify cognitive or learning disabilities by evaluating databases for individuals with diagnostic codes for unspecified delays, behavioral disorders, language or speech problems [7,8], or through IQ and achievement tests [4,5]. Because these studies examine generalized learning problems, they contribute minimally to our understanding of the memory processes that underlie the cognitive impairment.

An important challenge in the study of anesthetic neurotoxicity is developing a model by which cognitive effects in animals can be translated to humans. Memory processing is highly conserved across rodent and human species [9]. In particular, hippocampal memory functions are very similar between rats and humans [9], and the hippocampus is crucial in spatial encoding, associative learning, and recognition memory in both rats and humans [9–12].

Rodent models therefore provide valuable insight into the types of memory that may be affected in humans. However, behavioral studies are prone to using overlapping models for evaluating learning and memory. Many studies use similar tests, such as the Morris water maze [2,13–15], because they have consistently identified a cognitive deficit. Identifying impairment in specific memory processes, such as recognition and associative memory, in animal models will provide insight into effects in humans and may help guide future assessments of learning and memory in children, as has recently been reported [6].

Recognition memory, which is a subtype of declarative memory, is crucial in humans for recalling different events, objects, and people [16,17]. It has been shown that animals also have episodic-like memory that can be demonstrated through tests involving memory for "what," "where," and "when" details of an event. This was first described in birds [18] and more recently in rodents [12,19–22], and models have since been developed to examine recognition memory in various ways [20,23–25]. Furthermore, many studies find that recognition memory processes rely on the hippocampus and thalamus [19,26], which are areas of neuronal degeneration following anesthesia [2,14].

The present study was designed to evaluate the effects of two commonly used volatile anesthetics – isoflurane and desflurane – on specific learning and memory processes following neonatal exposure. After delivering 1 Minimum Alveolar Concentration [27] of either anesthetic for 4 hours at postnatal day 7 (P7), subjects were evaluated in a set of recognition tasks involving associative memory, as well as social memory, that have been shown to be sensitive to lesions in hippocampal and thalamic circuits [19,28,29].

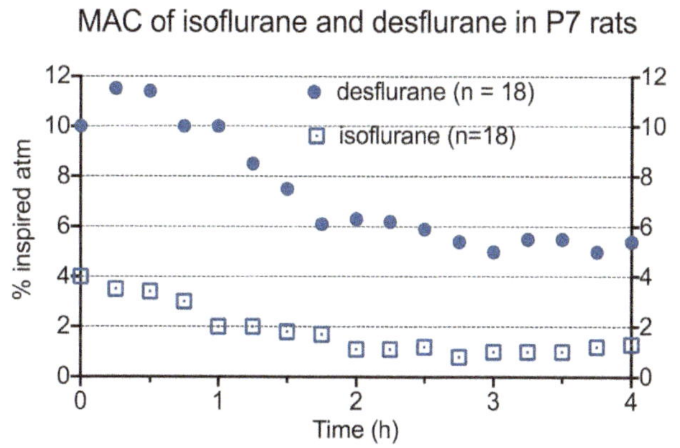

Figure 1. MAC of isoflurane and desflurane. Anesthetics were separately delivered to P7 rats in air and oxygen (FiO_2 50%) as previously described[6, 9]. Tail-clamping occurred every 15 minutes, and anesthetic concentration was adjusted to 1 MAC. As before[6, 9], MAC decreases with increasing duration of anesthesia for both agents.

Methods

Subjects

All experiments were conducted with approval from the Institutional Animal Care and Use Committee at the University of California, San Francisco. Five Sprague-Dawley dams with litters of postnatal day 6 (P6) pups from were obtained from Charles River Laboratories (Gilroy, CA). Each litter contained only males and was culled to ten pups. In total, the males were taken from at least ten different litters. On P7, animals from each litter were randomly assigned to control and treatment groups. They were weaned at P23 and housed three per cage under standard lab housing with 12 h light/dark cycle. Animals were food restricted (access to food only during light cycle) for tasks involving object recognition to increase activity and object exploration.

Anesthesia

Anesthesia was delivered as described previously [14,30,31]. Briefly, animals in the treatment groups received either isoflurane or desflurane as a single agent in air and oxygen ($FiO_2$50%) at 1 Minimum Alveolar Concentration [27] for four hours. MAC was determined by tail clamping every 15 minutes, and anesthetic concentration was adjusted accordingly, so that on average 50% of animals would move in response to clamping (Fig. 1). 12 out of 18 animals anesthetized with isoflurane survived to undergo behavioral testing, and 13 out of 18 animals anesthetized with desflurane survived and underwent behavioral testing. Control animals were concurrently placed in an anesthesia glove box of the same material and conditions without being exposed to anesthesia or tail clamping. Animals were kept on a warming blanket, and temperatures were measured using an infrared laser thermometer and maintained with a goal of 35°C.

Histology

Brains from the two anesthetized groups and the control group (n = 10 per group) were assessed for acute neuronal death. Twelve hours after anesthesia, animals were transcardially perfused with cold 4% paraformaldehyde in phosphate-buffered saline and brains were removed, postfixed, and sunk in sucrose solution. They were then sliced into 60 micron-thick slices and every other slice was mounted and stained with FluoroJade C, a marker specific for neurodegeneration [32,33] (FJC, 0.001%, Millipore, Billerica, MA). FJ-positive cells were counted using Nikon Eclipse *80i* microscope under 20X magnification in each slice containing the structure of interest. Structures included in analysis were the anterodorsal (AD), anteroventral (AV), laterodorsal (LD), and anteromedial (AM) thalamic nuclei, as well as CA1-3 regions of the hippocampus and the dentate gyrus.

Object Recognition Tasks

Object recognition was assessed using similar arrangements as others [19,28]. Behavior testing occurred during the light phase of the circadian cycle between 0800 and 1700 hrs in two separate arenas, hereafter referred to as contexts, of identical size (61 cm square base, walls 50 cm high). Context 1 had yellow walls with a base covered in wood-effect vinyl lining, and context 2 had black walls with a black plastic base. Different visual cues were placed on the walls of each context. A video camera (SONY HDR-CX190) was mounted 2 meters above the testing area for recording and observing subjects. For each task, except the allocentric object-location task, subjects were placed into contexts in the same location and facing the south wall (away from the objects). Beginning at P42, subjects were habituated to the two contexts prior to testing by being placed individually into the context for 5 min per day for 4 consecutive days. All animals underwent all behavioral tasks. Subjects were tested on the same day for any given task and in the same sequence of tasks. All tasks were performed in the order presented in subsequent weeks, except for the first two (novel object and object-place) which were performed in the same week. The order of testing during the day was counterbalanced among groups.

Investigation of an object was defined as sniffing or placing the nose within 1 cm of and oriented toward the object. Subjects were recorded, and observers blinded to group assignment were used to determine investigation times. Object investigation times during the initial exposure for each task were compared to assess for possible confounding effects of varying investigation times on the ability to recognize objects. All objects and testing arenas were wiped with 70% ethanol between testing.

Novel Object Recognition. Testing began at P48 with novel object recognition. A single trial was performed for each animal consisting of "exposure" and "test" phases separated by a two-minute delay (Fig. 2A). During the exposure, subjects were placed into the context and allowed to explore two *identical* objects for four minutes. After the delay, they were placed into the same context for three minutes with one of the objects replaced with a

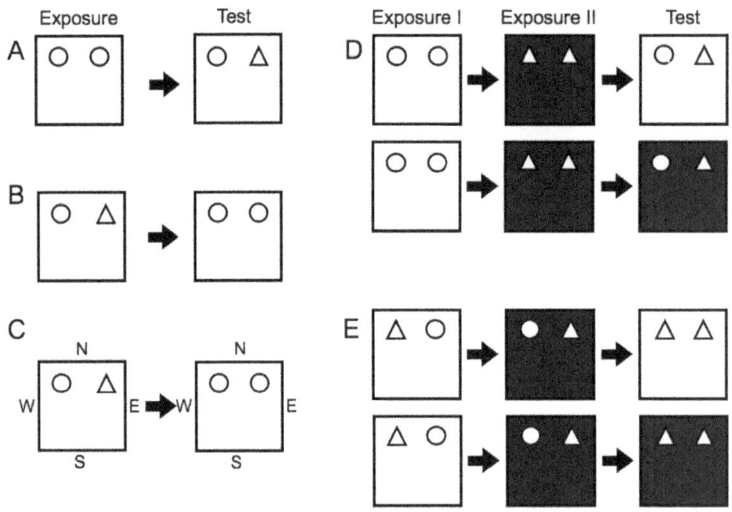

Figure 2. Object recognition. For each task, except allocentric object-place recognition, subjects are introduced at and facing the wall away from the objects. (A) *Novel object recognition.* Two identical objects are presented in the exposure, and one (right) is replaced with a novel object in the test phase. (B) *Object-place recognition.* Two different objects are presented, followed by two identical objects. In the test phase, the right object appears in a novel location within the context. (C) In the allocentric version of object-place recognition, subjects are again introduced at and facing the south wall (S) in the exposure. However, for the test phase, subjects are placed at and facing either the east (E) or west (W) wall. (D) *Object-context recognition.* Two different pairs of objects are presented in two different contexts, so each object is associated with a particular context. In the test phase, one object (right object, top row; left object, bottom row) appears within a context in which it has not been explored. (E) *Object-place-context recognition.* Two different objects are first presented in a context. The object locations are then reversed and presented in a different context. Thus, after two exposures, each object is seen in both contexts and both locations (left and right). In the test phase, two objects are presented in either context, so one (right object, top row; left object, bottom row) appears in a novel configuration of place and context.

novel object. Half of the subjects were tested in each context with the location (left or right) of the novel object counterbalanced among subjects.

Object-Place Recognition. Subjects were tested in their ability to recognize an object and its location. Two trials were performed, and investigation times were totaled for the two trials. In the exposure, two *different* objects were presented in a context for four minutes. After a two-minute delay, two *identical* copies of one of the previous objects were presented in the same context for three minutes (Fig. 2B). Both objects were equally familiar, but one now occupied a different location within the context.

Allocentric Object-Place Recognition. For the previous task, subjects were always introduced into the context facing the wall (south wall) opposite the two objects (Fig. 2C). In the allocentric version of the task, for the initial exposure, subjects were again placed into the context facing the south wall. In the test phase, however, the entry point was varied and half of the subjects were introduced facing either the east or west wall (Fig. 2C). Two trials were performed and the entry point was randomized among subjects.

Object-Context Recognition. Subjects were assessed in their ability to recognize an object with a particular context. The task required two separate exposures, each lasting four minutes and separated by a two-minute delay (Fig. 2D). In the first exposure, a pair of *identical* objects was presented in a context. Next, subjects were placed in a *different* context with a *different* pair of objects. In the test phase, lasting three minutes, subjects were placed into a context with one of each previously encountered object. Thus, one object was presented in the same context as before, while the other object appeared within a context in which it had not been explored. Two trials were conducted, and the test phase occurred in opposite contexts for each trial (Fig. 2D).

Object-Place-Context Recognition. Subjects were tested in their ability to recognize an object with its location and context (Fig. 2E). In the first exposure, two *different* objects were presented within a context. Next, subjects were placed in the opposite context with the *same* two objects and their locations reversed. Thus, after two exposures, each object was observed in both contexts and locations (left and right). In the test phase, two *identical* copies of either of the previous objects were presented in a context. The location and context associated with one object were familiar, while the other "displaced" object appeared in a location and context in which it had not been observed. Two trials were conducted with the test phase occurring in opposite contexts for each trial (Fig. 2E).

Social Behavior and Social Recognition

Following object recognition, animals were given unrestricted access to food. Social interaction and recognition were assessed using a discrimination paradigm one week after completing object recognition testing at P80. In the exposure, the subject was presented with a caged stimulus animal and a novel object for five minutes. This arrangement evaluates social behavior by determining whether subjects spend more time investigating the stimulus animal or object[7]. After a sixty-minute delay, subjects were presented simultaneously with the same "familiar" animal and a novel animal for three minutes. Recognition of the previously encountered animal was demonstrated by decreased investigation of the familiar target relative to the novel one.

Same-sex juvenile conspecifics were used as stimulus animals. Male pups five weeks of age were housed individually one week prior to testing. Investigation of the stimulus animal was defined as sniffing or direct contact with the subject's nose or paws. Investigation of the novel object was defined as sniffing or placing the nose within 1 cm of and oriented toward object.

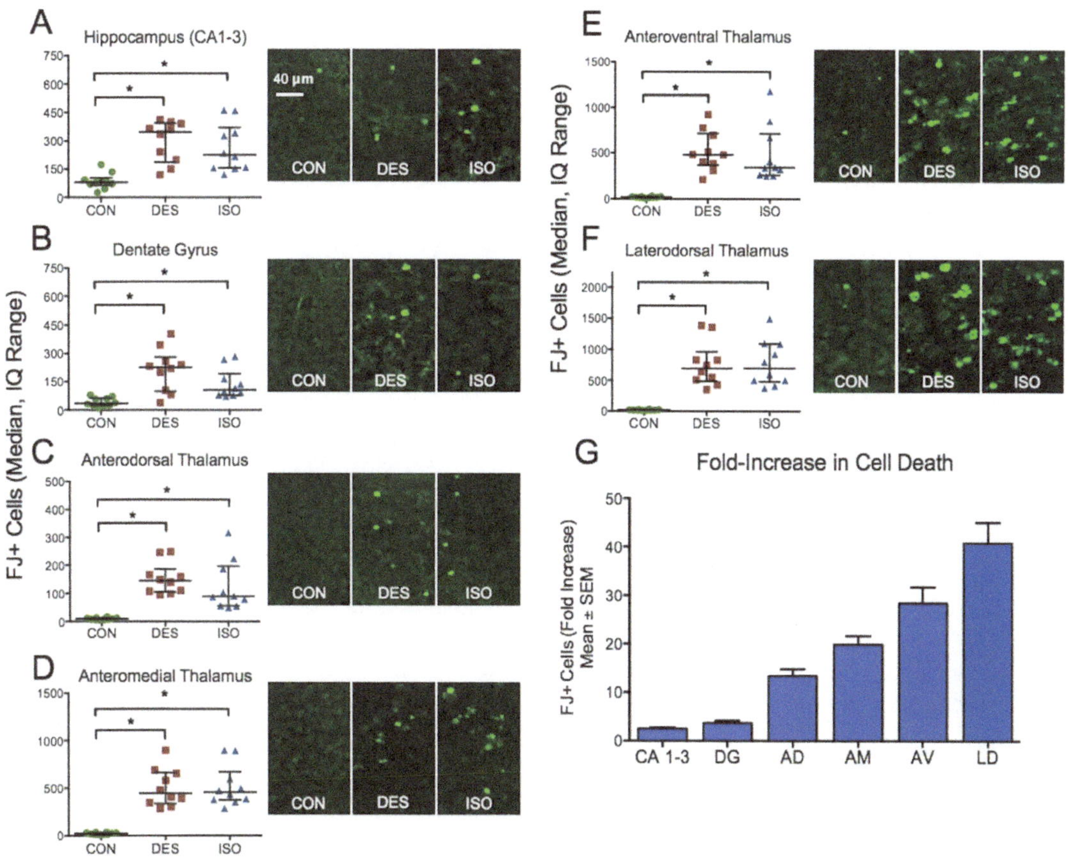

Figure 3. Neuronal death by group. A to F) Exposure to either anesthetic - desflurane or isoflurane - led to significantly increased neuronal death in each brain region. The degree of neurodegeneration was similar in desflurane and isoflurane-treated subjects. Sample images from brains at 20X magnification are shown alongside graphs comparing total cell death for each structure. **G)** The average increases in neuronal death relative to controls are shown. $^*P<0.05$.

Statistical Analysis

Data were analyzed using Prism 6 Software for Mac OSX (GraphPad Software Inc., San Diego, CA). Data were assessed for normal distribution using the D'Agostino and Pearson test. Parametric tests were used for normally distributed data; otherwise, nonparametric tests were used for analysis. All comparisons used a two-tail test and a P value less than 0.05 was considered statistically significant.

Total FluoroJade-positive cells for each brain region were compared among the groups – control, desflurane, isoflurane – using one-way ANOVA for parametric data or the Kruskal-Wallis test for nonparametric data. Bonferroni's post-test with multiple comparisons was used following one-way ANOVA, and Dunn's post-test was used with the Kruskal-Wallis test. The fold-increase in neuronal death was determined for each structure by dividing the total FJ-positive cells for all anesthetized animals ($n = 20$) by the average number of FJ-positive cells per structure for control animals ($n = 10$).

Recognition tasks were first assessed by comparing the investigation times of each target using paired tests for each group. Paired t-test was used for normally distributed data, and nonparametric data were analyzed with the Wilcoxon matched-pairs rank test. Also, to identify possible confounding effects of varying investigation times on subsequent object/animal recognition, the times during the exposure phase were compared between the groups using either one-way ANOVA with Bonferroni's post-test or the Kruskal-Wallis test with Dunn's post-test.

In addition, a "discrimination index" (DI) was calculated and represents the relative time spent exploring each target (eg. Familiar versus Novel). To calculate DI, the time spent investigating the familiar target was subtracted from the time spent on the novel target, and this was divided by the total time spent investigating the two (eg. DI = (Novel-Familiar)/(Total Time)). This value was compared to a theoretical value of zero using one sample t-test to assess whether a preference was shown for one of the objects, and a positive DI indicates preference for the novel aspect of the task. For each task, DI of control animals was compared against DI of all anesthetized animals. Also, within the group of anesthetized animals, the DI of desflurane-treated subjects was compared with that of isoflurane-treated subjects. These comparisons were made using either unpaired t-test for parametric data or the Mann Whitney test for nonparametric data.

Results

Increased neuronal death occurs similarly in desflurane and isoflurane-treated animals

There was increased neuronal death in each brain region in animals exposed to either desflurane or isoflurane relative to the control animals (Fig. 3). No difference in the extent of cell death was identified between the two anesthetized groups. Anesthetic exposure resulted in significantly increased cell death in the hippocampus (P = 0.0001, one-way ANOVA; control vs. des P = 0.0002, control vs. iso P = 0.0015, des vs. iso P = 0.99, Bonferroni), dentate gyrus (P = 0.0003, one-way ANOVA; control vs. des P = 0.0002, control vs. iso P = 0.03, des vs. iso P = 0.16, Bonferroni), anterodorsal thalamus (P<0.0001, one-way ANOVA; control vs. des P<0.0001, control vs. iso P = 0.0007, des vs. iso P = 0.98, Bonferroni), anteromedial thalamus (P<0.0001, one-way ANOVA; control vs. des P<0.0001, control vs. iso P<0.0001, des vs. iso P = 0.99, Bonferroni), anteroventral thalamus (P<0.0001, Kruskal-Walli test; control vs. des P<0.0001, control vs. iso P = 0.001, des vs. iso P = 0.99, Dunn's), and laterodorsal thalamus (P<0.0001, one-way ANOVA; control vs. des P<0.0001, control vs. iso P<0.0001, des vs. iso P = 0.99, Bonferroni). The relative fold-increase in cell death for each brain region is shown in Figure 3G.

Novel Object and Object-Place Recognition are Unaffected

Subjects from each group were able to distinguish familiar and novel objects, revealed by increased investigation times of the novel object (control P = 0.006, desflurane P = 0.01, isoflurane P = 0.0003; paired t-test familiar vs. novel, Fig. 4A). Object-place recognition was also intact in each group, and animals spent more time with the object in a novel location (control P = 0.006, desflurane P = 0.001, isoflurane P = 0.0008, paired t-test familiar vs. novel location, Fig. 4C). There was no difference in object exploration times among groups during the exposure for either task (novel object P = 0.5, one-way ANOVA, object-place P = 0.2, Kruskal-Wallis).

Discrimination Indexes [3] for all subjects were greater than zero for both novel object recognition (control P = 0.007, desflurane P = 0.002, isoflurane P = 0.002, one sample t-test, Fig. 4B) and object-place recognition (control P = 0.01, desflurane P = 0.001, isoflurane P = 0.001, one sample t-test, Fig. 4D). No differences in DI were identified between control and anesthetized subjects (novel object P = 0.9, unpaired t-test; object-place P = 0.3, Mann Whitney test) or between desflurane and isoflurane subjects (novel object P = 0.83, unpaired t-test; object-place P = 0.64, Mann Whitney test).

Isoflurane but not desflurane treated animals are impaired in object-context and social recognition

Only the isoflurane group was impaired in the ability to associate an object with its context and spent similar amounts of time with each object in this task (control P = 0.001, Wilcoxon test familiar vs. novel context; desflurane P = 0.006, isoflurane P = 0.2, paired t-test, Fig. 5A). DIs of control and desflurane subjects were greater than zero but not in isoflurane-treated subjects (control P = 0.004, desflurane P = 0.04, isoflurane P = 0.95, one sample t-test, Fig. 5B). Comparison of DI between control and anesthetized subjects did not reveal a difference (P = 0.094, unpaired t-test, Fig. 5B). Within the anesthetized group, DI did not differ significantly between desflurane and isoflurane-treated subjects (P = 0.32, unpaired t-test). Exploration times in the exposure phases of the object-context task were similar for the three groups (P = 0.6, one-way ANOVA).

Isoflurane animals also had impaired social memory while desflurane animals were unaffected when comparing social target investigation times (control P = 0.0009, desflurane P = 0.002, isoflurane P = 0.08; paired t-test familiar vs. novel animal, Fig. 5C). DIs of control and desflurane subjects were greater than zero (control P = 0.0009, desflurane P = 0.002, one sample t-test, Fig. 5D), although isoflurane DI did not differ significantly from zero (P = 0.064, one sample t-test, Fig. 5D). No difference between DI was identified in control vs. anesthetized groups (P = 0.84, unpaired t-test). In the subset of anesthetized subjects, the isoflurane DI was lower than desflurane DI although it did not reach statistical significance (P = 0.17, unpaired t-test). In the exposure of the social recognition task, animals from all groups displayed normal social behavior and spent significantly greater time investigating the social target relative to the object (all P< 0.0001, paired t-test object vs. social target).

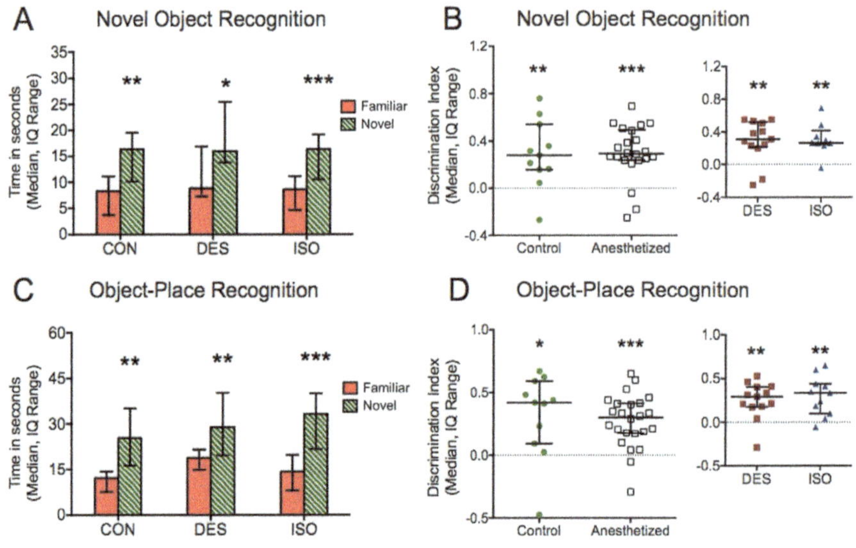

Figure 4. Novel object and object-place recognition. A) Subjects all demonstrated successful object recognition and preferentially explored the novel object. B) Each group's DI was significantly greater than zero, and there was no difference in DIs. C) Subjects were also able to identify an object in a novel location, demonstrated by a relative increase in investigation of that object. D) Again, DIs for all subjects were greater than zero with no differences identified. *P<0.05, **P<0.01, ***P<0.001, CON = control, DES = desflurane, ISO = isoflurane.

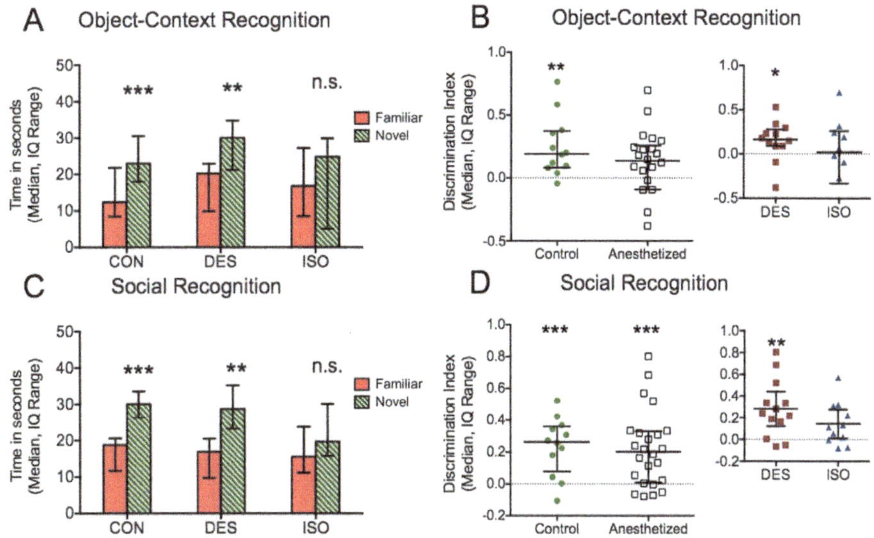

Figure 5. Object-context and social recognition. A) Isoflurane-treated animals were impaired in associating an object with a particular context. Animals exposed to desflurane, on the other hand, recognized when an object appeared in a different context and spent more time with that object. B) The DI for anesthetized subjects in this task did not differ from zero, and, within this group, only the desflurane DI significantly exceeded zero. C) Desflurane-treated subjects also had no change in social recognition ability, spending more time with the novel animal, while isoflurane-treated animals had deficient social memory. D) DI for both control and anesthetized animals exceeded zero, although DI for the subset of isoflurane-treated subjects did not. *P<0.05, **P<0.01, ***P<0.001, n.s. = not significant.

Anesthetized subjects are impaired in allocentric object-place and object-place-context recognition

Animals from both isoflurane and desflurane groups were impaired in object recognition when the entry site was varied in the allocentric version of the object-place task (control P = 0.001, desflurane P = 0.08, paired t-test familiar vs. novel; isoflurane P = 0.2, Wilcoxon test, Fig. 6A). The control DI was greater than zero (P = 0.0004, one sample t-test, Fig. 6B), while neither desflurane nor isoflurane DI differed from zero (desflurane P = 0.094, isoflurane P = 0.31, one sample t-test, Fig. 6B). DI of control animals was also significantly greater than that of anesthetized subjects (P = 0.024, unpaired t-test), although no difference was detected in the subset of desflurane and isoflurane-treated animals (P = 0.95, unpaired t-test).

Anesthetized subjects from both groups were also unable to distinguish objects in the object-place-context task (control P = 0.04, desflurane P = 0.5, paired t-test familiar vs. displaced; isoflurane P = 0.8, Wilcoxon test, Fig. 6C). Only the control DI exceeded zero in this task (control P = 0.021, desflurane P = 0.71, isoflurane P = 0.7, one sample t-test, Fig. 6D). Control DI was again significantly greater than DI for anesthetized subjects (P = 0.04, unpaired t-test), and no difference was found between desflurane and isoflurane DIs (P = 0.59, unpaired t-test). Investigation times during the exposures were similar between groups for each task (allocentric object-place P = 0.1, object-place-context P = 0.7, one-way ANOVA). The summary of all behavioral testing is presented in Table 1, where each group is evaluated whether they demonstrate a preference for the novel portion of the task by recognizing a familiar set of stimuli.

Discussion

The main finding of this study is that exposure to the volatile anesthetics isoflurane and desflurane causes impairment in tasks relying on specific cognitive processes of associative learning and recognition memory. After exposure to 1 MAC of either anesthetic for 4 hours during the early postnatal period, adult subjects could identify a novel object and recognize changes in an object's spatial location. However, anesthetized animals were unable to recognize an object's location when they entered the testing arena from a different vantage point or perform a complex task requiring the integration of object, place, and context details. In addition, isoflurane-treated subjects were impaired in context-specific object recognition and exhibited deficient social memory.

The behaviors assessed in this study provide valuable insight into the types of learning affected by neonatal anesthesia exposure. The object recognition tasks performed here rely on spatial memory, but they also require associative processing to encode the relationships among distinct elements encountered during a given exposure [28,34,35]. Both control and treatment animals easily recognize a novel object, but animals that were anesthetized on P7 begin to show impairment when presented with objects that were previously in a different location or context, suggesting problems with associative learning. The impairment in the allocentric object-place task may also be related to spatial memory, because the animals are able to identify objects when relying on egocentric cues but struggle when forced to rely on allocentric cues.

Episodic memory is associative in nature, and memory formation relies in large part on our ability to link new experiences and items with closely related ideas, facts, and the environment or context in which we learn them [36]. Clearly, a problem forming associations and relationships would affect memory encoding over time. Furthermore, within the broad domain of episodic memory, recognition memory is a specific type of memory that, according to the dual process model, is comprised of recollection and familiarity [26,36]. It is likely that impairment in the object recognition and associative memory tasks could also result from a deficit in recollection, a process underlying recognition memory [19,28]. We recently reported deficits in recollection in both rodents and children after anesthesia at an early age [6]. Persistent problems with associative and recognition memory in children would have important consequences for learning and development throughout

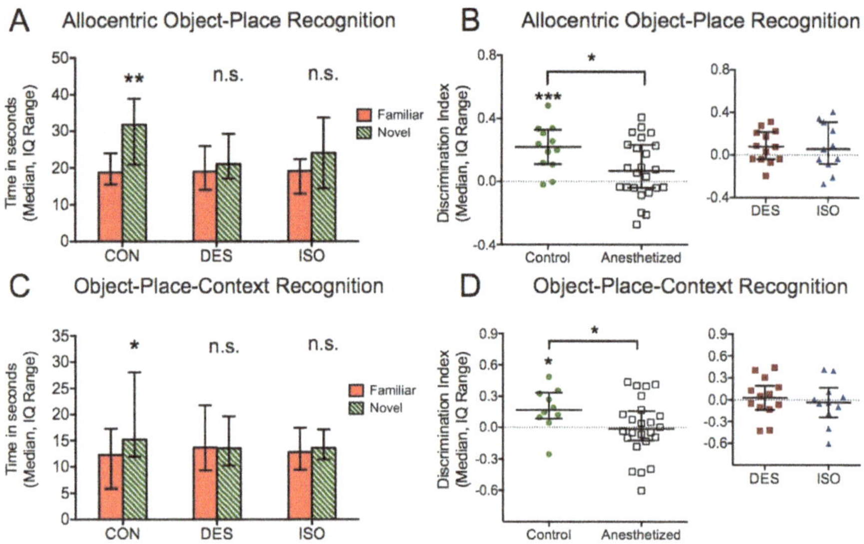

Figure 6. Allocentric object-place and object-place-context recognition. A) Exposure to isoflurane or desflurane led to impairment in identifying an object's location when the site of entry into the context was changed. The varied entry points forced subjects to rely on allocentric cues to identify the object's location. B) DI of control animals was significantly greater than that of anesthetized subjects. Neither desflurane nor isoflurane DI significantly exceeded zero. C) Isoflurane and desflurane-treated subjects were also impaired in recognition of an object that required association of its place and context. D) Again, control DI was greater than anesthetized DI. Neither subset of anesthetized subjects - desflurane or isoflurane - had DI greater than zero. *$P<0.05$, **$P<0.01$, n.s. = not significant.

adolescence. The precise cognitive domains that may be impaired in children and how these effects manifest later in life is still unclear, and these are important areas of future investigation.

Isoflurane has been used in numerous studies to investigate the effects of anesthesia and many labs have reported cell death and behavioral changes after isoflurane exposure [1–3,14,30]. The effects associated with desflurane, though, are less well described. Similar to other volatile anesthetics, desflurane in neonates has been shown to induce cell death [37,38]. However, few studies of behavior have been performed, and only one of these has demonstrated cognitive impairment [38]. Kodama and colleagues found that mice exposed to desflurane later developed problems with short-term and long-term memory [38]. In our present study, we demonstrate impairment in desflurane-treated animals using two separate tasks that involve associative learning. Together, these behavioral results show that desflurane, like isoflurane [2,14,30] and sevoflurane [13,30,39], alters long-term cognitive behavior.

Isoflurane-treated animals were impaired in two additional behavioral tasks, suggesting a distinct outcome from those anesthetized with desflurane. Others have also identified distinct outcomes using different anesthetic agents [37,38,40,41], although the reason underlying these behavioral findings is unclear. The types of memory involved in this series of behavioral testing are processed in the medial temporal lobe [19,28], including hippocampus and dentate gyrus, as well as the anterior thalamus and prefrontal cortex [26],[42], and we identified increased neurodegeneration in each of these brain regions. However, the observation of distinct behavioral outcomes occurred in the setting of a similar extent of neuronal injury. The discrepancy between histologic and behavioral findings suggest that, although neuronal death may play a role in determining behavioral phenotype, other effects on neural development likely contribute, as well. In fact, there is evidence that volatile anesthetics can alter synaptogenesis and dendritic spine density even in the absence of cell death [43]. In addition, anesthetics have been shown to result in significant

Table 1. Summary of behavioral testing.

	Discrimination Index for task greater than zero?		
	Control	**DES**	**ISO**
Novel Object Recognition	Yes	Yes	Yes
Object-Place Recognition	Yes	Yes	Yes
Object-Context Recognition	Yes	Yes	***No***
Social Recognition	Yes	Yes	***No***
Allocentric Object-Place Recognition	Yes	***No***	***No***
Object-Place-Context Recognition	Yes	***No***	***No***

For each test, recognition of a familiar set of stimuli results in preferential exploration of the novel aspect of the task. Discrimination Index (DI) represents the time spent with the novel object or animal relative to the familiar one, and DI significantly greater than zero demonstrates successful recognition in the task.

neuroinflammation [41], changes in cell signaling [44], and stem cell proliferation [45,46]. It is likely that anesthetic effects on these processes of brain development contribute to the ultimate cognitive outcome.

Isoflurane-treated animals also had difficulty with social recognition which is more likely related to long-term memory processes than their capacity for social interaction. Unlike previous reports [39], we found all animals behaved similarly during the exposure portion of the test, spending much more time with a novel animal than an object. In fact, throughout these experiments none of the treatment groups demonstrated a difference in exploration time during the exposure phase. This suggests anesthetic exposure does not alter investigatory or social behavior, motivation, or attention.

Limitations

The purpose of this study is to evaluate two separate anesthetics using outcomes of cell death and behavior. We cannot make conclusive remarks regarding mechanisms underlying cognitive impairment, and separate studies are needed to better understand these processes. Also, a comprehensive analysis of neuronal death was not undertaken, and it is possible that other brain regions show a difference. The hippocampus and thalamus were chosen, however, because of their underlying role in the investigated behavior.

Social recognition is based on olfaction in rodents [47] and we did not perform a separate experiment to exclude impaired olfaction as the basis for deficient social recognition in our subjects. However, we have previously determined that anesthetic exposure does not impair olfaction [6]. Isoflurane-treated subjects displayed typical social behavior in each part of the test, suggesting impaired recognition was due to effects on memory rather than interest, motivation, or olfaction. Also, although the rats were tested serially, they did not show any signs of decreasing interest with the objects as we used objects that appeared novel to the subjects in each trial. In fact, the exploration times remained very similar across the tests from first to last.

There are numerous studies documenting effects of gestational and early life stress on long-term behavior [48,49]. Because the animals were shipped, rather than bred in the housing facility, it is possible that they were exposed to early life stress that may affect aspects of behavior. Although effects of stress are likely evenly distributed amongst behavior groups, these considerations should be taken into account when interpreting behavioral results.

Finally, the cognitive outcomes from the two anesthetics appear to be different; however, it is possible that the two anesthetics were not entirely equal in depth in spite of being adjusted to 1 MAC. This must be taken into consideration when attempting to make direct comparisons between the two volatile anesthetics.

Conclusion

Neonatal exposure to isoflurane and desflurane led to impairment in object recognition tasks relying on spatial and associative memory. These findings provide evidence that anesthetics can affect distinct cognitive processes that are fundamental to learning and memory in rodents, as well as humans.

Author Contributions

Conceived and designed the experiments: BHL JTC OH LV JWS. Performed the experiments: BHL JTC OH LV JWS. Analyzed the data: BHL JTC OH LV JWS. Contributed reagents/materials/analysis tools: BHL JTC OH LV JWS. Contributed to the writing of the manuscript: BHL JTC OH LV JWS.

References

1. Gentry KR, Steele LM, Sedensky MM, Morgan PG (2013) Early developmental exposure to volatile anesthetics causes behavioral defects in Caenorhabditis elegans. Anesth Analg 116: 185–189.
2. Jevtovic-Todorovic V, Hartman RE, Izumi Y, Benshoff ND, Dikranian K, et al. (2003) Early exposure to common anesthetic agents causes widespread neurodegeneration in the developing rat brain and persistent learning deficits. J Neurosci 23: 876–882.
3. Brambrink AM, Evers AS, Avidan MS, Farber NB, Smith DJ, et al. (2010) Isoflurane-induced neuroapoptosis in the neonatal rhesus macaque brain. Anesthesiology 112: 834–841.
4. Flick RP, Katusic SK, Colligan RC, Wilder RT, Voigt RG, et al. (2011) Cognitive and behavioral outcomes after early exposure to anesthesia and surgery. Pediatrics 128: e1053–1061.
5. Wilder RT, Flick RP, Sprung J, Katusic SK, Barbaresi WJ, et al. (2009) Early exposure to anesthesia and learning disabilities in a population-based birth cohort. Anesthesiology 110: 796–804.
6. Stratmann G, Lee J, Sall JW, Lee B, Alvi BS, et al. (2014) Effect of general anesthesia in infancy on long-term recognition memory in humans and rats. Neuropsychopharmacology 39. EPub ahead of print.
7. DiMaggio C, Sun LS, Kakavouli A, Byrne MW, Li G (2009) A retrospective cohort study of the association of anesthesia and hernia repair surgery with behavioral and developmental disorders in young children. J Neurosurg Anesthesiol 21: 286–291.
8. DiMaggio C, Sun LS, Li G (2011) Early childhood exposure to anesthesia and risk of developmental and behavioral disorders in a sibling birth cohort. Anesth Analg 113: 1143–1151.
9. Bunsey M, Eichenbaum H (1996) Conservation of hippocampal memory function in rats and humans. Nature 379: 255–257.
10. Eichenbaum H, Yonelinas AP, Ranganath C (2007) The medial temporal lobe and recognition memory. Annu Rev Neurosci 30: 123–152.
11. Burgess N, Maguire EA, O'Keefe J (2002) The human hippocampus and spatial and episodic memory. Neuron 35: 625–641.
12. Fortin NJ, Wright SP, Eichenbaum H (2004) Recollection-like memory retrieval in rats is dependent on the hippocampus. Nature 431: 188–191.
13. Shih J, May LD, Gonzalez HE, Lee EW, Alvi RS, et al. (2012) Delayed environmental enrichment reverses sevoflurane-induced memory impairment in rats. Anesthesiology 116: 586–602.
14. Stratmann G, May LD, Sall JW, Alvi RS, Bell JS, et al. (2009) Effect of hypercarbia and isoflurane on brain cell death and neurocognitive dysfunction in 7-day-old rats. Anesthesiology 110: 849–861.
15. Boscolo A, Ori C, Bennett J, Wiltgen B, Jevtovic-Todorovic V (2013) Mitochondrial protectant pramipexole prevents sex-specific long-term cognitive impairment from early anaesthesia exposure in rats. Br J Anaesth.
16. Yonelinas AP (2001) Components of episodic memory: the contribution of recollection and familiarity. Philos Trans R Soc Lond B Biol Sci 356: 1363–1374.
17. Brown MW, Aggleton JP (2001) Recognition memory: what are the roles of the perirhinal cortex and hippocampus? Nat Rev Neurosci 2: 51–61.
18. Clayton NS, Dickinson A (1998) Episodic-like memory during cache recovery by scrub jays. Nature 395: 272–274.
19. Eacott MJ, Norman G (2004) Integrated memory for object, place, and context in rats: a possible model of episodic-like memory? J Neurosci 24: 1948–1953.
20. Eacott MJ, Easton A, Zinkivskay A (2005) Recollection in an episodic-like memory task in the rat. Learn Mem 12: 221–223.
21. Dere E, Huston JP, De Souza Silva MA (2005) Episodic-like memory in mice: simultaneous assessment of object, place and temporal order memory. Brain Res Brain Res Protoc 16: 10–19.
22. Kart-Teke E, De Souza Silva MA, Huston JP, Dere E (2006) Wistar rats show episodic-like memory for unique experiences. Neurobiol Learn Mem 85: 173–182.
23. Eichenbaum H, Fortin N, Sauvage M, Robitsek RJ, Farovik A (2010) An animal model of amnesia that uses Receiver Operating Characteristics (ROC) analysis to distinguish recollection from familiarity deficits in recognition memory. Neuropsychologia 48: 2281–2289.
24. Easton A, Eacott MJ (2010) Recollection of episodic memory within the medial temporal lobe: behavioural dissociations from other types of memory. Behav Brain Res 215: 310–317.
25. Sauvage MM (2010) ROC in animals: uncovering the neural substrates of recollection and familiarity in episodic recognition memory. Conscious Cogn 19: 816–828.
26. Aggleton JP, Dumont JR, Warburton EC (2011) Unraveling the contributions of the diencephalon to recognition memory: a review. Learn Mem 18: 384–400.
27. Macbeth AH, Edds JS, Young WS 3rd (2009) Housing conditions and stimulus females: a robust social discrimination task for studying male rodent social recognition. Nat Protoc 4: 1574–1581.

28. Langston RF, Wood ER (2010) Associative recognition and the hippocampus: differential effects of hippocampal lesions on object-place, object-context and object-place-context memory. Hippocampus 20: 1139–1153.
29. Cross L, Brown MW, Aggleton JP, Warburton EC (2012) The medial dorsal thalamic nucleus and the medial prefrontal cortex of the rat function together to support associative recognition and recency but not item recognition. Learn Mem 20: 41–50.
30. Ramage TM, Chang FL, Shih J, Alvi RS, Quitoriano GR, et al. (2013) Distinct long-term neurocognitive outcomes after equipotent sevoflurane or isoflurane anaesthesia in immature rats. Br J Anaesth.
31. Stratmann G, Sall JW, Eger EI 2nd, Laster MJ, Bell JS, et al. (2009) Increasing the duration of isoflurane anesthesia decreases the minimum alveolar anesthetic concentration in 7-day-old but not in 60-day-old rats. Anesth Analg 109: 801–806.
32. Schmued LC, Stowers CC, Scallet AC, Xu L (2005) Fluoro-Jade C results in ultra high resolution and contrast labeling of degenerating neurons. Brain Res 1035: 24–31.
33. Wang L, Liu YH, Huang YG, Chen LW (2008) Time-course of neuronal death in the mouse pilocarpine model of chronic epilepsy using Fluoro-Jade C staining. Brain Res 1241: 157–167.
34. Aggleton JP, Sanderson DJ, Pearce JM (2007) Structural learning and the hippocampus. Hippocampus 17: 723–734.
35. Mumby DG, Gaskin S, Glenn MJ, Schramek TE, Lehmann H (2002) Hippocampal damage and exploratory preferences in rats: memory for objects, places, and contexts. Learn Mem 9: 49–57.
36. Mayes A, Montaldi D, Migo E (2007) Associative memory and the medial temporal lobes. Trends Cogn Sci 11: 126–135.
37. Istaphanous GK, Howard J, Nan X, Hughes EA, McCann JC, et al. (2011) Comparison of the neuroapoptotic properties of equipotent anesthetic concentrations of desflurane, isoflurane, or sevoflurane in neonatal mice. Anesthesiology 114: 578–587.
38. Kodama M, Satoh Y, Otsubo Y, Araki Y, Yonamine R, et al. (2011) Neonatal desflurane exposure induces more robust neuroapoptosis than do isoflurane and sevoflurane and impairs working memory. Anesthesiology 115: 979–991.
39. Satomoto M, Satoh Y, Terui K, Miyao H, Takishima K, et al. (2009) Neonatal exposure to sevoflurane induces abnormal social behaviors and deficits in fear conditioning in mice. Anesthesiology 110: 628–637.
40. Liang G, Ward C, Peng J, Zhao Y, Huang B, et al. (2010) Isoflurane causes greater neurodegeneration than an equivalent exposure of sevoflurane in the developing brain of neonatal mice. Anesthesiology 112: 1325–1334.
41. Shen X, Dong Y, Xu Z, Wang H, Miao C, et al. (2013) Selective anesthesia-induced neuroinflammation in developing mouse brain and cognitive impairment. Anesthesiology 118: 502–515.
42. Aggleton JP, Hunt PR, Nagle S, Neave N (1996) The effects of selective lesions within the anterior thalamic nuclei on spatial memory in the rat. Behav Brain Res 81: 189–198.
43. Briner A, De Roo M, Dayer A, Muller D, Habre W, et al. (2010) Volatile anesthetics rapidly increase dendritic spine density in the rat medial prefrontal cortex during synaptogenesis. Anesthesiology 112: 546–556.
44. Masaki E, Kawamura M, Kato F (2004) Attenuation of gap-junction-mediated signaling facilitated anesthetic effect of sevoflurane in the central nervous system of rats. Anesth Analg 98: 647–652, table of contents.
45. Sall JW, Stratmann G, Leong J, McKleroy W, Mason D, et al. (2009) Isoflurane inhibits growth but does not cause cell death in hippocampal neural precursor cells grown in culture. Anesthesiology 110: 826–833.
46. Lin N, Moon TS, Stratmann G, Sall JW (2013) Biphasic change of progenitor proliferation in dentate gyrus after single dose of isoflurane in young adult rats. J Neurosurg Anesthesiol 25: 306–310.
47. Tang AC, Reeb BC, Romeo RD, McEwen BS (2003) Modification of social memory, hypothalamic-pituitary-adrenal axis, and brain asymmetry by neonatal novelty exposure. J Neurosci 23: 8254–8260.
48. Koenig JI, Elmer GI, Shepard PD, Lee PR, Mayo C, et al. (2005) Prenatal exposure to a repeated variable stress paradigm elicits behavioral and neuroendocrinological changes in the adult offspring: potential relevance to schizophrenia. Behav Brain Res 156: 251–261.
49. Weinstock M (2001) Alterations induced by gestational stress in brain morphology and behaviour of the offspring. Prog Neurobiol 65: 427–451.

3

Heat Hyperalgesia and Mechanical Hypersensitivity Induced by Calcitonin Gene-Related Peptide in a Mouse Model of Neurofibromatosis

Stephanie White[1¶], Blanca Marquez de Prado[1,2¶], Andrew F. Russo[2], Donna L. Hammond[1,3]*

1 Department of Anesthesia, University of Iowa, Iowa City, Iowa, United States of America, 2 Department of Molecular Physiology and Biophysics, University of Iowa, Iowa City, Iowa, United States of America, 3 Department of Pharmacology, University of Iowa, Iowa City, Iowa, United States of America

Abstract

This study examined whether mice with a deficiency of neurofibromin, a Ras GTPase activating protein, exhibit a nociceptive phenotype and probed a possible contribution by calcitonin gene-related peptide. In the absence of inflammation, *Nf1*$^{+/-}$ mice (B6.129S6 Nf1<tm1Fcr>/J) and wild type littermates responded comparably to heat or mechanical stimuli, except for a subtle enhanced mechanical sensitivity in female *Nf1*$^{+/-}$ mice. Nociceptive phenotype was also examined after inflammation induced by capsaicin and formalin, which release endogenous calcitonin gene-related peptide. Intraplantar injection of capsaicin evoked comparable heat hyperalgesia and mechanical hypersensitivity in *Nf1*$^{+/-}$ and wild type mice of both genders. Formalin injection caused a similar duration of licking in male *Nf1*$^{+/-}$ and wild type mice. Female *Nf1*$^{+/-}$ mice licked less than wild type mice, but displayed other nociceptive behaviors. In contrast, intraplantar injection of CGRP caused greater heat hyperalgesia in *Nf1*$^{+/-}$ mice of both genders compared to wild type mice. Male *Nf1*$^{+/-}$ mice also exhibited greater mechanical hypersensitivity; however, female *Nf1*$^{+/-}$ mice exhibited less mechanical hypersensitivity than their wild type littermates. Transcripts for calcitonin gene-related peptide were similar in the dorsal root ganglia of both genotypes and genders. Transcripts for receptor activity-modifying protein-1, which is rate-limiting for the calcitonin gene-related peptide receptor, in the spinal cord were comparable for both genotypes and genders. The increased responsiveness to intraplantar calcitonin gene-related peptide suggests that the peripheral actions of calcitonin gene-related peptide are enhanced as a result of the neurofibromin deficit. The analgesic efficacy of calcitonin gene-related peptide receptor antagonists may therefore merit investigation in neurofibromatosis patients.

Editor: Claudia Sommer, University of Würzburg, Germany

Funding: This work was supported by the Department of Defense through Grant NF073016 to DLH and Grant NF100114 to BMdP. The funders had no role in study design, data collection and analysis, decision to publish, or preparation of the manuscript.

Competing Interests: The authors have declared that no competing interests exist.

* Email: Donna-hammond@uiowa.edu

¶ SW and BMdP are co-first authors on this work.

Introduction

Neurofibromatosis 1 (NF1) is an autosomal dominant disorder that results in reduced levels of neurofibromin, a GTPase activating protein (GAP) involved in the regulation of Ras signaling (i.e. a Ras-GAP). This genetic disorder affects one in 3500 births worldwide – an incidence that equates to ~90,000 Americans and a million persons worldwide [1–4]. Nearly half of these cases result from new mutations. As such, *Nf1* has one of the highest rates of new mutations for any known single gene disorder [3,5]. One in four individuals with NF1 experience chronic bodily pain, as well as migraine and headache pain, over periods of months to years [1,6,7]. Severe pain also results from neurofibromas on spinal roots and malignant peripheral nerve sheath tumors [3]. The chronic nature of the pain, as well as its lancinating and paroxysmal character, contribute to the poor quality of life for patients with NF [8]. There is a great need for mechanistic based pharmacotherapies for the relief of pain in this patient population.

Early studies by Hingtgen and colleagues focused attention on the possible role of calcitonin gene-related peptide (CGRP) in pain associated with NF1. CGRP is a key factor in peripheral inflammation and in the production of nociception both in the spinal cord and in the periphery [9–12]. Interestingly, high densities of CGRP-immunoreactive fibers are present in neurofibromas in patients [13]. Using a rodent model of NF1 (*Nf1*$^{+/-}$ mice), Hingtgen and colleagues determined that haploid insufficiency of neurofibromin is associated with an increased release of CGRP from cultured dorsal root ganglion (DRG) neurons and spinal cord slices [14], as well as increased excitability of primary afferent neurons that convey pain [15,16]. More recent studies determined that the DRG of *Nf1*$^{+/-}$ mice have increased transcripts for Nav1.7 and Nav1.8, which are likely to underlie the enhanced excitability of primary afferent neurons [17], as well as increased N-type calcium currents that could contribute to enhanced release of neurotransmitter [18]. Collectively, these data suggest that an increased release of CGRP and decreased thresholds for activation of sensory neurons may underlie pain in NF1.

The aim of this study was to determine whether *Nf1*$^{+/-}$ mice exhibit a nociceptive phenotype and could serve as a model of pain in NF1, potentially facilitating the development of new therapies.

Nociceptive responsiveness of male and female *Nf1*$^{+/-}$ mice to heat and mechanical stimuli was determined in the absence of inflammation and after inflammation induced by exogenous administration of CGRP or by formalin or capsaicin, two agents that can release CGRP in the spinal cord and periphery. Ancillary studies quantitated levels of transcript for CGRP in the DRG and receptor activity-modifying protein-1 (RAMP1) in the spinal cord. RAMP1 associates with the calcitonin-like receptor to form the CGRP receptor [19], and is rate limiting for the activity of CGRP [20]. The results indicate that *Nf1*$^{+/-}$ mice are not a robust animal model for the pain experienced by NF patients, a conclusion that was also reached by O'Brien et al. [21]. Nonetheless, the finding that neurofibromin deficit is associated with an enhanced effect of CGRP in the periphery suggests that CGRP receptor antagonists may merit investigation for the treatment of pain in NF patients.

Materials and Methods

Experimental model

Mutation of *Nf1* in one allele is sufficient for expression and nearly complete penetrance of the disorder in humans. These studies therefore used *Nf1*$^{+/-}$ mice as a rodent model of NF1. These mice exhibit an increased predisposition to develop tumors as they age [22,23]. Use of homozygous null mutant mice was not feasible as the mutation is embryonic lethal [22,24]. Moreover, no definitive examples of patients homozygous for mutation of *Nf1* have been identified [25].

Litter-matched wild type (WT) and *Nf1*$^{+/-}$ (B6.129S6 Nf1<tm1Fcr>/J) mice of both genders (Jackson, Bar Harbor, Maine) weighing 23–30 grams were used. Female mice were tested randomly throughout the estrous cycle. Mice were housed in groups of five on SoftZorb paper enrichment bedding in a temperature controlled room on a 12-hr light/dark cycle. All testing occurred during the light cycle from 9:00 to 15:00 hr. Mice were euthanized at the conclusion of the experiments by CO_2 inhalation. These experiments were approved by the University of Iowa Animal Care and Use Committee (ACURF 0711237) and were conducted in accordance with the guidelines of the National Institutes of Health Guide for the Care and Use of Laboratory Animals and the guidelines of the International Association for the Study of Pain. With the exception of the capsaicin test, mice were used once and received only one dose of an agent. Every effort was made to minimize the number of mice used and their suffering. In all experiments, the investigator was blinded to the genotype. Blinding to intraplantar (ipl) treatment was not possible because capsaicin and formalin both produce spontaneous pain behaviors, while CGRP produces erythema and inflammation upon injection.

Heat threshold

Experiments were conducted to determine responsiveness to noxious heat, and whether heat hyperalgesia produced by ipl injection of CGRP or capsaicin differed by genotype or gender. Mice were acclimated to the testing environment for several hrs on two successive days and then allowed to move freely for one hr within a small Plexiglas enclosure that rested on an elevated glass surface maintained at 25°C. On the third day, the mice were acclimated to the environment for two more hrs and again allowed to acclimate to the testing chambers for another 30 min. A high intensity beam of light was then positioned under each hindpaw, and the latency to withdraw the hindpaw from the heat stimulus was recorded (UARD group, La Jolla, CA). If the mouse did not withdraw its paw within 20 sec, the test was terminated to prevent tissue injury. Care was taken to ensure that the surface of the hindpaw was flush with glass to avoid a heat-sink effect [26].

The first set of experiments assessed basal sensitivity to a noxious heat stimulus. The radiant heat stimulus was delivered at two different rates, 2.5°C/sec and 6.5°C/sec, as measured at the surface. These rates corresponded to 0.6°C/sec and 1.0°C/sec, as measured within the tissue. For both stimuli, the subdermal temperature at which withdrawal occurred was 40–41°C, in agreement with similar studies in the rat [27–29]. The lower rate of heating, which likely preferentially activates C-fibers, was used in the second set of experiments that assessed heat hyperalgesia. After determination of baseline paw withdrawal latency, an ipl injection of 5 µg CGRP, 0.01% capsaicin, or PBS was made into a hind paw. Paw withdrawal latency was redetermined 15, 30, 45, and 60 min after CGRP and 15 min after capsaicin.

Data were expressed as the mean ± S.E.M. Baseline paw withdrawal latencies were compared using a two-way analysis of variance (ANOVA) in which genotype was one factor and intensity was the second factor. The effects of CGRP or capsaicin were compared to their vehicle using a two-way repeated measures ANOVA in which one factor was genotype and the repeated factor was time. The Holm-Sidak test was used to make comparisons among mean values for the different treatment groups. A $P<0.05$ was considered significant in these and all subsequent analyses.

Mechanical threshold

Additional experiments determined mechanical threshold and examined whether mechanical hypersensitivity after ipl injection of CGRP or capsaicin differed by genotype or gender. Mice were acclimated to the testing environment for several hrs on two successive days. On the third day, the mice were acclimated for two more hrs to the environment and then allowed to move freely for a further 30 min within a small Plexiglas enclosure with a mesh floor. Mechanical hypersensitivity was assessed with a series of von Frey filaments that ranged from 1.65–4.31 log mN (0.0008–2 g). The filaments were applied to the plantar surface of each hindpaw between the pads. Care was taken to vary the site of application in this area. Testing was initiated by a two-sec application of the 3.84 filament before and the 3.22 filament after ipl injection of CGRP or capsaicin with enough pressure to cause the filament to bend slightly. If the mouse withdrew or lifted the paw, filaments of successively lower force were applied until one that produced no response to five applications was identified. The next higher force filament was then applied for a total of five times and the percentage of responses was recorded for that filament. Filaments of successively higher force were applied in this manner until a filament was reached that produced withdrawal on all five presentations or the 4.31 filament was reached. Higher filaments were not used because they lifted the hindpaw before the filament bent. After determination of basal threshold, either 5 µg CGRP, 0.001 or 0.01% capsaicin or their respective vehicles were injected. Mechanical hypersensitivity was redetermined 5 and 15 min after CGRP or PBS, and 15 min after capsaicin or vehicle by which time capsaicin's associated spontaneous pain behaviors had subsided.

Force-response curves were generated for both hindpaws and fit by non-linear regression to determine an EF_{50} with 95% confidence limits (CL) using Graphpad Prism. The minimum and maximum values were constrained to 0 and 100, respectively. Comparisons of EF_{50} values were made by F-test using Graphpad Prism version 5.0.

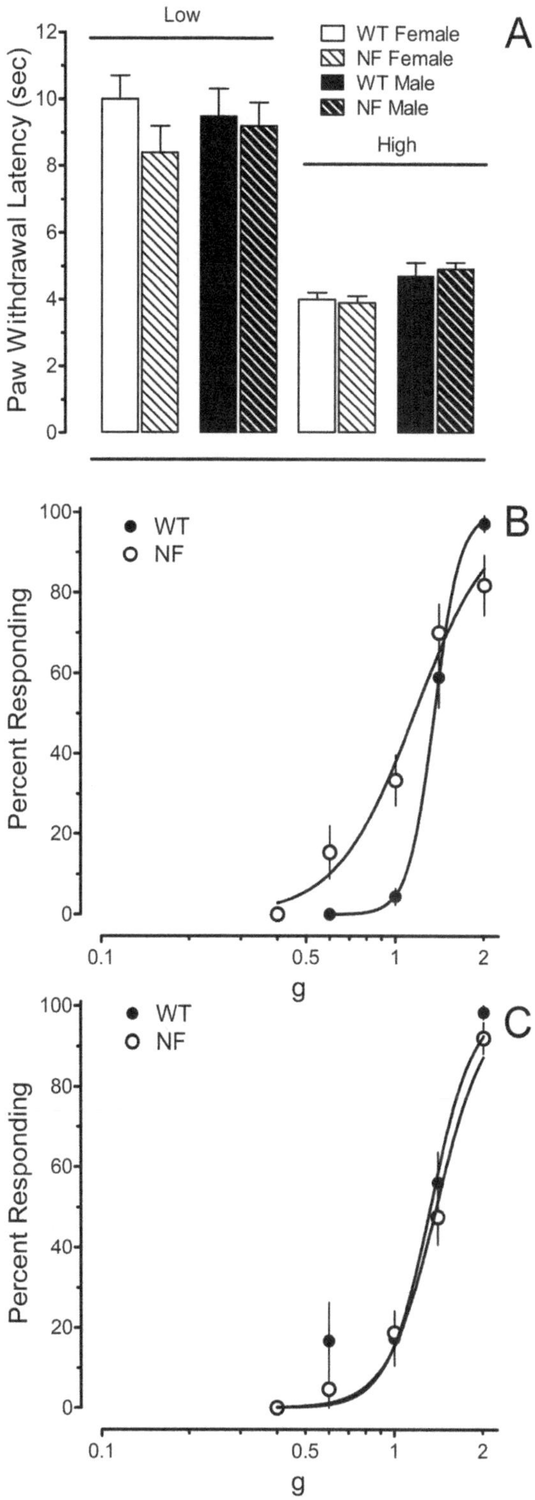

Figure 1. Assessment of acute nociception in $Nf1^{+/-}$ mice and WT littermates. In the absence of injury, $Nf1^{+/-}$ mice did not exhibit robust differences in sensitivity to noxious heat or tactile stimuli applied to the plantar surface of the hindpaw. (A) Paw withdrawal latency to low or high heating rates did not differ among genotypes or genders. Response latencies for both hindpaws were averaged to yield a single value for each mouse. Data are mean ± SEM of 6–8 mice. (B) Mechanical sensitivity was slightly greater in female $Nf1^{+/-}$ mice than wild type (WT) littermates (N = 18 in each group). (C) Male $Nf1^{+/-}$ and WT mice did not differ in their mechanical sensitivity (n = 16 and 15, respectively). Panels B and C were constructed using baseline data for the ipsilateral hindpaw of mice in the capsaicin and CGRP treatment groups. Data are expressed as the mean ± SEM.

Spontaneous pain behavior

Spontaneous pain behaviors evoked by ipl injection of 0.01% capsaicin or 2% formalin in one hindpaw were also quantified. In the case of capsaicin, the amount of time spent licking the injected paw was recorded in 5 min epochs for 15 min; spontaneous pain behaviors were essentially absent after 15 min. In the interest of making efficient use of each mouse and because the licking evoked by capsaicin was highly variable, each mouse received an injection of capsaicin in the left and right hindpaw, separated by a month. The duration of licking of each hindpaw was then averaged for that mouse. In the case of formalin, spontaneous pain behaviors were recorded for 90 min with a video camera and analyzed offline. The amount of time spent licking the paw, as well as the percentage of mice that exhibited guarding, flinching or unweighting of the injected paw, were quantified in 5 min epochs.

Duration of licking after capsaicin was expressed as the mean ± S.E.M. and compared between genotypes by two-way ANOVA for repeated measures. The Holm-Sidak test was used to compare group mean values. The duration of licking after formalin was analyzed in the same manner. In addition, the total time spent licking during phase one (0–5 min), phase two (15–50 min) and phase three (55–90 min) of the formalin test was calculated and compared by two-way ANOVA for repeated measures. Finally, guarding, flinching or unweighting of the injected paw after formalin were collectively scored as either present or absent. The percentage of mice that exhibited these behaviors was averaged over time for each of the three phases of the formalin test and compared by ANOVA.

Quantitation of CGRP and RAMP1 mRNA

Mice were euthanized by CO_2 inhalation followed by decapitation. The entire spinal cord and all DRG were rapidly removed from each mouse and stored in RNAlater (Ambion, Austin, TX). Total RNA was isolated from the tissue using the RNeasy kit according to the manufacturer's directions (Qiagen, Valencia, CA) and DNA contamination removed by digestion with Amp Grade DNase I (Invitrogen, Carlsbad, CA). Briefly, less than 30 mg of tissue was disrupted and homogenized in RTL buffer containing β-mercaptoethanol using a Tissue Tearor. The lysate was then centrifuged and the supernatant saved in a clean tube. The RNA was precipitated using 1 volume of 70% ethanol and loaded on the column. After one wash, 40 μl of buffer containing 1 unit DNase I was applied to the column and allowed to incubate for 15 min. The DNase was then removed by extensive washing. The RNA was eluted using RNase free water, and RNA concentration was determined by spectrometry. The RNA integrity number was determined for a subset of samples, and ranged between 8.1 and 8.6. Reverse transcription was performed using the Taqman RT-PCR mix (Applied Biosystems, Carlsbad, CA) with 0.5 μg RNA, 1X RT buffer, 5.5 mM $MgCl_2$, 0.5 mM dNTP, 4 units RNase inhibitor, 2.5 μM random hexamers, 12.5 units Multiscribe reverse transcriptase in 10 μl at 25°C for 10 min, 48°C for 30 min and 95°C for 5 min. Q-PCR was performed using 50 ng cDNA, 670 nM each primer (67 nM for CGRP primers) and 1X IQ^{tm} SYB Green Supermix (BioRad, Hercules, CA) in 15 μl. The cycle conditions were: 95°C for 10 min, followed by 40 cycles of 95°C for 15 s and annealing/extension at 60°C for 30 s and 72°C for 45 sec. Reactions were performed in triplicate and analyzed using a Bio-Rad MY-IQ thermocycler. At the end of amplifica-

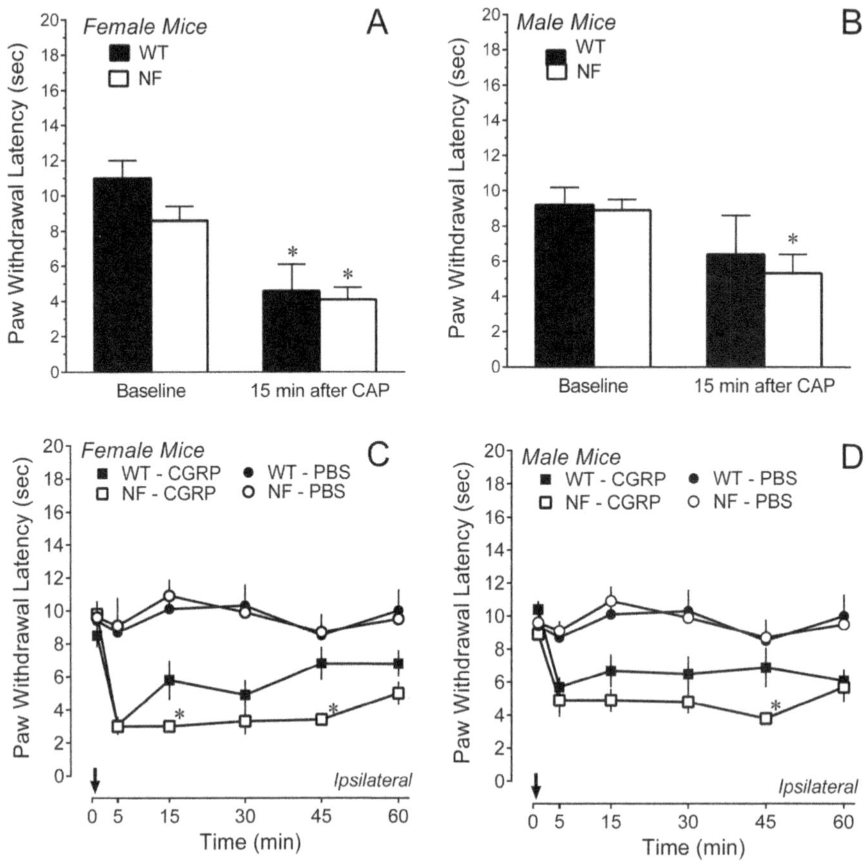

Figure 2. Intraplantar injection of 0.01% capsaicin or 5 µg CGRP induced heat hyperalgesia. (A, B) The magnitude of heat hyperalgesia determined 15 min after injection of capsaicin did not differ between genotypes in either females or males. * P<0.05 compared to baseline. (C, D) Paw withdrawal latency was decreased within 5 min of injection (arrow) of CGRP, but not PBS in females and males of both genotypes. Heat hyperalgesia in female and male *Nf1*$^{+/-}$ mice was greater than their WT littermates. The data for PBS are the pooled responses of two female and two male mice of each genotype. * P<0.05 compared to WT at the same time point. Data in all panels are expressed as the mean ± SEM of determinations in 6–8 mice of each gender and genotype.

tion, a thermal melt curve was generated. The one sample that that did not yield a homogenous melt curve was excluded. Primers for mRAMP1, CGRP, mGAPDH and β-actin have been described [20]. During this work, it was discovered that the description of the reverse primer for mRAMP1 in Zhang et al. (2007) contained a typographical error and an extraneous nucleotide. Although the correct primer (5′GCACTTGCT-GAAGTATCGATGG3′) was used for that work, the textual errors were replicated when ordering primer for this study. Nonetheless, the PCR product yielded the correct cDNA as verified by sequence analysis. Cycle thresholds (C_T) for mRAMP1, CGRP, GAPDH and β-actin were converted to absolute numbers using standard curves generated with serial dilutions of pGEM-QmRAMP1, pQmCGRP, pQmGAPDH and pQmβ-actin plasmids, respectively. For RAMP1, the mean efficiency of the PCR was 99.1±1.1% with a mean slope of −3.35±0.03. For β-actin, the mean efficiency was 94.8±1.0% with a mean slope of −3.43±0.03. For CGRP, the efficiency of the PCR was 93.2% with a mean slope of −3.299 and for GAPDH the efficiency of the PCR was 101.0% with a mean slope of −3.496.

Drugs and Vehicle Controls

All drugs were purchased from (Sigma, St Louis, MO) and prepared fresh each day. Calcitonin gene-related peptide was dissolved in PBS, which served as its vehicle control. Capsaicin was dissolved in 5% Tween 80 and 5% ethanol and brought to volume with PBS. In the von Frey experiments, a few mice received PBS as the control and others received PBS with 5% Tween 80 and 5% ethanol as the control. As there was no difference in the effects of either vehicle, the data were pooled for statistical analysis. Formalin was diluted to 2% using PBS. All drugs were injected in the plantar surface of one hindpaw with a 33-gauge stainless steel injector needle. Formalin was injected in a volume of 20 µl, while capsaicin or CGRP was injected in a volume of 10 µl. Drug delivery was monitored by following the movement of an air bubble in the tubing that connected the injector to the syringe pump.

Results

Nociceptive thresholds in the absence of injury

No differences in paw withdrawal latency were evident between the genotypes or by gender at either heating rate (Fig. 1A). With respect to mechanical sensitivity, the EF_{50} (95% CL) values for female WT and *Nf1*$^{+/-}$ mice were 1.35 (1.30−1.40) g and 1.16 (1.04–1.28) g, respectively (P<0.01). The small, but significant increase in mechanical sensitivity of female *Nf1*$^{+/-}$ mice could be attributed to an enhanced responsiveness to lower force filaments

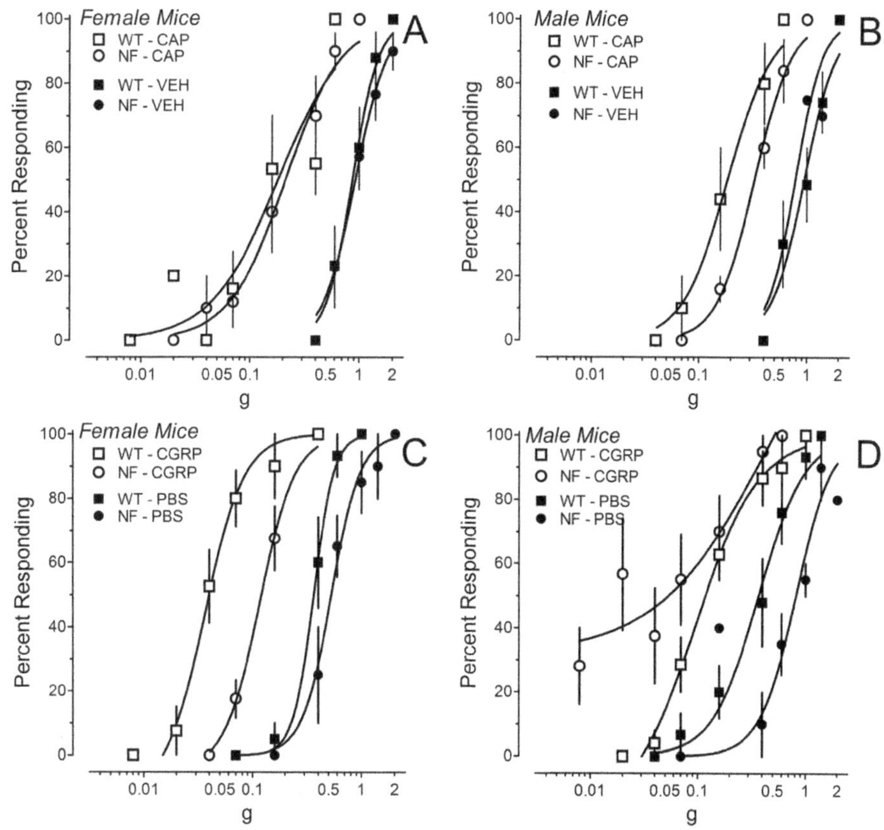

Figure 3. Mechanical hypersensitivity induced by intraplantar injection of 0.001% capsaicin (CAP) or 5 µg CGRP. (A, B) Force-response curves for the ipsilateral hindpaw after injection of CAP or vehicle (VEH) in $Nf1^{+/-}$ (circles) or WT (squares) mice. Data are the mean ± SEM of responses by 5–7 mice of each gender and genotype. (C, D) Force-response curves for the ipsilateral hindpaw after injection of CGRP or PBS in $Nf1^{+/-}$ (circles) or WT (squares) mice. Data in panels C-D are the mean ± SEM of responses by 4–8 mice of each gender and genotype, with the exception of CGRP in $Nf1^{+/-}$ mice where 11 mice were tested.

(Fig. 1B). The EF_{50} (95% CL) values for male WT and male $N1f^{+/-}$ mice were 1.32 (1.23–1.42) and 1.38 (1.30–1.48) g, respectively (P>0.5; Fig. 1C). Thus, with the exception of a small increase in mechanical sensitivity in female $Nf1^{+/-}$ mice, responsiveness to heat and mechanical stimuli did not differ between the genotypes or between the genders. Subsequent experiments examined whether $Nf1^{+/-}$ mice differed from their WT littermates in their responses to inflammatory agents.

Table 1. Capsaicin evokes mechanical hypersensitivity in both wildtype and $Nf1^{+/-}$ mice.

Female	**WT**		$Nf1^{+/-}$	
	Vehicle [6]	**Capsaicin [6]**	**Vehicle [7]**	**Capsaicin [5]**
Baseline	1.43 (1.37–1.50)	1.37 (1.31–1.44)	1.57 (1.46–1.69)	1.52 (1.29–1.79)
After	0.87 (0.73–1.03)[‡]	0.18 (0.11–0.29)[‡**]	0.92 (0.77–1.10)[‡]	0.21 (0.15–0.29)[‡**]
Male	**WT**		$Nf1^{+/-}$	
	Vehicle [6]	**Capsaicin [5]**	**Vehicle [4]**	**Capsaicin [4]**
Baseline	1.42 (1.36–1.48)	1.40 (1.29–1.52)	1.51 (1.40–1.63)	1.49 (1.36–1.63)
After	0.95 (0.78–1.15)[‡]	0.18 (0.12–0.27)[‡**]	0.78 (0.60–1.01)[‡]	0.32 (0.28–0.39)[‡**a]

EF_{50} and 95% confidence limits (g) of force–response curves for the ipsilateral hindpaw before and 15 min after intraplantar injection of 0.001% capsaicin or vehicle. Curves were fit by non-linear regression with minimum constrained to 0 and maximum to 100. Numbers of mice in each group appear in brackets.

*P<0.05,

** P<0.01 compared to vehicle at corresponding time point.

†P<0.05,

‡P<0.01 compared to baseline value.

aP<0.05 compared to WT at corresponding time point.

Table 2. Calcitonin gene-related peptide evokes mechanical hypersensitivity in both wildtype and Nf1$^{+/-}$ mice.

Female	**WT**		*Nf1$^{+/-}$*	
	PBS [4]	**CGRP [8]**	**PBS [4]**	**CGRP [8]**
Baseline	1.51 (1.38–1.67)	1.25 (1.16–1.35)	1.17 (0.86–1.59)^{a}	0.98 (0.88–1.05)^{aa}
After	0.36 (0.29–0.45)‡	0.04 (0.03–0.05)‡**	0.53 (0.44–0.64)^{‡aa}	0.12 (0.10–0.15)$^{‡**\ aa}$
Male	**WT**		*Nf1$^{+/-}$*	
	PBS [5]	**CGRP [8]**	**PBS [5]**	**CGRP [11]**
Baseline	1.38 (1.16–1.65)	1.22 (1.07–1.41)	1.40 (1.27–1.55)	1.29 (1.18–1.41)
After	0.37 (0.28–0.48)‡	0.12 (0.10–0.16)‡**	0.82 (0.66–1.00)^{‡aa}	0.04 n.d.

EF_{50} and 95% confidence limits (g) determined for force-response curves for the ipsilateral hindpaw before and 15 min after intraplantar injection of 5 µg CGRP or PBS Curves were fit by non-linear regression with minimum constrained to 0 and maximum to 100. Numbers of mice in each group appear in brackets.
*P<0.05,
** P<0.01 compared to vehicle at corresponding time point.
†P<0.05,
‡P<0.01 compared to baseline value.
^{a}P<0.05,
^{aa}P<0.01 compared to WT at corresponding time point.

Heat hyperalgesia evoked by capsaicin or CGRP

Injection of 0.01% capsaicin in the hindpaw decreased paw withdrawal latency to a similar extent in female *Nf1*$^{+/-}$ and WT mice (Fig. 2A). Capsaicin also significantly decreased paw withdrawal latency in male *Nf1*$^{+/-}$ mice, but did not significantly decrease paw withdrawal latency in male WT mice (P = 0.13; Fig. 2B). Nonetheless, male WT and *Nf1*$^{+/-}$ mice had comparable paw withdrawal latencies after capsaicin (P>0.5). These results indicate that the magnitude of capsaicin-induced heat hyperalgesia was comparable in both genotypes and genders.

Intraplantar injection of CGRP produced heat hyperalgesia in *Nf1*$^{+/-}$ mice and WT littermates of both genders. Female *Nf1*$^{+/-}$ mice exhibited a significantly greater decrease in paw withdrawal latency than female WT mice 15 and 45 min after injection (Fig. 2C). Male *Nf1*$^{+/-}$ mice exhibited a significantly greater decrease in paw withdrawal latency than male WT mice 45 min after injection (Fig. 2D). Intraplantar injection of PBS did not alter paw withdrawal latency of the ipsilateral hindpaw of either gender or genotype. Thus, unlike the heat hyperalgesia induced by capsaicin, the heat hyperalgesia induced by CGRP was greater in both male and female *Nf1*$^{+/-}$ mice compared to their corresponding WT controls.

Mechanical sensitivity after capsaicin or CGRP

Injection of 0.01% capsaicin in the hindpaw dramatically shifted the force-response curves to the left such that the lowest filament (0.008 g, 1.65 log mN) elicited responses on more than 50% of its presentations in most mice. Although mechanical hypersensitivity did not differ between genotypes or gender, a ceiling effect could have disguised subtle differences. Fifteen min after injection of a ten-fold lower dose of capsaicin (0.001%) female *Nf1*$^{+/-}$ and WT mice exhibited equivalent mechanical hypersensitivity, while male *Nf1*$^{+/-}$ mice exhibited less mechanical hypersensitivity than male WT mice (Fig. 3B, Table 1). Injection of vehicle also produced a very small, but statistically significant leftward shift in the force-response curves compared to baseline (Table 1). Thus, in female mice, capsaicin induced an equivalent mechanical hypersensitivity in both genotypes, whereas male *Nf1*$^{+/-}$ mice were less affected.

Intraplantar injection of CGRP or PBS also produced mechanical hypersensitivity of the ipsilateral hindpaw. Five min after ipl injection of PBS or 5 µg CGRP, force-response curves for the ipsilateral paw were shifted left in both genotypes and genders (data not shown). The shift by CGRP was much greater than that by PBS (data not shown). Fifteen min later, the shift in force-response curves by PBS was greatly diminished but still significantly to the left of baseline values (Table 2 and Fig. 3C, D). In contrast, the dramatic leftward shift produced by CGRP was sustained through 15 min (Table 2). In female *N1f*$^{+/-}$ mice, CGRP induced less mechanical hypersensitivity than female WT mice (Fig. 3C). However, male *Nf1*$^{+/-}$ mice exhibited greater mechanical hypersensitivity than male WT mice at very low filament forces (Fig. 3D). These results indicate that peripheral injection of CGRP produced mechanical hypersensitivity in both genotypes, and that the magnitude was a function of gender.

Spontaneous behavior after acute inflammatory stimuli

Injection of inflammatory agents such as capsaicin and formalin produced a variety of spontaneous pain behaviors. In the case of 0.01% capsaicin, the predominant behavior measured in the first 15 min was licking of the hindpaw. Female *Nf1*$^{+/-}$ and WT mice did not differ statistically in the duration of licking (simple main effect for genotype: P = 0.066; Fig. 4A). Male mice of each genotype exhibited comparable durations of licking (P>0.6; Fig. 4B). Similar conclusions were reached when the data were converted to area under the curve for the 15 min period. Thus, a deficit in neurofibromin neither facilitated nor inhibited capsaicin-induced spontaneous pain behaviors.

In the case of formalin, a constellation of behaviors was observed over 90 min that included guarding behaviors and unweighting of the affected hindpaw, as well as licking or flinching of the ipsilateral hindpaw. Interestingly, the duration of licking in female *Nf1*$^{+/-}$ mice was significantly lower in the second phase compared to female WT mice (Fig. 4C, E). There was no difference in the time spent licking in male mice of either genotype (Fig. 4D, F). Analysis of guarding, unweighting and flinching behaviors revealed that female *Nf1*$^{+/-}$ mice exhibited a much higher incidence of these behaviors than female WT mice during the second and third phase (Fig. 5A). These behaviors are likely to

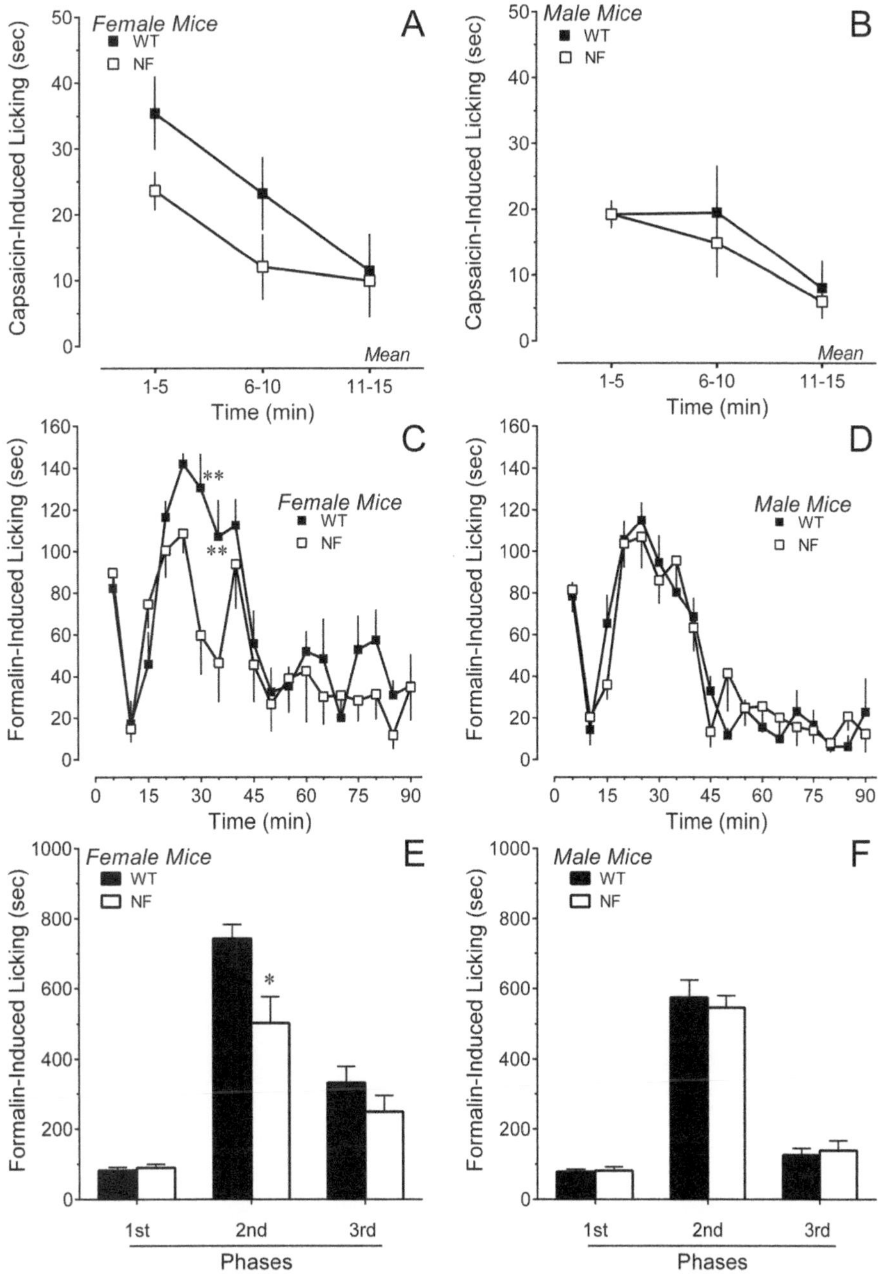

Figure 4. Duration of licking of the ipsilateral hindpaw after intraplantar injection of inflammatory irritants. Panels A and B illustrate the time course of licking after intraplantar injection of 0.01% capsaicin in the hindpaw of female or male mice, respectively. Panels C and D illustrate the time course of licking after intraplantar injection of 2% formalin in female or male mice, respectively. Panels E and F present the total duration of licking in phases 1 (0–5), 2 (15–55 min) and 3 (55–90 min) of the formalin test in female and male mice, respectively. Data are the mean ± S.E.M. of determinations in 6–8 mice of each gender and genotype. * P<0.05, ** P<0.01 compared to corresponding WT littermates.

have interfered with licking. There was no significant difference in the incidence of these behaviors between male $Nf1^{+/-}$ and WT mice (Fig. 5B, D). Formalin increased paw thickness by the same extent in all genotypes and genders (by 0.8±0.1, 0.9±0.1, 0.9±0.1 and 0.7±0.1 mm, n = 8 each group; P>0.5). Contralateral paw thickness ranged between 1.3 and 1.4 mm.

CGRP and RAMP1 Transcripts

Figure 6A illustrates levels of CGRP mRNA in the DRG of $Nf1^{+/-}$ mice and their WT littermates. There were no significant differences when the genders were combined for analysis (All; P = 0.2 Student's t-test). Two-way analysis indicated that CGRP transcript levels did not differ between genotypes within a gender, or between genders within a genotype (P>0.2 each factor). Figure 6B illustrates levels of RAMP1 mRNA in the spinal cord of $Nf1^{+/-}$ and WT littermates (Fig. 6B). Levels of RAMP1 transcript did not differ between genotypes when genders were combined for analysis (All; P>0.1; Student's t-test). Two-way analysis indicated that RAMP1 transcript levels did not differ between genotypes within a gender, or between genders within a genotype (P>0.05

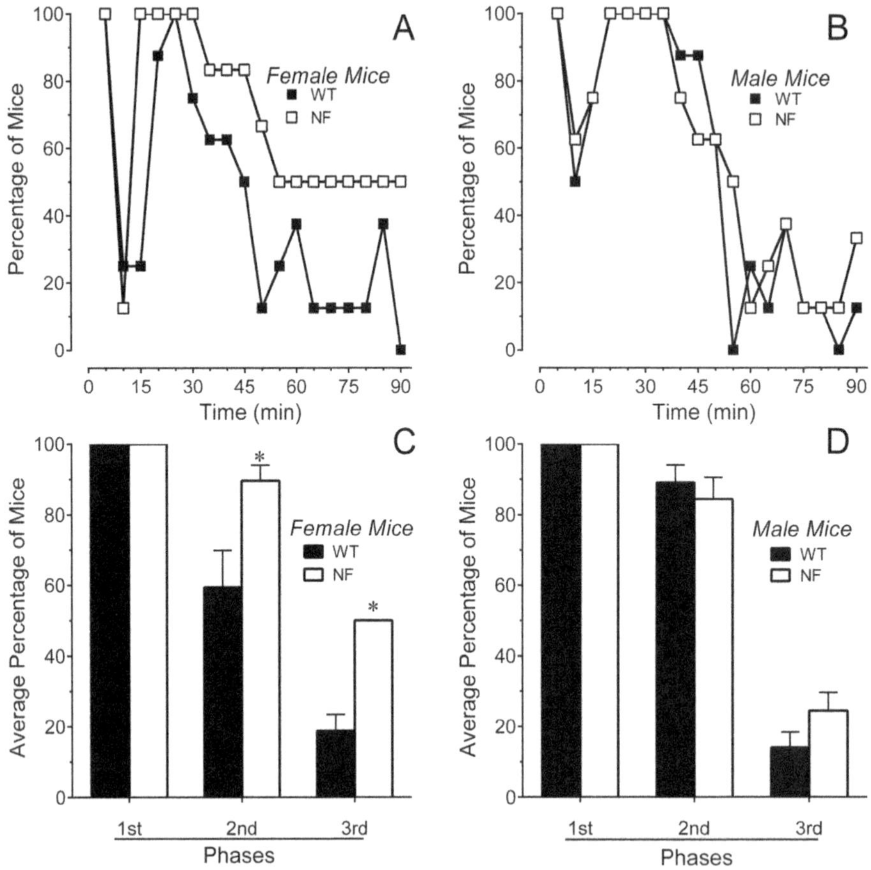

Figure 5. Intraplantar injection of formalin induced spontaneous pain behaviors in both genders and genotypes. Time course of guarding, flinching or unweighting of the hindpaw after intraplantar injection of formalin in (A) female or (B) male mice. The percentage of female $Nf1^{+/-}$ mice that exhibited these behaviors was higher than WT littermates, but did not differ in male mice of either genotype. Percentage of (C) female or (D) male mice exhibiting guarding, flinching or unweighting of the hindpaw averaged for the first phase (0–5 min), second phase (15–55 min) and third phase (55–90 min) of the formalin test. Six to eight mice of each gender and genotype were tested. * $P<0.05$, ** $P<0.01$ compared to corresponding WT littermate.

each factor). The difference between male $Nf1^{+/-}$ and WT mice was not statistically significant ($P = 0.1$; Student's t-test).

Discussion

This extensive characterization of the nociceptive responses of male and female $Nf1^{+/-}$ mice was prompted by (1) the enhanced excitability of primary afferent neurons in $Nf1^{+/-}$ mice [16], (2) the increased release of CGRP from sensory neurons of $Nf1^{+/-}$ mice [14], and (3) the well-established role of CGRP as a nociceptive neurotransmitter in the periphery and spinal cord [9–12]. The results indicate that $Nf1^{+/-}$ mice did not differ from WT mice in responsiveness to acute heat stimuli delivered at a rate that preferentially activated either Aδ- or C-fibers [27,28]. They also did not differ from WT mice in responsiveness to innocuous mechanical stimuli with the exception of a subtle enhanced mechanical sensitivity in female $Nf1^{+/-}$ mice. Given that neither content nor the basal release of CGRP from cultured DRG neurons and spinal cord slices differed between WT and $Nf1^{+/-}$ mice [14], it is perhaps not unexpected that WT and $Nf1^{+/-}$ mice did not differ in their responsiveness to brief heat or mechanical stimuli in the absence of inflammation. O'Brien et al. reached a similar conclusion in their recent survey of the responsiveness of $Nf1^{+/-}$ mice to noxious heat or itch-producing stimuli [21].

Nociceptive phenotype in inflammatory models

Intraplantar injection of capsaicin releases CGRP from the central and peripheral terminals of primary afferent neurons [14,30–33]. Neither female nor male $Nf1^{+/-}$ mice differed from their WT littermates with respect to heat hyperalgesia induced by ipl capsaicin. Female $Nf1^{+/-}$ mice also did not differ from their WT littermates in the magnitude of mechanical hypersensitivity that developed, and male $Nf1^{+/-}$ mice exhibited only slightly less mechanical hypersensitivity than WT littermates. These findings were unexpected given that capsaicin evokes greater release of CGRP from the terminals of nociceptive afferents in $Nf1^{+/-}$ mice than WT mice [14].

The formalin test was used to assess nociceptive phenotype in a model of more prolonged inflammation and as a non-reflexive measure of nociceptive behaviors. Formalin-evoked pain behaviors are also dependent on CGRP [34]. Formalin directly activates transient receptor potential (TRP), subfamily A, member 1 channels (TRPA1) [35,36], and TRP channel, subfamily V, member 1 (TRPV1) channels [37] in DRG neurons. In mice, many TRPV1-immunoreactive primary afferent neurons coexpress TRPA1 [38,39]. Formalin is therefore likely to cause a central and peripheral release of CGRP similar to that caused by capsaicin. Indeed, male $Nf1^{+/-}$ mice did not differ from WT littermates in either the duration of licking or other nociceptive

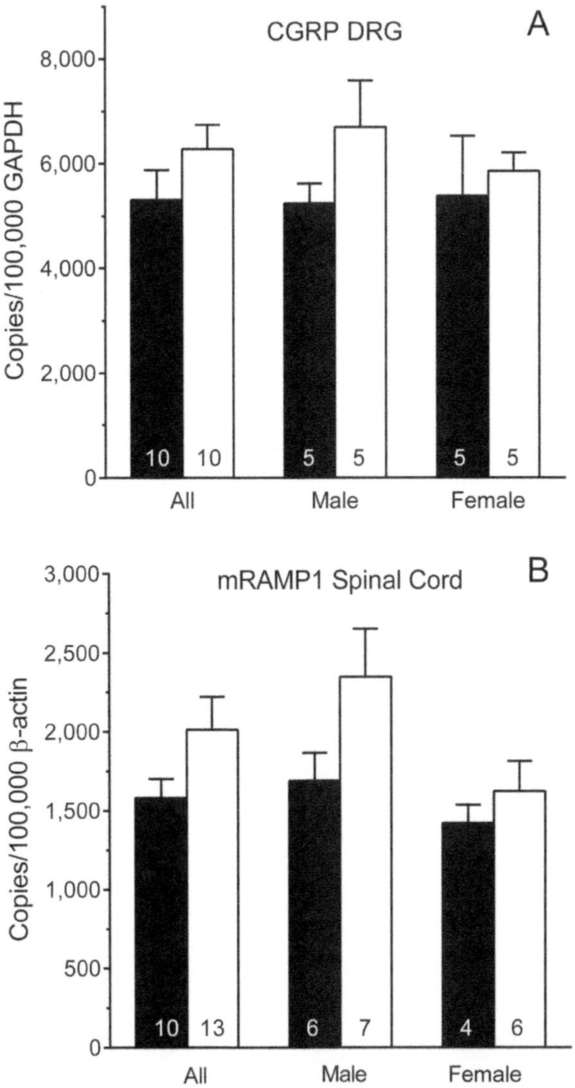

Figure 6. Levels of CGRP mRNA and RAMP1 mRNA. (A) Levels of CGRP mRNA in the dorsal root ganglion (DRG) of *Nf1*$^{+/-}$ and WT mice did not differ by genotype or gender. (B) Levels of RAMP1 mRNA in the spinal cord of *Nf1*$^{+/-}$ and WT mice did not differ by gender or genotype. Data are expressed as mean ± SEM copies normalized to 100,000 GAPDH for the DRG and to 100,000 β-actin for spinal cord. Numbers in the columns are the number of mice. * $P<0.05$ compared to corresponding WT littermates. *Nf1*$^{+/-}$ mice (open bars); WT mice (solid bars)

behaviors in agreement with the report by O'Brien et al. [21]. Female *Nf1*$^{+/-}$ mice showed less licking than WT mice, but this observation is not necessarily indicative of a reduced nociception because these mice also exhibited additional competing behaviors that suggested that formalin was more noxious.

Subsequent experiments injected CGRP into the hindpaw to limit the site of action to the periphery. A more consistent phenotype of exacerbated nociception emerged in this model. Both male and female *Nf1*$^{+/-}$ mice exhibited greater heat hyperalgesia than their respective WT littermates after ipl injection of CGRP. Male *Nf1*$^{+/-}$ mice also exhibited greater mechanical hypersensitivity their WT littermates, although female *Nf1*$^{+/-}$ mice exhibited less mechanical hypersensitivity than their WT littermates. It is well established that CGRP increases its own synthesis, and most likely its own release from sensory neurons [20,40]. Although levels of transcript (this study) and protein [14] for CGRP were equivalent in the DRG of *Nf1*$^{+/-}$ and WT mice, an enhanced release of endogenous CGRP from the peripheral terminals of primary afferents in *Nf1*$^{+/-}$ mice cannot be excluded. Another mechanism that may be responsible for the enhanced nociceptive effects of peripherally administered CGRP in *Nf1*$^{+/-}$ mice involves invading macrophages and the subsequent release of inflammatory cytokines [41]. Macrophages in *Nf1*$^{+/-}$ mice may express increased numbers of the CGRP receptor or RAMP1, or receptors of higher affinity or efficacy upon activation leading to increased release of cytokines. Additional studies will be required to test this hypothesis.

Nociceptive Phenotypes of Other Ras-GAP Deficient Mice

Recently, the nociceptive phenotype of another Ras-GAP deficient mouse was investigated. Mice with a heterozygous mutation for Synaptic GAP (SynGAP), a neuronal Ras-GAP, also did not differ from WT mice in their responsiveness to heat or mechanical stimuli in the absence of inflammation [42]. As observed with *Nf1*$^{+/-}$ mice, ipl injection of capsaicin induced equivalent mechanical hypersensitivity in *SynGAP* deficient and WT mice [42]. Although capsaicin induced greater heat hyperalgesia in *SynGAP* deficient mice than WT mice, this result can be attributed to the finding that *SynGAP* mice have three-fold higher levels of TRPV1 in the DRG [42]. It is not known whether the DRG of *Nf1*$^{+/-}$ mice have higher levels of TRPV1 than WT mice. However, given that the magnitude of capsaicin-induced heat hyperalgesia was similar in both genotypes, this is considered unlikely.

Conclusions

The results of this study do not support the hypothesis that a reduction in neurofibromin is associated with enhanced acute or inflammatory nociception, and confirm the conclusions of another recent comprehensive analysis of male *Nf1*$^{+/-}$ mice. [21]. The present study extends this conclusion to additional models of inflammatory injury and also includes female *Nf1*$^{+/-}$ mice. Gender is an important consideration given that many chronic pain conditions such as migraine and fibromyalgia are more prevalent in women than men [43,44].

This study also provides new information relevant to the 'CGRP hypothesis' posited by Hingtgen and colleagues. It determined that levels of transcript for CGRP were unchanged in the DRG of *Nf1*$^{+/-}$ mice, as were levels of transcript for RAMP1 in the spinal cord. The finding of enhanced heat hyperalgesia in both genders and of mechanical hypersensitivity in male *Nf1*$^{+/-}$ mice after ipl injection of CGRP suggests that the peripheral actions of CGRP may be enhanced as a result of neurofibromin deficit. This exacerbation may be the result of increased peripheral release of neurotransmitter from primary afferent neurons or the expression of CGRP receptors by invading macrophages that release proinflammatory cytokines in response to CGRP. As noted earlier, high densities of CGRP-immunoreactive fibers are present in neurofibromas in patients [13]. Thus, consideration should be given to testing the efficacy of CGRP receptor antagonists developed for relief of migraine [45] in diminishing bodily pain and pain associated with nerve sheath tumors in NF patients.

Acknowledgments

We thank Dr. Christina Winford and Dr. Roxanne Walder for their assistance with troubleshooting the RT-qPCR experiments.

Author Contributions

Conceived and designed the experiments: DLH AFR. Performed the experiments: SW BMdP. Analyzed the data: DLH SW BMdP. Contributed reagents/materials/analysis tools: AFR. Wrote the paper: DLH BMdP.

References

1. Riccardi VM (1992) Type 1 neurofibromatosis and the pediatric patient. Curr Probl Pediatr 22: 66–106; discussion 107.
2. Lakkis MM, Tennekoon GI (2000) Neurofibromatosis type 1. I. General overview. J Neurosci Res 62: 755–763.
3. Lee MJ, Stephenson DA (2007) Recent developments in neurofibromatosis type 1. Current Opin Neurol 20: 135–141.
4. McClatchey AI (2007) Neurofibromatosis. Ann Rev Pathol 2: 191–216.
5. Theos A, Korf BR (2006) Pathophysiology of neurofibromatosis type 1. Ann Intern Med 144: 842–849.
6. Creange A, Zeller J, Rostaing-Rigattieri S, Brugieres P, Degos JD, et al. (1999) Neurological complications of neurofibromatosis type 1 in adulthood. Brain 122: 473–481.
7. Drouet A, Wolkenstein P, Lefaucheur JP, Pinson S, Combemale P, et al. (2004) Neurofibromatosis 1-associated neuropathies: a reappraisal. Brain 127: 1993–2009.
8. Wolkenstein P, Zeller J, Revuz J, Ecosse E, Leplege A (2001) Quality-of-life impairment in neurofibromatosis type 1: a cross-sectional study of 128 cases. Arch Dermatol 137: 1421–1425.
9. Seybold VS (2009) The role of peptides in central sensitization. Hdbk Exper Pharmacol 451–491.
10. Yu L-C, Hou J-F, Fu F-H, Zhang Y-X (2009) Roles of calcitonin gene-related peptide and its receptors in pain-related behavioral responses in the central nervous system. Neurosci & Biobehav Rev 33: 1185–1191.
11. Van Rossum D, Hanisch U-K, Quirion R (1997) Neuroanatomical localization, pharmacological characterization and functions of CGRP, related peptides and their Receptors. Neurosci & Biobehav Rev 21: 649–678.
12. Benemei S, Nicoletti P, Capone JG, Geppetti P (2009) CGRP receptors in the control of pain and inflammation. Cur Opin Pharmacol 9: 9–14.
13. Vaalasti A, Suomalainen H, Kuokkanen K, Rechardt L (1990) Neuropeptides in cutaneous neurofibromas of von Recklinghausen's disease. J Cutaneous Pathol 17: 371–373.
14. Hingtgen CM, Roy SL, Clapp DW (2006) Stimulus-evoked release of neuropeptides is enhanced in sensory neurons from mice with a heterozygous mutation of the Nf1 gene. Neuroscience 137: 637–645.
15. Wang Y, Duan JH, Hingtgen CM, Nicol GD (2010) Augmented sodium currents contribute to the enhanced excitability of small diameter capsaicin-sensitive sensory neurons isolated from Nf1+/mice. J Neurophysiol 103: 2085–20894.
16. Wang Y, Nicol GD, Clapp DW, Hingtgen CM (2005) Sensory neurons from Nf1 haploinsufficient mice exhibit increased excitability. J Neurophysiol 94: 3670–3676.
17. Hodgdon KE, Hingtgen CM, Nicol GD (2012) Dorsal root ganglia isolated from Nf1+/− mice exhibit increased levels of mRNA expression of voltage-dependent sodium channels. Neuroscience 206: 237–244.
18. Duan JH, Hodgdon KE, Hingtgen CM, Nicol GD (2014) N-type calcium current, Cav2.2, is enhanced in small-diameter sensory neurons isolated from $Nf1^{+/-}$ mice. Neuroscience 270: 192–202.
19. Hay DL, Poyner DR, Sexton PM (2006) GPCR modulation by RAMPs. Pharmacol & Ther 109: 173–197.
20. Zhang Z, Winborn CS, Marquez de Prado B, Russo AF (2007) Sensitization of calcitonin gene-related peptide receptors by receptor activity-modifying protein-1 in the trigeminal ganglion. J Neurosci 27: 2693–2703.
21. O'Brien DE, Brenner DS, Gutmann DH, Gereau RWt (2013) Assessment of pain and itch behavior in a mouse model of neurofibromatosis type 1. J Pain 14: 628–637.
22. Jacks T, Shih TS, Schmitt EM, Bronson RT, Bernards A, et al. (1994) Tumour predisposition in mice heterozygous for a targeted mutation in Nf1. Nat Genetics 7: 353–361.
23. Riccardi VM, Womack JE, Jacks T (1994) Neurofibromatosis and related tumors. Natural occurrence and animal models. Am J Pathol 145: 994–1000.
24. Brannan CI, Perkins AS, Vogel KS, Ratner N, Nordlund ML, et al. (1994) Targeted disruption of the neurofibromatosis type-1 gene leads to developmental abnormalities in heart and various neural crest-derived tissues. Genes & Develop 8: 1019–1029.
25. Vance JM, Pericak-Vance MA, Yamaoka LH, Speer MC, Rosenwasser GO, et al. (1989) Genetic linkage mapping of chromosome 17 markers and neurofibromatosis type I. Am J Human Gen 44: 25–29.
26. Hirata H, Pataky A, Kajander K, LaMotte RH, Collins JG (1990) A model of peripheral mononeuropathy in the rat. Pain 42: 253–255.
27. Yeomans DC, Proudfit HK (1994) Characterization of the foot withdrawal response to noxious radiant heat in the rat. Pain 59: 85–94.
28. Yeomans DC, Proudfit HK (1996) Nociceptive responses to high and low rates of noxious cutaneous heating are mediated by different nociceptors in the rat: electrophysiological evidence. Pain 68: 141–150.
29. McMullan S, Simpson DA, Lumb BM (2004) A reliable method for the preferential activation of C- or A-fibre heat nociceptors. J Neurosci Methods 138: 133–139.
30. Lundberg JM, Franco-Cereceda A, Alving K, Delay-Goyet P, Lou Y-P (1992) Release of Calcitonin Gene—Related Peptide from Sensory Neurons. Ann NY Acad Sci 657: 187–193.
31. Li D, Ren Y, Xu X, Zou X, Fang L, et al. (2008) Sensitization of primary afferent nociceptors induced by intradermal capsaicin involves the peripheral release of calcitonin gene-related Peptide driven by dorsal root reflexes. J Pain 9: 1155–1168.
32. Sun R-Q, Lawand NB, Willis WD (2003) The role of calcitonin gene-related peptide (CGRP) in the generation and maintenance of mechanical allodynia and hyperalgesia in rats after intradermal injection of capsaicin. Pain 104: 201–208.
33. Kilo S, Harding-Rose C, Hargreaves KM, Flores CM (1997) Peripheral CGRP release as a marker for neurogenic inflammation: a model system for the study of neuropeptide secretion in rat paw skin. Pain 73: 201–207.
34. Salmon AM, Damaj MI, Marubio LM, Epping-Jordan MP, Merlo-Pich E, et al. (2001) Altered neuroadaptation in opiate dependence and neurogenic inflammatory nociception in alpha CGRP-deficient mice. Nat Neurosci 4: 357–358.
35. McNamara CR, Mandel-Brehm J, Bautista DM, Siemens J, Deranian KL, et al. (2007) TRPA1 mediates formalin-induced pain. Proc Natl Acad Sci U S A 104: 13525–13530.
36. Macpherson LJ, Xiao B, Kwan KY, Petrus MJ, Dubin AE, et al. (2007) An ion channel essential for sensing chemical damage. J Neurosci 27: 11412–11415.
37. Tian LJ, Du YR, Xiao Y, Lv ZM, Yu YQ, et al. (2009) Mediating roles of the vanilloid receptor TRPV1 in activation of rat primary afferent nociceptive neurons by formaldehyde. Acta physiol Sin 61: 404–416.
38. Story GM, Peier AM, Reeve AJ, Eid SR, Mosbacher J, et al. (2003) ANKTM1, a TRP-like channel expressed in nociceptive neurons, is activated by cold temperatures. Cell 112: 819–829.
39. Malin S, Molliver D, Christianson JA, Schwartz ES, Cornuet P, et al. (2011) TRPV1 and TRPA1 function and modulation are target tissue dependent. J Neurosci 31: 10516–10528.
40. Segond von Banchet G, Pastor A, Biskup C, Schlegel C, Benndorf K, et al. (2002) Localization of functional calcitonin gene-related peptide binding sites in a subpopulation of cultured dorsal root ganglion neurons. Neuroscience 110: 131–145.
41. Ma W, Quirion R (2006) Increased calcitonin gene-related peptide in neuroma and invading macrophages is involved in the up-regulation of interleukin-6 and thermal hyperalgesia in a rat model of mononeuropathy. J Neurochem 98: 180–192.
42. Duarte DB, Duan JH, Nicol GD, Vasko MR, Hingtgen CM (2011) Reduced expression of SynGAP, a neuronal GTPase-activating protein, enhances capsaicin-induced peripheral sensitization. J Neurophysiol 106: 309–318.
43. Fillingim RB, King CD, Ribeiro-Dasilva MC, Rahim-Williams B, Riley JL 3rd (2009) Sex, gender, and pain: a review of recent clinical and experimental findings. J Pain 10: 447–485.
44. Bartley EJ, Fillingim RB (2013) Sex differences in pain: a brief review of clinical and experimental findings. Br J Anaesth 111: 52–58.
45. Moore EL, Salvatore CA (2012) Targeting a family B GPCR/RAMP receptor complex: CGRP receptor antagonists and migraine. Br J Pharmacol 166: 66–78.

Bone Morphogenetic Protein 6 Polymorphisms Are Associated with Radiographic Progression in Ankylosing Spondylitis

Young Bin Joo[1]◑, So-Young Bang[1]◑, Tae-Hwan Kim[1]*, Seung-Cheol Shim[2], Seunghun Lee[3], Kyung Bin Joo[3], Jong Heon Kim[4], Hye Joon Min[5], Proton Rahman[6], Robert D. Inman[7]

1 Department of Rheumatology, Hanyang University Hospital for Rheumatic Diseases, Seoul, Republic of Korea, **2** Division of Rheumatology, Daejeon Rheumatoid & Degenerative Arthritis Center, Chungnam National University Hospital, Daejeon, Republic of Korea, **3** Department of Radiology, Hanyang University Hospital for Rheumatic Diseases, Seoul, Republic of Korea, **4** Department of Orthopedics, Hanyang University Hospital for Rheumatic Diseases, Seoul, Republic of Korea, **5** Department of anthropology, Cornell University, Ithaca, New York, United States of America, **6** Department of Rheumatology, Memorial University, St. Clare's Mercy Hospital, St. John's, Newfoundland, Canada, **7** Division of Rheumatology, University of Toronto, Toronto Western Hospital, Toronto, Ontario, Canada

Abstract

Background and Object: Nearly 25 genetic loci associated with susceptibility to ankylosing spondylitis (AS) have been identified by several large studies. However, there have been limited studies to identify the genes associated with radiographic severity of the disease. Thus we investigated which genes involved in bone formation pathways might be associated with radiographic severity in AS.

Methods: A total of 417 Korean AS patients were classified into two groups based on the radiographic severity as defined by the modified Stoke' Ankylosing Spondylitis Spinal Score (mSASSS) system. Severe AS was defined by the presence of syndesmophytes and/or fusion in the lumbar or cervical spine ($n = 195$). Mild AS was defined by the absence of any syndesmophyte or fusion ($n = 170$). A total of 251 single nucleotide polymorphisms (SNPs) within 52 genes related to bone formation were selected and genotyped. Odds ratios (OR) and 95% confidence interval (95% CI) were analysed by multivariate logistic regression controlling for age at onset of symptoms, sex, disease duration, and smoking status as covariates.

Results: We identified new loci of bone morphogenetic protein 6 (*BMP6*) associated with radiographic severity in patients with AS that passed false discovery rate threshold. Two SNPs in *BMP6* were significantly associated with radiologic severity [*rs270378* (OR 1.97, $p = 6.74 \times 10^{-4}$) and *rs1235192* [OR 1.92, $p = 1.17 \times 10^{-3}$]) adjusted by covariates.

Conclusion: This is the first study to demonstrate that *BMP6* is associated with radiographic severity in AS, supporting the role wingless-type like/BMP pathway on radiographic progression in AS.

Editor: Shervin Assassi, University of Texas Health Science Center at Houston, United States of America

Funding: The authors have no support or funding to report.

Competing Interests: The authors have declared that no competing interests exist.

* Email: thkim@hanyang.ac.kr

◑ These authors contributed equally to this work.

Introduction

Ankylosing spondylitis (AS) is a chronic inflammatory disease that preferentially affects the axial structures causing spinal ankylosis [1]. The process of ankylosis is closely associated with permanent work disability as well as decreased quality of life [2]

AS is a highly heritable (>90%), and human leukocyte antigen B27 (HLA-B27) is the strongest genetic association with AS, with >80% of patients being positive for HLA-B27 [3,4]. However, HLA-B27 contributes only 16–50% of genetic risk [5], reflecting the fact that other non-HLA-B27 variants likely influence disease susceptibility. Recently, the International Genetics of Ankylosing Spondylitis Consortium confirmed the association of 25 loci at genome-wide significance in addition to HLA-B27. This included 12 of the 13 previously reported loci associated with AS in Europeans and 13 additional loci [1].

Although radiologic severity is also largely heritable (>60%) [6], there has been limited studies addressing the genetic influence on severity in contrast to studies of susceptibility to AS. A few studies confirmed the positive association with severity of AS, which have reported that that large multifunctional peptidase (LMP) 2, major histocompatibility complex and in endoplasmic reticulum amino-peptidases (ERAP) 1 have been reported to affect radiographic severity in AS [7–11]. These studies generally used candidate

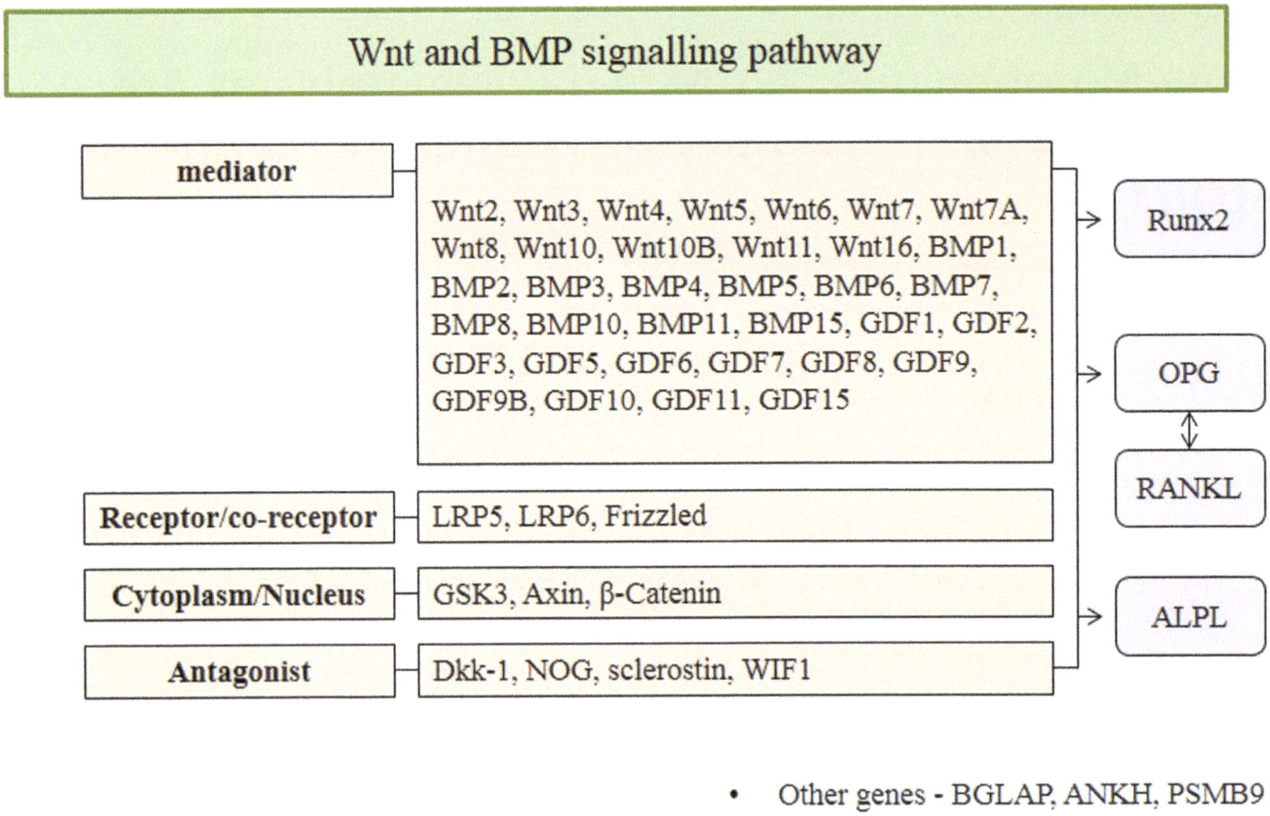

Figure 1. 52 Gene lists analyzed in our study. Genes were selected from public databases including the SNP database of the National Centre for Biotechnology Information (NCBI; http://www.ncbi.nlm.nih.gov/SNP/) and the International HapMap Project (http://www.hapmap.org/).

susceptibility gene of AS for analysis of possible associated genetic markers with severity. Two studies did not identify any significant genetic markers showing significant association with radiographic severity in AS [12,13].

Underlying mechanism of new bone formation in AS remain incompletely understood. Current concepts propose a complex interaction between chronic inflammation and wingless-type like (WNT) pathway [14]. A recent study demonstrated that uncoupled interaction of WNT pathway with inflammation may play a key role in the development of new bone formation in AS. The effect of anti-tumor necrosis factor alpha agents on radiographic progression in AS has led to differing conclusions [15,16]. The effect of increased C-reactive protein (CRP) or erythrocyte sedimentation rate (ESR) on structural change in AS is also inconclusive; some report its positive relationship [17,18], but others are not, especially in longstanding AS [19,20]. Some studies showed Dickkopf-1 and sclerostin is associated with radiographic severity independently inflammation, implicating complex molecular mechanisms, which can directly inhibit or enhance the WNT pathway, and which could be significantly impacting new bone formation in AS [21–23].

Based on these data, we hypothesized that genetic factors related to bone formation could be responsible for differential radiographic severity amongst AS. To test this hypothesis, we investigated the potential association of radiographic severity with the polymorphisms of genes involved in bone formation in Korean patients with AS.

Materials and Methods

Study Population and Clinical Data

We included a total of 417 patients with AS who are all of Korean ethnicity, recruited from the Hanyang University Hospital for Rheumatic Disease. All patients with AS satisfied the 1984 modified New York criteria for AS [24]. Clinical data collected included age, gender, age at disease onset, which means the onset age of axial symptoms, disease duration, smoking status, nonsteroidal anti-inflammatory drugs (NSAIDs) dose and duration used, HLA-B27 positivity, baseline ESR, and CRP. NSAIDs used was scored by the method which Dougados et al. suggested [25].

Radiographic Scoring

The modified Stoke Ankylosing Spondylitis Spinal Score (mSASSS), which is considered the standard for quantification of chronic spinal changes in AS, was used for assessing radiographic severity. [26,27] In mSASSS, scoring evaluates the anterior radiographic changes of the lumbar spine and cervical spine in lateral radiographic view: 0 - normal, 1 - erosion, squaring, or sclerosis, 2 -syndesmophyte or 3– bridging syndesmophyte (maximum 72) [28] In the cases with less than 3 vertebral site missing, the missing scores were substituted by the mean score of the vertebra of the same spinal segment of the patients. Two expert radiologists (SL, KBJ) scored independently. Then, discordant scores were reevaluated by both readers. Their interclass and intraclass correlation coefficients were 0.95 and 0.97, respectively.

Table 1. Clinical characteristics of study cohort.

	All patients (n = 365)	Severe AS (n = 195)	Mild AS (n = 170)	*p*
Age at onset, year	37.0±8.6	41.6±8.1	33.0±6.8	<0.001
Male	340 (93.2)	174 (89.2)	166 (97.6)	0.001
Disease duration, year	14.1±6.8	16.7±7.3	11.9±5.4	<0.001
Smoker (n = 322)	201 (62.4)	114 (74.0)	87 (51.8)	<0.001
HLA-B27 (n = 344)	334 (97.1)	151 (98.7)	183 (95.8)	0.195
ESR, mm/hr (n = 197)	20.5±23.9	23.2±26.4	18.1±21.4	0.135
CRP, mg/dL (n = 194)	1.2±2.2	1.4±2.7	1.1±1.6	0.381
mSASSS, range 0–72				
Cervical spine	12.2±11.0	19.4±12.5	6.0±2.7	<0.001
Lumbar spine	10.8±13.1	21.9±11.5	1.2±2.1	<0.001
Total	23.1±21.9	41.5±19.7	7.2±3.6	<0.001
*Continuous NSAID intake (n = 161)	44 (27.3)	24 (33.3)	20 (22.5)	0.124

Data were shown to mean ± SD or n (%).
*Continuous NSAID intake was defined as 70 or more the score. AS; ankylosing spondylitis, HLA-B27: human leukocyte antigen-B27; ESR: erythrocyte sedimentation rate; CRP: C-reactive protein; Msasss: modified stokes AS spine score; NSAID: non-steroidal anti-inflammatory drugs.

Severity Classification

The patients with AS are classified into two groups-mild or severe-based on the radiographic severity as follows. Within the measurement error of mSASSS, that scores of 1 is intermediate, and perhaps of indeterminate significance. Also, since a syndesmophyte at only 1 level can be seen in other state than AS, severe AS was defined by three or more syndesmophytes and/or fusion at the lumbar spine or cervical spine. Mild AS was defined by the absence of any syndesmophyte. Patients who had only 1 or 2 syndesmophytes or fusion were excluded from the analysis to allow a clear differentiation of severity between mild and severe.

Genotyping

In this study, 52 candidate genes (see **Figure 1** and **Table S1**) associated with involved in bone formation pathways were selected from public databases including the SNP database of the National Centre for Biotechnology Information (NCBI; http://www.ncbi.nlm.nih.gov/SNP/) and the International HapMap Project (http://www.hapmap.org/). SNP genotyping using the Sequenom MassARRAY® system (iPLEX GOLD) was performed according to the manufacturer's instructions (Sequenom, San Diego, CA, USA). Briefly, PCR and single-base extension (SBE) primers were designed using MassARRAY assay design software (Sequenom, San Diego, CA, USA). Manufacturer's instructions for the multiplex reaction were followed for the PCR amplification, the shrimp alkaline phosphatase (SAP) enzyme treatment, the SBE reactions using an iPLEX GOLD assay, and the clean-up with a resin kit (Sequenom, San Diego, CA, USA). The multiplex assays were designed using Sequenom's Assay Design Suite 1.0. Only 251 SNPs of 52 genes were genotyped due to problems inherent with designing multiplex reactions. PCR and SBE primers sequences and all protocols are available upon request. Reaction products were dispensed onto a SpectroCHIP bioarray (Sequenom, San Diego, CA, USA) using a MassARRAY nanodispenser (Sequenom, San Diego, CA, USA) and assayed on the MassARRAY platform (Sequenom, San Diego, CA, USA). Differences in mass were detected with matrix-assisted laser desorption/ionization time-of-flight mass spectrometry (MALDI-TOF MS). MassARRAY Workstation software was used to process and analyse the iPLEX SpectroCHIP bioarray. Typer Analyzer software was used to analyse all genotypes obtained from the assays.

Statistical Analysis

We eliminated SNPs that had insufficient call rates (<90% and minor allele frequency <1%) in cases and controls, Hardy-Weinberg disequilibrium in controls ($p<1\times10^{-5}$), and samples that were less than 90% sequenced. To determine the association of respective SNPs with radiologic severity, odds ratio (OR) and 95% confidence interval were calculated using logistic analysis (allelic model), controlling for age of disease onset, sex, disease duration, and smoking status. Given the large number of tests, there was high potential for false discovery. Thus, we used a false discovery rate (FDR) method to control the error inherent in multiple comparisons [29]. The association of genotype of significant genes with total mSASSS was analyzed using Kruskal-Wallis test with Mann Whitney P. Statistical analyses were conducted in PLINK v1.07 and SPSS17 software (Chicago, IL, USA).

Ethics Statement

The Institutional Review Board of Hanyang University approved the protocol. All patients gave written informed consent.

Results

Clinical Characteristics of Patients with AS

In this study, we included the AS patient with longstanding disease; the mean disease duration from symptoms onset to the time when radiograph was taken was 14.1±6.8 years, and the mean score of mSASSS was 23.1±21.9 **(Table 1)**. After excluding the patients who had only 1 or 2 syndesmophyte or fusion, a total of 365 patients were classified into 2 groups such as severe (n = 195) or mild AS (n = 170). Patients with severe AS were older at onset of symptoms (41.6±8.1 vs 33.0±6.8), had higher percentage of males (97.6 vs 89.2) and smokers (74.0 vs 51.8), and had longer disease duration (16.7±7.3 vs 11.9±5.4) compared with those with mild AS. The percentage of HLA-B27, NSAID used, ESR, and CRP were not significantly different between the two groups. Total mSASSS (range 0–72) was 41.5±19.7 in

Table 2. Significant association between polymorphism associated with bone formation in AS patients.

SNP	Gene	Chr	Position	Risk Allele	Allele Freq. (Cases)	Allele Freq. (Controls)	OR	95% CI	p	FDR thresholds
rs270378	BMP6	6	7762715	C	0.585	0.497	1.97	1.33 - 2.90	6.74×10^{-4}	1.56×10^{-3}
rs1235192	BMP6	6	7867046	G	0.716	0.606	1.92	1.30–2.86	1.17×10^{-3}	1.61×10^{-3}

AS: ankylosing spondylitis; SNP: single nucleotide polymorphism; Chr: chromosome; Freq: frequency; OR: odds ratio; CI: confidence interval; FDR: false discovery rate; BMP6: bone morphogenetic protein 6.

patients with severe AS, and 7.2±3.6 in that with mild AS ($p<$ 0.001).

Associations of SNPs Related to Bone Formation Mechanism with Radiologic Severity

To control the clinical differences between two groups, logistic regression analysis was adjusted for age at onset of symptoms, sex, disease duration, and smoking status. Among 52 genes analyzed, only BMP6-related SNPs were associated with radiographic severity **(Table 2 and Table S2)**. SNP *rs270378* of BMP6 showed the strongest association with severe AS (OR 1.97, $p=6.74\times10^{-4}$, Table 2). *rs1235192* of BMP6 was also associated with severe AS (OR 1.92, $p=1.17\times10^{-3}$), although these SNPs did not reach significance after Bonferroni correction. These two SNPs were not in linkage disequilibrium (LD) ($R2=0.004$, $D'=0.106$, Distance: 104 kb).

Association of Allele Frequency (Genotype) of BMP6 with Total mSASSS

We looked at the trend of the allele with the actual mSASSS. In this study, it appears that the presence of risk allele in *rs1235192* was associated with markedly increased total mSASSS. As shown in **figure 2**, mSASSS in the group with G (TG or GG) was much higher than that in the group without it ($p=0.046$). But the allele difference of SNP rs270378 for mSASSS was not statistically significant ($P>0.05$).

Discussion

Our results highlight the role of certain biological pathways in the pathogenesis of AS. Recently, new hypothesis have been proposed that WNTs and BMPs are likely to play an important role in new bone formation in AS [14]. However, genetic studies that were examined this hypothesis are few, although genetic factors are likely playing a key role in defining new bone formation [14]. In this study, we specifically examined SNPs of genes related to bone formation, and most of which were related to WNTs and BMPs pathways. Among them, risk alleles at *rs270378* and *rs1235192* in *BMP6* were found to increase the risk of syndesmophyte formation. These relationships remained significant even after adjusted *P* value by FDR was applied to the multiple comparisons. We demonstrated for the first time that SNPs in *BMP6* likely play a contributory role in syndesmophyte formation or ankylosis in AS.

Recently, several genetic association studies were done to identify the risk variant for radiographic severity in AS. Haroon et al reported that *LMP2* variants in Caucasian AS affected baseline mSASSS, but not radiographic progression [7]. ERAP1 variants was reported to be associated with syndesmophyte formation in Taiwanese patients with AS, as reported by Wang et al [8]. This study compared the polymorphisms of genes between patients with at least one syndesmophyte vs those with no syndesmophytes. Two studies have suggested that prediction of radiographic severity was improved by genetic variants by showing prediction model of radiographic severity using the bath ankylosing spondylitis radiology index (BASRI) [10,30].

Our results add to the knowledge about the genetic factors of AS radiographic severity in above results. The present study used the mSASSS to define severe AS, since the mSASSS had been accepted as the optimal method for quantification of chronic spinal changes [26] Other method such as BASRI is difficult to differentiate less or more severe spinal disease as its ceiling effect, But the mSASSS method could. The study addressed specifically severe cases, thereby eliminating cases of intermediate severity

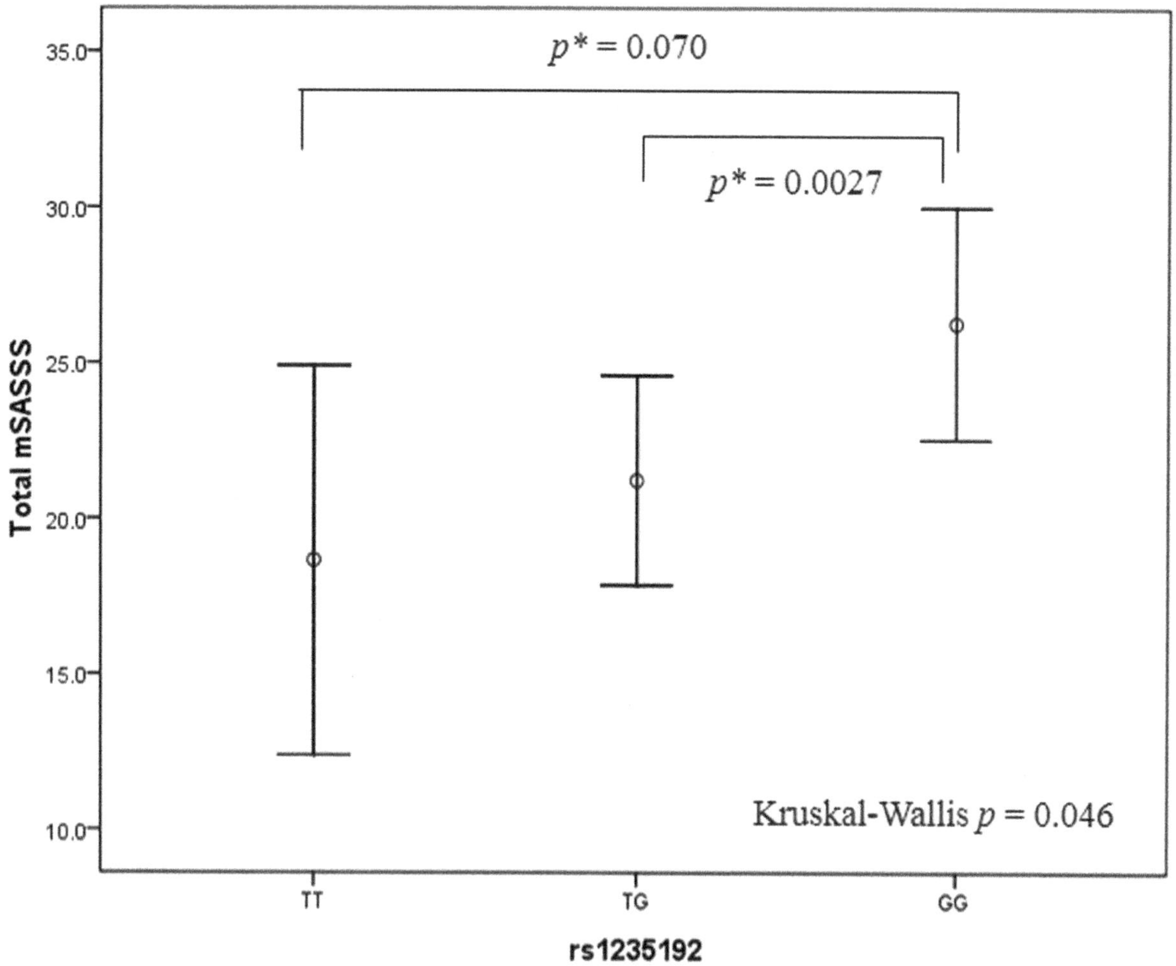

Figure 2. Association of genotype of BMP6 with total mSASSS. Data represent mean (95% CI). p = 0.046 by the Kruskal-Wallis test. *Mann Whitney P.

which may confound clear stratification for severity. There are reports of successfully identifying the risk variant using extremely high or low levels of interest [31,32]. We also adjusted for smoking status, which is known to important environmental risk factor for radiographic progression, as well as age, sex, and disease duration. These points considered in our study may lead to accurate prediction of genetic markers of radiographic severity.

We found that the two (rs270378 and rs1235192) SNPs in BMP6 are associated with increased risk of syndesmophyte formation. These SNPs were not in LD ($R2 = 0.004$, $D' = 0.106$, Distance: 104 kb). Interestingly, stronger effect on syndesmophytes was found in the group carrying double risk SNPs, rs270378 C and rs1235192 G ($P = 3.48 \times 10{-}4$). There were two separate signals at this locus. The association at each SNP in the locus was with a common variant. All these findings suggest that these two SNPs confer the risk for syndesmophytes through independent contribution.

In this study, it appears that the presence of risk allele in rs1235192 was associated with markedly increased total mSASSS. As shown in figure 2, the mSASSS score in the group with G was much higher than that in the group without it ($P = 0.046$). But the allele difference of SNP rs270378 for mSASSS score was not statistically significant ($P > 0.05$).

BMPs play an important role in bone morphogenesis and remodeling in health and disease. BMPs, including BMP6, are important in bone metabolism and can induce ectopic osteogenesis [33]. It has been known that *BMP6* messenger RNA is localized in hypertrophic cartilage [34], and *BMP6* has an important role in the maintenance and repair of human articular cartilage [35]. Polymorphisms in *BMP6* were independently associated with risk for sickle cell osteonecrosis [36,37], pulmonary hypertension in sickle cell disease, [38] breast cancer growth and progression [39]. However, there was no report about variants in *BMP* genes and their association with new bone formation in AS.

In AS, two process of endochondral and direct bone formation contribute to ankylosis process. WNTs and BMP signaling play a role in endochondral bone formation and WNTs also play in direct bone formation [14]. In WNT pathway, WNT bind to low-density lipoprotein receptor-related protein 5 and 6 (LRP5 and 6) on mesenchymal cells followed by activation of intracellular β-catenin involve in bone formation proceeds. During this process, other key molecules such as BMP, axin, glycogen synthase kinase 3 beta (GSK3β), pronounced like the toy Frisbee (FRZB) interact each other to enhance or inhibit to bone formation [14]. WNT signaling elements such as Wnt3a and Wnt10b are associated with direct membranous bone formation, whereas, over-expression of β-catenin in late stage of chondrogenesis is associated with endochondral bone formation through stimulation of the chondrocytes maturation [40]. We investigated the polymorphisms in genes associated with WNT pathway but we did not identify the risk variant affecting the differential radiographic severity in AS.

BMPs are also important for signaling in bone formation process in AS. In the presence of BMPs, progenitor cells first differentiate into chondrocytes building a cartilaginous template that is subsequently replaced by bone [41–43]. Three specific BMPs have been studied in human AS. The levels of BMP2, BMP4, and BMP7 increased in AS patients with spinal fusion compared with patients without fusion [44]. However, these changes in BMP2 and BMP7 are not specific to AS, since BMP2 and BMP7 also increased in RA patients [45]. Until now, there is no report regarding to the level of BMP6 and its association with radiographic severity in human AS.

An Interesting observation on ankylosis in experimental models was seen in the study of Lories et al. [46]. They demonstrated that different BMPs are expressed during the process of ankylosis in male DBA/1 mice. BMP2 was induced in the early stage, BMP7 affects prehypertrophic chondrocytes, and BMP6 affects to hypertrophic chondrocytes in later stage. By immunohistochemistry staining, BMP6 was positive in hypertrophic chondrocyte-like cell showing later stage of endochondral bone formation in ankylosing enthesitis. This is interpreted as indicating that BMP6 is necessary to complete bone formation. This finding supports to our results that polymorphisms of BMP6 could affect to the bone formation, especially syndesmophyte formation in AS. However, further study investigating human histologic finding is needed to demonstrate the biologic role of BMP6 in syndesmophyte or ankylosis formation in human AS.

There is some limitation in this study. We used the cross-sectional data not longitudinal data. To determine the radiographic severity, it would be optimal to compare the radiographs between baseline and later follow-up. To address this in part, we selected primarily longstanding AS patients. The mean disease duration is 14.1±6.8 years, and more than 75% had disease duration of 10 years or more. Considering that significant radiographic progression commonly occurs in the first 10 years of disease [47] and that the strongest predictor of radiologic spinal progression is the presence of syndesmophytes at baseline [19,48–50], mild AS patients who have no syndesmophyte over a course of 11.9±5.4 years of disease are likely to how minimal progression over time. In contrast, patients with severe AS who have already three more syndesmophytes at entry to the clinic are likely to show increased radiographic progression during further follow-up. We had not included functional data in the study. However, our result was supported by the experimental study of Lories et al discussed above [46]. As mentioned above, BMP6, which was associated with increased risk of development of syndesmophyte in our study, has been found in the early course of bone formation in animal immunohistochemistry study. However, future functional study in patients with AS is needed for better understanding of the role of BMP6 in bone formation. Finally, type 1 error of our result was controlled with the FDR method, not Bonferroni correction as our sample size was small. Despite the perception of small sample size, this is the largest racially and ethinically homogeneous AS population with mSASSS reported to date. Thus our results are meaningful and acceptable as type 1 error of result was controlled with the FDR method.

In summary, we show that certain BMP6 polymorphisms, especially *rs270378* and *rs1235192,* are possible risk factors for the development of syndesmophyte and ankylosis in AS. These variants could be excellent candidates for further investigation although replication in larger sample and in different ethnic groups is needed.

Supporting Information

Table S1 This table contains the 366 single nucleotide polymorphisms (SNPs) analyzed in our study.
(DOCX)

Table S2 SNPs Association between polymorphism associated with bone formation in AS patients ($p<0.05$, adjusted by age at onset of symptom, sex, disease duration, and smoking).
(DOCX)

Author Contributions

Conceived and designed the experiments: YBJ SYB THK SCS JHK. Performed the experiments: HJM PR RDI KBJ SHL. Analyzed the data: SYB YBJ THK. Contributed reagents/materials/analysis tools: THK PR RDI. Contributed to the writing of the manuscript: YBJ SYB SCS THK.

References

1. Cortes A, Hadler J, Pointon JP, Robinson PC, Karaderi T, et al. (2013) Identification of multiple risk variants for ankylosing spondylitis through high-density genotyping of immune-related loci. Nat Genet 45: 730–738.
2. Chen HA, Chen CH, Liao HT, Lin YJ, Chen PC, et al. (2011) Factors associated with radiographic spinal involvement and hip involvement in ankylosing spondylitis. Semin Arthritis Rheum 40: 552–558.
3. Brown MA, Kennedy LG, MacGregor AJ, Darke C, Duncan E, et al. (1997) Susceptibility to ankylosing spondylitis in twins: the role of genes, HLA, and the environment. Arthritis Rheum 40: 1823–1828.
4. Brown MA (2008) Breakthroughs in genetic studies of ankylosing spondylitis. Rheumatology (Oxford) 47: 132–137.
5. Khan MA, Ball EJ (2002) Genetic aspects of ankylosing spondylitis. Best Pract Res Clin Rheumatol 16: 675–690.
6. Brophy S, Hickey S, Menon A, Taylor G, Bradbury L, et al. (2004) Concordance of disease severity among family members with ankylosing spondylitis? J Rheumatol 31: 1775–1778.
7. Haroon N, Maksymowych WP, Rahman P, Tsui FW, O'Shea FD, et al. (2012) Radiographic severity of ankylosing spondylitis is associated with polymorphism of the large multifunctional peptidase 2 gene in the Spondyloarthritis Research Consortium of Canada cohort. Arthritis Rheum 64: 1119–1126.
8. Wang CM, Ho HH, Chang SW, Wu YJ, Lin JC, et al. (2012) ERAP1 genetic variations associated with HLA-B27 interaction and disease severity of syndesmophytes formation in Taiwanese ankylosing spondylitis. Arthritis Res Ther 14: R125.
9. Lian Z, Chai W, Shi LL, Chen C, Liu J, et al. (2013) Analysis of PPARGC1B, RUNX3 and TBKBP1 Polymorphisms in Chinese Han Patients with Ankylosing Spondylitis: A Case-Control Study. PLoS One 8: e61527.
10. Bartolome N, Szczypiorska M, Sanchez A, Sanz J, Juanola-Roura X, et al. (2012) Genetic polymorphisms inside and outside the MHC improve prediction of AS radiographic severity in addition to clinical variables. Rheumatology (Oxford) 51: 1471–1478.
11. Szczypiorska M, Sanchez A, Bartolome N, Arteta D, Sanz J, et al. (2011) ERAP1 polymorphisms and haplotypes are associated with ankylosing spondylitis susceptibility and functional severity in a Spanish population. Rheumatology (Oxford) 50: 1969–1975.
12. Pimentel-Santos FM, Ligeiro D, Matos M, Mourao AF, Vieira de Sousa E, et al. (2012) ANKH and susceptibility to and severity of ankylosing spondylitis. J Rheumatol 39: 131–134.
13. Seo JS, Lee SS, Kim SI, Ryu WH, Sa KH, et al. (2005) Influence of VEGF gene polymorphisms on the severity of ankylosing spondylitis. Rheumatology (Oxford) 44: 1299–1302.
14. Lories RJ, Luyten FP, de Vlam K (2009) Progress in spondylarthritis. Mechanisms of new bone formation in spondyloarthritis. Arthritis Res Ther 11: 221.
15. van der Heijde D, Salonen D, Weissman BN, Landewe R, Maksymowych WP, et al. (2009) Assessment of radiographic progression in the spines of patients with ankylosing spondylitis treated with adalimumab for up to 2 years. Arthritis Res Ther 11: R127.
16. van der Heijde D, Landewe R, Einstein S, Ory P, Vosse D, et al. (2008) Radiographic progression of ankylosing spondylitis after up to two years of treatment with etanercept. Arthritis Rheum 58: 1324–1331.
17. Ramiro S, van der Heijde D, van Tubergen A, Stolwijk C, Dougados M, et al. (2014) Higher disease activity leads to more structural damage in the spine in

ankylosing spondylitis: 12-year longitudinal data from the OASIS cohort. Ann Rheum Dis.
18. Poddubnyy D, Haibel H, Listing J, Marker-Hermann E, Zeidler H, et al. (2012) Baseline radiographic damage, elevated acute-phase reactant levels, and cigarette smoking status predict spinal radiographic progression in early axial spondylarthritis. Arthritis Rheum 64: 1388–1398.
19. van Tubergen A, Ramiro S, van der Heijde D, Dougados M, Mielants H, et al. (2012) Development of new syndesmophytes and bridges in ankylosing spondylitis and their predictors: a longitudinal study. Ann Rheum Dis 71: 518–523.
20. Kroon F, Landewe R, Dougados M, van der Heijde D (2012) Continuous NSAID use reverts the effects of inflammation on radiographic progression in patients with ankylosing spondylitis. Ann Rheum Dis 71: 1623–1629.
21. Heiland GR, Appel H, Poddubnyy D, Zwerina J, Hueber A, et al. (2012) High level of functional dickkopf-1 predicts protection from syndesmophyte formation in patients with ankylosing spondylitis. Ann Rheum Dis 71: 572–574.
22. Appel H, Ruiz-Heiland G, Listing J, Zwerina J, Herrmann M, et al. (2009) Altered skeletal expression of sclerostin and its link to radiographic progression in ankylosing spondylitis. Arthritis Rheum 60: 3257–3262.
23. Schett G, Rudwaleit M (2010) Can we stop progression of ankylosing spondylitis? Best Pract Res Clin Rheumatol 24: 363–371.
24. van der Linden S, Valkenburg HA, Cats A (1984) Evaluation of diagnostic criteria for ankylosing spondylitis. A proposal for modification of the New York criteria. Arthritis Rheum 27: 361–368.
25. Dougados M, Braun J, Szanto S, Combe B, Geher P, et al. (2012) Nonsteroidal antiinflammatory drug intake according to the Assessment of SpondyloArthritis International Society Score in clinical trials evaluating tumor necrosis factor blockers: example of etanercept in advanced ankylosing spondylitis. Arthritis Care Res (Hoboken) 64: 290–294.
26. Wanders AJ, Landewe RB, Spoorenberg A, Dougados M, van der Linden S, et al. (2004) What is the most appropriate radiologic scoring method for ankylosing spondylitis? A comparison of the available methods based on the Outcome Measures in Rheumatology Clinical Trials filter. Arthritis Rheum 50: 2622–2632.
27. van der Heijde D, Landewe R (2005) Selection of a method for scoring radiographs for ankylosing spondylitis clinical trials, by the Assessment in Ankylosing Spondylitis Working Group and OMERACT. J Rheumatol 32: 2048–2049.
28. Creemers MC, Franssen MJ, van't Hof MA, Gribnau FW, van de Putte LB, et al. (2005) Assessment of outcome in ankylosing spondylitis: an extended radiographic scoring system. Ann Rheum Dis 64: 127–129.
29. Benjamini Y, Drai D, Elmer G, Kafkafi N, Golani I (2001) Controlling the false discovery rate in behavior genetics research. Behav Brain Res 125: 279–284.
30. Ward MM, Hendrey MR, Malley JD, Learch TJ, Davis JC Jr, et al. (2009) Clinical and immunogenetic prognostic factors for radiographic severity in ankylosing spondylitis. Arthritis Rheum 61: 859–866.
31. Edmondson AC, Braund PS, Stylianou IM, Khera AV, Nelson CP, et al. (2011) Dense genotyping of candidate gene loci identifies variants associated with high-density lipoprotein cholesterol. Circ Cardiovasc Genet 4: 145–155.
32. Bandarian F, Hedayati M, Daneshpour MS, Naseri M, Azizi F (2013) Genetic Polymorphisms in the APOA1 Gene and their Relationship with Serum HDL Cholesterol Levels. Lipids 48: 1207–1216.
33. Jane JA, Jr., Dunford BA, Kron A, Pittman DD, Sasaki T, et al. (2002) Ectopic osteogenesis using adenoviral bone morphogenetic protein (BMP)-4 and BMP-6 gene transfer. Mol Ther 6: 464–470.
34. Gitelman SE, Kobrin MS, Ye JQ, Lopez AR, Lee A, et al. (1994) Recombinant Vgr-1/BMP-6-expressing tumors induce fibrosis and endochondral bone formation in vivo. J Cell Biol 126: 1595–1609.
35. Bobacz K, Gruber R, Soleiman A, Erlacher L, Smolen JS, et al. (2003) Expression of bone morphogenetic protein 6 in healthy and osteoarthritic human articular chondrocytes and stimulation of matrix synthesis in vitro. Arthritis Rheum 48: 2501–2508.
36. Baldwin C, Nolan VG, Wyszynski DF, Ma QL, Sebastiani P, et al. (2005) Association of klotho, bone morphogenic protein 6, and annexin A2 polymorphisms with sickle cell osteonecrosis. Blood 106: 372–375.
37. Ulug P, Vasavda N, Awogbade M, Cunningham J, Menzel S, et al. (2009) Association of sickle avascular necrosis with bone morphogenic protein 6. Ann Hematol 88: 803–805.
38. Ashley-Koch AE, Elliott L, Kail ME, De Castro LM, Jonassaint J, et al. (2008) Identification of genetic polymorphisms associated with risk for pulmonary hypertension in sickle cell disease. Blood 111: 5721–5726.
39. Slattery ML, John EM, Torres-Mejia G, Herrick JS, Giuliano AR, et al. (2013) Genetic variation in bone morphogenetic proteins and breast cancer risk in hispanic and non-hispanic white women: The breast cancer health disparities study. Int J Cancer 132: 2928–2939.
40. Macsai CE, Foster BK, Xian CJ (2008) Roles of Wnt signalling in bone growth, remodelling, skeletal disorders and fracture repair. J Cell Physiol 215: 578–587.
41. Carter S, Braem K, Lories RJ (2012) The role of bone morphogenetic proteins in ankylosing spondylitis. Ther Adv Musculoskelet Dis 4: 293–299.
42. Urist MR (1965) Bone: formation by autoinduction. Science 150: 893–899.
43. Hall BK, Miyake T (2000) All for one and one for all: condensations and the initiation of skeletal development. Bioessays 22: 138–147.
44. Chen HA, Chen CH, Lin YJ, Chen PC, Chen WS, et al. (2010) Association of bone morphogenetic proteins with spinal fusion in ankylosing spondylitis. J Rheumatol 37: 2126–2132.
45. Park MC, Park YB, Lee SK (2008) Relationship of bone morphogenetic proteins to disease activity and radiographic damage in patients with ankylosing spondylitis. Scand J Rheumatol 37: 200–204.
46. Lories RJ, Derese I, Luyten FP (2005) Modulation of bone morphogenetic protein signaling inhibits the onset and progression of ankylosing enthesitis. J Clin Invest 115: 1571–1579.
47. Carette S, Graham D, Little H, Rubenstein J, Rosen P (1983) The natural disease course of ankylosing spondylitis. Arthritis Rheum 26: 186–190.
48. Baraliakos X, Listing J, Rudwaleit M, Haibel H, Brandt J, et al. (2007) Progression of radiographic damage in patients with ankylosing spondylitis: defining the central role of syndesmophytes. Ann Rheum Dis 66: 910–915.
49. Maksymowych WP, Landewe R, Conner-Spady B, Dougados M, Mielants H, et al. (2007) Serum matrix metalloproteinase 3 is an independent predictor of structural damage progression in patients with ankylosing spondylitis. Arthritis Rheum 56: 1846–1853.
50. Baraliakos X, Listing J, von der Recke A, Braun J (2009) The natural course of radiographic progression in ankylosing spondylitis–evidence for major individual variations in a large proportion of patients. J Rheumatol 36: 997–1002.

5

The Association between GP Consultations for Non-Specific Physical Symptoms in Children and Parents: A Case-Control Study

Mujahed Shraim[1,2,3], Milisa Blagojevic-Bucknall[1], Christian D. Mallen[1], Kate M. Dunn[1]*

1 Arthritis Research UK Primary Care Centre, Keele University, Keele, United Kingdom, **2** Work Environment Department, University of Massachusetts Lowell, Lowell, Massachusetts, United States of America, **3** Center for Disability Research, Liberty Mutual Research Institute for Safety, Hopkinton, Massachusetts, United States of America

Abstract

Background: Non-specific physical symptoms (NSPS) such as abdominal pain, headache and musculoskeletal pain are widespread in the community, and are common reasons for visiting a general practitioner (GP). Causes of NSPS are multifactorial, but may include parental influences.

Objective: To investigate associations between GP consultations for NSPS in parents and their children.

Methods: Matched case-control study using GP consultation data from 12 GP practices in the United Kingdom. Participants were 1328 children who consulted a GP for NSPS in 2009 (cases), 3980 controls who consulted a GP in 2009 but not for NSPS, plus parents of cases and controls (n = 8354). Primary outcome measure: child consultation status for NSPS.

Results: Maternal consultation for NSPS was associated with significantly increased odds of their child consulting for NSPS (odds ratio (OR) 1.51, 95% confidence intervals (CI) 1.33, 1.73); there was no significant association with paternal consultations (OR 0.87, 95% CI 0.71, 1.08). Each additional maternal consultation for NSPS was associated with an increase in the rate ratio for number of consultations for NSPS in the child by 1.03 (95% CI 1.01, 1.05). This overall association was clearest in maternal-child consultations for painful NSPS and for specific bodily systems including gastrointestinal, musculoskeletal and neurologic symptoms.

Conclusions: Maternal GP consultation for NSPS is associated with increased odds of GP consultations for NSPS in children. This study included a large sample of children and parents and used medical records data which is not subject to recall bias. However, analysis was based on medical records, thus the presence of NSPS not leading to consultations is unknown. Medical practitioners managing children with NSPS need to be aware of this association.

Editor: Martin Chalumeau, Université Paris Descartes; AP-HP, Groupe Hospitalier Cochin-Saint-Vincent-de-Paul, France

Funding: MS was funded by NHS Research and Development Support for New Medical Schools. CDM is funded by a Clinician Scientist Fellowship (19634) from Arthritis Research UK. KMD is funded through a Research Career Development Fellowship from the Wellcome Trust (083572). MB is supported by a NIHR National School for Primary Care Research Fellowship. CiPCA is funded by the North Staffordshire Primary Care Research Consortium and Keele University Research Institute for Primary Care and Health Sciences. The funders had no role in study design, data collection and analysis, decision to publish, or preparation of the manuscript.

Competing Interests: The authors have declared that no competing interests exist.

* Email: k.m.dunn@keele.ac.uk

Introduction

Non-specific physical symptoms (NSPS), such as musculoskeletal pain, abdominal pain, and headache are common in children [1,2]. Annually, about one third of children consult a general practitioner (GP) for NSPS [3,4]. NSPS among children are associated with functional impairment and negative impact on quality of life [5,6]. This represents a significant burden on health care services through frequent general practitioner (GP) consultations, diagnostic testing, and referrals to secondary care services [7–9]. The causes of NSPS in children are yet to be fully explained, but are likely to be multifactorial, including genetic and psychosocial factors, such as parental influence on childhood illness and health-seeking behavior [3,10,11].

A recent systematic review found evidence of an association between GP consultations for NSPS in parents and children, but its findings were limited by the methodology used in the empirical studies, including the use of cross-sectional designs, reliance on self-reported data by either parents or children, and including children from specific age groups only [12]. Further research using documented GP consultation data may provide more precise information about the impact of parental NSPS on the child's health and GP consulting behavior for NSPS.

The objective of this study was to investigate the association between GP consultations for NSPS in parents and their children, assess whether this is different for mothers and fathers, and identify gradients of association for any observed associations.

Methods

Ethics statement

Ethical approval for the Consultations in Primary Care Archive (CiPCA) database was given by the North Staffordshire and Staffordshire Research Ethics Committees (UK), who gave permission to download and store anonymised medical record information for research use from participating general practices. All general practices participating in CiPCA inform their patient populations that their anonymised records will be used in this way and all patients are offered the opportunity to withdraw their records from inclusion in CiPCA.

Study design and setting

This was a matched case-control study of children and their parents registered with UK GP practices. The setting was GP practices contributing to CiPCA, a primary care research database containing all recorded primary care consultations occurring at a subset of GP practices in Staffordshire, UK. In 2007, 12 GP practices contributed to the CiPCA database. The total population registered with these practices at mid-year 2009 was 104,911. CiPCA is a high quality, anonymized, and validated database, and the contributing practices have regular cycles of training, assessment and feedback with respect to the quality of coded clinical data [13]. Data from CiPCA on the annual consultation prevalence for musculoskeletal conditions are comparable to data from larger national primary care databases [14].

Participants

Eligible participants were children and their parents registered with CiPCA practices between January 2007 and December 2009. We randomly selected only one child per household for inclusion in the study, because the main exposure of interest was parental consultation for NSPS, which would be the same for siblings; this thereby avoids over representing families with more than one child. Cases were defined as children, aged 2 to 16 years in 2009, who had at least one recorded GP consultation for NSPS between 1 January and 31 December 2009 (inclusive). We used the same criteria to define controls except that controls had at least one GP consultation, but not for NSPS.

We matched controls to cases on sex, maternal age group, and GP practice. We included between one to four controls per case (depending on the availability of suitable controls). If more than four controls per case were available, four were randomly selected. The sample size was calculated for 80% study power and 95% confidence using EpiCalc 2000 [15]. Sample size calculations showed that 535 children were required (107 cases and 428 controls) for each analysis (within mothers and children, and within fathers and children) to be able to detect an association between GP consultation for NSPS in parents and children with an odds ratio (OR) of 2, assuming the proportion exposed in the control group is 20%, and with 1:4 ratio of cases to controls.

Study variables

Outcome measures were the child's GP consultation status for NSPS and stratified by type of NSPS (painful and not-painful), different body systems, and single NSPS (see table 1), number of GP consultations for NSPS, and number of different NSPS consulted for.

Ascertainment of child GP consultations for NSPS

We identified GP consultations for NSPS by using a comprehensive list of standardized diagnostic Read codes referring to the list of NSPS presented in table 1. This list includes 33 NSPS from the diagnostic criteria in the third revision of Diagnostic and Statistical Manual of Mental Disorders for Somatization Disorder [16] and nine NSPS from the somatization factor of the Hopkins Symptom Checklist [17]. These NSPS were included in previous studies of Children's Somatization Inventory [18,19] and other epidemiological studies investigating NSPS in children and adolescents [1,20].

Read codes are a hierarchy of morbidity, symptoms and process codes that are used to record all electronic morbidity data in primary care in the UK [21]. We developed this list of Read codes by reviewing all Read codes referring to signs and symptoms in Read coding system. The full list of Read codes for included NSPS is available upon request from the authors. We classified GP consultations for NSPS as such if the reason for encounter was coded by the GP using any Read codes from our list. Also, one reviewer (MS) reviewed all free-text records for these consultations to ensure that the cause of symptoms (in the opinion of the GP) was not-specific: (a) not due to trauma or pregnancy (in mothers) (b) no recorded abnormalities on physical examination and/or diagnostic testing. If no information indicating (a) or (b) was available in the free-text records, we classified such consultations as consultations for NSPS.

Assessment of exposure to parental consultations for NSPS

Within the CiPCA database, household identification codes were used to link household members, then date of birth was used to determine parents of included children. A mother/father of a randomly selected child within each household was defined as being a female/male aged 17 to 45 years at the birth of the child. All GP consultations made by parents between 1 January 2007 and 31 December 2008 were extracted from the CiPCA database. Maternal and paternal GP consultation status for NSPS between 2007 and 2008 were identified using the same method as described above for children. In children with GP consultation data on both parents, parental GP consultation status for NSPS was grouped into four categories. These comprised: both parents consulted for NSPS, only mother consulted for NSPS, only father consulted for NSPS, and neither parent consulted for NSPS. We also measured the total number of GP consultations for NSPS, and number of different NSPS in consulting parents during 2007-8. We also measured NSPS in parents sorted by painful and not-painful NSPS, body system, and single NSPS (table 1).

Measurement of other independent variables

Besides variables used for case-control matching, we also obtained child's age, paternal age group, child birth order, household member count, index of multiple deprivation (IMD) 2007 scores for residential area level deprivation for included children, and parental history of anxiety or depressive disorders.

Children's age was split into tertiles (2–6, 7–11 and 12–16) and parents' age into quartiles (19–28, 29–39, 40–50 and 51–61 for mothers and 22–29, 30–40, 41–51 and 52–62 for fathers). Parents' age in 2009 rather than 2007 was used to reflect their age at the time of children's consultation. For example, mothers in the age group 19–28 years were two years younger at the time of their consultation in 2007.

Younger siblings for index children were defined as persons from the same household born after the index child, whereas older siblings were defined as persons from the same household and aged 16 or less at the birth of the index child. The birth order of the child was classified as "first" if the child had no siblings or if the child was the oldest child in the household (with no other household members' meeting the definition for a sibling).

Table 1. List of NSPS and their distribution in children and parents.

Non-specific physical symptoms	Case-children (n = 1328)	All mothers (n = 5308)	All fathers (n = 3058)
Musculoskeletal symptoms			
Pain in extremities	99 (7.5)	253 (4.8)	124 (4.1)
Back pain	59 (4.4)	460 (8.6)	237 (7.8)
Joint pain	209 (15.7)	627 (11.8)	148 (4.8)
Muscle soreness	5 (0.4)	15 (0.3)	7 (0.2)
Gastrointestinal symptoms			
Abdominal pain	346 (26.1)	547 (10.3)	130 (4.3)
Vomiting	146 (11.0)	39 (0.7)	13 (0.4)
Nausea	20 (1.5)	60 (1.1)	9 (0.3)
Bloating	3 (0.2)	37 (0.7)	6 (0.2)
Diarrhea	83 (6.3)	56 (1.1)	28 (0.9)
Constipation	132 (9.9)	59 (1.1)	10 (0.3)
Multiple food intolerance	0	0	0
Globus (lump in the throat)	0	7 (0.1)	0
Dysphagia (difficulty swallowing)	0	0	0
Cardiopulmonary symptoms			
Palpitations	9 (0.7)	17 (0.3)	34 (1.1)
Chest pain	62 (4.7)	211 (4.0)	119 (3.9)
Hyperventilation or Dyspnea	44 (3.3)	63 (1.2)	12 (0.4)
Hot or cold spells	1 (0.1)	17 (0.3)	4 (0.1)
Urogenital symptoms			
Pain during urination	1 (0.1)	0	0
Difficulty urinating (Dysuria)	77 (5.8)	4 (0.1)	3 (0.1)
Burning sensation in sexual organs or rectum	0	0	0
Dysmenorrhea (painful menstruation)	0	28 (0.5)	**
Metrorrhagia (irregular menstrual periods)	0	99 (1.9)	**
Menorrhagia (heavy menstrual bleeding)	0	210 (4.0)	**
Sexual indifference (decreased libido)*	*	16 (0.3)	16 (0.5)
Dyspareunia (pain during intercourse)*	*	26 (0.5)	**
Neurologic symptoms			
Dizziness/fainting (syncope)	22 (1.7)	168 (3.2)	43 (1.4)
Transient Amnesia (loss of memory)	0	4 (0.1)	1 (0.0)
Transient Aphonia (loss of voice)	0	0	0
Transient deafness	0	0	0
Transient Diplopia (double vision)	0	0	0
Transient blurred vision	1 (0.1)	4 (0.1)	0
Transient blindness	0	0	0
Transient seizure or convulsion	11 (0.8)	0	0
Transient Ataxia (trouble walking)	0	0	0
Transient Paresis (paralysis)	0	0	0
Headache	167 (12.6)	454 (8.6)	90 (2.9)
Paresthesia (numbness or tingling sensation)	4 (0.3)	58 (1.1)	33 (1.1)
Weakness in parts of the body	0	0	0
Heavy feelings in arms or legs	1 (0.1)	0	0
General symptoms			
Fatigue	68 (5.1)	225 (4.2)	58 (1.9)

NSPS = non-specific physical symptoms; values are numbers (%); * = Symptoms were excluded from analysis for children; ** = Not Applicable.

Table 2. Baseline characteristics of children.

	Cases (n = 1328) n(%)[a]	Controls (n = 3980) n(%)[a]	*p*-value
Child gender (Female)[b]	739 (55.6)	2073 (52.1)	0.99
Child age[c]	10 (9)	8 (8)	<0.01
Child age group [b]			
2–6 years	428 (32.2)	1688 (42.4)	
7–11 years	325 (24.5)	1114 (28.0)	
12–16 years	575 (43.3)	1178 (29.6)	
Child birth order [b]			
First	63 (57.5)	2083 (52.3)	<0.01
Not first	565 (42.5)	1897 (47.7)	
Household members' count	4 (1)	4 (1)	0.02
Household member count [b]			
≤3	691 (52.0)	1908 (47.9)	
>3	637 (48.0)	2072 (52.1)	
IMD 2007 score[c]	22.4 (22.9)	23.1 (22.9)	0.93
IMD 2007quartiles [b]			
I	272 (20.5)	819 (20.6)	
II	262 (19.7)	785 (19.7)	
III	263 (19.8)	792 (19.9)	
IV	280 (21.1)	809 (20.3)	
V	244 (18.4)	759 (19.1)	
Missing IMD score [b]	7 (0.5)	16 (0.4)	
Mother age[c]	39 (11)	38 (9)	<0.01
Mother age group [b]			
19–29 years	216 (16.3)	722 (18.1)	
30–40 years	604 (45.5)	1972 (49.5)	
41–51 years	475 (35.8)	1227 (30.8)	
52–62 years	33 (2.5)	59 (1.5)	
Father age[c]	41 (10)	40 (9)	<0.01
Father age group[b]			
22–32 years	101 (13.2)	378 (16.6)	
33–43 years	381 (49.9)	1241 (54.4)	
44–54 years	246 (32.2)	590 (25.9)	
55–65 years	36 (4.7)	73 (3.2)	
Mother history of anxiety or depressive disorder 2007–2008 [b]			
No	993 (74.8)	3188 (80.1)	<0.01
Yes	335 (25.2)	792 (19.9)	
Father history of anxiety or depressive disorder 2007–2008[b,d]			
No	699 (91.4)	2110 (92.4)	0.39
Yes	65 (8.5)	172 (7.5)	

[a]Percentages may not total 100 due to rounding; [b]Number (%); [c]Median (Interquartile range) Index of Multiple Deprivation 2007; [d]564 (42.5%) of cases and 1698 (42.7%) of controls had no paternal records. Controls were matched to cases on sex, maternal age group, and GP practice.

The child household member count was dichotomized into households with three members or less and households with more than three households. Households with 13 or more members were excluded to prevent including families living in shared households. The IMD 2007 scores were constructed by the Department of Communities and Local Government, and conceptualized as a weighted area level aggregation of scores for seven domains of deprivation including income; employment; health deprivation and disability; education, skills and training; barriers to housing and services; crime; living environment [22]. IMD 2007 scores range from 0% to 100% where higher scores indicate greater deprivation [22]. IMD 2007 scores were also presented as quintiles with "1" representing the most affluent and "5" representing the most deprived. Maternal and paternal history of anxiety or depressive disorders status (yes, no) was identified by searching parental electronic primary care records between 2007 and 2008 using a list of symptom and diagnostic Read codes referring to anxiety and depressive disorders (this list is available on request from the authors).

Statistical methods

Chi-squared tests and Mann-Whitney U tests were performed to test for significant baseline differences between cases and controls. We performed univariable analyses to examine crude associations between the independent variables and the child GP consultation status for NSPS using Cox regression. Effect size estimates were summarised using odds ratios (OR) with 95% confidence intervals (CI). We included all independent variables in the multivariable Cox regression to obtain adjusted associations between parental and child consultation for NSPS. In separate multivariable analyses, we also tested for any interaction effects between parental GP consultations for NSPS and other independent variables on the child GP consultation for NSPS.

In order to test for any potential gradient in associations, logistic regression was used to model effect of increasing number of paternal GP consultations for NSPS, and increasing number of different NSPS a parent consults for, on whether a child consults for NSPS. Similar analyses tested the relationship between consultation for multiple NSPS in parents and children. Furthermore, using Poisson regression we investigated whether there was a relationship between number of maternal consultations for NSPS and number of NSPS consultations in children.

In analyses for associations for painful and not-painful NSPS, body system, and single NSPS we adopted an unmatched case-control approach using logistic regression because relatively small number of cases have consulted for these symptoms categories. All analyses were carried out using SPSS (version 20.0) [23] and STATA (version 12) [24].

Results

Characteristics of cases and controls

5308 children were included (1328 cases and 3980 controls). The mothers of all children were identified. The fathers of 42.5% of cases and 42.7% of controls were unknown based on GP registration data, leaving 766 cases and 2292 controls with identifiable fathers. This may be because fathers were registered with other GP practices or were not registered with any practice at all, or because children were living with single-mothers. The baseline characteristics of all study participants are shown in table 2. Cases and controls differed significantly on all variables except for IMD 2007 scores and father history of anxiety or depressive disorders. Median age for cases was 10 years (Interquartile range 9) and 8 (8) years for controls (table 2). Maternal age was significantly different in cases and controls despite matching them on maternal age group. The most common single NSPS in children were abdominal pain, joint pain and headache. Abdominal pain, joint pain and back pain were the most common symptoms in parents (table 1).

The association between GP consultations for NSPS in parents and children

Overall, 52% of cases and 41% of controls had a maternal history of consultation for NSPS, and 30% of cases and controls (with available paternal records) had paternal history of consultation for NSPS.

Initially, analyses included all children, irrespective of whether both parents were identified. Univariable analysis revealed that cases were more likely than controls to have a history of maternal GP consultation for NSPS (crude OR 1.55, 95% CI 1.37, 1.76), a finding which persisted in multivariable analysis (adjusted OR 1.51, 95% CI 1.33, 1.73) after adjustment for child age group, father age group, child birth order, household members' count, and maternal history of anxiety and depressive disorders. We found no significant association between GP consultation for NSPS in fathers and children (table 3). Subsequently, analyses included only those children who had both parents identified in the study sample (764 cases and 2183 controls).

We found that in instances where only a mother consulted for NSPS, the odds of a child having a GP consultation for NSPS was 1.38 (95% CI 1.14, 1.69) as compared to a child with neither parent consulting for NSPS. We found no significant association between GP consultations for NSPS in fathers and children (see Table 4). However, GP consultation for NSPS in both parents was associated with increased odds of child consulting for NSPS (adjusted OR 1.57, 95% CI 1.23, 2.01).

No significant interaction effects were identified between parental consultation for NSPS and other independent variables on the child GP consultation status for NSPS.

Gradients association between GP consultations for NSPS in parents and children

Analyses for gradients association were restricted to mother-child pairs because we found no significant associations between GP consultations for NSPS in fathers and children. Logistic regression analysis showed a significant increase in the odds of child consulting for NSPS with increasing number of GP consultations for NSPS and number of different NSPS consulted for in the mother (see table 5). Children whose mother consulted only once had odds of consulting almost 1.4 times higher than children whose mother didn't consult. These odds increased to 2.14 (95% CI 1.68, 2.72) for those children whose mother consulted more than three times.

Restricting the analysis only to cases, Poisson regression showed that each additional one maternal GP consultation for NSPS was associated with increase in the rate ratio for number of consultations for NSPS in the child by 1.03 (95% CI 1.01, 1.05). Additionally, using logistic regression, we found that cases whose mothers consulted with multiple NSPS (two or more NSPS) had increased odds of consulting with multiple NSPS as compared to cases whose mothers did not consult for NSPS (adjusted OR 2.24, 95% CI 1.68, 2.99).

The association between GP consultations for NSPS groups and single NSPS in parents and children

As shown in table 6, we found significant associations between consultations for painful NSPS in mothers and children (OR 1.49, 95% CI 1.28, 1.74), but not for not-painful NSPS (OR 1.11, 95% CI 0.88, 1.40). Logistic regression analysis showed significant associations between maternal and child consultations for musculoskeletal, gastrointestinal, and neurologic symptoms, but not for cardiopulmonary and urogenital symptoms (table 6). Additionally, the association between maternal and child consultations for single NSPS was statistically significant for abdominal pain, joint pain, extremities pain, headache, and vomiting (table 6)

Discussion

This study found statistically significant associations between GP consultations for NSPS in mothers (but not fathers) and their children. The association between parental and child consultation was stronger when both parents consulted for NSPS. We also found a statistically significant gradient of association between the number of GP consultations for NSPS and the number of NSPS in mothers and children. Additionally, we found significant associ-

Table 3. Associations between consultations for NSPS in either parant and children.

	Cases (n = 1328) n(%)	Controls (n = 3980) n(%)	Crude OR (95% CI)	Adjusted OR (95% CI)
Maternal consultation history for NSPS 2007–2008				
Yes	695 (52.3)	1642 (41.3)	1.55 (1.37, 1.76)	1.51 (1.33, 1.73)
No	633 (47.7)	2338 (58.7)	1	1
Paternal consultation history for NSPS 2007–2008				
Yes	228 (29.9)	692 (30.4)	0.89 (0.73, 1.09)	0.87 (0.71, 1.08)
No	536 (70.1)	1590 (69.6)	1	1

NSPS = non-specific physical symptoms; OR = odds ratio; CI = confidence intervals; 564 (42.5%) of cases and 1698 (42.7%) of controls had no paternal records. ORs were adjusted for child age, father age, child birth order; household members' count, Index of Multiple Deprivation 2007 scores; maternal and paternal anxiety or depressive disorder.

ations between maternal and child consultation for painful symptoms, specific body systems, and single NSPS.

The observed associations between GP consultations for NSPS in mothers and children are consistent with the findings of a systematic review which found evidence of an association between GP consultations for NSPS in parents and children [12]. However, that review found only eight studies, and the majority of studies used self-reported data by either parents or children and used cross-sectional designs. One study reported that the associations between GP consultations for abdominal pain or headache were greater for mother-child pairs than father-child pairs [3]. Another study found maternal GP consultations NSPS more predictive of the child consultations for gastrointestinal NSPS than those of fathers [25].

With respect to the significant association between maternal and child consultation for painful NSPS, but not for not-painful symptoms, it may be that consulting behavior is influenced by level of pain severity and perceived seriousness of the symptoms [26,27]. For example, parents may perceive painful NSPS in themselves and in their children as more serious than not-painful NSPS, which influences their GP consultation rates for these NSPS.

One possible explanation for these associations is an inherited genetic predisposition to NSPS. There is some evidence that genetic effects contribute to the onset of some NSPS and syndromes, such as headache and irritable bowel syndrome [28,29]. However, it is seems unlikely for genetic factors to fully explain this, because only maternal (and not paternal) consultations for NSPS were associated with the child consulting for NSPS. Another explanation is shared exposure of family members to certain social and environmental factors (e.g. stressful events, lack of social support, socioeconomic circumstances, and poor family functioning) which have been found to be associated with greater reporting of NSPS [30,31] and GP consultations for NSPS in parents and children [7]. One plausible explanation is the childhood social learning of illness behavior, which has been hypothesised to play an important role in the development of illness and healthcare seeking behavior among children [32–34]. A number of studies have suggested that parental responses and attitudes toward the child illness (reinforcement) and parental coping mechanisms with their own illness (role modelling) may influence symptom frequency, disability days, and healthcare consultations in their children [35,36]. We would expect social learning and role modeling to increase with child's age. However, we found no significant interaction effects between the child age group (or other independent variables) and maternal consultations for NSPS on the child GP consultation status for NSPS. This suggests that the maternal effect on child consultations for NSPS through "reinforcement" is present at all ages and represent a more important influence.

Strengths and limitations

The main limitations of the previous few studies that examined the association between GP consultations for NSPS in parents and children were the use of self-reported data which is prone to recall bias, including children from specific age groups, and the use of cross-sectional designs that are unable to distinguish the direction of associations. Strengths of our study therefore include the fact that we used documented GP consultations, which are more precise source of information on attendance in primary care than relying on self-reported data by children or their parents that may be prone to recall bias [37]. Additionally, we included a large sample (n = 5308) and relied on documented GP attendance from

Table 4. Associations between consultations for NSPS in both parents and children.

	Cases (n = 764) n(%)	Controls (n = 2183) n(%)	Crude OR (95% CI)	Adjusted OR (95% CI)
Both parents did not consult for NSPS	276 (36.1)	989 (45.3)	1	1
Only father consulted for NSPS	78 (10.2)	335 (15.3)	0.82 (0.63, 1.08)	0.83 (0.63, 1.10)
Only mother consulted for NSPS	260 (34.0)	568 (26.0)	1.44 (1.20, 1.74)	1.38 (1.14, 1.69)
Both parents consulted for NSPS	150 (19.6)	291 (13.3)	1.63 (1.29, 2.06)	1.57 (1.23, 2.01)

NSPS = non-specific physical symptoms; OR = odds ratio; CI = confidence intervals. ORs were adjusted for child age, father age, child birth order; household members' count, Index of Multiple Deprivation 2007 scores; maternal and paternal anxiety or depressive disorder.

Table 5. Associations between number of consultations for NSPS and number of different NSPS in mother and child consultation for NSPS.

NSPS	Cases n = 1328 n(%)	Controls n = 3980 n(%)	Crude OR (95% CI)	Adjusted OR (95% CI)
Maternal number of consultations for NSPS				
0	633 (47.7)	2338 (58.7)	1	1
1	300 (22.6)	809 (20.3)	1.37 (1.17, 1.61)	1.38 (1.17, 1.63)
2	156 (11.7)	406 (10.2)	1.41 (1.14, 1.73)	1.36 (1.10, 1.68)
3	96 (7.2)	198 (5)	1.77 (1.36, 2.31)	1.69 (1.28, 2.22)
>3	143 (10.8)	229 (5.8)	2.24 (1.78, 2.82)	2.14 (1.68, 2.72)
Maternal number of different NSPS				
0	663 (47.7)	2338 (58.7)	1	1
1–2	601 (45.3)	1494 (37.5)	1.47 (1.29, 1.68)	1.45 (1.27, 1.66)
>2	94 (7.1)	148 (3.7)	2.37 (1.79, 3.12)	2.24 (1.68, 2.99)

OR = odds ratio; CI = confidence intervals. ORs were adjusted for child age, child birth order; household members' count, Index of Multiple Deprivation 2007 scores; maternal anxiety or depressive disorder.

12 practices which increases the internal and external validity of our findings. Also, as described in the methods section, CiPCA is a high quality validated database, which enhances the validity of our findings. For example, 97% of all GP consultations that occurred in the CiPCA practices in 2006 were given a morbidity code [38]. Another important strength is that parental consultation status for NSPS was ascertained using parental consultations data in the two years preceding the child consultation, which provides a clear temporal relationship. Additionally, the observed associations were supported by evidence of gradients of association.

One limitation is the potential for diagnostic misclassification, which is a common problem in primary care [39]. However, diagnostic misclassification is unlikely to completely explain the associations found in this study due to the high quality of coded clinical data within CiPCA practices. Additionally, the current classification system used in primary care allows for coding definitive diagnoses (e.g. urinary tract infection) as well as symptoms' diagnoses (e.g. abdominal pain) when a definitive diagnosis is not established, which reduces the potential for diagnostic misclassification. One potential limitation is the lack of blinding of GPs to symptoms in parents and children at time of consultation. However, we believe that this is minimal and not systematic because it does not explain differences in associations between mothers and fathers, and that our findings were based on association between parents' consultations in 2007–2008 and the child's consultations in 2009. Another limitation is that, based on GP practice registered population data, we were not able to examine whether our findings are different for children living or not living in the same house as their mother and father. Also, paternal consultations status for NSPS was unknown for 43% of children. However, this was distributed equally between cases and controls. Additionally, it is unlikely that the lack of significant associations between GP consultations for NSPS in fathers and children is entirely attributed to low study power as the numbers of children with paternal consultation data were more than those needed based on sample size calculations. Although we matched controls and cases on maternal age group, they differed significantly on maternal age. However, it is unlikely for this to lead to significant changes in our ORs estimates because we also found statistically significant associations for single NSPS in mother and children after adjustment for maternal age in unmatched analyses.

Although this study set out to examine the association between consultation patterns for NSPS in parents and children, GP consultation data only provides a measure of health problems for which practice registered populations have consulted. Thus, the presence of other NSPS which did not result in GP consultation remains unknown.

Generalizability

In the UK over 97% of the population is registered with a GP practice, which usually provides first point access to non-emergency healthcare [40]. We used a large population-based sample of families registered with GP practices from Staffordshire. This area is more deprived than England as a whole, but we found no significant associations between child GP consultation for NSPS and area level deprivation in either univariable or multivariable analyses. Although the healthcare setting in UK may be different from other healthcare settings, similar associations for specific symptoms between parents and children were reported in different countries [3,25,41].

Implications for clinical practice and future research

These findings indicate that GPs and other medical practitioners managing children with NSPS in secondary care settings should be aware of the association between consultations for NSPS in parents and children, as such insights might direct medical practitioners toward alternative management approaches. For example, a recent randomized controlled trial has demonstrated that cognitive behavioral therapy (CBT) targeting children's coping responses to recurrent abdominal pain and parents' responses to pain in their children was associated with significant reduction in pain and gastrointestinal symptoms severity in children at six month follow-up [42]. It is not clear whether CBT had an impact on the consultation behavior of children for NSPS. There is some evidence from literature on adults that CBT, pharmacological therapy, and aerobic exercise for patients presenting with NSPS in primary care and general outpatient clinics are effective in reducing frequency of symptoms, the number of consultations, and related psychological distress [43–46]. Potentially, such interventions for parents could impact on the illness and healthcare seeking behavior of both parents and their children, but no studies exist to confirm or refute this. This provides a rationale for future research to focus on development of

Table 6. Associations between consultation for specific symptoms in mothers & children.

	NSPS in the child			
NSPS in the mother	**Yes**	**No**	**Crude OR (95% CI)**	**Adjusted OR (95% CI)**
Painful NSPS				
Yes	376	1441	1.53 (1.32, 1.77)	1.49 (1.28, 1.74)
No	509	2982	1	1
Not-painful NSPS				
Yes	111	843	1.21 (0.97, 1.50)	1.11 (0.88, 1.40)
No	429	3925	1	1
Musculoskeletal NSPS				
Yes	130	1128	1.53 (1.23, 1.90)	1.41 (1.22, 1.75)
No	284	3766	1	1
Gastrointestinal NSPS				
Yes	112	576	1.51 (1.21, 1.89)	1.40 (1.12, 1.76)
No	527	493	1	1
Neurological NSPS				
Yes	44	558	1.92 (1.36, 2.69)	2.10 (1.46, 3.02)
No	186	4520	1	1
Cardiopulmonary NSPS				
Yes	5	210	1.62 (0.65, 4.04)	1.27 (0.50, 3.25)
No	74	5019	1	1
Urogenital NSPS				
Yes	5	352	0.96 (0.39, 2.40)	0.90 (0.36, 2.26)
No	72	4879	1	1
Abdominal pain				
Yes	59	488	1.89 (1.40, 2.53)	1.81 (1.34, 2.44)
No	287	4474	1	1
Joint pain				
Yes	37	590	1.64 (1.14, 2.37)	1.55 (1.07, 2.25)
No	172	4509	1	1
Headache				
Yes	23	431	1.75 (1.11, 2.74)	2.02 (1.26, 3.24)
No	144	4710	1	1
Vomiting				
Yes	6	33	6.67 (2.75, 16.15)	4.98 (2.00, 12.40)
No	140	5129	1	1
Constipation				
Yes	1	58	0.67 (0.09, 4.90)	0.60 (0.08, 4.40)
No	131	5118	1	1
Pain in extremities				
Yes	10	243	2.30 (1.18, 4.47)	2.12 (1.08, 4.16)
No	89	4966	1	1
Diarrhea				
Yes	2	54	2.36 (0.57, 9.86)	2.17 (0.51, 9.36)
No	81	5171	1	1
Fatigue				
Yes	2	223	0.68 (0.17, 2.80)	0.70 (0.17, 2.89)
No	66	5017	1	1
Back pain				
Yes	8	452	1.67 (0.79, 3.53)	1.42 (0.66, 3.05)
No	51	4797	1	1

Table 6. Cont.

	NSPS in the child			
NSPS in the mother	**Yes**	**No**	**Crude OR (95% CI)**	**Adjusted OR (95% CI)**
Fainting/dizziness				
Yes	1	167	0.54 (0.08, 3.95)	0.52 (0.07, 3.86)
No	56	5084	1	1

OR = odds ratio; CI = confidence intervals. ORs were adjusted for child age, child sex, mother age, child birth order; household members' count, Index of Multiple Deprivation 2007 scores; maternal anxiety or depressive disorder, and GP practice.

appropriate clinical guidelines on management of parents and children with consultations for NSPS. Additionally, more prospective and qualitative research is required to fully explain the exact mechanisms underlying the association between GP consultations for NSPS in mothers and children. Such research may shed light on interventions that may help in preventing the development or recurrence of consultations for NSPS in children.

Conclusions

This study suggests that exposure to maternal GP consultations for NSPS is a significant risk factor for similar consultations in the child. This finding was strengthened by evidence of gradients of association between number of GP consultations for NSPS and number of NSPS in mothers and children as well as associations for specific type symptom groups and single NSPS especially painful NSPS. This study adds further evidence that children may learn their illness and consultation behavior from their mothers, and that recurrent consultation for NSPS in children should be viewed within a family context.

Acknowledgments

The Keele GP Research Partnership and the Informatics team at the Arthritis Research UK Primary Care Centre.

MS is funded by NHS Research and Development Support for New Medical Schools. MB is supported by a NIHR National School for Primary Care Research Fellowship. CDM is funded by a Clinician Scientist Fellowship (19634) from Arthritis Research UK. KMD is funded through a Research Career Development Fellowship from the Wellcome Trust [083572]. CiPCA is funded by the North Staffordshire Primary Care Research Consortium and Keele University Institute for Primary Care and Health.

Author Contributions

Conceived and designed the experiments: MS CDM KMD. Analyzed the data: MS MB. Contributed reagents/materials/analysis tools: MS MB CDM KMD. Wrote the paper: MS MB CDM KMD.

References

1. Eminson M, Benjamin S, Shortall A, Woods T, Faragher B (1996) Physical symptoms and illness attitudes in adolescents: An epidemiological study. J Child Psychol Psychiatry 37: 519–528.
2. Perquin CW, Hazebroek-Kampschreur AA, Hunfeld JA, Bohnen AM, van Suijlekom-Smit LW, et al. (2000) Pain in children and adolescents: A common experience. Pain 87: 51–58.
3. Cardol M, van den Bosch WJ, Spreeuwenberg P, Groenewegen PP, van Dijk L, et al. (2006) All in the family: Headaches and abdominal pain as indicators for consultation patterns in families. Ann Fam Med 4: 506–511.
4. van Eekelen FC, Perquin CW, Hunfeld JA, Hazebroek-Kampschreur AA, van Suijlekom-Smit LW, et al. (2002) Comparison between children and adolescents with and without chronic benign pain: Consultation rate and pain characteristics. Br J Gen Pract 52: 211–213.
5. Roth-Isigkeit A, Thyen U, Raspe HH, Stoven H, Schmucker P (2004) Reports of pain among German children and adolescents: An epidemiological study. Acta Paediatr 93: 258–263.
6. Domenech-Llaberia E, Jane C, Canals J, Ballespi S, Esparo G, et al. (2004) Parental reports of somatic symptoms in preschool children: Prevalence and associations in a Spanish sample. J Am Acad Child Adolesc Psychiatry 43: 598–604.
7. Little P, Somerville J, Williamson I, Warner G, Moore M, et al. (2001) Family influences in a cross-sectional survey of higher child attendance. Br J Gen Pract 51: 977–81, 984.
8. Jackson JL, Kroenke K (2008) Prevalence, impact, and prognosis of multisomatoform disorder in primary care: A 5-year follow-up study. Psychosom Med 70: 430–434.
9. Reid S, Wessely S, Crayford T, Hotopf M (2001) Medically unexplained symptoms in frequent attenders of secondary health care: Retrospective cohort study. BMJ 322: 767.
10. El-Metwally A, Mikkelsson M, Stahl M, Macfarlane GJ, Jones GT, et al. (2008) Genetic and environmental influences on non-specific low back pain in children: A twin study. Eur Spine J 17: 502–508.
11. Levy RL, Jones KR, Whitehead WE, Feld SI, Talley NJ, et al. (2001) Irritable bowel syndrome in twins: Heredity and social learning both contribute to etiology. Gastroenterology 121: 799–804.
12. Shraim M, Mallen CD, Dunn KM (2013) GP consultations for medically unexplained physical symptoms in parents and their children: A systematic review. Br J Gen Pract 63: e318–25.
13. Porcheret M, Hughes R, Evans D, Jordan K, Whitehurst T, et al. (2004) Data quality of general practice electronic health records: The impact of a program of assessments, feedback, and training. J Am Med Inform Assoc 11: 78–86.
14. Jordan K, Clarke AM, Symmons DP, Fleming D, Porcheret M, et al. (2007) Measuring disease prevalence: A comparison of musculoskeletal disease using four general practice consultation databases. Br J Gen Pract 57: 7–14.
15. Gilman J, Myatt M (1998) EpiCalc 2000. 1.02.
16. American Psychiatric Association (1987) Diagnostic and statistical manual of mental disorders. Washington, DC: American Psychiatric Association.
17. Derogatis LR, Lipman RS, Rickels K, Uhlenhuth EH, Covi L (1974) The Hopkins symptom checklist (HSCL): A self-report symptom inventory. Behav Sci 19: 1–15.
18. Walker LS, Beck JE, Garber J, Lambert W (2009) Children's somatization inventory: Psychometric properties of the revised form (CSI-24). J Pediatr Psychol 34: 430–440.
19. Garber J, Walker LS, Zeman J (1991) Somatization symptoms in a community sample of children and adolescents: Further validation of the children's somatization inventory. Psychological Assessment 3: 588–595.
20. Rask CU, Olsen EM, Elberling H, Christensen MF, Ornbol E, et al. (2009) Functional somatic symptoms and associated impairment in 5-7-year-old children: The Copenhagen child cohort 2000. Eur J Epidemiol 24: 625–634.
21. Chisholm J (1990) The Read clinical classification. BMJ 300: 1092.
22. Department for Communities and Local Government (2007) The English indices of deprivation 2007. London: Department for Communities and Local Government.
23. IBM Corp (2011) IBM SPSS statistics for windows. 20.0.
24. Stata Corp (2011) Stata statistical software. 12.
25. Levy RL, Whitehead WE, Von Korff MR, Feld AD (2000) Intergenerational transmission of gastrointestinal illness behavior. Am J Gastroenterol 95: 451–456.
26. Perquin CW, Hunfeld JA, Hazebroek-Kampschreur AA, van Suijlekom-Smit LW, Passchier J, et al. (2001) Insights in the use of health care services in chronic benign pain in childhood and adolescence. Pain 94: 205–213.

27. Masiero S, Carraro E, Sarto D, Bonaldo L, Ferraro C (2010) Healthcare service use in adolescents with non-specific musculoskeletal pain. Acta Paediatr 99: 1224–1228.
28. Larsson B, Bille B, Pedersen NL (1995) Genetic influence in headaches: A Swedish twin study. Headache 35: 513–519.
29. Morris-Yates A, Talley NJ, Boyce PM, Nandurkar S, Andrews G (1998) Evidence of a genetic contribution to functional bowel disorder. Am J Gastroenterol 93: 1311–1317.
30. Kashikar-Zuck S, Lynch AM, Slater S, Graham TB, Swain NF, et al. (2008) Family factors, emotional functioning, and functional impairment in juvenile fibromyalgia syndrome. Arthritis Rheum 59: 1392–1398.
31. Groholt EK, Stigum H, Nordhagen R, Kohler L (2003) Recurrent pain in children, socio-economic factors and accumulation in families. Eur J Epidemiol 18: 965–975.
32. Levy RL, Langer SL, Whitehead WE (2007) Social learning contributions to the etiology and treatment of functional abdominal pain and inflammatory bowel disease in children and adults. World J Gastroenterol 13: 2397–2403.
33. Cardol M, van Dijk L, van den Bosch WJ, Spreeuwenberg P, de Bakker DH, et al. (2007) Striking variations in consultation rates with general practice reveal family influence. BMC Fam Pract 8: 4.
34. Craig TK, Cox AD, Klein K (2002) Intergenerational transmission of somatization behaviour: A study of chronic somatizers and their children. Psychol Med 32: 805–816.
35. Whitehead WE, Crowell MD, Heller BR, Robinson JC, Schuster MM, et al. (1994) Modeling and reinforcement of the sick role during childhood predicts adult illness behavior. Psychosom Med 56: 541–550.
36. Walker LS, Zeman JL (1992) Parental response to child illness behavior. J Pediatr Psychol 17: 49–71.
37. Jordan K, Jinks C, Croft P (2006) Health care utilization: Measurement using primary care records and patient recall both showed bias. J Clin Epidemiol 59: 791–797.
38. Jordan KP, Kadam UT, Hayward R, Porcheret M, Young C, et al. (2010) Annual consultation prevalence of regional musculoskeletal problems in primary care: An observational study. BMC Musculoskelet Disord 11: 144-2474-11-144.
39. de Lusignan S (2005) The barriers to clinical coding in general practice: A literature review. Med Inform Internet Med 30: 89–97.
40. Department of Health (2011) Andrew Lansley: Moving forward on modernising the NHS. Available: http://www.dh.gov.uk/en/MediaCentre/Pressreleases/DH_128162. Accessed 2012 April 24.
41. Campo JV, Bridge J, Lucas A, Savorelli S, Walker L, et al. (2007) Physical and emotional health of mothers of youth with functional abdominal pain. Arch Pediatr Adolesc Med 161: 131–137.
42. Levy RL, Langer SL, Walker LS, Romano JM, Christie DL, et al. (2010) Cognitive-behavioral therapy for children with functional abdominal pain and their parents decreases pain and other symptoms. Am J Gastroenterol 105: 946–956.
43. Husain K, Browne T, Chalder T (2007) A review of psychological models and interventions for medically unexplained somatic symptoms in children. Child & Adolescent Mental Health 12: 2–8.
44. Sumathipala A, Hewege S, Hanwella R, Mann AH (2000) Randomized controlled trial of cognitive behaviour therapy for repeated consultations for medically unexplained complaints: A feasibility study in sri lanka. Psychol Med 30: 747–757.
45. Speckens AE, van Hemert AM, Spinhoven P, Hawton KE, Bolk JH, et al. (1995) Cognitive behavioural therapy for medically unexplained physical symptoms: A randomised controlled trial. BMJ 311: 1328–1332.
46. Peters S, Stanley I, Rose M, Kaney S, Salmon P (2002) A randomized controlled trial of group aerobic exercise in primary care patients with persistent, unexplained physical symptoms. Fam Pract 19: 665–674.

6

Carbamazepine Potentiates the Effectiveness of Morphine in a Rodent Model of Neuropathic Pain

Michael R. Due[1], Xiao-Fang Yang[2], Yohance M. Allette[3], Aaron L. Randolph[1], Matthew S. Ripsch[1], Sarah M. Wilson[4], Erik T. Dustrude[3], Rajesh Khanna[2,5], Fletcher A. White[1,5]*

1 Department of Anesthesia, Indiana University School of Medicine, Indianapolis, Indiana, United States of America, **2** Department of Pharmacology, College of Medicine, University of Arizona, Tucson, Arizona, United States of America, **3** Department of Cell Biology and Anatomy, Indiana University School of Medicine, Indianapolis, Indiana, United States of America, **4** Program in Medical Neurosciences, Paul and Carole Stark Neurosciences Research Institute, Indiana University School of Medicine, Indianapolis, Indiana, United States of America, **5** Department of Pharmacology and Toxicology, Indiana University School of Medicine, Indianapolis, Indiana, United States of America

Abstract

Approximately 60% of morphine is glucuronidated to morphine-3-glucuronide (M3G) which may aggravate preexisting pain conditions. Accumulating evidence indicates that M3G signaling through neuronal Toll-like receptor 4 (TLR4) may be central to this proalgesic signaling event. These events are known to include elevated neuronal excitability, increased voltage-gated sodium (NaV) current, tactile allodynia and decreased opioid analgesic efficacy. Using an *in vitro* ratiometric-based calcium influx analysis of acutely dissociated small and medium-diameter neurons derived from lumbar dorsal root ganglion (DRG), we observed that M3G-sensitive neurons responded to lipopolysaccharide (LPS) and over 35% of these M3G/LPS-responsive cells exhibited sensitivity to capsaicin. In addition, M3G-exposed sensory neurons significantly increased excitatory activity and potentiated NaV current as measured by current and voltage clamp, when compared to baseline level measurements. The M3G-dependent excitability and potentiation of NaV current in these sensory neurons could be reversed by the addition of carbamazepine (CBZ), a known inhibitor of several NaV currents. We then compared the efficacy between CBZ and morphine as independent agents, to the combined treatment of both drugs simultaneously, in the tibial nerve injury (TNI) model of neuropathic pain. The potent anti-nociceptive effects of morphine (5 mg/kg, i.p.) were observed in TNI rodents at post-injury day (PID) 7–14 and absent at PID21–28, while administration of CBZ (10 mg/kg, i.p.) alone failed to produce anti-nociceptive effects at any time following TNI (PID 7–28). In contrast to either drug alone at PID28, the combination of morphine and CBZ completely attenuated tactile hyperalgesia in the rodent TNI model. The basis for the potentiation of morphine in combination with CBZ may be due to the effects of a latent upregulation of NaV1.7 in the DRG following TNI. Taken together, our observations demonstrate a potential therapeutic use of morphine and CBZ as a combinational treatment for neuropathic pain.

Editor: Thiago Mattar Cunha, University of Sao Paulo, Brazil

Funding: This work was supported by NIH NIDA R01DA026040 and NIDDK DK100905. The funders had no role in study design, data collection and analysis, decision to publish, or preparation of the manuscript.

Competing Interests: The authors have declared that no competing interests exist.

* Email: fawhite@iupui.edu

Introduction

Morphine is the cornerstone of pain management in a number of pain conditions. However, therapeutic administration of morphine or morphine equivalents for neuropathic pain is limited to the second or third line of medication due to multiple adverse effects including incomplete efficacy [1], respiratory depression, and induction of sedation, constipation, nausea, vomiting, addiction and tolerance [2]. It has also been reported both experimentally and clinically that exposure to morphine can elicit a paradoxical pain in regions of the body unrelated to the initial pain complaint, aggravating preexisting pain; opioid-induced hyperalgesia (OIH) [3]. However, the molecular mechanisms of OIH are largely unknown. Numerous groups have suggested that OIH may be due to tonic, descending facilitation in the spinal cord [4,5] or in the spinal cord dorsal horn [6,7] through changes in activity of NMDA receptors. Though neither of these modes of action can be completely ruled out, an alternative OIH mechanism involves functional activation of the innate immune receptor Toll-like receptor 4 (TLR4) known to exhibited by a subpopulation of nociceptive neurons [8,9].

TLR4 is a member of a fundamental family of receptors known for their ability to recognize pathogen-associated molecular patterns and facilitate the production of pro-inflammatory cytokines. TLR4 activation is not limited to pathogen detection; recent publications suggest that opioids and their glucuronide metabolites, among other ligands, can elicit TLR4-dependent activation in glial and neuronal cells [9,10,11,12,13,14]. Moreover, both pharmacological blockade of TLR4 signaling and the use of TLR4 knockout mice serve to prevent behavioral hyperalgesia due to morphine tolerance and potentiate acute morphine analgesia *in vivo* [9,15,16].

Molecular modeling of opioid receptors has provided key information regarding the affinity of a variety of opioid ligands. Yet relatively little is known regarding the opioid-mediated TLR4 receptor action on neurons associated with the nociceptive pathway. A recent investigation using the morphine metabolite, morphine-3-glucuronide (M3G) to study TLR4-mediated activation in small diameter nociceptive neurons revealed that the there is a substantial increase in the current density for voltage-gated sodium channels (NaV), NaV1.6, NaV1.7 and NaV1.9, but not NaV1.8. [9]. The fact that these Na^+ currents were influenced by a TLR4 agonist suggests that pharmacological targeting may provide mechanistic insights into both OIH and neuropathic disorders.

A suitable candidate to potentially diminish the neuronal TLR4 agonist-mediated signaling increases in excitation via sodium current modulation, is the anti-epileptic drug carbamazepine (CBZ) [17]. CBZ, a state-dependent channel blocker that inhibits sodium current within seconds when applied externally, [18] is known to stabilize the inactivated current state of NaV1.3, NaV1.7, and NaV1.8 without targeting resurgent sodium current [19,20]. Though the degree to which sodium channel blockade impacts TLR4 agonist-mediated effects is largely unknown, Black and colleagues have shown that phenytoin and tetrodotoxin substantially reduces phagocytic activity of microglia cells activated with the TLR4 agonist, lipopolysaccharide (LPS) [21]. Taken together, these TLR4-agonist-mediated events demonstrate that sodium channels may be possibly affiliated with TLR4 signaling as well as instrumental to the rapid induction of cellular activity in both immune cells and nociceptive sensory neurons.

The aim of this study was to assay the degree to which CBZ administration can diminish M3G/TLR4-induced neuronal activity *in vitro* and to characterize the potency of morphine, alone or in combination, with CBZ in the tibial nerve injury (TNI) model of neuropathic pain over time. We also determined the degree to which expression levels of NaV1.7 change following TNI paralleled changes in diminished morphine efficacy.

Materials and Methods

Pathogen-free, adult female and male Sprague-Dawley (S/D) rats (150–200 g; Harlan Laboratories, Madison, WI) were housed in temperature (23±3°C) and light (12-h light: 12-h dark cycle; lights on at 07:00 h) controlled rooms with standard rodent chow and autoclaved tap water available. Experiments were performed during the light cycle. Animals were randomly assigned to the treatment groups. All animal experiments were approved by the Institutional Animal Care and Use Committees of Indiana University School of Medicine and College of Medicine, University of Arizona. All procedures were conducted in accordance with the Guide for Care and Use of Laboratory Animals published by the National Institutes of Health and the ethical guidelines established by the International Association for the Study of Pain.

Tibial Nerve Injury

All rodents were anesthetized during the procedure with isoflurane (4% induction, 2% maintenance). To model neuropathic pain we performed a tibial nerve injury (TNI) as previously described [22,23,24,25]. Rodents were anesthetized using isoflurane at 4% induction and 2% maintenance. Under anesthesia, the right sciatic nerve was isolated under aseptic surgical conditions by blunt dissection of the femoral biceps muscle, without damaging the epimycium. The sciatic nerve and its three branches were isolated: the sural, common peroneal and tibial nerves and only the tibial nerve was tightly-ligated with 5-0 silk and transected distal to the ligation. The removal of an additional 2–4 mm of distal nerve stump was removed to prevent re-innervation by the proximal nerve. The overlying muscle and skin was then sutured in two separate layers.

Behavioral assessment

All rodents were habituated to testing chambers which were transparent plastic cages with a floor of wire mesh with ~1 cm×1 cm openings for at least two days and baseline testing occurred for each of three days before TNI to establish force threshold necessary for paw withdrawal using previously described techniques [26,27]. The incidence of foot withdrawal was expressed as a percentage of the 6 applications of each stimulus and the percentage of withdrawals was then plotted as a function of force. The von Frey withdrawal threshold was defined as the force that evoked a minimum detectable withdrawal observed on 50% of the tests given at the same force level. Following TNI, animal behavioral thresholds were assayed at least 30 minutes prior to drug administration and tested again following reagent administration.

Drugs and Administration

Carbamazepine (CBZ) was purchased from Sigma (St. Louis, MO). Morphine sulfate salt and morphine-3-glucuronoide (M3G) was provided by NIDA Drug Supply Program (Rockville, MD). For *in vitro* studies, a 75 mM solution of CBZ was made up in dimethyl sulphoxide (DMSO). A 2.67-µl aliquot was taken directly from this stock and put into the 2 ml of bathing solution for the population data to obtain a final concentration of 100 µM [DMSO, 0.1% (v/v)]. For *in vivo* studies, CBZ was suspended in 5% DMSO (% of final volume) in saline (0.9%). Morphine was freshly prepared on the day of the experiment in saline such that the final dose was dissolved in 1 mL and administered by intraperitoneal (i.p.) injections.

RNA isolation and RT-qPCR

Lumbar dorsal root ganglia (DRG; L4-L5) were dissected from adult Sprague Dawley rats, frozen in liquid nitrogen, and maintained at −80°C until processed for RNA extraction. Total RNA was extracted from the samples using the RNeasy RNA extraction and purification kit (Qiagen). Single stranded cDNA was synthesized using reverse transcriptase (Bioline) with oligo-dT primers. Quantitative PCR was performed as previously described [28]. Briefly, resultant cDNA samples were amplified on an ABI PRISM 7900 HT Sequence Detection System (Applied Biosystems) using the reporter, SYBR Green. The PCR reaction was as follows: 1x, 50°C, 2 min; 1x, 95°C, 10 min; 45x, 95°C, 15 s, 60°C, 1 min; 1x, 25°C, hold. To check for DNA contamination, PCR was run using an L27 (ribosomal housekeeping gene) primer pair, whose PCR product crosses an intron. The mRNA level for each gene (x) relative to L27 mRNA (internal control) was calculated using the following equation where Ct refers to threshold cycles: mRNA (x%) = $2^{Ct(L27)-Ct(x)} \times 100$.

Nav 1.7 For GAGAGCGGAGAGATGGATTC

Nav 1.7 Rev GCTTCAGTGGTTGTGATG

Preparation of acutely dissociated dorsal root ganglion neurons

The L4–L6 DRGs were acutely dissociated using methods described by Ma and LaMotte [29]. Briefly, L4–L6 DRGs were removed from naive animals. The cells were then dissociated by mechanical trituration in culture media containing 1 mg/ml bovine serum albumin and trypsin inhibitor (Worthington Biochemical, Lakewood, NJ). The culture media was Ham's F-12 mixture, DMEM, supplemented with 10% fetal bovine serum, penicillin and streptomycin (100 µg/ml and 100 U/ml) and N2 (Life Technologies). The cells were then plated on coverslips coated with poly-L lysine and laminin (BD bioscience) and incubated for 2–3 h before more culture media was added to the wells. The cells were then allowed to sit undisturbed for 12–15 h to adhere at 37°C (with 5% CO2).

Intracellular calcium imaging

Acute dissociation of lumbar DRG and ratiometric Fura 2-AM based intracellular calcium imaging was performed between 20–26°C using methods previously described [27]. Sterile solution was applied to cells prior to LPS followed by M3G application, and any cells that responded to buffer alone were not used. Compounds were applied directly into the coverslip bathing solution as a static solution. LPS (1 µg/mL) was applied first, followed by M3G (3 µM), after which capsaicin (3 nM; Sigma-Aldrich) was added (at least 100 cells were assayed from three rodents). Additional experiments utilizing at least 50 cells reversed the order of LPS and M3G. Only calcium imaging traces that reflected at least a 50% increase over baseline were included in the analysis. At least three minutes were allowed to pass between ligand inductions in order to allow neurons to return to a manifested baseline of calcium flux, to maintain the integrity of the results. If the neuron was unable to return to a baseline level, it was omitted from the study. All data were analyzed by two independent analyzers and only responses that were in agreement between the two individuals were used in the responsive cell counts.

Electrophysiology

Sharp-electrode intracellular recordings were obtained from 4 to 18 hours after acute dissociation of lumbar DRG and current clamp protocols were performed using methods previously described [9,22]. A neuron was accepted for study only when it exhibited a resting membrane potential (RMP) more negative than −45 mV. For each neuron isolated for study, a continuous recording was obtained for 1 minute without the delivery of any external stimulus. Neuronal excitability of small and medium diameter dissociated DRG sensory neurons was measured by injecting 1-s current pulses into the soma every 30 s. Current was adjusted in order to elicit 1–2 action potentials per current injection under baseline conditions. Following control current injections, M3G (3 µM) was applied to the coverslip and current injections continued every 30 s. Neuronal excitability was measured as number of action potentials elicited per current pulse before and immediately after addition of M3G (15 and 45 s, respectively). If M3G increased neuronal excitability, CBZ (2 mM) or vehicle was added to the bath to determine if M3G-elicited neuronal excitation could be reversed.

Whole cell voltage-clamp recordings were made from small- and medium-diameter DRG neurons (25 µm<DRG diameter < 45 µm) using HEKA EPC10 amplifier (Germany). Electrodes were pulled from Warner Instruments thin walled borosilicate glass (Hamden, CT) with a Sutter P-97 electrode puller (Novato, CA) to produce 1–2 megaohm resistant pipets when filled with internal solutions. Recordings were performed in a reduced sodium solution to ensure fidelity of the voltage-clamp. External solution concentrations (in mM): 70 NaCl, 60 Choline-Cl, 30 TEA-Cl, 3 KCl, 1$CaCl_2$, 1 $MgCl_2$, 0.05 $CdCl_2$, 10 HEPES, 10 Glucose (pH 7.3) (310–320 mOsm/L). Internal solution concentrations (in mM): 140 CsCl, 5 $MgSO_4$, 10 EGTA, 4 ATP Na_2-ATP, 25 HEPES (pH 7.2) (290–310 mOsm/L). Whole cell capacitance and series resistance were compensated by the amplifier, and linear leak currents were digitally subtracted by P/4. Analysis was performed using HEKA FitMaster (Germany) and Origin 9.1 (Northhampton, MA).

Statistics

GraphPad Software (LaJolla, CA) was used to determine the statistical significance. Results were expressed as mean ± SEM. When only two groups were compared, Student t test was used. Multiple comparisons were evaluated by Tukey's multiple comparison tests after one-way ANOVA. $p<0.05$ was considered to be statistically significant.

Results

TLR4 agonist-induced intracellular calcium mobilization in dissociated sensory neurons

It is known that LPS can elicit excitation in sensory neurons in culture [9] and can contribute to the release of CGRP from capsaicin sensitive neurons [30]. Some reports suggest that this relatively fast neuronal activation may be dependent on both TLR4 and TRPV1 channels [8]. We therefore examined the effects of the known TLR4 agonists, LPS and M3G on $[Ca^{2+}]_i$ in cultured rat DRG neurons as a screen for the presence of functional receptors. Calcium mobilization was used in this instance strictly as an indication of TLR4 receptor activation and does not necessarily imply a role for this phenomenon in the other physiological effects of TLR4 agonists. The concentration of M3G and LPS used in this experiment was based on our previous observations of their effects on Ca mobilization in sensory neurons [9]. The application of vehicle at the beginning of experiment (i.e., 10 µl of 0.1% BSA/PBS in 1 ml of BSS) did not alter $[Ca^{2+}]_i$ (data not shown). Bath application of M3G followed by LPS exposure increased $[Ca^{2+}]_i$ in a large number of DRG neurons (**Fig 1** and **Table 1**). Many of these DRG neurons also responded to capsaicin (**Table 1**). These observations were maintained and

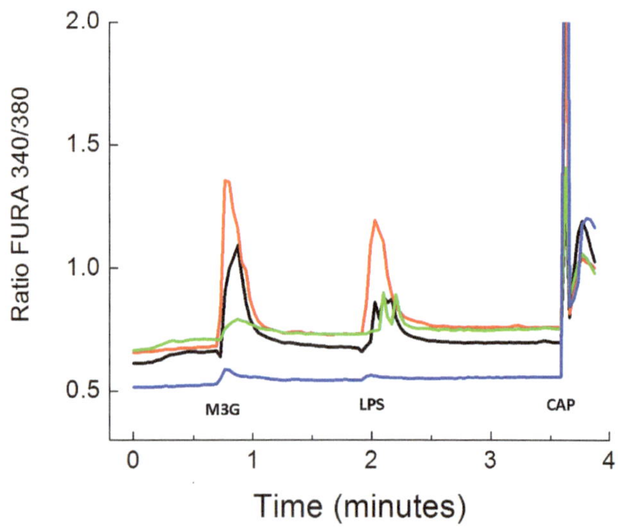

Figure 1. Description of calcium imaging. LPS-induced calcium flux in acutely dissociated small to medium diameter sensory neurons. Fura-2 loaded primary afferent neurons were stimulated with bath applications of morphine metabolite, morphine 3 glucuronide (M3G), the TLR4 agonist LPS, and capsaicin (CAP). [Ca2+]I levels were measured as ratio fluorscence of excitation at 340/380 nm over time. Four cells were assayed in this experiment and were represented by the blue, black green and red traces. The red and black traces clearly exhibited significant calcium flux after both M3G and LPS exposure while the green and blue traces exhibited only mild to moderate responses to these exogenous stimuli. All four traces exhibited robust calcium flux responses to capsaicin.

Table 1.

Total Number of cells: 122

Treatment	Cell Number	Percentage
LPS responsive cells	(45/122)	36.89%
LPS/Capsaicin-sensitive cells	(21/45)	46.67%
M3G responsive cells	(19/122)	15.57%
M3G/LPS responsive cells	(18/19)	94.73%
M3G/LPS + Capsaicin-sensitive cells	(7/18)	38.88%

supported regardless of whether the cells were first subjected to M3G followed by LPS, or vice versa.

Morphine-3-glucuronide-induced sensory neuron excitation *in vitro* is blocked by carbamazepine

Activation of TLR4-mediated neuronal excitation by M3G selectively elicits increased density in the voltage-gated sodium currents NaV1.6, NaV1.7 and NaV1.9 [9] and CBZ is known to produce a differential block of NaV1.7 [20]. To investigate the degree to which M3G-induced neuronal excitation is affected by exposure to CBZ, we subjected sensory neurons to bath-applied M3G, followed by administration of CBZ. Not unlike our previous published observations [9], repeated current pulse combined with M3G administration produced a significant increase in the excitability of small- to medium-diameter sensory neurons when compared to baseline levels. Less than 18% of total neurons responded to M3G administration. We also observed 1.53±0.2 APs in cells under control conditions compared to 5.75±0.5 APs in cells subjected to M3G (n = 28) (Fig. 2A). Subsequent treatment with CBZ completely blocked M3G-dependent excitability in all sensory neurons that responded to M3G (1.13±0.3 APs for CBZ, n = 10; ANOVA, interaction F = 45.35, $p<0.05$; Dunnett's multiple comparison test, $P<0.05$) (Fig. 2B).

Morphine-3-glucuronide-induced potentiation is dependent on voltage-gated sodium channels

Treatment with M3G potentiates currents in dorsal root ganglia cells [9]. CBZ has also been shown to inhibit voltage-gated sodium channel currents via hyperpolarizing shift in the voltage dependence of steady-state fast inactivation [20]. Here, we verify that the observed potentiation is dependent on voltage-gated sodium channels using whole-cell patch clamp technique and voltage step depolarizations from −80 mV to record isolated sodium currents and current densities from primary afferent sensory neurons (**Fig. 3A**). Sensory neurons were treated with an exposure to vehicle, 500 ug CBZ, 3 μM M3G, or a combination of both 3 μM M3G and 500 ug CBZ and current densities were compared between treatment groups (**Fig. 3B**; n = 24). CBZ treated cells measured 95.7±15.2 pA/pF, a ~70% decrease in current density (**Fig. 3C**). M3G treated cells measured 430.0±48.3 pA/pF compared to 283.0±38.8 pA/pF for vehicle treated cells, a ~50% increase in current density (**Fig. 3C**). Treatment with both M3G and CBZ measured 111.3±25.1 pA/pF, a ~60% decrease in current density (**Fig. 3C**). Potentiation and reduction of current density by all treatment groups was measured to be statistically significant by one-way ANOVA and Tukey's post-hoc test. Thus, the potentiation of voltage gated sodium current mediated by M3G was attenuated by treatment with CBZ. Treatment with CBZ produced a characteristic hyperpolarizing shift in the voltage dependence of steady-state fast inactivation, −82.9±3.6 mV compared to −50.3±1.5 mV in vehicle treated cells (**Fig. 3C**). Treatment with both M3G and CBZ prevented this shift (**Table 2**).

Effect of Morphine on TNI-induced tactile allodynia at post-injury day 7–28

Opioids such as morphine are the most effective broad spectrum analgesics available for moderate to severe pain acute pain

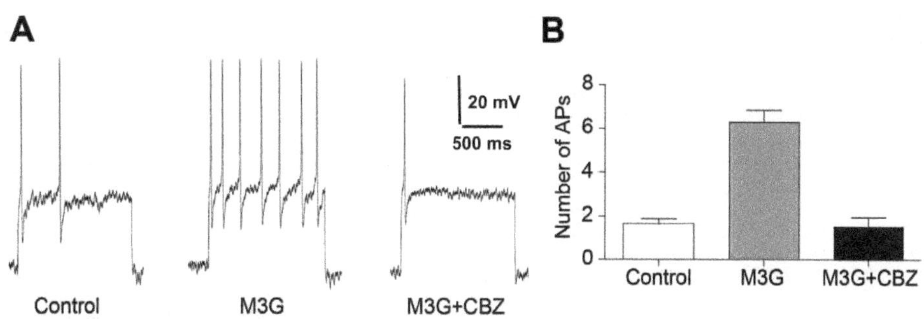

Figure 2. Morphine-3-glucuronide (M3G) increased excitability of nociceptive dorsal root ganglion neurons is reversed in the presence of carbamazepine (CBZ). (A) Current clamp recordings were performed on small (≥30 μm) to medium (≥40 μm) dorsal root ganglion (DRG) neurons (L1-6) from naïve rats. Firing of two to four action potentials (APs) was elicited by a 1 second depolarizing current injection (ranging from 0.1 to 0.6 nA depending on the cell) every 30 seconds. Representative recordings demonstrating that application of 3 μg/mL M3G increases the number of elicited APs. Bath applied CBZ reversed the effect of M3G-increased excitability. (B) Group data showing that M3G caused a significant increase in DRG AP firing that is reversed by CBZ (*$P<0.05$).

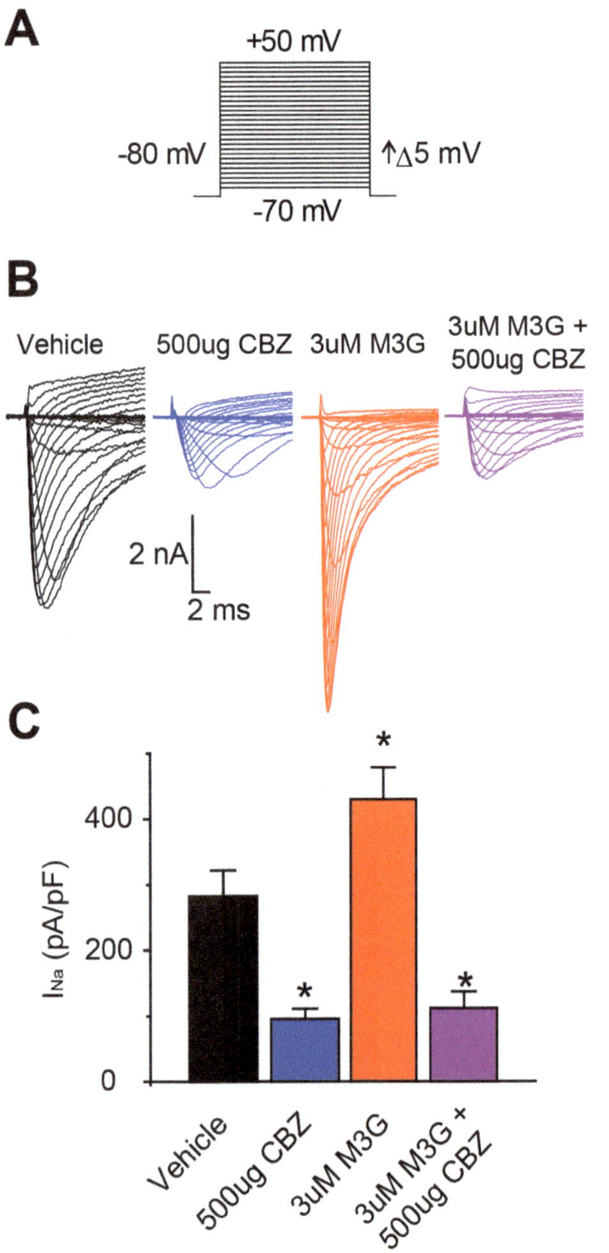

Figure 3. Morphine-3-glucuronide (M3G) potentiation of sodium currents is blocked by carbamazepine (CBZ). A, currents were elicited by performing voltage steps from a holding potential of −80 mV, in 5 mV increments, from −70 mV to +50 mV. B, representative traces from dorsal root ganglia cells treated with either 0.1% DMSO (Vehicle), 500 ug CBZ, 3 µM M3G, or both 3 µM M3G and 500 ug CBZ. C, peak currents (pA) were normalized to cell capacitance (pF) to measure current density (pA/pF). Asterisks indicate statistically significant differences between treatment groups and vehicle group (*P<0.05, one way ANOVA with Tukey's post-hoc test). Bars represent mean ± S.E.

conditions, however neuropathic pain tends to be less responsive to opioids. The ability of morphine to evoke pain relief diminishes over time and may be partially due to the ability of the opioid and the metabolite M3G to act through non-classic opioid receptors [31]. To identify the limits of morphine to reduce hypernociception following induction of a rodent neuropathic pain model, rats were subjected to a TNI procedure and tested at post-injury day 7 (PID7). All tested animals demonstrated signs of mechanical allodynia with ipsilateral threshold values of 28.7±2.5 mN compared with pre-surgery withdrawal threshold values of 72.1±5.0 mN (n = 64; p<0.001) (**Fig. 4A**). The injured animals continued to exhibit mechanical allodynia for as long as they were monitored. Body weight and general welfare (grooming/socialization) of the animals were routinely observed and appeared to be unaffected by the nerve injury.

The dose-response function for the morphine reversal of TNI pain at PID7 was determined using a within-subjects design. Rats were habituated and baseline testing conducted as described in the methods. Not unlike previous work by Erichsen and Blackburn-Monro [32], systemic administration of low dose morphine (0.5 or 1 mg/kg, i.p.) had no effect on withdrawal threshold up to 120 min post-injection for the ipsilateral hindlimb compared with either the pre-injection withdrawal threshold or with vehicle-treated animals at the corresponding time points. In contrast, i.p. injection of morphine at 5 mg/kg significantly increased withdrawal threshold of the ipsilateral hindlimb 30 min after injection to 73±1.6 mN ($F = 12.81$, $p<0.05$), compared with baseline and vehicle), and this effect continued up to 90 min, before returning to a level of sensitivity comparable with baseline and vehicle at 120 min (**Fig. 4A**).

To test the degree to which the 5 mg/kg (i.p.) concentration of morphine is effective for the reversal of TNI-induced tactile allodynia across time, independent groups of injured rats at PID 14 (n = 8), 21 (n = 8), and 28 (n = 8) were also assayed for mechanical allodynia following morphine administration. At a dosage of 5 mg/kg of morphine in the rodents, tactile allodynia was reversed in PID 14 animals. However, this dosage proved ineffective at PID 21 or 28, with no significant differences in pain behavior ($F = 48.14$, $p<0.05$, **Fig. 4B**).

Combination of morphine and carbamazepine reverses TNI-induced tactile allodynia at post-injury day 28 in a dose dependent manner

It is known that administration of M3G can induce tactile allodynia through a TLR4-mediated mechanism in the absence of nerve injury [9]. That neuronal exposure to M3G and the associated potentiation of NaV currents in vitro can be reversed by CBZ suggests a potential benefit of a combination pharmacotherapy approach using morphine and CBZ *in vivo* for TNI-induced tactile allodynia. To first determine whether CBZ alone is effective for TNI-induced tactile allodynia, we administered CBZ 10 mg/kg i.p. to TNI rodents at PID28 and compared the outcomes to similar injections of morphine 5 mg/kg i.p. at PID 28. Neither drug negated the injury-induced behavior ($F = 19.2$, $p<0.05$, **Fig. 5A**).

The potential impact of NaV1.7 in the injured peripheral nervous system may be pain syndrome specific as determined by NaV1.7 knockout mouse strains [33] and gain of NaV1.7 function appears to result in congenital insensitivity to pain or lead to severe familial pain disorders [34]. However diminishing the off-target effects of morphine directly or via its metabolite M3G may offer increased analgesic value for the widely used clinical opioid. As a proof-of-concept, morphine was combined with CBZ to produce a novel combination pharmacotherapy. In the 2-drug-combination studies, morphine plus CBZ completely attenuated mechanical allodynia at 5 mg/kg and 1 mg/kg concentration ($F = 19.2$, $p< 0.05$, **Fig. 5B**). Additional analysis revealed that there was increased efficacy with the combination pharmacotherapy of 5 mg/kg morphine and 10 mg/kg CBZ as PWTs following administration of both drugs did not return to pre-injury levels for

Table 2.

Condition	Activation		Fast Inactivation	
	V1/2	k	V1/2	k
Vehicle	−17.4±2.1 (n = 4)	6.7±0.7 (n = 4)	−50.3±1.5 (n = 4)	14.8±1.4 (n = 4)
500 ug CBZ	−12.4±1.7 (n = 5)	5.4±0.5 (n = 5)	−82.9±3.6 (n = 4)	17.7±2.7 (n = 4)
3 μM M3G	−17.0±2.1 (n = 5)	6.7±0.7 (n = 5)	−52.7±1.9 (n = 5)	18.5±2.3 (n = 5)
3 μM M3G + 500 ug CBZ	−21.4±0.4 (n = 3)	3.0±0.3 (n = 3)	−45.7±3.0 (n = 3)	11.1±2.1 (n = 3)

at least 240 minutes in the PID28 rodent group. Similar observations were present in age-matched male rodents subjected to TNI (data not shown; n = 6–8 per post injury time point).

Increased NaV1.7 expression following tibial nerve injury by post-injury day 28

Given the relative selectivity of CBZ for the NaV1.7 current state [20] and a recent report by Laedermann and colleagues which describes spared nerve injury-induced increases in NaV1.7 [35,36], we sought to determine the degree to which TNI changes in NaV1.7 correspond with morphine efficacy across time. Based on a quantitative real time PCR analysis, it appears that rodents subjected to TNI exhibited substantial increases in NaV1.7 mRNA by day 28 compared to naïve tissue levels, whereas post-injury day 14 values did not reach statistical significance (**Fig. 6**; n = 4, ANOVA, F = 5.571; $p<0.05$).

Discussion

It is known that opioids such as morphine and opioid metabolites induce glial-associated inflammatory responses within the brain and spinal cord via the non-classical opioid receptor, TLR4 [12]. Ligand activation of neuronal TLR4 has also been observed in the nervous system [8,10,37] and may play a direct role in the diminished efficacy of opioids in neuropathic pain conditions. The present set of multidisciplinary studies provide converging lines of evidence that TLR4-mediated increased neuronal excitation is likely dependent upon the CBZ-sensitive sodium current, and that the latent increase in NaV1.7 mRNA expression in sensory ganglia following TNI contributes to decreased opioid efficacy in a rodent model of neuropathic pain.

The use of opioids such as morphine to treat neuropathic pain is controversial due to the mixed results of clinical studies and is considered to be a second or third tier of treatment at best [38] [39]. Pre-clinical evidence indeed supports the observation that the analgesic effects of morphine are greatly diminished in the setting of neuropathic pain and quite often necessitates greater concentrations of morphine to provide pain relief. The mechanisms associated with these changes in opioid efficacy are often attributed to opioid tolerance. However, clear examples of the loss of morphine analgesia are evident in models of neuropathic pain such as spared nerve injury. Erichsen and Blackburn-Monro first demonstrated that this type of injury model required systemic doses of up to 6 mg/kg morphine for nociceptive pain relief at day 7 [32]. In contrast, doses of morphine as high as 10–30 mg/kg are necessary to provide relief for neuropathic pain at post-injury day 14 [40,41]. A comparison of the opioid dose needed to reverse mechanical allodynia in the present study appear to parallel these previous observations as the efficacy of the morphine dose that provided opioid analgesia up to day 14 was completely lacking at injury day 21 or 28. Together, these data readily indicate that the efficacy of morphine alone in attenuation of tactile allodynia is refractory over time following injury-induced changes in the neurobiology of the rodent.

Though the analgesic mechanism of opioids is largely thought to modulate transmission of pain sensation at the level of the spinal cord or by altering the perception of painful stimulus/stimulus-independent pain at cortical regions [42], it is conceivable that cell membrane bound receptors other than opioid receptors in either the spinal cord or the peripheral nervous system may contribute to the diminished efficacy of opioids in neuropathic pain conditions over time. For example, numerous lines of evidence suggest that the pathogenesis of neuropathic pain is dependent in part on abnormal spontaneous activity within sensory neurons [29,43,44]. As this spontaneous activity is likely dependent on NaVs for the generation and conduction of action potentials, it is conceivable that neuronal hyperexcitability after injury is dependent on injury-induced changes in specific isoforms of NaV channels including NaV1.7 [45]. Molecular mechanisms which may contribute to the latent changes in sodium channel expression include the ubiquitin protein ligase known as neuronal precursor cell expressed developmentally downregulated-4 type 2 or NEDD4-2 [35]. NEDD4-2 was recently identified as a posttranslational regulator of a number of different sodium channels including NaV1.7 [35]. Subsequently reduced levels of NEDD4-2 due to peripheral nerve injury may contribute to the development of both neuropathic pain disorders and diminished analgesic efficacy of opioids.

Expression of both Navl.7 and TLR4 may endow small nociceptive neurons with rapid repriming abilities that contribute to spontaneous discharge or hyperexcitability in the presence of opioids or opioid metabolites. To potentially control for the off-target effect of morphine or its metabolite M3G, we utilized CBZ in combination with morphine. CBZ is known to produce a substantial block of electrical activity associated with NaV current in sensory neurons and stably transfected human embryonic kidney 293 cells expressing wild-type NaV1.7 independent of resurgent currents [19,20]. Given the apparent effects of CBZ blockade of NaV current, it is reasonable to conclude that the combination of morphine with CBZ diminishes opioid-induced enhancement of electrical activity potentially associated with NaV1.7 in nociceptive sensory neurons while the central nervous system effects of morphine elicits analgesia sufficient to influence nociceptive behavior in the TNI model of neuropathic pain. However, evidence contained herein also suggests that responsive neurons elicit a range of current changes following exposure to M3G, all of which are greater that the averaged control value. This range of effects may be dependent on varying extents of expression of necessary pathway proteins in the heterogeneous system [9,46]. Although not tested in this study, it is unlikely that other anti-epileptic drugs such as gabapentin and pregabalin elicit

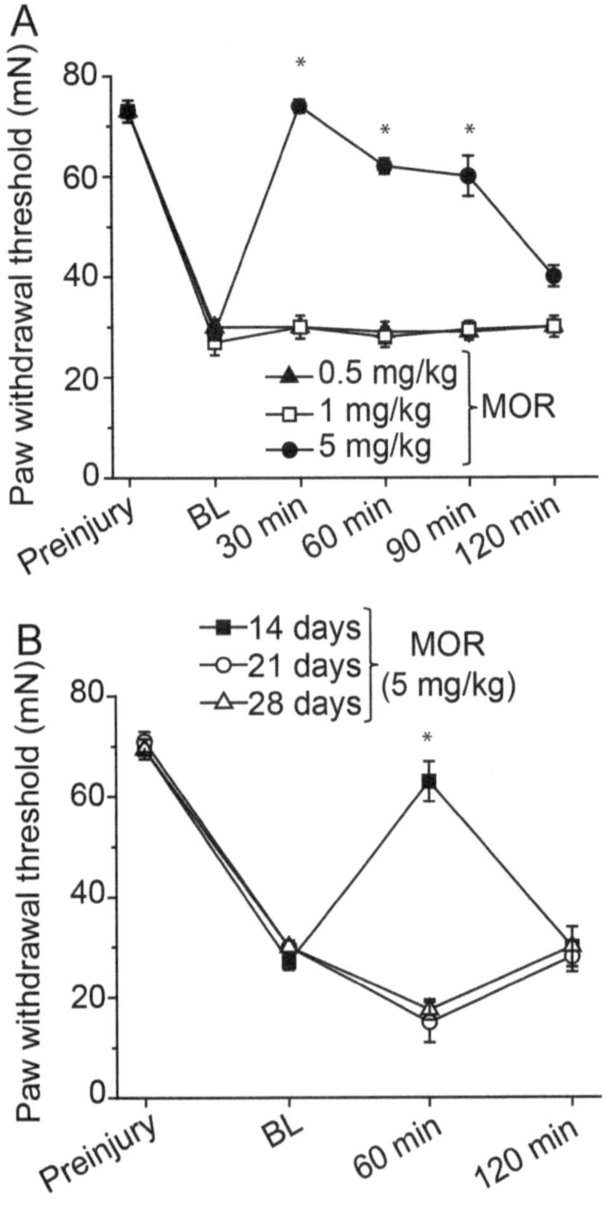

Figure 4. Dose- and time-effects of intraperitoneally administered morphine (MOR) on tactile allodynia in the tibial nerve injury (TNI) model at post-injury day 7. (A) The ability of MOR to attenuate tactile allodynia induced by TNI in a dose-dependent fashion was limited to 5 mg/kg. Each line represents the groups mean and SEM of 6–10 female rats. Drug group behavior at 30, 60, 90, or 120 minute vs TNI baseline (BL) behavior. (B) Time-dependent effects of intraperitoneally administered morphine (MOR) on tactile allodynia in the tibial nerve injury (TNI) model at post-injury day (PID) 14, 21 and 28. The ability of MOR to attenuate tactile allodynia induced by TNI was evident in PID 14 rats but not animals at PID21 or 28. Each line represents the groups mean and SEM of 6–10 rats. Drug group behavior at 60 minute or 120 minute vs TNI baseline (BL) behavior (*P<0.05).

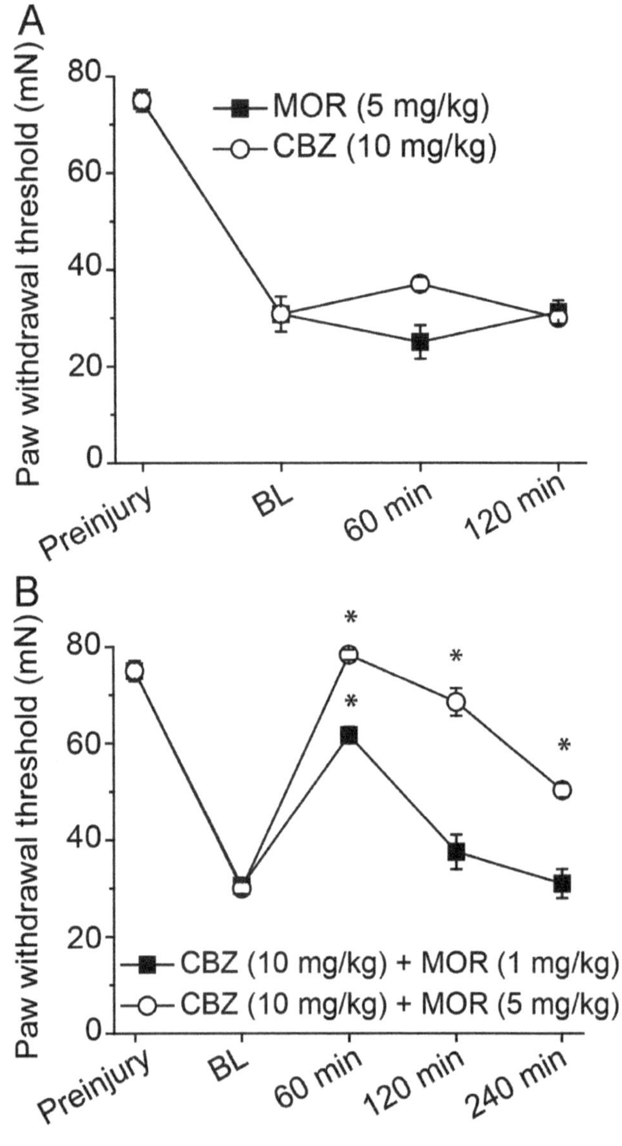

Figure 5. The effect of intraperitoneally administered morphine (MOR), carbamazepine (CBZ) or combination of MOR/CBZ on tactile allodynia in the tibial nerve injury (TNI) model at post-injury day (PID) 28. (A) Neither MOR or CBZ affect tactile allodynia induced by TNI. Each line represents the groups mean and SEM of 6–10 female rats. Drug group behavior at 60 minute or 120 minute vs TNI baseline (BL) behavior. (B) Effect of co-administered MOR and CBZ on tactile allodynia in the tibial nerve injury (TNI) model at post-injury day 28. The ability of MOR/CBZ to attenuate tactile allodynia induced by TNI was dose-dependent. Each line represents the groups mean and SEM of 6–10 rats. (*P<0.05; combination therapy group vs TNI baseline (BL) behavior).

similar effects as neither compound directly affects sodium current in a similar fashion [47].

The neuronal excitability mediated by opioids or their metabolites via TLR4 could also be influenced by signaling downstream of the receptor and may influence both capsaicin and non-capsaicin sensitive neurons. For example, it is possible that coordinated interactions between TLR4 ligands and sensory neurons could evoke TNFα-dependent tactile hypersensitivity and may be indicative of signaling dependent on the MyD88 signaling pathway [48]. Other proinflammatory cytokines which could conceivably be altered by the neuronal TLR4/MyD88 pathway including interleukin-1β [49] and deserves further investigation. However, the observed M3G-related neuronal signaling events are rapid and may be independent of signal transcription factors. Alternatively, the assembly of TLR adapter signaling proteins and activation of phospholipids in neurons may

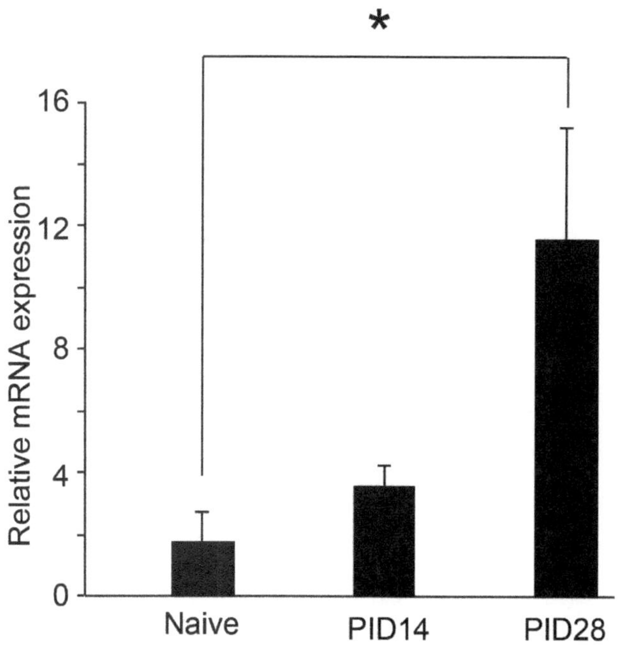

Figure 6. Tibal Nerve Injury (TNI) alters the expression of neuronal transcripts in rat dorsal root ganglion (DRG). RT-PCR analysis showing the mRNA expression profile of NaV1.7 in the DRG derived from naïve animal and at different time points following TNI; post injury day (PID) 14 and PID 28 (n = 3). RT-PCR data were analyzed using the Ct method and mRNA expression levels are expressed relative to L27- ribosomal housekeeping gene. (*$P<0.05$; TNI gene expression vs naive threshold baseline).

only require activation of a signal-transduction pathway leading to the observed increase in NaV current [50]. Additional studies are also underway to determine the degree to which hormonal regulation of neuronal TLR4 responses serve to influence neuropathic pain states alone or in combination with opioids [48,51].

The apparent lack of morphine efficacy *in vivo* may depend on the increased expression of NaV1.7 in the rat DRG following injury to the peripheral nerve. Given the negligible change of gene expression change up to PID14, morphine administration serves as an effective means by which to transiently reverse TNI-induced mechanical allodynia. However, the observed pronounced increase in NaV1.7 expression observed by PID28 in the rat supports the functional change in the inability of morphine to attenuate mechanical allodynia. The degree to which injury produces similar effects in murine spared nerve injury models is unknown and may vary from species to species [36].

It is likely that abnormal functioning of sodium channels in the peripheral nervous system is a key event in both the etiology of neuropathic pain [52] and opioid-induced hyperalgesia [9]. Subsequently, there are potential avenues for the use of morphine in combination with several FDA-approved partial seizure therapeutics currently known to affect the NaV1.7 current; lacosamide [20] or rufinamide [53] or possibly the anti-depressant duloxetine [54]. Oxcarbazepine, as a structural derivative of CBZ, may also affect NaV1.7 and serve as a suitable combinatorial therapeutic in combination with morphine for chronic pain (see Clinical Trials Registry No. NCT02078089). In contrast, anti-convulsive therapeutics that target focal seizure disorders by acting on voltage-sensitive calcium channels may not be able to diminish the off-target effects of opioids or provide enhanced opioid efficacy [55].

Together, the increased neuronal excitability via opioid-metabolite mediated neuronal TLR4 signaling increased NaV current in sensory neurons may serve as a robust signal to dampen the analgesic effects of morphine over time. However, here we show that the dampening of the analgesic effects of morphine on neuropathic pain behavior in vivo can be countered with the addition of CBZ. Thus, the same peripheral sensory neurons may possess opposing properties that elicit a critical interplay of mechanisms which may be central to the understanding of tolerance and paradoxical allodynia that can occur with opioid-based therapies.

Acknowledgments

We gratefully acknowledge Drs. Theodore Cummins and Zhiyong Tan for valuable discussion and critical reading of the manuscript. This work was supported by the NIH (DA026040 to FAW; DK100905 to FAW and RK); the National Scientist Development from the American Heart Association (SDG5280023 to RK); the Neurofibromatosis New Investigator Award from the DOD/CDMRP (NF1000099 to RK). Additional support for YMA as an Indiana CTSI Predoctoral trainee was provided by UL1 TR001107, NIH/NCATS (A. Shekhar, PI). The authors declare no conflicts of interest.

Author Contributions

Conceived and designed the experiments: MRD RK FAW. Performed the experiments: MRD XFY ALR MSR ETD YMA SMW. Analyzed the data: MRD YMA RK FAW. Contributed reagents/materials/analysis tools: YMA MRD RK FAW. Wrote the paper: MRD YMA RK FAW. Behavior/Physiology experiments: YMA MRD MSR XFY ETD SMW ALR.

References

1. Watson CP, Moulin D, Watt-Watson J, Gordon A, Eisenhoffer J (2003) Controlled-release oxycodone relieves neuropathic pain: a randomized controlled trial in painful diabetic neuropathy. Pain 105: 71–78.
2. Inturrisi CE, Lipman AG (2010) Opioid Analgesics; Fishman SM, Ballantyne JC, Rathmell JP, editors. Philadelphia: Lippincott Williams & Wilkins.
3. Angst MS, Clark JD (2006) Opioid-induced hyperalgesia: a qualitative systematic review. Anesthesiology 104: 570–587.
4. Ossipov MH, Lai J, King T, Vanderah TW, Malan TP Jr, et al. (2004) Antinociceptive and nociceptive actions of opioids. J Neurobiol 61: 126–148.
5. Vanderah TW, Suenaga NM, Ossipov MH, Malan TP Jr, Lai J, et al. (2001) Tonic descending facilitation from the rostral ventromedial medulla mediates opioid-induced abnormal pain and antinociceptive tolerance. J Neurosci 21: 279–286.
6. Drdla R, Gassner M, Gingl E, Sandkuhler J (2009) Induction of synaptic long-term potentiation after opioid withdrawal. Science 325: 207–210.
7. Heinl C, Drdla-Schutting R, Xanthos DN, Sandkuhler J (2011) Distinct mechanisms underlying pronociceptive effects of opioids. J Neurosci 31: 16748–16756.
8. Diogenes A, Ferraz CC, Akopian AN, Henry MA, Hargreaves KM (2011) LPS Sensitizes TRPV1 via Activation of TLR4 in Trigeminal Sensory Neurons. J Dent Res Jun; 90(6): 759–764.
9. Due MR, Piekarz AD, Wilson N, Feldman P, Ripsch MS, et al. (2012) Neuroexcitatory effects of morphine-3-glucuronide are dependent on Toll-like receptor 4 signaling. J Neuroinflammation 9: 200.
10. Maroso M, Balosso S, Ravizza T, Liu J, Aronica E, et al. (2010) Toll-like receptor 4 and high-mobility group box-1 are involved in ictogenesis and can be targeted to reduce seizures. Nat Med 16: 413–419.
11. Yaksh TL, Harty GJ, Onofrio BM (1986) High dose of spinal morphine produce a nonopiate receptor-mediated hyperesthesia: clinical and theoretic implications. Anesthesiology 64: 590–597.

12. Wang X, Loram LC, Ramos K, de Jesus AJ, Thomas J, et al. (2012) Morphine activates neuroinflammation in a manner parallel to endotoxin. Proc Natl Acad Sci U S A 109: 6325–6330.
13. Alfonso-Loeches S, Pascual-Lucas M, Blanco AM, Sanchez-Vera I, Guerri C (2010) Pivotal role of TLR4 receptors in alcohol-induced neuroinflammation and brain damage. J Neurosci 30: 8285–8295.
14. Lewis SS, Hutchinson MR, Zhang Y, Hund DK, Maier SF, et al. (2013) Glucuronic acid and the ethanol metabolite ethyl-glucuronide cause toll-like receptor 4 activation and enhanced pain. Brain Behav Immun 30: 24–32.
15. Hutchinson MR, Zhang Y, Shridhar M, Evans JH, Buchanan MM, et al. (2010) Evidence that opioids may have toll-like receptor 4 and MD-2 effects. Brain Behav Immun 24: 83–95.
16. Eidson LN, Murphy AZ (2013) Blockade of Toll-like receptor 4 attenuates morphine tolerance and facilitates the pain relieving properties of morphine. J Neurosci 33: 15952–15963.
17. Fischer TZ, Gilmore ES, Estacion M, Eastman E, Taylor S, et al. (2009) A novel Nav1.7 mutation producing carbamazepine-responsive erythromelalgia. Ann Neurol 65: 733–741.
18. Jo S, Bean BP (2014) Sidedness of carbamazepine accessibility to voltage-gated sodium channels. Mol Pharmacol 85: 381–387.
19. Theile JW, Cummins TR (2011) Inhibition of Navbeta4 peptide-mediated resurgent sodium currents in Nav1.7 channels by carbamazepine, riluzole, and anandamide. Mol Pharmacol 80: 724–734.
20. Sheets PL, Heers C, Stoehr T, Cummins TR (2008) Differential block of sensory neuronal voltage-gated sodium channels by lacosamide [(2R)-2-(acetylamino)-N-benzyl-3-methoxypropanamide], lidocaine, and carbamazepine. J Pharmacol Exp Ther 326: 89–99.
21. Black JA, Liu S, Waxman SG (2009) Sodium channel activity modulates multiple functions in microglia. Glia 57: 1072–1081.
22. Feldman P, Due MR, Ripsch MS, Khanna R, White FA (2012) The persistent release of HMGB1 contributes to tactile hyperalgesia in a rodent model of neuropathic pain. J Neuroinflammation 9: 180.
23. Wang Y, Wilson SM, Brittain JM, Ripsch MS, Salome C, et al. (2011) Merging Structural Motifs of Functionalized Amino Acids and alpha-Aminoamides Results in Novel Anticonvulsant Compounds with Significant Effects on Slow and Fast Inactivation of Voltage-gated Sodium Channels and in the Treatment of Neuropathic Pain. ACS Chem Neurosci 2: 317–322.
24. Lee BH, Won R, Baik EJ, Lee SH, Moon CH (2000) An animal model of neuropathic pain employing injury to the sciatic nerve branches. Neuroreport 11: 657–661.
25. Ju W, Li Q, Allette YM, Ripsch MS, White FA, et al. (2012) Suppression of pain-related behavior in two distinct rodent models of peripheral neuropathy by a homopolyarginine-conjugated CRMP2 peptide. J Neurochem Oct 26. doi: 10.1111/jnc.12070. [Epub ahead of print].
26. Ma C, Shu Y, Zheng Z, Chen Y, Yao H, et al. (2003) Similar Electrophysiological Changes in Axotomized and Neighboring Intact Dorsal Root Ganglion Neurons. J Neurophysiol 89: 1588–1602.
27. Bhangoo S, Ren D, Miller RJ, Henry KJ, Lineswala J, et al. (2007) Delayed functional expression of neuronal chemokine receptors following focal nerve demyelination in the rat: a mechanism for the development of chronic sensitization of peripheral nociceptors. Mol Pain 3: 38.
28. Brittain JM, Duarte DB, Wilson SM, Zhu W, Ballard C, et al. (2011) Suppression of inflammatory and neuropathic pain by uncoupling CRMP-2 from the presynaptic Ca(2)(+) channel complex. Nat Med 17: 822–829.
29. Ma C, LaMotte RH (2005) Enhanced excitability of dissociated primary sensory neurons after chronic compression of the dorsal root ganglion in the rat. Pain 113: 106–112.
30. Hou L, Wang X (2001) PKC and PKA, but not PKG mediate LPS-induced CGRP release and [Ca(2+)](i) elevation in DRG neurons of neonatal rats. J Neurosci Res 66: 592–600.
31. Hutchinson MR, Shavit Y, Grace PM, Rice KC, Maier SF, et al. (2011) Exploring the neuroimmunopharmacology of opioids: an integrative review of mechanisms of central immune signaling and their implications for opioid analgesia. Pharmacol Rev 63: 772–810.
32. Erichsen HK, Blackburn-Munro G (2002) Pharmacological characterisation of the spared nerve injury model of neuropathic pain. Pain 98: 151–161.
33. Minett MS, Falk S, Santana-Varela S, Bogdanov YD, Nassar MA, et al. (2014) Pain without nociceptors? Nav1.7-independent pain mechanisms. Cell Rep 6: 301–312.
34. Raouf R, Rugiero F, Kiesewetter H, Hatch R, Hummler E, et al. (2012) Sodium channels and mammalian sensory mechanotransduction. Mol Pain 8: 21.
35. Laedermann CJ, Cachemaille M, Kirschmann G, Pertin M, Gosselin RD, et al. (2013) Dysregulation of voltage-gated sodium channels by ubiquitin ligase NEDD4-2 in neuropathic pain. J Clin Invest 123: 3002–3013.
36. Laedermann CJ, Pertin M, Suter MR, Decosterd I (2014) Voltage-gated sodium channel expression in mouse DRG after SNI leads to re-evaluation of projections of injured fibers. Mol Pain 10: 19.
37. Ochoa-Cortes F, Ramos-Lomas T, Miranda-Morales M, Spreadbury I, Ibeakanma C, et al. (2010) Bacterial cell products signal to mouse colonic nociceptive dorsal root ganglia neurons. Am J Physiol Gastrointest Liver Physiol 299: G723–732.
38. O'Connor AB, Dworkin RH (2009) Treatment of neuropathic pain: an overview of recent guidelines. Am J Med 122: S22–32.
39. Eisenberg E, McNicol ED, Carr DB (2005) Efficacy and safety of opioid agonists in the treatment of neuropathic pain of nonmalignant origin: systematic review and meta-analysis of randomized controlled trials. JAMA 293: 3043–3052.
40. Miyazaki R, Yamamoto T (2012) The efficacy of morphine, pregabalin, gabapentin, and duloxetine on mechanical allodynia is different from that on neuroma pain in the rat neuropathic pain model. Anesth Analg 115: 182–188.
41. Decosterd I, Allchorne A, Woolf CJ (2004) Differential analgesic sensitivity of two distinct neuropathic pain models. Anesth Analg 99: 457–463.
42. Ossipov MH, Lai J, King T, Vanderah TW, Porreca F (2005) Underlying mechanisms of pronociceptive consequences of prolonged morphine exposure. Biopolymers 80: 319–324.
43. Devor M (2006) Sodium channels and mechanisms of neuropathic pain. J Pain 7: S3–S12.
44. Ma C, LaMotte RH (2007) Multiple sites for generation of ectopic spontaneous activity in neurons of the chronically compressed dorsal root ganglion. J Neurosci 27: 14059–14068.
45. Dib-Hajj SD, Yang Y, Black JA, Waxman SG (2013) The Na(V)1.7 sodium channel: from molecule to man. Nat Rev Neurosci 14: 49–62.
46. Allette YM, Due MR, Wilson SM, Feldman P, Ripsch MS, et al. (2014) Identification of a functional interaction of HMGB1 with Receptor for Advanced Glycation End-products in a model of neuropathic pain. Brain Behav Immun. 10.1016/j.bbi.2014.06.199.
47. Zhang JL, Yang JP, Zhang JR, Li RQ, Wang J, et al. (2013) Gabapentin reduces allodynia and hyperalgesia in painful diabetic neuropathy rats by decreasing expression level of Nav1.7 and p-ERK1/2 in DRG neurons. Brain Res 1493: 13–18.
48. Stokes JA, Cheung J, Eddinger K, Corr M, Yaksh TL (2013) Toll-like receptor signaling adapter proteins govern spread of neuropathic pain and recovery following nerve injury in male mice. J Neuroinflammation 10: 148.
49. Tse KH, Chow KB, Leung WK, Wong YH, Wise H (2014) Lipopolysaccharide differentially modulates expression of cytokines and cyclooxygenases in dorsal root ganglion cells via Toll-like receptor-4 dependent pathways. Neuroscience 267: 241–251.
50. Kagan JC, Medzhitov R (2006) Phosphoinositide-mediated adaptor recruitment controls Toll-like receptor signaling. Cell 125: 943–955.
51. Sorge RE, LaCroix-Fralish ML, Tuttle AH, Sotocinal SG, Austin JS, et al. (2011) Spinal cord Toll-like receptor 4 mediates inflammatory and neuropathic hypersensitivity in male but not female mice. J Neurosci 31: 15450–15454.
52. Waxman SG, Zamponi GW (2014) Regulating excitability of peripheral afferents: emerging ion channel targets. Nat Neurosci 17: 153–163.
53. Suter MR, Kirschmann G, Laedermann CJ, Abriel H, Decosterd I (2013) Rufinamide attenuates mechanical allodynia in a model of neuropathic pain in the mouse and stabilizes voltage-gated sodium channel inactivated state. Anesthesiology 118: 160–172.
54. Wang SY, Calderon J, Kuo Wang G (2010) Block of neuronal Na+ channels by antidepressant duloxetine in a state-dependent manner. Anesthesiology 113: 655–665.
55. Gilron I, Bailey JM, Tu D, Holden RR, Weaver DF, et al. (2005) Morphine, gabapentin, or their combination for neuropathic pain. N Engl J Med 352: 1324–1334.

7

Prevention Effect of Allopurinol on Post-Endoscopic Retrograde Cholangiopancreatography Pancreatitis

Wei-Li Cao[1,2]☙, Wen-Shan Yan[1,3]☙, Xiao-Hui Xiang[2], Kai Chen[2], Shi-Hai Xia[1,2]*

1 Postgraduate Training Base, Affiliated Hospital of Logistics University of the Chinese People's Armed Police Forces, Liaoning Medical University, Jinzhou, China, **2** Department of Hepatopancreatobiliary and Splenic Medicine, Affiliated Hospital of Logistics University of the Chinese People's Armed Police Forces, Tianjin, China, **3** Department of Endemic Area of Orthopedic Center Section III, Affiliated Hospital of Logistics University of the Chinese People's Armed Police Forces, Tianjin, China

Abstract

Background: Pancreatitis is the most common complication of endoscopic retrograde cholangiopancreatography (ERCP) which can be severe and cause death in approximately 10% of cases. Up to now, six randomized controlled trials (RCTs) have been found relevant to the effect of allopurinol on prevention of Post-ERCP pancreatitis (PEP). However, these results remained controversial.

Objective: To conduct a meta-analysis with RCTs published in full text to determine the effectiveness of prophylactic allopurinol of different dosages and administration time in the incidence and severity of PEP.

Methods: Literature search was performed in PubMed, Embase, Web of Science and Cochrane Library from databases inception to May 2014. RCTs comparing the effect of allopurinol with placebo on prevention of PEP were included. Statistical heterogeneity was quantitatively evaluated byχ^2 test with the significance set $P<0.10$ or $I^2>50\%$.

Results: Six RCTs consisting of 1974 participants were eventually included. The incidences of PEP in allopurinol group and placebo group were 8.4%(83/986) and 9.9%(98/988) respectively. Meta-analysis showed no evident prevention effect of allopurinol on the incidence of PEP (RR 0.75, 95%CI 0.39–1.42) with significant heterogeneity ($I^2=70.4\%$, $P=0.005$). When studies were stratified according to the dosages and administration time of allopurinol they applied, there was still no evident prevention effect of allopurinol on mild, moderate or severe PEP. However, statistically substantial heterogeneity was presented in the subgroup of moderate PEP when the effect of high dose of allopurinol was analyzed ($I_{moderate}^2=82.3\%$, $P_{moderate}=0.018$). Statistically significant heterogeneity was also observed in subgroup of mild PEP, when the effect of long adminstration time of allopurinol was investigated ($I_{mild}^2=62.8\%$, $P_{mild}=0.068$).

Conclusion: The prophylactic use of allopurinol in different dosages and administration time had no effect in preventing incidence and severity of PEP.

Editor: Juan Sastre, University of Valencia, Spain

Funding: The authors have no support or funding to report.

Competing Interests: The authors have declared that no competing interests exist.

* Email: xiash2014@sina.com

☙ These authors contributed equally to this work.

Introduction

Pancreatitis is the most common complication of endoscopic retrograde cholangiopancreatography (ERCP) with incidence being 3.5% in nonselected patients which presents as mild or moderate severity in roughly 90% of patients. However, it is severe and can cause death in approximately 10% of cases [1].

The mechanism of post-ERCP pancreatitis (PEP) remains unclear. Several studies show that free radicals play a great role in the pathogenesis of PEP. Oxygen radicals can lead to capillary endothelial injury, inducing the occurrence of acute pancreatitis [2,3,4,5]. Some free-radical scavengers (superoxide dismutase, catalase), protease inhibitors, and xanthine oxidase inhibitor have been investigated to prevent the frequency of PEP [2,4,6,7]. Allopurinol, a structural analog of the natural purine base hypoxanthine, is capable of inhibiting xanthine oxidase which can catalyze the transformation of hypoxanthine to xanthine and result in the production of oxygen-derived free radical [8]. So allopurinol may play a part in the prevention of PEP through the reduction of oxygen-derived free radical. Many studies in animal

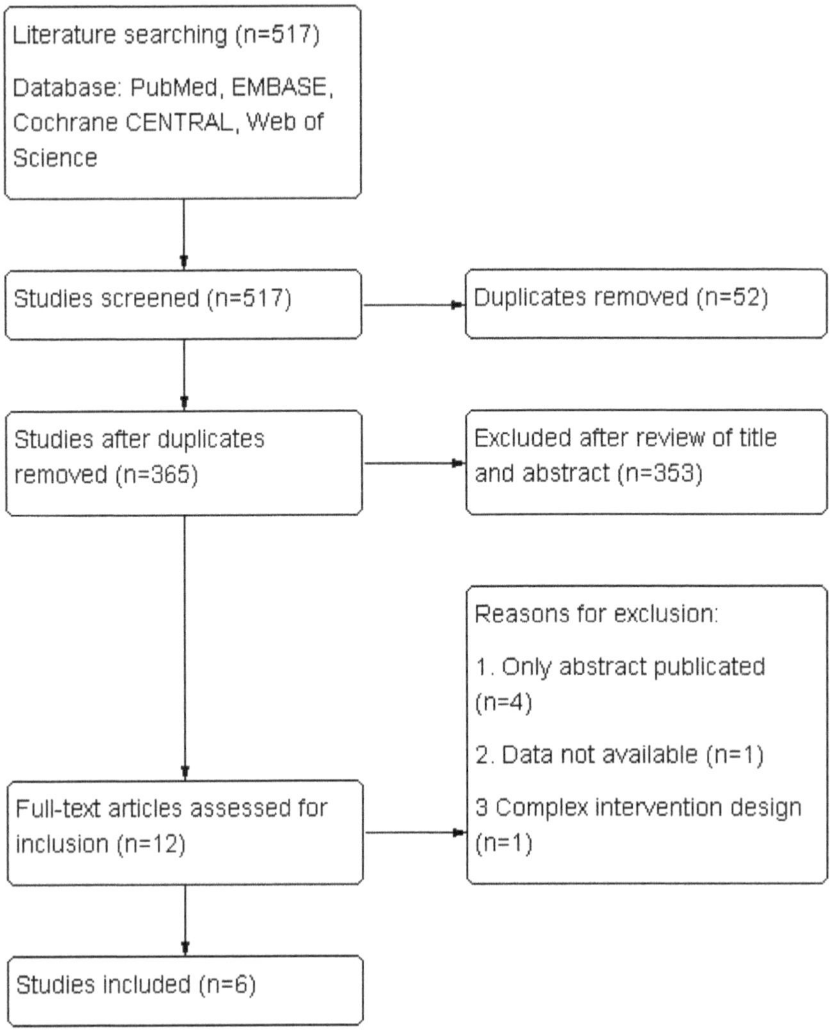

Figure 1. Flow chart of literature selection.

models have indicated that the degree of pancreatic inflammation and serum hyperamylasemia was decreased after pretreatment with allopurinol in pancreatography-induced pancreatitis [2,9].

In clinical trials, six randomized controlled trials (RCTs) have been published in full text about the effect of allopurinol on the prevention of PEP up to now [10,11,12,13,14,15]. These results remained controversial. Four prospective studies [10,11,13,15] have yielded negative results while another two studies [12,14] demonstrated that allopurinol could result in the alleviation of PEP. Katsinelos et al. [12] have indicated that the frequency of PEP was decreased after pretreatment with high-dose of allopurinol. Martinez-Torres et al. [14] have presented the result that the incidences of pancreatitis and hyperamylasemia were decreased after pretreated with allopurinol in patients under high-risk procedures. Two meta-analyses [16,17] published in 2008 displayed the same results that allopurinol was ineffective for the reduction of PEP. However, a few limits could be observed in previous meta-analyses such as lack of updated RCTs published within recent six years, less studies included and no stratification in terms of allopurinol dosage or adminstration time. Consequently, it is necessary to make a more comprehensive and latest meta-analysis which consists of all RCTs to estimate the effect of allopurinol on the PEP reduction.

The aim of this study is to determine the effectiveness of prophylactic allopurinol of different dosages and adminstration time in the incidence and severity of PEP in RCTs.

Materials and Methods

Literature and search strategy

Two reviewers cooperatively searched the following electronic databases: PubMed, Embase, Web of Science and Cochrane Library from databases inception to May 2014. The following related items were searched: allopurinol, placebo, post-endoscopic retrograde cholangiopancreatography pancreatitis, post-ERCP pancreatitis, PEP, randomized controlled trials. Searching strategy was constructed by combining the above items with "AND" or "OR". No restriction was applied to language. We had also screened reference lists of retrieved articles.

Study selection criteria

Two reviewers independently assessed the retrieved citations to determine whether they met the inclusion criteria. All disagreements were resolved by discussion with a third reviewer. To be included, the following criteria should be met: 1) patients were scheduled to undergo diagnostic or therapeutic ERCP; 2) random

Table 1. Characteristics of the included studies.

Reference	Country	Study design	No. patients	Patient inclusion creteria	Patient exclusion creteria	Allopurinol usage and dosage	Outcomes
Abbasinazari 2011	Iran	RCT	29/45	Patients who were to undergo diagnositic or therapeutic ERCP	1) any type of renal failure, 2) any type of anemia, 3) acute pancreatitis during 2 weeks before ERCP, 4) age lower than 20, 5) pregnancy, 6) patients under treatment with azathioprin, 7) refusal or inability to give informed consent.	300 mg at 3 h and 300 mg just before doing ERCP	Amylase concentration; abdominal pain; incidence of PEP
Martinez-Torres 2009	Mexico	RCT	85/85	Patients who were to undergo diagnositic or therapeutic ERCP	1) current pancreatitis or hyperamylasemia 2) non-steroidal anti-inflammatory drugs (NSAIDS) 3) failed ERCP in 12 months 4) previous endoscopic or surgical sphincterotomy 5)use of anticoagulants or platelet anti-aggregants 6) allergic to allopurinol 7) hemoglobin <8 g/dL, platelet count< 60 $\times 10^9$/L. 8) neutropenia; renal dysfunction; decompensated cirrhosis;9) known or suspected pregnancy or lactation;10) current or recent use of allopurinol or drugs with an interaction with allopurinol, 11) inability to swallow or absorb oral medication	300 mg at 15 h and 300 mg at 3 h before ERCP	Incidence of hyperamylasemia and PEP; ERCP morbidity
Romagnuolo 2008	Canada	RCT	293/293	Patients who were to undergo diagnositic or therapeutic ERCP	1) Haemoglobin level <8 g/dL; 2) platelet count of <60×10^9/ L; 3) relative neutropenia; significant renal dysfunction; decompensated cirrhosis; 4) allergic to allopurinol; 5) a known or suspected pregnancy or lactation; 6)current or recent use of allopurinol or drugs with a known interaction with allopurinol; 7) an inability to swallow or absorb oral medication; 8)recent acute pancreatitis	300 mg at 1 h before ERCP	proportion of PEP; proportion of patients with local complications of or the need for surgery
Katsinelos 2005	Greece	RCT	125/118	Patients who were to undergo diagnositic or therapeutic ERCP	1) acute pancreatitis ;2) age less than 18 years;3) history of allergy to allopurinol, 4) acute myocardial infarction with in 3 months before ERCP, 5) other severe systemic disease, 6) pregnancy or lactation, 7) refusal to participate.	600 mg at 15 h and 3 h before ERCP	Postprocedur e complica tions; incidence of PEP
Mosler 2005	United States	RCT	355/346	Patients who were to undergo diagnositic or therapeutic ERCP	1) less than 18 years; 2) intrauterine pregnancy; 3) mental disability; 4) incarceration in prison ; 5) active pancreatitis before the procedure; 6) allergy to allopurinol ; 7) actual treatment with allopurinol; 8) contrast allergy; 9) use of mercaptopurine, cyclosporine, chlorpromazine, dicumarol, azathioprine, ampicillin, amoxicillin, or thiazide diuretics; 10) impaired renal function 11) nursing mothers. 12)unable to undergo randomization within 4 hours of the procedure	600 mg at 4 h and 300 mg at 1 h before ERCP	Incidence of PEP
Budzynska 2001	Poland	RCT	99/101	Patients who were to undergo diagnositic or therapeutic ERCP	1) active acute pancreatitis,2) age under 18,3) severe systematic disease, 4) pregnancy or breast feeding, 5) contraindications to corticosteroid administration	200 mg at 15 h and 3 h before ERCP	Incidence of PEP; complications

Table 2. Number of patients in different stages.

Author	Patients in allopurinol group	PEP in allopurinol group	PEP classified by severity			Patients in placebo group	PEP in placebo group	PEP classified by severity		
			Mild	Moderate	Severe			Mild	Moderate	Severe
Abbasinazari 2011	29	3	2	1	0	45	5	3	2	0
Martinez-Torres 2009	85	2	2	0	0	85	8	8	0	0
Romagnuolo 2008	293	16	8	6	2	293	12	4	6	2
Katsinelos 2005	125	4	4	0	0	118	21	8	11	2
Mosler 2005	355	46	28	16	2	346	42	24	16	2
Budzynska 2001	99	12	9	2	1	101	8	5	3	0

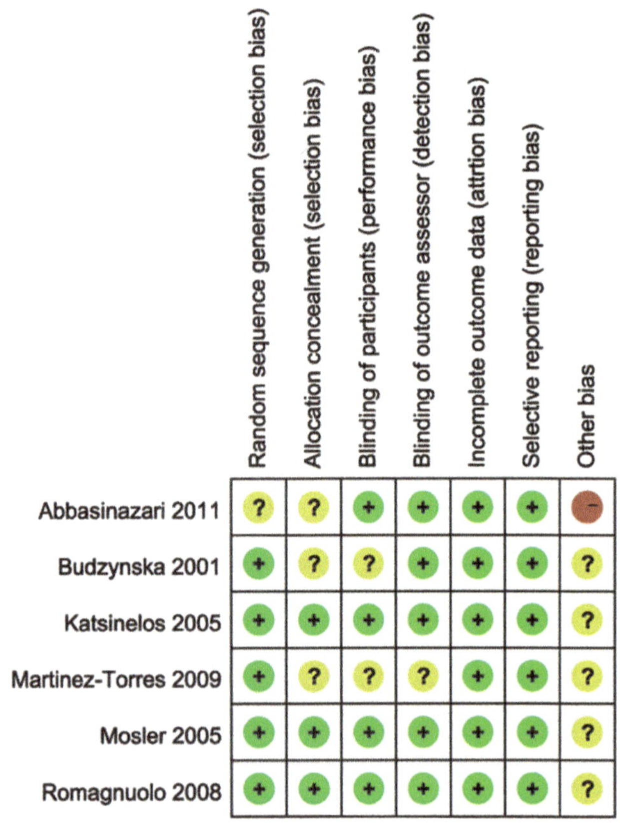

Figure 2. Risk of bias summary.

allocation of treatment; 3) the use of allopurinol in intervention group and placebo in control group. Exclusion criteria were: 1) Quasi-randomized clinical trials, retrospective studies, cohort studies and case-control studies; 2) other intervention instead of allopurinol 3) patients with the following characteristics: (i) current pancreatitis, hyperamylasemia, neutropenia, renal dysfunction, decompensated cirrhosis, pregnancy or lactation; (ii) use of anticoagulants, non-steroidal anti-inflammatory drugs (NSAIDS), platelet anti-aggregants or drugs with an interaction with allopurinol; (iii) allergic to allopurinol; (iv) platelet count$< 60 \times 10^9/L$; (v) unable to swallow or absorb oral medication; (vi) previous sphincterotomy.

Data extraction and quality assessment

Two reviewers independently conducted data extraction and study quality assessment. All discrepancies encountered were settled eventually by discussion until consensuses were reached. Data that extracted from the included studies consisted of study location, study design, number of patients in each group, inclusion and exclusion criteria of participants, intervention type, dosage of allopurinol used, administration time of allpurinol and PEP patients in different severity degrees. Quality of study was evaluated in six domains comprising sequence generation, allocation concealment, participants' blinding, assessors' blinding, incomplete data, selective reporting and other bias. Each study could be classified as unclear, low risk or high risk of bias for each domain on the ground of Cochrane Handbook 5.1.0 [18].

Statistical analysis

Statistical analyses were performed with the use of procedure STATA 12.0. Effect was presented by RR with 95%CI for

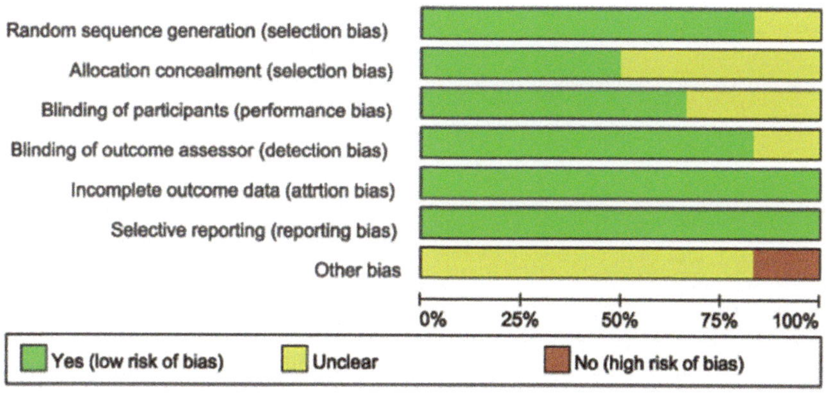

Figure 3. Risk of bias graph.

dichotomous variables. Statistical heterogeneity was quantitatively evaluated by χ^2 test with the significance set $P<0.10$ or $I^2>50\%$. Random effect model was used to analyze outcomes which presented significant heterogeneity among studies while fixed effect model to analyze those with non-significant heterogeneity. Publication bias was detected by funnel plot and Egger's test ($P<0.05$ indicated a significant publication bias).

Results

Literature search

The selection process of study was displayed in Fig. 1. Totally, 517 citations were searched online. After removing the duplicate, title and abstract screening and full text review, 6 RCTs were eventually met the inclusion criteria. No satisfied study was identified by examining the references of the six RCTs. Of all the participants from six RCTs, 986 were treated with allopurinol and

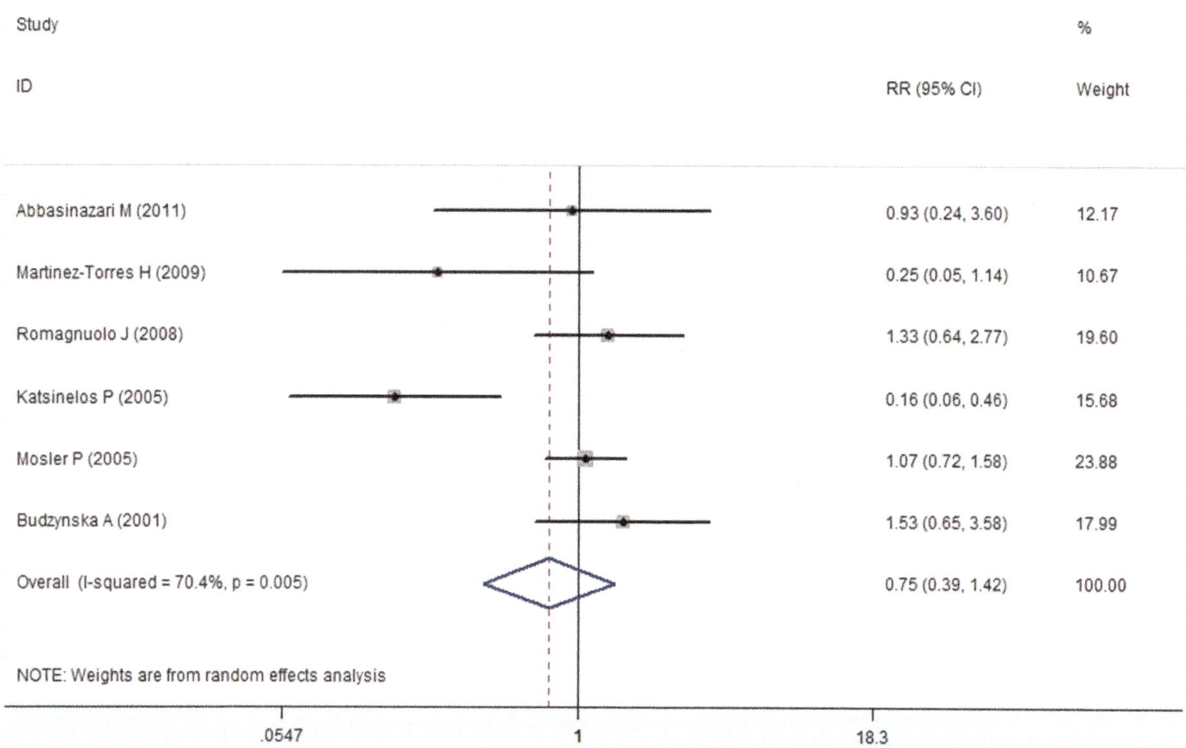

Figure 4. Prevention effect of allopurinol on PEP.

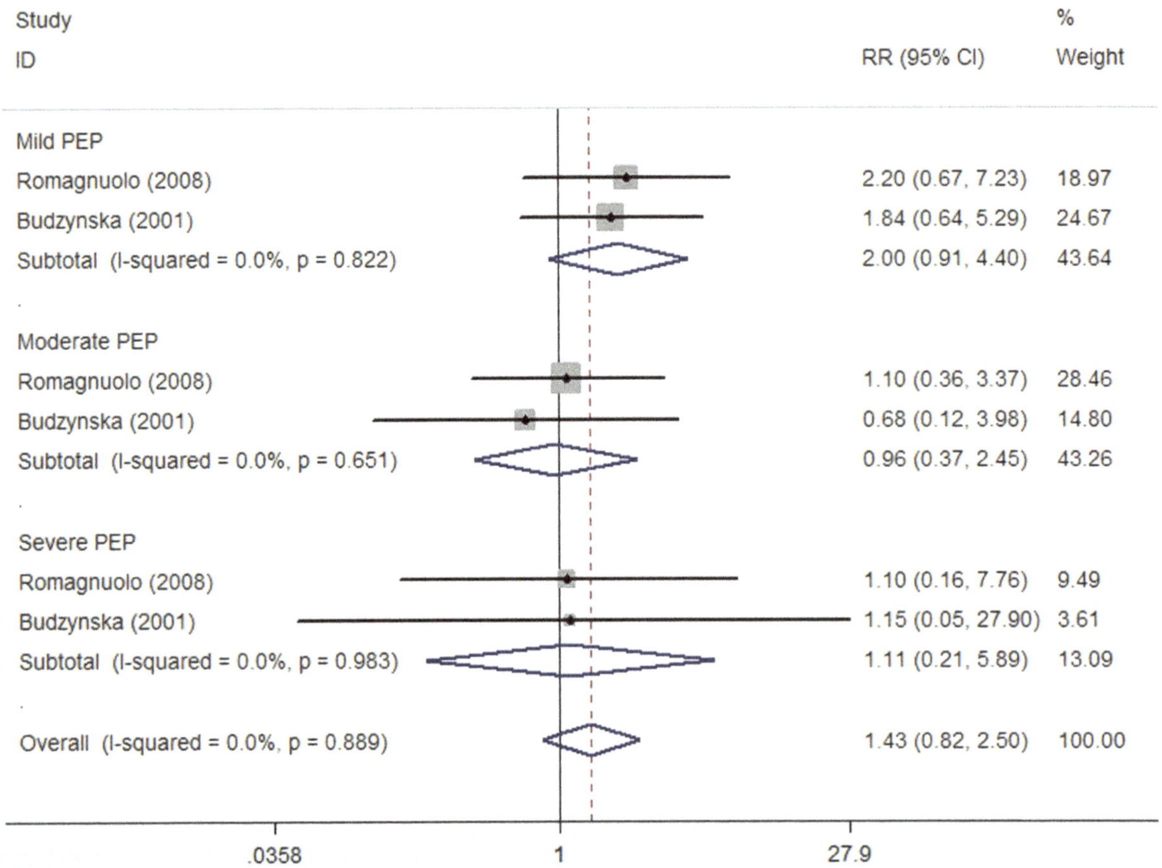

Figure 5. Prevention effect of low dose of allopurinol on PEP in different severity degrees.

988 with placebo. The characteristics of studies and numbers of patients in different stages were presented in Table 1 and Table 2.

Quality of the included studies

Among the six included trials [10,11,12,13,14,15], sequence generation which means a low risk of bias was clearly conducted and introduced in five studies [10,11,12,13,14]. Only one study [15] didn't describe the exact method of randomization in spite of simple description in title. Allocation concealment was done and described in three studies [11,12,13] with means like a blinded fashion by pharmacy staff, concealed envelopes and coded packets. The remaining three studies [10,14,15] shared no information about this domain. With regarding to participants' blinding, four trials [11,12,13,15] presented a low risk for they had illustrated and performed the blinding concretely, whereas in the remaining two trials [10,14], it remained unclear. In terms of outcome assessors' blinding, five studies [10,11,12,13,15] shared low risk and only one study [14] presented unclear for this domain. After carefully examining, all the six studies [10,11,12,13,14,15] shared low risk of bias regarding to incomplete outcome data. Similarly, all studies reported outcomes they planed previously, suggesting a low risk of bias. No other apparent bias was found among the included studies. Fig. 2 and Fig. 3 show the risk of bias summary.

Meta-analysis of allopurinol in prevention of developing PEP

Totally, six RCTs including 1974 participants were included in this meta-analysis. The PEP rates in allopurinol group and placebo group were 8.4% (83/986) and 9.9% (98/988) respectively. Pooled analysis showed no evident prevention effect of allopurinol on the frequency of PEP (RR 0.75, 95%CI 0.39–1.42) with significant heterogeneity ($I^2 = 70.4\%$, $P = 0.005$) and therefore random effect model was adopted (Fig. 4).

However, different dosages and administration time of allopurinol were applied in different studies and PEP could be classified as mild, moderate and severe as well. To identify whether allopurinol in various dosages and administration time could present different prevention effect on the severity of PEP, meta-analyses were performed respectively according to different dosages and administration time of allopurinol. (high moderate or low dose, long or short administration time with agreement of two reviewers).

Results of meta-analysis

Low dose of allopurinol. Two studies [10,13] investigated the prevention effect of low dose of allopurinol on the frequency of PEP, including 392 patients treated with allopurinol and 394 with

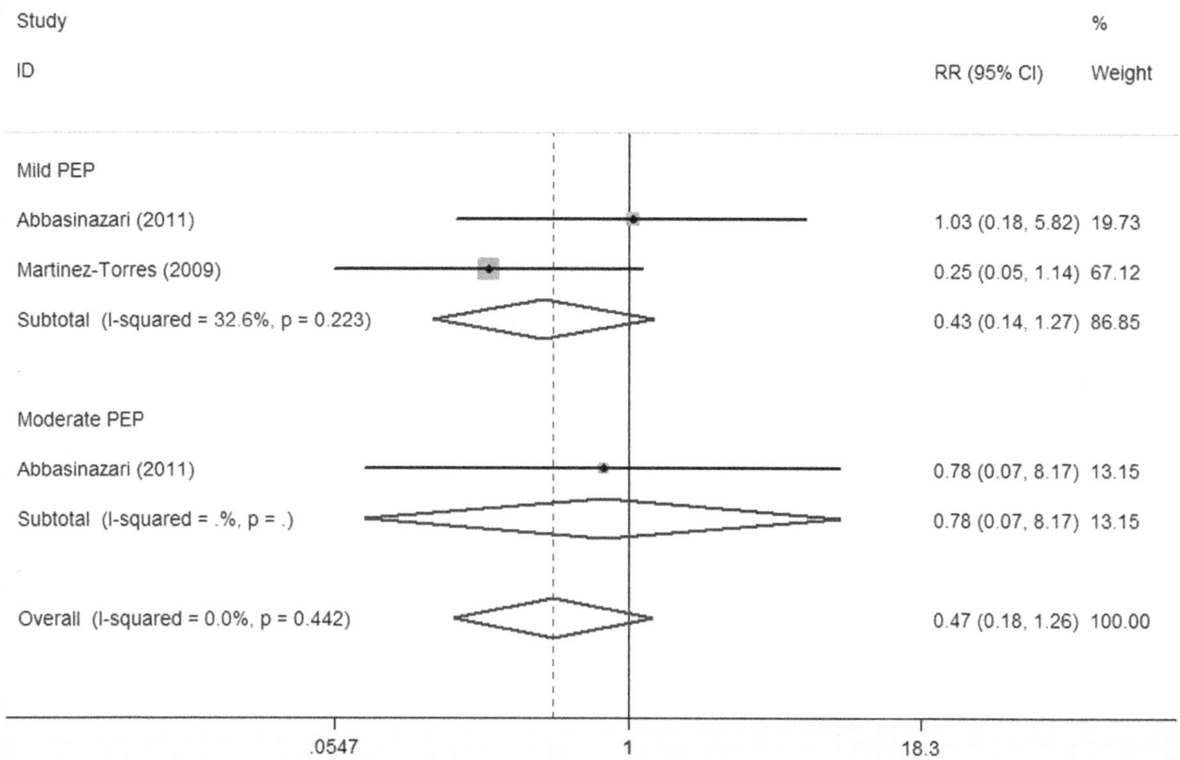

Figure 6. Prevention effect of moderate dose of allopurinol on PEP in different severity degrees.

placebo. Pooled analysis showed no significant prevention effect of allopurinol on mild (RR 2.00, 95%CI 0.91–4.40), moderate (RR 0.96, 95%CI 0.37–2.45) or severe PEP (RR 1.11, 95%CI 0.21–5.89) with no statistically substantial heterogeneity in any of the subgroups ($I_{mild}^2 = 0.0\%$, $P_{mild} = 0.822$, $I_{moderate}^2 = 0.0\%$, $P_{moderate} = 0.651$, and $I_{severe}^2 = 0.0\%$, $P_{severe} = 0.983$) (Fig. 5).

Moderate dose of allopurinol. The prevention effect of moderate dose of allopurinol on the severity of PEP was reported in two studies [14,15] which consisted of 114 patients treated with allopurinol and 130 with placebo. Subgroup analysis indicated no evident effect of allopurinol on mild (RR 0.43, 95%CI 0.14–1.27) or moderate PEP (RR 0.78, 95%CI 0.07–8.17) (Fig. 6). Notably, no severe PEP case was identified in either of the two trials. Fixed effect model was adopted due to non-significant heterogeneity of two studies ($I_{mild}^2 = 32.6\%$, $P_{mild} = 0.223$).

High dose of allopurinol. Two trials [11,12], comprising 480 patients in allopurinol group and 464 patients in placebo group, reported the prevention effect of high dose of allopurinol on PEP in different severity degrees. Subgroup analysis showed no substantial prevention effect of high dose of allopurinol on mild (RR 0.86, 95%CI 0.39–1.92), moderate (RR 0.26, 95%CI 0.01–7.70) or severe PEP (RR 0.60, 95%CI 0.12–3.11). Non-significant heterogeneity was observed in either mild PEP subgroup ($I^2 = 44.4\%$, $P = 0.180$) or severe PEP subgroup ($I^2 = 0.0\%$, $P = 0.366$). However, statistically evident heterogeneity was presented in subgroup of moderate PEP ($I^2 = 82.3\%$, $P = 0.018$) and therefore random effect model was applied (Fig. 7).

Long administration time of allopurinol. Three studies, including 309 patients treated with allopurinol and 304 with placebo, applied long administration time of allopurinol on the incidence of PEP. Pooled analysis showed no evident effect of allopurinol on mild (RR 0.65, 95%CI 0.20–2.11), moderate (RR 0.90, 95%CI 0.35–2.31) or severe PEP (RR 0.73, 95%CI 0.05–11.15). Non-significant heterogeneity was investigated in either moderate PEP subgroup ($I_{moderate}^2 = 0.0\%$, $P_{moderate} = 0.718$) or severe PEP subgroup ($I_{severe}^2 = 35.4\%$, $P_{severe} = 0.214$). However, statistically significant heterogeneity was observed in subgroup of mild PEP ($I_{mild}^2 = 62.8\%$, $P_{mild} = 0.068$) and therefore random effect model was used (Fig. 8).

Short administration time of allopurinol. The prevention effect of short administration time of allopurinol on the severity of PEP was reported in three studies including 677 patients treated with allopurinol and 684 with placebo. Subgroup analysis indicated no evident effect of allopurinol on mild (RR 1.24, 95%CI 0.78–1.97), moderate (RR 0.97, 95%CI 0.55–1.70) or severe PEP (RR 0.99, 95%CI 0.25–3.93). Fixed effect model was adopted due to non-significant heterogeneity among three studies ($I_{mild}^2 = 0.0\%$, $P_{mild} = 0.681$; $I_{moderate}^2 = 0.0\%$, $P_{moderate} = 0.981$; $I_{severe}^2 = 0.0\%$, $P_{severe} = 0.985$) (Fig. 9).

Publication bias. Funnel plot and Egger's test were performed to identify potential publication bias. Total prevention effect of allopurinol on PEP evaluated from the six included studies was used as index for funnel plot which presented symmetrical (Fig. 10). Egger's test indicated non-significant publication bias ($P = 0.457$).

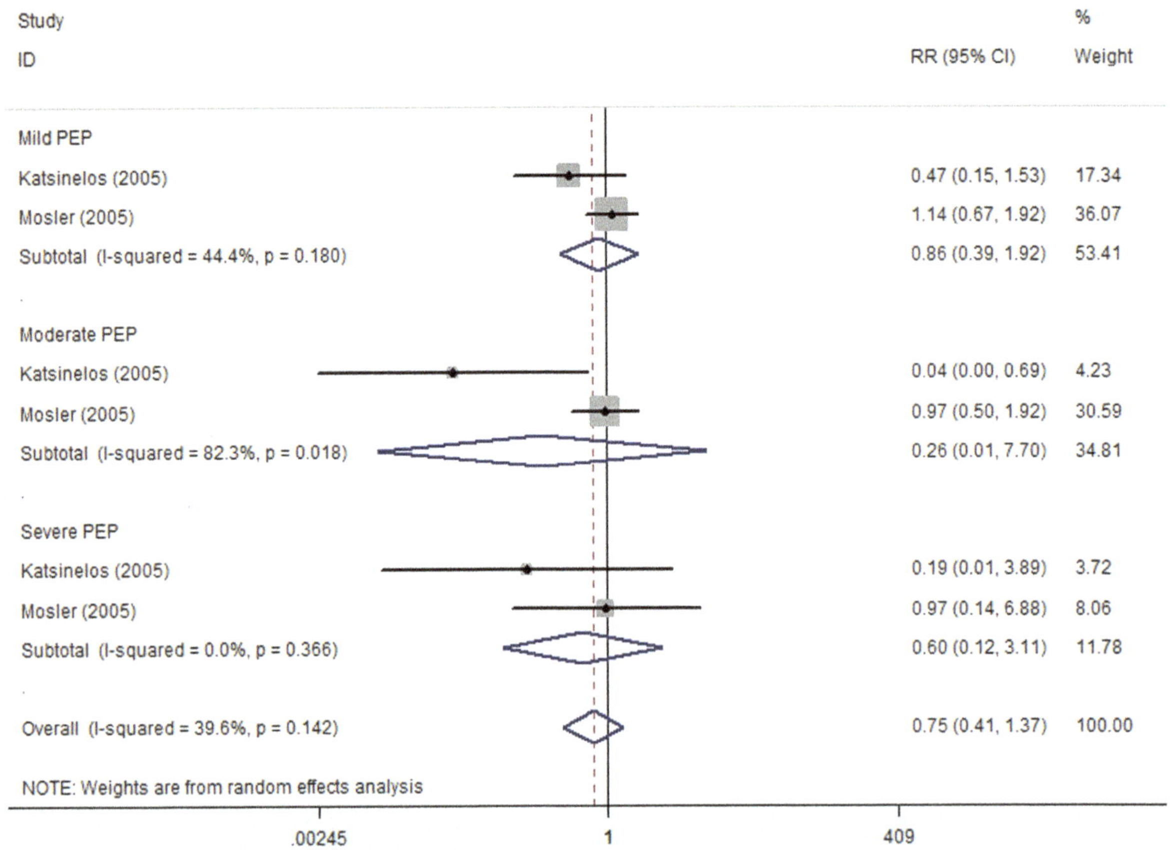

Figure 7. Prevention effect of high dose of allopurinol on PEP in different severity degrees.

Discussion

Meta-analysis of the six included RCTs [10,11,12,13,14,15] indicated that no significant prevention effect of allopurinol on the frequency of PEP. When studies were stratified according to the dosage of allopurinol, there was still no statistically evident prevention effect of allopurinol on mild, moderate and severe PEP. Five doses of allopurinol were applied in the trials (300 mg, 400 mg, 600 mg, 900 mg and 1200 mg) which had been divided into three levels: low (300 mg, 400 mg), moderate (600 mg) and high (900 mg and 1200 mg) after two reviewers' discussion and agreement.

Two RCTs [10,13] applied a low dosage of allopurinol. Budzynska et al. [10] showed that allopurinol did not play a significant role in the incidence and severity of PEP. Similarly, Romagnuolo et al. [13] concluded that the overall risk of PEP did not decrease after pretreated with allopurinol. However, it might have potential benefit in high-risk group but potential harm (PEP rates: allopurinol 5.4% vs. placebo 1.5%) in non–high-risk group. The mechanism with regard to this harm is unclear and it could be owing to an idiosyncratic reaction to this medicine [13], nevertheless, no evidence was observed to prove this presumption. Romagnuolo et al. [13] found that the percentage of patients with pancreatic duct injections was significantly higher in allopurinol group(allopurinol 129 vs. placebo 102, P = 0.02), which might result in higher occurrence of PEP in non–high-risk subgroup.

Two studies [14,15] investigated the prevention effect of moderate dosage of allopurinol. Martinez-Torres et al. [14] indicated that pretreatment with allopurinol decreased the incidences of hyperamylasemia and PEP in patients under high-risk procedures. However, Abbasinazari et al. [15] drew the opposite conclusion with the same dose of allopurinol that there was no difference between allopurinol and placebo for the occurrence of PEP (P = 0.97). According to our analysis, moderate dosage of allopurinol did not have any influence on the prevention of PEP. However, difference could be found in the administration time of the two RCTs. In Martinez-Torres' research, subjects were administrated with allopurinol at 15 h and 3 h before ERCP, while at 3 h and just before doing ERCP in Abbasinazari' study. It is necessary to assess whether administration time plays a part in the effect of allopurinol.

Two trials [11,12], both published in 2005, applied a high dose of allopurinol in research. Mosler et al. [11] reached the result that the overall frequency of pancreatitis was 12.55%. (allopurinol 12.96% vs. placebo 12.14%; P = 0.52). Besides, there was also no significant difference in mild (allopurinol 7.9% vs. placebo 6.9%), moderate (allopurinol 4.5% vs. placebo 4.6%) or severe (allopurinol 0.6% vs. placebo 0.6%) PEP. On the contrary, Katsinelos

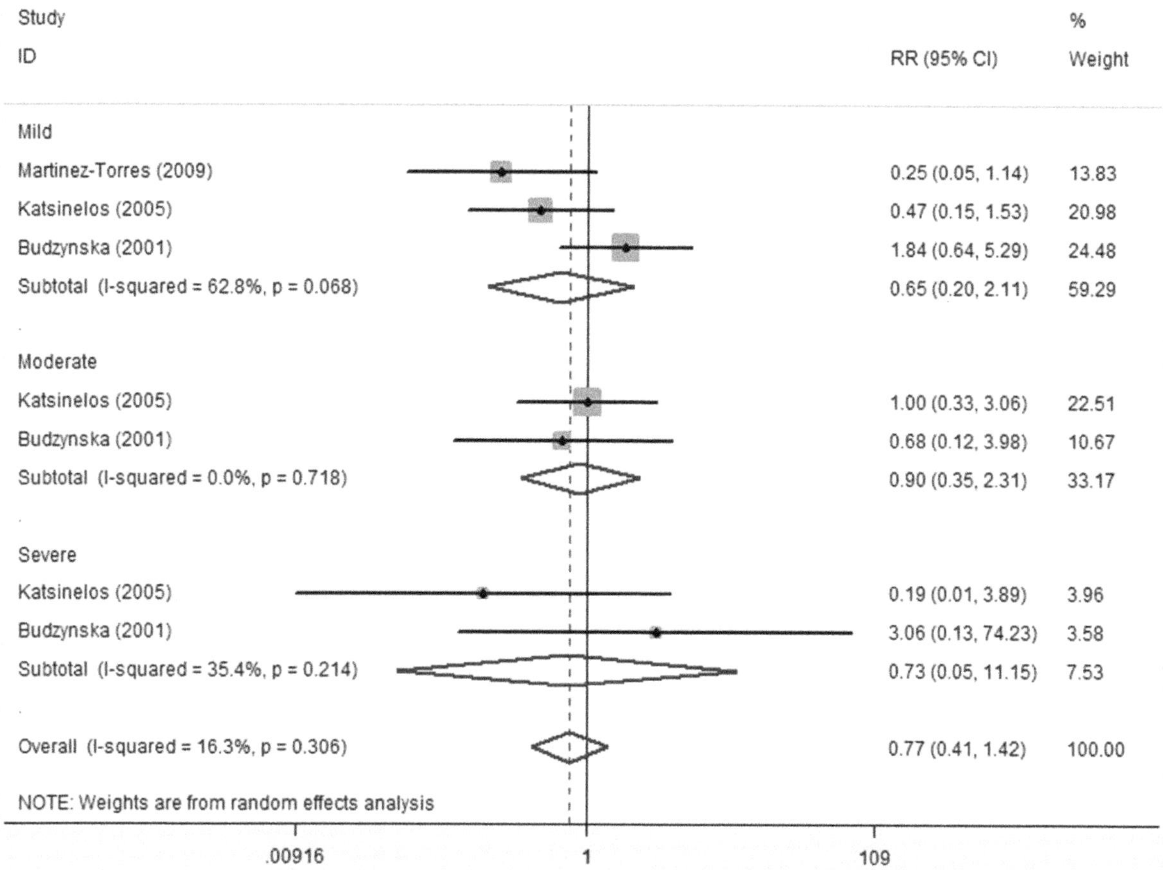

Figure 8. Prevention effect of long adminstration time of allopurinol on PEP in different severity degrees.

et al. [12] held the view that the risk of PEP decreased with the highest dosage(1200 mg) of allopurinol. Administration time of the two studies was not the same, as well. Patients were administrated with allopurinol at 15 h and 3 h before ERCP in Katsinelos' study, while at 4 h and 1 h before ERCP in Mosler' work. So next we tried to investigate whether the effect of allopurinol could be influenced by administration time.

Allopurinol, to our knowledge, can be absorbed approximately 90% in the gastrointestinal tract. It has a rapid onset and 70% of which can transform into a long-lasting active metabolite oxypurinol in liver. Peak plasma levels of allopurinol and oxypurinol can be observed at 1.5 hours and 4.5 hours, respectively. The half life of allopurinol is 1 to 2 hours and that of oxypurinol is about 15 hours [19,20]. To identify whether the prevention effect of allopurinol could be influenced by administration time, we classified the administration time into two levels: long (15 h and 3 h before ERCP) and short (4 h and 1 h before ERCP, 3 h and just before ERCP, 1 h before ERCP) after two reviewers discussion and agreement.

Long administration time of allopurinol was applied in three RCTs [10,12,14]. No evident effect of allopurinol can be observed on mild, moderate or severe PEP in Fig. 8. The metabolite of allopurinol (oxypurinol) was mainly examined in the plasma at 15 h and 3 h before ERCP. Administration of allopurinol at the two time points was long enough to ensure the role of allopurinol for PEP, however, there was no effect of allopurinol observed. We concluded that long administration time of allopurinol played no role in the prevention of PEP. In the three RCTs [10,12,14], Budzynska et al. [10] held the view that allopurinol had no effect in preventing PEP, while Katsinelos and Martinez-Torres et al. [12,14] insisted that allopurinol played a significant role in reducing the incidence of PEP. Katsinelos et al. [12] indicated that their patients group could be considered as a low risk group owing to a small number of patients with sphincter of Oddi dysfunction or previous acute pancreatitis and no pancreatic duct manipulations needed. Martinez-Torres et al. [14] concluded that allopurinol decreased the incidences of PEP in patients under high-risk procedures. The patients were classified into low-risk and high-risk subgroups. Precut sphincterotomy, pancreatic duct manipulation and multiple procedures were considered as risk factors for PEP by Martinez-Torres [14]. Although the results of these two studies by Katsinelos and Martinez-Torres [12,14] were positive, some differences could be examined. Allopurinol was effective in low risk group of Katsinelos' study [12], while it was effective in high-risk group of Martinez-Torres' study [14]. Therefore, we speculated that it might be the risk factors that affected the results. However, the risk factors were inconsistent with each other among the studies, what is more, the PEP data

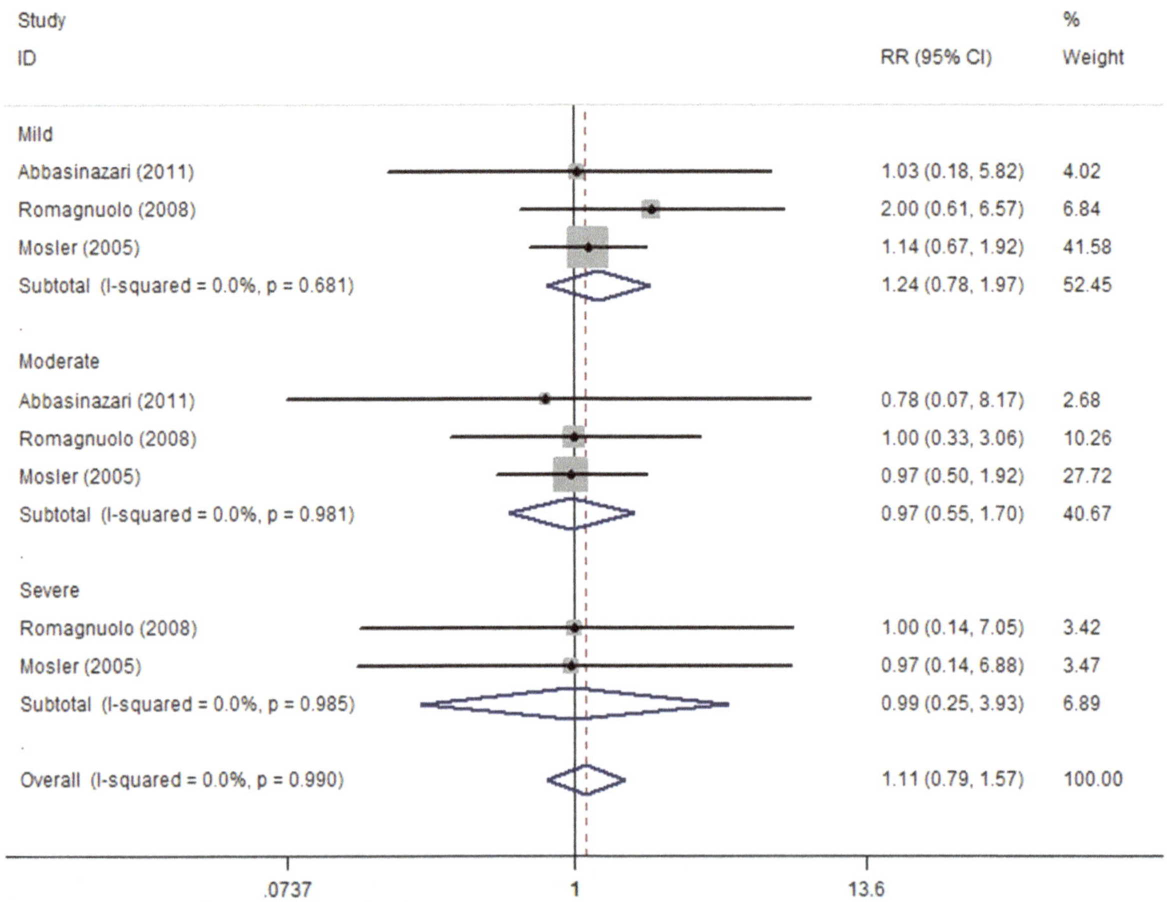

Figure 9. Prevention effect of short adminstration time of allopurinol on PEP in different severity degrees.

about risk factors were too limited to analyze whether risk factors affected the role of allopurinol.

Three trials [11,13,15] reported short administration time of allopurinol. Subgroup analysis indicated no statistically evident effect of allopurinol on mild, moderate or severe PEP. In Mosler' study [11], allopurinol was administrated at 4 h and 1 h before ERCP. At this time, allopurinol and oxypurinol were both presented with high levels in the plasma. However, Mosler et al. [11] drew the conclusion that allopurinol was ineffective in the prevention of PEP. Romagnuolo et al. [13] using the lowest dose (300 mg) of allopurinol at 1 h before ERCP held the view that allopurinol did not appear to decrease the overall risk of PEP; however, it might be beneficial in high-risk group but potential harm in non–high-risk group. It seems that administration at 1 h before ERCP was just enough to guarantee the work of allopurinol. Abbasinazari et al. [15] indicated that allopurinol did not exert function in occurrence of PEP. In their study, there were total 74 patients undergoing ERCP of which 29 in allopurinol group and 45 in placebo group and therefore the result might be affected by the small number of patients.

Yet there were still some limitations in the above RCTs [10,11,12,13,14,15]. Firstly, Katsinelos et al. [12] reported relatively high incidence of PEP in the placebo group (17.8%) which might affect the positive result. This could be attributed to the following aspects: high rate of pancreatic-duct opacification (72.9%), biliary sphincterotomy (73.7%) and pre-cut sphincterotomy (14.4%); varieties of criteria used to define pancreatitis; the comprehensive follow-up [12]. Secondly, the risk factors were inconsistent in above RCTs [10,11,12,13,14,15]. For example, male gender, days of hospitalization and administration of allopurinol were considered as risk factors in Katsinelos'study [12], while previous PEP, pancreatic injection and pancreatic therapy were predictors of PEP compared with non-significant risk factors such as sex, number of pancreatic injections, biliary sphincterotomy and pancreatic stent placement in Romagnuolo's study [13]. Thirdly, two trials [14,15] reported the outcome about amylase, however, we could not analyze it, because Martinez-Torres [14] et al. showed the number of patients with hyperamylasemia, whereas Abbasinazari et al. [15] displayed amylase concentration. Fourthly, it was worth noting that Abbasinazari et al. [15] distinguished the effect between allopurinol and oxypurinol, we considered it unnecessary to make this distinction before making sure the prevention effect of allopurinol.

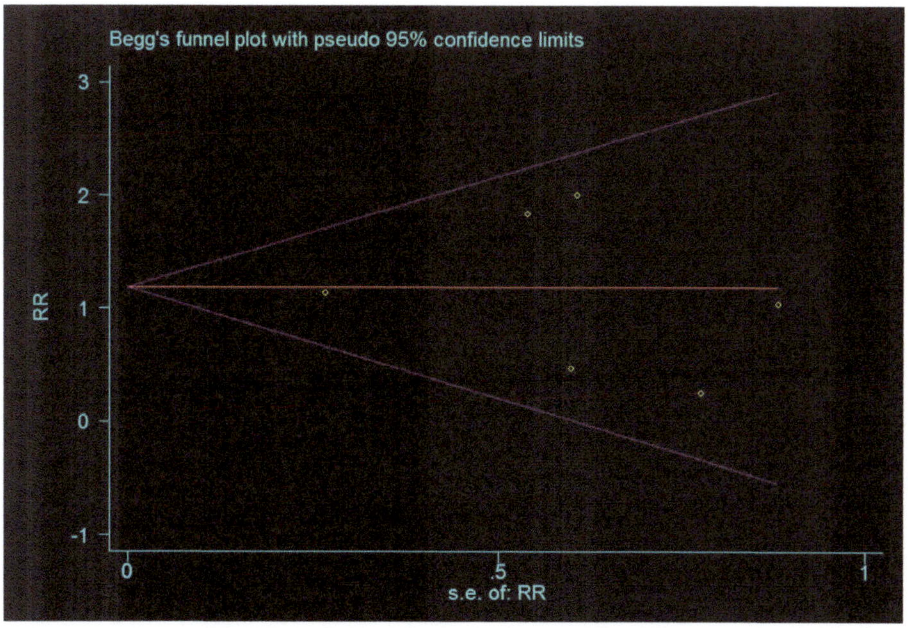

Figure 10. Funnel plot of the included studies assessed the effect of allopurinol on PEP.

In terms of the above problems, we recommended the following: in the first place, it was suggested that risk factors in all future RCTs should be classified into patient-related risk factors and procedure-related risk factors. Definite patient-related risk factors (suspected SOD, female gender and previous pancreatitis) and definite procedure-related risk factors (precut sphincterotomy and pancreatic injection) were listed in the table in European guideline which could act as a guide to the future research [21]. In the next place, the reported form related to amylase should remain the same in future study.

Procedural and pharmacological prophylaxes were usually used to prevent the frequency of PEP. The procedural interventions such as guide-wire cannulation [22] and pancreatic stent placement [23] were beneficial in high-risk group. However, pancreatic stenting required a skilled endoscopist and it could act as a high risk of PEP once failed [24]. As for pharmacological prophylaxis, it was possible that non-steroidal anti-inflammatory drugs (NSAIDs) might be useful [25]. Using 100 mg of diclofenac or indomethacin administered rectally would be effective in preventing the incidence of PEP [21]. Two promising agents for decreasing the frequency of PEP,gabexate mesilate and somatostatin, had some problems such as the long time infusion and the cost-effectiveness, particularly in outpatients [26].

A perfect agent should be safe for patients, well tolerated, relatively affordable and have a short administration time and therefore allopurinol seems to be a good choice. It was a safe and useful agent to treat gout and tumor-lysis syndrome and for the reduction of complications such as myocardial infarction, postoperative arrhythmias and mortality after cardiovascular surgery [27]. However, our meta-analysis did not show any evident effect of allopurinol in different dosages and adminstration time on mild to severe PEP. Additionally, an adverse event of allopurinol was reported recently. A 46-year-old man was treated with allopurinol for asymptomatic hyperuricemia. However, pancreatitis and the allopurinol hypersensitivity syndrome which characterized by rash, fever, and internal organ involvement occurred in the patient [28]. Consequently, investigators should be cautious and further examine the role of allopurinol in the prevention of PEP. Although our result was similar to the previous meta-analysis published in 2008 [16,17], it was more systematic, comprehensive and novel. Additionally, there was no publication bias.

In conclusion, this meta-analysis showed that the prophylactic use of allopurinol in different dosages and administration time had no effect in preventing incidence and severity of PEP. Further well-designed placebo-controlled RCTs are warranted to confirm the effect of allopurinol in preventing PEP.

Supporting Information

Checklist S1 PRISMA Checklist.
(DOC)

Author Contributions

Conceived and designed the experiments: SHX WLC WSY. Performed the experiments: WLC WSY XHX. Analyzed the data: WLC WSY KC. Contributed reagents/materials/analysis tools: WLC WSY XHX. Contributed to the writing of the manuscript: WLC WSY XHX KC.

References

1. Dumonceau JM, Andriulli A, Deviere J, Mariani A, Rigaux J, et al. (2010) European Society of Gastrointestinal Endoscopy (ESGE) Guideline: prophylaxis of post-ERCP pancreatitis. Endoscopy 42: 503–515.
2. Nordback IH, Cameron JL (1993) The mechanism of conversion of xanthine dehydrogenase to xanthine oxidase in acute pancreatitis in the canine isolated pancreas preparation. Surgery 113: 90–97.
3. Sanfey H, Bulkley GB, Cameron JL (1984) The role of oxygen-derived free radicals in the pathogenesis of acute pancreatitis. Ann Surg 200: 405–413.
4. Sanfey H, Bulkley GB, Cameron JL (1985) The pathogenesis of acute pancreatitis. The source and role of oxygen-derived free radicals in three different experimental models. Ann Surg 201: 633–639.
5. Sanfey H, Cameron JL (1984) Increased capillary permeability: an early lesion in acute pancreatitis. Surgery 96: 485–491.

6. Masci E, Cavallini G, Mariani A, Frulloni L, Testoni PA, et al. (2003) Comparison of two dosing regimens of gabexate in the prophylaxis of post-ERCP pancreatitis. Am J Gastroenterol 98: 2182–2186.
7. Cavallini G, Tittobello A, Frulloni L, Masci E, Mariana A, et al. (1996) Gabexate for the prevention of pancreatic damage related to endoscopic retrograde cholangiopancreatography. Gabexate in digestive endoscopy-Italian Group. N Engl J Med 335: 919–923.
8. Kountouras J, Chatzopoulos D, Zavos C (2001) Reactive oxygen metabolites and upper gastrointestinal diseases. Hepatogastroenterology 48: 743–751.
9. Guan W, Osanai T, Kamada T, Hanada H, Ishizaka H, et al. (2003) Effect of allopurinol pretreatment on free radical generation after primary coronary angioplasty for acute myocardial infarction. J Cardiovasc Pharmacol 41: 699–705.
10. Budzynska A, Marek T, Nowak A, Kaczor R, Nowakowska-Dulawa E (2001) A prospective, randomized, placebo-controlled trial of prednisone and allopurinol in the prevention of ERCP-induced pancreatitis. Endoscopy 33: 766–772.
11. Mosler P, Sherman S, Marks J, Watkins JL, Geenen JE, et al. (2005) Oral allopurinol does not prevent the frequency or the severity of post-ERCP pancreatitis. Gastrointest Endosc 62: 245–250.
12. Katsinelos P, Kountouras J, Chatzis J, Christodoulou K, Paroutoglou G, et al. (2005) High-dose allopurinol for prevention of post-ERCP pancreatitis: a prospective randomized double-blind controlled trial. Gastrointest Endosc 61: 407–415.
13. Romagnuolo J, Hilsden R, Sandha GS, Cole M, Bass S, et al. (2008) Allopurinol to prevent pancreatitis after endoscopic retrograde cholangiopancreatography: a randomized placebo-controlled trial. Clin Gastroenterol Hepatol 6: 465–471; quiz 371.
14. Martinez-Torres H, Rodriguez-Lomeli X, Davalos-Cobian C, Garcia-Correa J, Maldonado-Martinez JM, et al. (2009) Oral allopurinol to prevent hyperamylasemia and acute pancreatitis after endoscopic retrograde cholangiopancreatography. World J Gastroenterol 15: 1600–1606.
15. Abbasinazari M, Mohammad AAH, Moshiri K, Pourhoseingholi MA, Zali MR (2011) Does allopurinol prevent post endoscopic retrograde cholangiopancreatography pancreatitis? A randomized double blind trial. Acta Med Iran 49: 579–583.
16. Zheng M, Chen Y, Bai J, Xin Y, Pan X, et al. (2008) Meta-analysis of prophylactic allopurinol use in post-endoscopic retrograde cholangiopancreatography pancreatitis. Pancreas 37: 247–253.
17. Bai Y, Gao J, Zhang W, Zou D, Li Z (2008) Meta-analysis: allopurinol in the prevention of postendoscopic retrograde cholangiopancreatography pancreatitis. Aliment Pharmacol Ther 28: 557–564.
18. Higgins JPT, Green S (editors) (2011) Cochrane Handbook for Systematic Reviews of Interventions Version 5.1.0 [updated March 2011]. The Cochrane Collaboration.
19. Kountouras J, Chatzopoulos D, Zavos C (2001) Reactive oxygen metabolites and upper gastrointestinal diseases. Hepatogastroenterology 48: 743–751.
20. Pacher P, Nivorozhkin A, Szabo C (2006) Therapeutic effects of xanthine oxidase inhibitors: renaissance half a century after the discovery of allopurinol. Pharmacol Rev 58: 87–114.
21. Dumonceau JM, Andriulli A, Deviere J, Mariani A, Rigaux J, et al. (2010) European Society of Gastrointestinal Endoscopy (ESGE) Guideline: prophylaxis of post-ERCP pancreatitis. Endoscopy 42: 503–515.
22. Cheung J, Tsoi KK, Quan WL, Lau JY, Sung JJ (2009) Guidewire versus conventional contrast cannulation of the common bile duct for the prevention of post-ERCP pancreatitis: a systematic review and meta-analysis. Gastrointest Endosc 70: 1211–1219.
23. Sofuni A, Maguchi H, Itoi T, Katanuma A, Hisai H, et al. (2007) Prophylaxis of post-endoscopic retrograde cholangiopancreatography pancreatitis by an endoscopic pancreatic spontaneous dislodgement stent. Clin Gastroenterol Hepatol 5: 1339–1346.
24. Freeman ML, Overby C, Qi D (2004) Pancreatic stent insertion: consequences of failure and results of a modified technique to maximize success. Gastrointest Endosc 59: 8–14.
25. Arata S, Takada T, Hirata K, Yoshida M, Mayumi T, et al. (2010) Post-ERCP pancreatitis. J Hepatobiliary Pancreat Sci 17: 70–78.
26. Freeman ML, Guda NM (2004) Prevention of post-ERCP pancreatitis: a comprehensive review. Gastrointest Endosc 59: 845–864.
27. Pacher P, Nivorozhkin A, Szabo C (2006) Therapeutic effects of xanthine oxidase inhibitors: renaissance half a century after the discovery of allopurinol. Pharmacol Rev 58: 87–114.
28. Fathallah N, Ben SC, Slim R, Kaabia N, Letaief A, et al. (2010) Fatal allopurinol-induced hypersensitivity syndrome associated with pancreatic abnormalities. J Clin Rheumatol 16: 170–171.

8

The Association of Depression and Anxiety with Pain: A Study from NESDA

Eric W. de Heer[1,2]*, Marloes M. J. G. Gerrits[3], Aartjan T. F. Beekman[3,4], Jack Dekker[5,6], Harm W. J. van Marwijk[7], Margot W. M. de Waal[8], Philip Spinhoven[9,10], Brenda W. J. H. Penninx[3], Christina M. van der Feltz-Cornelis[1,2,11]

1 TopClinical Center for Body, Mind, and Health, GGz Breburg Tilburg, Tilburg, The Netherlands, **2** Tilburg School of Behavioral and Social Sciences, Tranzo Department, University of Tilburg, Tilburg, The Netherlands, **3** Department of Psychiatry, EMGO Institute for Health and Care research, VU University Medical Centre, Amsterdam, The Netherlands, **4** GGZ inGeest, Mental Health Institute, Amsterdam, The Netherlands, **5** Arkin, Mental Health Institute, Amsterdam, The Netherlands, **6** Department of Clinical Psychology, VU University, Amsterdam, The Netherlands, **7** Department of General Practice, EMGO Institute for Health and Care Research, VU University Medical Centre, Amsterdam, The Netherlands, **8** Department of Public Health and Primary Care, Leiden university Medical Centre, Leiden, The Netherlands, **9** Institute of Psychology, Leiden University, Leiden, The Netherlands, **10** Department of Psychiatry, Leiden University Medical Centre, Leiden, The Netherlands, **11** Trimbos Institute, Utrecht, the Netherlands

Abstract

Chronic pain is commonly co-morbid with a depressive or anxiety disorder. Objective of this study is to examine the influence of depression, along with anxiety, on pain-related disability, pain intensity, and pain location in a large sample of adults with and without a depressive and/or anxiety disorder. The study population consisted of 2981 participants with a depressive, anxiety, co-morbid depressive and anxiety disorder, remitted disorder or no current disorder (controls). Severity of depressive and anxiety symptoms was also assessed. In separate multinomial regression analyses, the association of presence of depressive or anxiety disorders and symptom severity with the Chronic Pain Grade and location of pain was explored. Presence of a depressive (OR = 6.67; P<.001), anxiety (OR = 4.84; P<.001), or co-morbid depressive and anxiety disorder (OR = 30.26; P<.001) was associated with the Chronic Pain Grade. Moreover, symptom severity was associated with more disabling and severely limiting pain. Also, a remitted depressive or anxiety disorder showed more disabling and severely limiting pain (OR = 3.53; P<.001) as compared to controls. A current anxiety disorder (OR = 2.96; p<.001) and a co-morbid depressive and anxiety disorder (OR = 5.15; P<.001) were more strongly associated with cardio-respiratory pain, than gastro-intestinal or musculoskeletal pain. These findings remain after adjustment for chronic cardio respiratory illness. Patients with a current and remitted depressive and/or anxiety disorder and those with more severe symptoms have more disabling pain and pain of cardio-respiratory nature, than persons without a depressive or anxiety disorder. This warrants further research.

Editor: H. Sunny Sun, National Cheng Kung University Medical College, Taiwan

Funding: The infrastructure for the NESDA study is funded through the Geestkracht program of the Netherlands Organisation for Health Research and Development (Zon-MW, grant number 10-000-1002) and is supported by participating universities and mental health care organisations (VU University Medical Center, GGZ inGeest, Arkin, Leiden University Medical Center, GGZ Rivierduinen, University Medical Center Groningen, Lentis, GGZ Friesland, GGZ Drenthe, IQ Healthcare, Netherlands Institute for Health Services Research [NIVEL], and the Netherlands Institute of Mental Health and Addiction [Trimbos]. The funders had no role in study design, data collection and analysis, decision to publish, or preparation of the manuscript.

Competing Interests: The authors of this manuscript have read the journal's policy and have the following competing interests: ATFB reports grants from Eli Lilly, grants from Astra Zeneca, grants from Jansen, grants from Shire, personal fees (as a speaker) from Eli Lilly, and personal fees (as a speaker) from Lundbeck, outside the submitted work. JD and CMFC report grants from Eli Lilly, outside the submitted work. BWJHP reports grants from Dutch government, ministry of Health (ZonMw), during the conduct of the study. This does not alter their adherence to PLOS ONE policies on sharing data and materials, except those mentioned in the data availability statement.

* Email: e.deheer@ggzbreburg.nl

Introduction

Chronic pain is common in up to 70% of patients with depressive and anxiety disorders [1–9]. Chronic pain and depression most likely have a bidirectional association: depression is a predictor of persistent pain and pain is a predictor of the persistence of depression [1,3,10]. A possible explanation is that impaired functioning caused by pain can lead to social isolation, which in turn can lead to a negative effect on depressive symptoms, and vice versa [11,12]. Furthermore, different brain areas, such as the amygdala and hypothalamus, play a role in both depression and pain [13,14]. Also, when depression and chronic pain are co-morbid, recognition and treatment of depression are less effective, as patients mostly only present their physical complaints and receive treatment accordingly [1].

Most studies up to now have only considered the relationship of pain with depression, whereas its association with anxiety disorders has been less examined. It is likely that the association of pain and anxiety is equally important, as depression and anxiety commonly appear together. Pain may cause feelings of anxiety, which in turn can make one more sensitive to pain, with persistence of the pain experience as a consequence [15]. Furthermore, anxiety disorders and chronic pain share underlying cognitive and behavioural processes, such as increased attention towards threat and anxious avoidance of physical exertion [16,17]. Fear avoidance can play a role in chronic pain, with the (acute) pain experience leading to pain catastrophising and pain-related fear which in turn will lead to greater disability and persistent pain experience [15]. Therefore, we need more comprehensive insight by studying both depression and anxiety in concert (separately and as co-morbid problems) with pain [18–20]. Another reason to study the cross-sectional relationship between depressive and anxiety disorders and pain is that pain also has a negative impact on the prognosis of psychopathology and psychiatric treatment outcome, with pain leading to more treatment resistance [2,21–23]. Pain may be a marker of a more difficult-to-treat disorder, and lead to a longer time before remission [24].

Pain is a common presenting symptom in depression and anxiety and several studies have explored this association for specific pain symptoms, such as back pain [25–27] or neck pain [27,28]. However, pain symptoms often occur in more than one location and thus may be clustered; clustering of (medically unexplained) physical symptoms was examined by Wessely et al. [29], Nimnuan et al. [30], and Fink et al. [31]. These studies found different clusters of pain symptoms, the most prominent being musculoskeletal, gastro-intestinal, and cardio-respiratory pain. Associations were found between depressive, but mostly anxiety symptoms and cardio-respiratory pain, musculoskeletal pain and gastro-intestinal pain. However, the strength of these associations and the correlation with pain-related disability has not yet been explored [32–34]. Therefore, this study will explore the association of clustered locations of pain (musculoskeletal, gastro-intestinal, and cardio-respiratory) with depression and anxiety, while taking severity of pain and pain-related disability into account.

We aim to examine and compare the impact of current and remitted depressive, anxiety and co-morbid disorders on different pain-variables in a large sample of individuals with depressive and/or anxiety disorders versus normal controls. We will explore if severity of depressive or anxiety symptoms is associated with severity of pain and pain-related disability, and whether these associations are stronger for certain clustered pain locations. We expect that not only a depressive disorder will have a strong association with abovementioned pain-variables, but that an anxiety disorder will show a comparably strong association, with comorbid depression and anxiety showing the strongest association.

Methods

Sample

The present study used data from the Netherlands Study of Depression and Anxiety (NESDA): an ongoing longitudinal cohort study in which 2981 participants, recruited from the community, general practice and secondary mental health care, are monitored to investigate the long-term course and consequences of depressive and anxiety disorders. Penninx et al. [35] provide a detailed description of the NESDA study design and sampling procedures. NESDA was designed to include patients with depressive and anxiety disorders at different stages of development of their disorder. In order to achieve this, participants were recruited from the community, in primary care and in specialised mental health care [35]. At baseline, healthy controls, persons with a prior history, and persons with a current depressive and/or anxiety disorder, between 18 and 65 years old, were included. The sample was stratified for setting (community, primary care, and specialised mental health). Furthermore, the sample includes a range of psychopathology: from those without a depressive or anxiety disorder (controls) to those with a current, first or recurrent (in the past 6 months) depressive or anxiety disorder and those with a remitted disorder (at baseline, a depressive and/or anxiety disorder was diagnosed in the past, but no diagnoses were present at 6 months before baseline). The disorders included dysthymia, major depressive disorder, general anxiety disorder, panic disorder, social phobia, and agoraphobia. Exclusion criteria were not being fluent in Dutch and a primary diagnosis of psychotic, obsessive compulsive, bipolar or severe addiction disorder. The research protocol was approved by the Ethical Committee of participating universities and written informed consent was obtained from all participants. Interviews were conducted by specially trained research staff.

The sample consists of 2329 persons with a current diagnosis of depression (n = 396) or anxiety disorder (n = 543), a remitted disorder (n = 628) and 652 persons without a history of depressive and/or anxiety disorder and no current diagnosis of depression or anxiety disorder. All 2981 participants were interviewed, by specially trained clinical research staff, for depression and/or anxiety in the baseline interview using the DSM IV based Composite International Diagnostic Interview (CIDI, version 2.1), a reliable and valid instrument for assessing depressive and anxiety disorders [36].

The baseline measurement of NESDA, collected between September 2004 and February 2007, was used for this study. Next to the structured interview to assess mental health, self-report questionnaires were used to assess physical health (such as chronic disease, pain, and severity of mental health).

Measures

Pain assessment. Pain was assessed using the 7-item Chronic Pain Grade (CPG) Scale by von Korff [37]. The CPG is a reliable and valid instrument for chronic pain populations and the general population [37,38]. The CPG is a good instrument for measuring pain-related variables and for making a hierarchical classification of pain intensity and pain-related disability. It has good internal consistency (with a Cronbach's alpha of 0.91) and the item-total correlations are all high, ranging from .69 to .83.

The CPG grades (chronic) pain using pain intensity and pain-related disability. Pain intensity is based on the mean of the average, worst, and present pain on a scale of 0–100. Pain-related disability is based on the mean of interference with usual activities, work/household activities, and family/social activities on a scale of 0–100, and the number of days (0–180) one is unable to carry out usual activities due to pain in the previous 6 months. To create 5 grades for chronic pain, the following calculations were used: pain intensity was divided into low intensity (score <50) and high intensity (score ≥ 50). To calculate the score of pain-related disability, an overall score of 0–6 was created by assigning 0–3 points for disability score (0–29 = 0; 30–49 = 1; 50–69 = 2; 70–100 = 3) and adding 0–3 points for number of disability days (0–6 days = 0; 7–14 days = 1; 15–30 days = 2; >30 days = 3). With these scores, 5 grades of chronic pain can be calculated:

grade 0 (no pain symptoms);
grade 1 (low pain intensity (<50) – low disability (<3 points));
grade 2 (high intensity (≥ 50) – low disability (<3 points));

Table 1. Baseline characteristics of total NESDA sample (N = 2981).

		N (%)	Mean (SD)
Demographics			
Female gender		1979 (66.4)	
Age in years			41.9 (13.1)
Level of education	Basic	199 (6.7)	
	Intermediate	1736 (58.2)	
	High	1046 (35.1)	
Partner or married		2066 (69.3)	
Psychopathology characteristics			
No psychopathology		652 (21.9)	
Remitted disorder		628 (21.0)	
	# of depressive episodes		1.73 (5.9)
Current depressive disorder		396 (13.3)	
	# of depressive episodes		10.29 (71.3)
Current anxiety disorder		543 (18.2)	
Current depressive and anxiety disorder		762 (25.6)	
	# of depressive episodes		9.88 (72.6)
Severity of depression (QIDS)*	None	1121 (37.6)	
	Mild	820 (27.5)	
	Moderate	627 (21.0)	
	(Very) Severe	374 (12.5)	
Severity of anxiety (BAI)**	Normal	1477 (49.5)	
	Mild	758 (25.4)	
	Moderate	493 (16.5)	
	Severe	218 (7.3)	
Other characteristics			
Musculoskeletal chronic disease		648 (21.7)	
Gastro-intestinal chronic disease		335 (11.2)	
Cardio respiratory chronic disease		775 (26.0)	
Antidepressant use		785 (26.4)	
Use of other psychotropic drugs		700 (23.5)	

*39 missing.
**35 missing.

grade 3 (high disability – moderately limiting (3–4 disability points, regardless of intensity));

grade 4 (high disability – severely limiting (5–6 disability points, regardless of intensity)).

Along with the CPG, we also assessed the specific pain location. To locate the specific pain location, an inventory was made, with a self-report questionnaire, of pain symptoms in the back, neck, head, stomach, joints, chest, and face. Participants could report one or more of these pain locations, and were asked which of these pain locations bothered them the most in the last six months. We then categorised these pain locations as musculoskeletal (back, neck, head, joints, face), gastro-intestinal (stomach), and cardio respiratory (chest) pain symptoms. Participants could report multiple pain symptoms across the categories.

Depression and anxiety. The presence of a depressive or anxiety disorder was established using the CIDI. In this study, psychopathology profiles were made for each participant. A participant either had no psychopathology (n = 652), a remitted disorder (depression and/or anxiety) (n = 628), a current depressive disorder (n = 396), a current anxiety disorder (n = 543) or a current co-morbid depressive and anxiety disorder (n = 762) (in the past 6 months).

In addition to this categorical approach of disorders (yes/no), we also assessed severity of depressive and anxiety symptoms. Severity of depressive symptoms was assessed with the Quick Inventory of Depressive Symptomatology-Self-Report (QIDS-SR) [39], in which no pain items are included. The QIDS-SR is the shortened version of the self-rated Inventory of Depressive Symptomatology (IDS-SR) [40] and is a 16-item questionnaire with a range of 0 to 27 with high internal consistency (Cronbach's α = 0.86). A score of 0–5 refers to none to mild depressive symptoms, a score of 6–10 refers to mild severity, a score of 11–15 refers to moderate severity, and a score of 16 or higher refers to (very) severe depressive symptoms. Severity of anxiety symptoms was assessed with the Beck Anxiety Inventory (BAI) [41], which also does not include any pain items. The BAI is a 27-item questionnaire ranging from 0 to 63 also with high internal

Table 2. Baseline pain characteristics divided by psychopathology.

		Total	No psychopathology	Remitted disorder	Current depressive disorder	Current anxiety disorder	Current depressive and anxiety disorder
		N = 2981	N = 652	N = 627	N = 396	N = 543	N = 762
CPG*	Grade 0, N (%)	170 (5.7)	82 (12.6)	33 (5.3)	19 (4.8)	23 (4.2)	13 (1.7)
	Grade 1, N (%)	1635 (54.8)	441 (67.6)	379 (60.4)	194 (49.0)	315 (58.0)	306 (40.2)
	Grade 2, N (%)	605 (20.3)	81 (12.4)	134 (21.4)	86 (21.7)	118 (21.7)	186 (24.4)
	Grade 3, N (%)	311 (10.4)	29 (4.4)	48 (7.7)	60 (15.2)	52 (9.6)	122 (16.0)
	Grade 4, N (%)	259 (8.7)	19 (2.9)	33 (5.3)	37 (9.3)	35 (6.4)	135 (17.7)
Pain location	No pain, N (%)	170 (5.7)	82 (12.6)	33 (5.3)	19 (4.8)	23 (4.2)	13 (1.7)
	Musculoskeletal, N (%)	2753 (92.4)	552 (84.7)	586 (93.3)	374 (94.4)	507 (93.4)	734 (96.3)
	Gastro-intestinal, N (%)	1432 (48.0)	207 (31.7)	250 (39.8)	216 (54.5)	278 (51.2)	481 (63.1)
	Cardio respiratory, N (%)	764 (25.6)	77 (11.8)	117 (18.6)	101 (25.5)	156 (28.7)	313 (41.1)

*1 missing.

consistency (Cronbach's $\alpha = 0.92$). A score of 0–9 refers to normal severity, whereas a score of 10–18 refers to mild severity, a score of 18–29 refers to moderate severity, and a score higher than 29 refers to severe anxiety symptoms [42].

Covariates. Covariates were selected a priori based on previous research on the association of depression and anxiety with pain. Socio-demographic factors included gender, age, level of education, and partner status. Furthermore, the presence of chronic diseases was taken into account as a covariate. Based on self-report during the initial interview, the presence of a chronic disease was assessed. These chronic diseases were then categorised, by a physician, into cardio respiratory disease (coronary heart disease, angina pectoris, heart failure, chronic nonspecific lung disease, stroke, hypertension), gastro-intestinal disease (diabetes, (gastro-intestinal) ulcer, ulcerative colitis or Crohn's disease, liver cirrhosis, hepatitis) and musculoskeletal disease (arthritis, osteoarthritis, rheumatism). Because medication can have an analgesic influence on pain, the use of antidepressants and other psychotropic drugs were also selected as covariates. Also, the number of depressive episodes was taken into account as a covariate.

Statistical Analyses. All statistical analyses were performed in SPSS 19 for Windows. Descriptive analyses were used to assess baseline characteristics across the total sample. To assess the associations of type of disorder with the CPG, we used multinomial logistic regression analyses. For the pain outcome variable (the CPG) we used the group with no pain (CPG0) as a reference category. For type of disorder, the healthy control group without depression or anxiety was selected as a reference category. In this analysis we controlled for all the covariates.

We used adjusted multinomial analyses to assess the association of severity of depressive and anxiety symptoms with the outcome variable CPG, with the lowest severity category as the reference category.

Furthermore, we used four separate logistic regression analyses to examine the association of depression and/or anxiety with the outcome variable of location of pain (1. no pain, 2. musculoskeletal pain (controlling for the presence of musculoskeletal disease), 3. gastro-intestinal pain (controlling for the presence of gastro-intestinal disease), and 4. cardio respiratory pain (controlling for the presence of cardio respiratory disease)). Here also, having no depressive or anxiety disorder was used as a reference category.

Results

Table 1 presents the baseline characteristics of the total population. Of the total sample, 652 participants reported no psychopathology, and slightly less participants (628) reported a remitted depressive and/or anxiety disorder (with a mean of 1.73 depressive episodes). The least participants had a current depressive disorder (with a mean of 10.29 depressive episodes), followed by a current anxiety disorder. Most participants reported a current comorbid depressive and anxiety disorder, with a mean of almost 10 depressive episodes. 26.4% of the total sample used antidepressant medication. Of the 2981 participants, 170 (5.7%) reported no pain symptoms. Most participants (92.4%) reported having musculoskeletal pain, followed by gastro-intestinal pain (1432 participants), and cardio respiratory pain (764 participants). Table 2 shows the pain characteristics, separated in no psychopathology, remitted disorder, current depressive disorder, current anxiety disorder, and current depressive and anxiety disorder. Of the total sample and of each of the abovementioned groups, most participants had low intensity and low pain-related disability (CPG1), and pain of musculoskeletal origin. Especially when a depressive disorder is comorbid with an anxiety disorder, more

Table 3. Associations of presence of current depressive disorder, current anxiety disorder, current co-morbid depression and anxiety and remitted depression or anxiety with the Chronic Pain Grade, with no depression and/or anxiety disorder as a reference category.

	CPG1[a,b]	CPG2[a,b]	CPG3[a,b]	CPG4[a,b]
	OR (95% CI)	*OR (95% CI)*	*OR (95% CI)*	*OR (95% CI)*
No psychopathology	reference	reference	reference	reference
Remitted depression/anxiety	1.87 (1.17–2.97)*	3.45 (2.02–5.87)**	3.49 (1.81–6.73)**	3.53 (1.67–7.43)*
Depression current	1.35 (0.72–2.55)	3.53 (1.76–7.08)**	7.14 (3.28–15.54)**	6.67 (2.81–15.88)**
Anxiety current	2.10 (1.25–3.54)*	4.06 (2.26–7.30)**	5.15 (2.57–10.31)**	4.84 (2.22–10.57)**
Co-morbid depression and anxiety current	3.13 (1.56–6.25)*	10.18 (4.87–21.26)**	19.72 (8.77–44.35)**	30.26 (12.68–72.23)**

*p<.05;
**p<.001.
[a]reference category is no pain.
[b]adjusted for age, gender, level of education, partner status, antidepressant use, use of other psychotropic drugs, chronic diseases, and number of depressive episodes.

participants report highly disabling and severely limiting pain (CPG4).

Association of depression and/or anxiety with the CPG

Table 3 shows results from the adjusted multinomial logistic regression analysis assessing the association of depression and/or anxiety with the CPG. The results show a significant association and the odds ratios (ORs) rise per CPG level. For all CPG levels, the ORs were significantly elevated compared to the reference group. Having a co-morbid depressive and anxiety disorder, as compared to having no disorder, showed the strongest association (OR = 30.26; 95% CI = 12.68–72.23). Also, when compared to having no depression or anxiety, there is still a high odds of having disabling pain symptoms when the depressive or anxiety disorder is remitted (CPG1: OR = 1.87; 95% CI = 1.17–2.97; CPG4: OR = 3.53; 95% CI = 1.67–7.43). However, the confidence intervals do overlap. Therefore, four sensitivity analyses were performed, each with an other psychopathology group (remitted disorder, current depressive disorder, current anxiety disorder, comorbid depression and anxiety) as a reference category, in order to examine the possible differences in associations between pain and various depressive and anxiety disorder categories (Tables 4–7). With a current depressive disorder or anxiety disorder as reference group, the results show no significant differences between these disorders on the CPG. A current anxiety disorder and a current depressive disorder also show no significant difference with a remitted disorder. Only a co-morbid depressive and anxiety disorder had a significantly higher association with the CPG compared to a remitted, current depressive, and current anxiety disorder. These findings were similar to those in the analysis with the reference group of healthy controls. The unadjusted results did not differ from the adjusted results.

Because the reference group for pain (CPG0) was small (N = 170), another sensitivity analysis was conducted where CPG0 and CPG1 were combined to form the reference category (Table 8). This analysis showed that the association between type of disorder and CPG mostly remains: as can be seen in table 8, all associations became less strong after combining CPG0 and CPG1 as a reference category, but remained significant.

Association of severity of depressive and anxiety symptoms with the CPG

Table 9 shows the association of the severity of depressive symptoms (as measured with the QIDS) and anxiety symptoms (as measured with the BAI) with the CPG. Similar to the main finding, as the severity of the depressive symptoms increases, the odds of having highly disabling and severely limiting pain increases as well. The same accounts for the association between severity of anxiety symptoms and the CPG. The unadjusted results did not differ from the adjusted results.

Table 4. Associations of presence of current depressive disorder, current anxiety disorder, current co-morbid depression and anxiety and remitted depression or anxiety with the Chronic Pain Grade, with remitted disorder as a reference category.

	CPG1[a,b]	CPG2[a,b]	CPG3[a,b]	CPG4[a,b]
	OR (95% CI)	*OR (95% CI)*	*OR (95% CI)*	*OR (95% CI)*
Remitted depression/anxiety	reference	reference	reference	reference
No psychopathology	.54 (.34–.85)*	.29 (.17–.50)**	.29 (.15–.55)**	.28 (.14–.60)*
Depression current	.72 (.39–1.36)	1.03 (.52–2.01)	2.04 (.98–4.25)	1.89 (.85–4.20)
Anxiety current	1.13 (.64–2.00)	1.18 (.64–2.18)	1.47 (.74–2.94)	1.37 (.65–2.91)
Co-morbid depression and anxiety current	1.68 (.84–3.36)	2.95 (1.43–6.09)*	5.65 (2.61–12.22)**	8.58 (3.84–19.21)**

*p<.05;
**p<.001.
[a]reference category is no pain.
[b]adjusted for age, gender, level of education, partner status, antidepressant use, use of other psychotropic drugs, chronic diseases, and number of depressive episodes.

Table 5. Associations of presence of current depressive disorder, current anxiety disorder, current co-morbid depression and anxiety and remitted depression or anxiety with the Chronic Pain Grade, with current depressive disorder as a reference category.

	CPG1[a,b]	CPG2[a,b]	CPG3[a,b]	CPG4[a,b]
	OR (95% CI)	*OR (95% CI)*	*OR (95% CI)*	*OR (95% CI)*
Depression current	reference	reference	reference	reference
No psychopathology	.74 (.39–1.40)	.28 (.14–.57)**	.14 (.0–31)**	.15 (.06–.36)**
Remitted depression/anxiety	1.38 (.74–2.59)	.98 (.50–1.91)	.49 (.24–1.02)	.53 (.24–1.17)
Anxiety current	1.56 (.79–3.05)	1.15 (.56–2.35)	.72 (.34–1.54)	.73 (.32–1.65)
Comorbid depression and anxiety current	2.31 (1.10–4.85)*	2.88 (1.34–6.21)*	2.76 (1.25–6.09)*	4.53 (2.00–10.30)**

*p<.05;
**p<.001.
[a]reference category is no pain.
[b]adjusted for age, gender, level of education, partner status, antidepressant use, use of other psychotropic drugs, chronic diseases, and number of depressive episodes.

Because the reference group for pain (CPG0) was small (N = 170), a sensitivity analysis was conducted where CPG0 and CPG1 were combined to form the reference category (table 10). This analysis showed that the association found between severity of depressive and anxiety symptoms and CPG mostly remains, with more severe depressive or anxiety symptoms being more strongly associated with more disabling and limiting pain, when CPG0 and CPG1 were combined to have a larger reference group. Here also, all associations were less strong, with some associations (especially the association of severe anxiety symptoms with the CPG2 and CPG4) remaining statistically significant, while other associations (e.g. the association of mild and moderate anxiety symptoms with CPG3) becoming non-significant.

Association of depression and/or anxiety with musculoskeletal, gastro-intestinal, and cardio respiratory pain symptoms

Table 11 shows the multinomial logistic regression analyses assessing the association of depression and/or anxiety with three clustered pain locations. For those with pain, the highest ORs are seen in co-morbid depression and anxiety. The ORs for musculoskeletal pain range from 2.28 (95% CI = 1.53–3.42) for a depressive or anxiety disorder in remission to 3.88 (95% CI = 2.33–6.47) for a co-morbid depressive and anxiety disorder. For gastro-intestinal pain, the ORs range from 1.40 (95% CI = 1.10–1.78) for a depressive or anxiety disorder in remission to 3.31 (95% CI = 2.57–4.27) for a co-morbid depressive and anxiety disorder. Cardio respiratory pain shows a range in ORs from 1.74 (95% CI = 1.27–2.40) for a depressive or anxiety disorder in remission to 5.15 (95% CI = 3.80–6.98) for co-morbid depressive and anxiety disorder. The unadjusted results did not differ from the adjusted results.

Discussion

The high proportion of participants with anxiety and depressive disorders in this study reflects the sampling strategy for including sufficient numbers of respondents to examine individuals at different stages of development and severity of depression and anxiety. This study demonstrates considerable associations between presence of depressive and anxiety disorders (current and remitted) and symptom severity with different pain dimensions, namely pain-related disability, pain intensity, and the location of pain symptoms (musculoskeletal, gastro-intestinal, and cardio respiratory).

Presence and severity of depressive or anxiety disorder

Our results show that having a mood or anxiety disorder increases the odds of highly disabling and severely limiting pain. Also, the severity of the depressive and anxiety symptoms are significantly associated with pain-related disability and limiting

Table 6. Associations of presence of current depressive disorder, current anxiety disorder, current co-morbid depression and anxiety and remitted depression or anxiety with the Chronic Pain Grade, with current anxiety disorder as a reference category.

	CPG1[a,b]	CPG2[a,b]	CPG3[a,b]	CPG4[a,b]
	OR (95% CI)	*OR (95% CI)*	*OR (95% CI)*	*OR (95% CI)*
Anxiety current	reference	reference	reference	reference
No psychopathology	.48 (.28–.80)*	.25 (.14–.44)**	.19 (.10–.39)**	.21 (.10–.45)**
Remitted depression/anxiety	.89 (.450–1.57)	.85 (.46–1.57)	.68 (.34–1.35)	.73 (.34–1.54)
Depression current	.64 (.33–1.26)	.87 (.43–1.78)	1.39 (.65–2.97)	1.38 (.61–3.13)
Comorbid depression and anxiety current	1.49 (.72–3.06)	2.51 (1.18–5.30)*	3.83 (1.74–8.42)*	6.25 (2.76–14.15)**

*p<.05;
**p<.001.
[a]reference category is no pain.
[b]adjusted for age, gender, level of education, partner status, antidepressant use, use of other psychotropic drugs, chronic diseases, and number of depressive episodes.

Table 7. Associations of presence of current depressive disorder, current anxiety disorder, current co-morbid depression and anxiety and remitted depression or anxiety with the Chronic Pain Grade, with comorbid depressive- and anxiety disorder as a reference category.

	CPG1[a,b]	CPG2[a,b]	CPG3[a,b]	CPG4[a,b]
	OR (95% CI)	*OR (95% CI)*	*OR (95% CI)*	*OR (95% CI)*
Comorbid depression and anxiety current	reference	reference	reference	reference
No psychopathology	.32 (.16–.64)*	.10 (.05–.21)**	.05 (.02–.11)**	.03 (.01–.08)**
Remitted depression/anxiety	.60 (.30–1.20)	.34 (.16–.70)*	.18 (.08–.38)**	.12 (.05–.26)**
Depression current	.43 (.21–.91)*	.35 (.16–.75)*	.36 (.16-.80)*	.22 (.10–.50)**
Anxiety current	.67 (.33–1.39)	.40 (.19–.85)*	.26 (.12–.57)*	.16 (.07–.36)**

*p<.05;
**p<.001.
[a]reference category is no pain.
[b]adjusted for age, gender, level of education, partner status, antidepressant use, use of other psychotropic drugs, chronic diseases, and number of depressive episodes.

pain, with more severe symptoms having higher odds for highly disabling and severely limiting pain.

Depressive and anxiety disorders may add to pain as they increase the likelihood of social isolation, increased attention towards threat and avoidance of physical exertion [11,12,16,17]. Depression and anxiety disorders also share the same pathophysiological pathways as pain [43–45]. They facilitate the central modulation of the pain response, in the periaqueductal gray, amygdala, and hypothalamus [1,13,14], and when deficits occur in these areas, modulation of signals from the body are disturbed, leading to a more severe experience of pain. Although these brain areas all play a role in depression, anxiety, and pain, not every individual responds the same to pain stimuli [46–48]. Some individuals are more sensitive to pain than others. The use of EEG may help in identifying neuronal markers for sensitivity to pain [46], and whether there are differences between depressive and anxious individuals. Furthermore, depression and anxiety induce stress and increases the production of pro-inflammatory cytokines [49–51], which may increase pain [52,53]. The finding showing higher pain-related disability in co-morbid depression and anxiety in our study is similar to findings from the STAR*D studies [54–56].

Depressive or anxiety disorder in remission

Regarding the association of a remitted disorder and pain, we expected persons with remitted depression or anxiety to have similar pain symptoms as controls without depression or anxiety. However, this is not the case. Persons with a remitted depressive or anxiety disorder still showed high odds on the pain outcomes when compared to those that have no such disorder. This is remarkable, because this means that having a remitted disorder is not the same as having no disorder with regards to pain. This raises several questions.

First, pain symptoms may be residual symptoms in depressive and anxiety disorder. This finding may suggest that pain in patients with remitted depressive or anxiety disorder might be indicative of a risk for recurrence, as disability in life (e.g. disability to fulfil his or her role at home) is an important risk factor for the recurrence of anxiety disorders [57], and our results show that those with a remitted diagnosis still have high odds of having pain symptoms and pain-related disability.

Another explanation for the high odds of pain symptoms in remitted depression or anxiety might be that treatment, if it was provided, for the depressive or anxiety disorder is not effective for pain symptoms, or treatment should be different when pain is co-morbid with the depressive or anxiety disorder. For example, it has been suggested that patients with depression and pain are a

Table 8. (Results from sensitivity analysis, with CPG0 and CPG1 combined) Associations of presence of current depressive disorder, current anxiety disorder, current co-morbid depression and anxiety and remitted depression or anxiety with the Chronic Pain Grade, with no depression and/or anxiety disorder as a reference category.

	CPG2[a,b]	CPG3[a,b]	CPG4[a,b]
	OR (95% CI)	*OR (95% CI)*	*OR (95% CI)*
No psychopathology	reference	reference	reference
Remitted depression/anxiety	1.99 (1.45–2.73)**	2.01 (1.22–3.30)*	2.03 (1.10–3.73)*
Depression current	2.78 (1.93–4.01)**	5.61 (3.39–9.29)**	5.23 (2.77–9.85)**
Anxiety current	2.09 (1.50–2.92)**	2.65 (1.61–4.35)**	2.48 (1.34–4.59)*
Comorbid depression and anxiety current	3.63 (2.61–5.04)**	7.01 (4.38–11.23)**	10.72 (6.07–18.96)**

*p<.05;
**p<.001.
[a]reference category is no pain.
[b]adjusted for age, gender, level of education, partner status, antidepressant use, use of other psychotropic drugs, chronic diseases, and number of depressive episodes.

Table 9. Association of severity of depressive symptoms and anxiety symptoms with the Chronic Pain Grade.

		CPG1[a,b]	CPG2[a,b]	CPG3[a,b]	CPG4[a,b]
		OR (95% CI)	*OR (95% CI)*	*OR (95% CI)*	*OR (95% CI)*
QIDS[b]	None	reference	reference	reference	reference
	Mild	2.59 (1.55–4.34)**	3.72 (2.13–6.49)**	3.99 (2.13–7.49)**	4.05 (1.99–8.23)**
	Moderate	1.10 (0.59–2.02)	1.56 (.91–3.40)	3.32 (1.62–6.80)*	2.91 (1.31–6.48)*
	(Very) Severe	1.11 (.43–2.87)	2.18 (.81–5.87)	4.66 (1.65–13.16)*	7.93 (2.70–23.35)**
BAI[c]	Normal	reference	reference	reference	reference
	Mild	1.76 (.59–12.51)	2.41 (1.36–4.29)*	2.66 (1.42–4.97)*	3.07 (1.54–6.12)*
	Moderate	2.23 (.99–5.03)	4.22 (1.82–9.79)*	3.89 (1.60–9.45)*	6.69 (2.66–16.84)**
	Severe	2.73 (1.02–3.02)*	6.70 (1.44–31.20)*	8.29 (1.73–39.59)*	13.32 (2.73–64.97)*

*p<.05;
**p<.001.
[a]reference category is no pain.
[b]adjusted for age, gender, level of education, partner status, chronic diseases, antidepressant use, use of other psychotropic drugs, number of depressive episodes, and severity of anxiety symptoms.
[c]adjusted for age, gender, level of education, partner status, chronic diseases, antidepressant use, use of other psychotropic drugs, number of depressive episodes, and severity of depressive symptoms.

distinctively other group of patients than those with depression without pain, with the former having a focus on health and the latter having a focus on a negative view of the self [58,59]. If that is the case, the treatment should be different for depressive disorder with pain and depressive disorder without pain. The same could possibly apply to patients with an anxiety disorder with or without pain. This finding warrants further research, to examine if having a depressive or anxiety disorder in remission may be a possible risk factor for subsequent long lasting chronic pain.

Pain location

Of the total sample, 92.4% reported pain symptoms of musculoskeletal nature, followed by 48% reporting gastro-intestinal pain and 25.6% of cardio respiratory pain. Because musculoskeletal pain has by far the highest prevalence in this study, we expected that this pain location would have the highest association with depression and anxiety. However, this expectation was not confirmed. Our findings show that those with a current depressive disorder or a remitted depressive or anxiety disorder have high odds for having musculoskeletal pain, but the odds for having pain of cardio respiratory origin are also large when compared to having no depressive or anxiety disorder. Furthermore, persons having a current anxiety or co-morbid depressive and anxiety disorder show high odds for having cardio respiratory pain. These findings remain after adjustment for chronic cardio respiratory illness.

In a review by Celano & Huffman [60], depressive disorder was associated with cardiac disease, such as coronary artery disease. This also applies to anxiety which appears to be a risk factor for coronary heart disease and cardiac mortality [61]. The finding

Table 10. (Results of sensitivity analysis, with CPG0 and CPG1 combined) Association of severity of depressive symptoms and anxiety symptoms with the Chronic Pain Grade.

		CPG2[a,b]	CPG3[a,b]	CPG4[a,b]
		OR (95% CI)	*OR (95% CI)*	*OR (95% CI)*
QIDS[b]	None	reference	reference	reference
	Mild	1.55 (1.18–2.02)*	1.65 (1.11–2.46)*	1.67 (1.00–2.80)*
	Moderate	1.67 (1.21–2.33)*	3.14 (2.04–4.83)**	2.75 (1.58–4.78)**
	(Very) Severe	2.05 (1.36–3.09)*	4.37 (2.61–7.33)**	7.42 (4.08–13.649)**
BAI[c]	Normal	reference	reference	reference
	Mild	1.42 (1.09–1.85)*	1.57 (1.09–2.24)*	1.81 (1.14–2.87)*
	Moderate	1.99 (1.44–2.75)**	1.83 (1.19–2.81)*	3.15 (1.91–5.19)**
	Severe	2.59 (1.63–4.13)**	3.12 (1.86–5.53)**	5.16 (2.83–9.41)**

*p<.05;
**p<.001.
[a]reference category is no pain.
[b]adjusted for age, gender, level of education, partner status, chronic diseases, antidepressant use, use of other psychotropic drugs, number of depressive episodes, and severity of anxiety symptoms.
[c]adjusted for age, gender, level of education, partner status, chronic diseases, antidepressant use, use of other psychotropic drugs, number of depressive episodes, and severity of depressive symptoms.

Table 11. Associations of remitted psychopathology, current depressive disorder, current anxiety disorder, and current co-morbid depression and anxiety with pain location, with no depression and/or anxiety as reference category.

	No pain[a]	Musculoskeletal[a]	Gastro-intestinal[a]	Cardio respiratory[a]
	OR (95% CI)	*OR (95% CI)*	*OR (95% CI)*	*OR (95% CI)*
No psychopathology	reference	reference	reference	reference
Remitted depression/anxiety	.47 (.30–.75)*	2.28 (1.53–3.42)**	1.40 (1.10–1.78)*	1.74 (1.27–2.40)*
Depression current	.52 (.28–.97)*	2.64 (1.53–4.56)**	2.43 (1.84–3.22)**	2.63 (1.86–3.70)**
Anxiety current	.39 (.24–.66)**	2.29 (1.49–3.51)**	2.08 (1.61–2.68)**	2.96 (2.16–4.04)**
Co-morbid depression and anxiety current	.19 (.10–.38)**	3.88 (2.33–6.47)**	3.31 (2.57–4.27)**	5.15 (3.80–6.98)**

*p<.05;
**p<.001.
a = adjusted for age, gender, level of education, partner status, antidepressant use, use of other psychotropic drugs, number of depressive episodes, and chronic disease.

that anxiety shows such high odds for cardio respiratory pain symptoms, even when we controlled for cardio respiratory disease, could be due to the fact that anxious patients with chest pain are more sensitive to bodily sensations [62]; in that case, the experience of pain would be centrally modulated in such a way as to elevate the odds for experiencing pain. However, another explanation might be possible as well; stress induced anxiety has an elevating effect on cytokines [49], and elevated cytokines lead to pain symptoms. This might explain our findings.

In the STAR*D study, depressed patients (with less sleep quality and sympathetic arousal) showed an association with higher cardiac risk, which may be similar to our findings [63] whereby having a depressive disorder had higher odds for having cardio respiratory pain when compared to having no depressive or anxiety disorder. Even when we controlled for having a chronic disease of cardio respiratory origin, the association remained strong and significant. Previous research showed that having a mental illness is a possible risk factor for cardiovascular disease [64,65]. Our finding that a depression/anxiety, whether or not in remission, shows a strong association with cardiac pain is worth exploring in further longitudinal research to explore a possible causal relation of depression and/or anxiety (current or in remission) with cardiac disease, of which cardio respiratory pain might be an early indicator.

Strengths of the study

A strength of this study is the large sample size. Also, because patients with a depressive or anxiety disorder often report pain in multiple locations, the categorisation of pain locations makes these results clinically relevant and widely applicable. Moreover, this study not only examines the association of pain with depressive or anxiety disorder, but also with co-morbid depression and anxiety, as well as with remitted disorders. Additionally, in the analyses of the pain symptoms, the no pain group was the reference category which is new compared to earlier studies that compared low pain with high pain – which is subject to interpretation bias as pain is a subjective experience. In our study, we had a healthy control group with no pain in which better contrasts could be made with those who had pain.

Limitations

This study also has some limitations. First, it is not possible to make inferences about causality because this was a cross-sectional observational study. Second, some of the subgroups of our sample were smaller than the other groups, such as those with no pain symptoms (CPG0, N = 170). However, a sensitivity analysis revealed that the association between severity of depressive and anxiety symptoms and CPG mostly remains, with more severe depressive or anxiety symptoms being more strongly associated with more disabling and limiting pain when CPG0 and CPG1 were combined to have a larger reference group. Therefore, these associations can be considered valid and of clinical relevance as they indicate a clear difference in association with depression or anxiety between patients with and without pain. Another possible limitation is the self-reporting of physical illness, which might lead to overreporting or underreporting of chronic physical illness; however, a study by Kriegsman et al. [66] shows that patients report their physical illness fairly accurately when compared to the reports of their general practitioner, even when taking depressive symptomatology into account. Furthermore, no information was available whether a physical illness was organic or functional, which may have its effect on pain. For example, individuals with an organic disease describe their pain as consistent, whereas those without an organic disease describe their pain as variable and diffuse [67]. Also, PTSD has been linked to increased risk for pain [68,69]. Therefore, future research that examines the association of anxiety disorders with pain should also include PTSD.

Conclusion

This study shows that depressive and anxiety disorders have a similar and very strong association with the CPG (which includes pain-related disability and pain intensity) and musculoskeletal pain, cardio respiratory pain, and gastro-intestinal pain compared to a control group without depressive or anxiety disorder. Depression and anxiety share the same pathophysiological pathways as pain and can have a reciprocal effect on each other, which could explain these associations. Moreover, even a remitted disorder has a strong association with pain. This might mean that patients with depression or anxiety and pain are a different group and need different treatment than patients that do not have pain accompanying their depression or anxiety. Depression and anxiety also have a strong association with cardio respiratory pain, and this association remained after correction for cardiovascular or respiratory illness. This strong association between depression/anxiety (current or in remission) with cardio respiratory pain is an interesting finding, which warrants further longitudinal research to examine a possible causal relation of cardiac pain and a mental disorder (current or in remission) with cardiac disease.

Author Contributions

Conceived and designed the experiments: BWJHP ATFB PS HWJM. Performed the experiments: BWJHP ATFB PS HWJM. Analyzed the data: EH MMJGG BWJHP HWJM MWMW PS. Contributed reagents/materials/analysis tools: BWJHP ATFB PS HWJM. Contributed to the writing of the manuscript: EH MMJGG ATFB JD BWJHP HWJM MWMW PS CMFC.

References

1. Bair MJ, Robinson RL, Katon W, Kroenke K (2003) Depression and pain comorbidity: a literature review. Arch Intern Med 163: 2433–2445.
2. Demyttenaere K, Bruffaerts R, Lee S, Posada-Villa J, Kovess V, et al. (2007) Mental disorders among persons with chronic back or neck pain: results from the World Mental Health Surveys. Pain 129: 332–342.
3. Gureje O, Von Korff M, Kola L, Demyttenaere K, He Y, et al. (2008) The relation between multiple pains and mental disorders: results from the World Mental Health Surveys. Pain 135: 82–91.
4. Gureje O, Von Korff M, Simon GE, Gater R (1998) Persistent pain and well-being: a World Health Organization Study in Primary Care. JAMA 280: 147–151.
5. Means-Christensen AJ, Roy-Byrne PP, Sherbourne CD, Craske MG, Stein MB (2008) Relationships among pain, anxiety, and depression in primary care. Depress Anxiety 25: 593–600.
6. Stahl S, Briley M (2004) Understanding pain in depression. Hum Psychopharmacol 19: S9–S13.
7. Wise TN, Fishbain DA, Holder-Perkins V (2007) Painful physical symptoms in depression: a clinical challenge. Pain Med 8: S75–82.
8. Burloux G, Forestier P, Dalery J, Guyotat J (1989) Chronic pain and posttraumatic stress disorders. Psychother Psychosom 52: 119–124.
9. Ayuso Mateos JL, Bayon Perez C, Santo-Domingo Carrasco J, Olivares D (1989) Atypical chest pain and panic disorder. Psychother Psychosom 52: 92–95.
10. Ohayon MM, Schatzberg AF (2003) Using chronic pain to predict depressive morbidity in the general population. Arch Gen Psychiatry 60: 39–47.
11. Saito T, Kai I, Takizawa A (2012) Effects of a program to prevent social isolation on loneliness, depression, and subjective well-being of older adults: a randomized trial among older migrants in Japan. Arch Gerontol Geriatr 55: 539–547.
12. Jang Y, Haley WE, Small BJ, Mortimer JA (2002) The role of mastery and social resources in the associations between disability and depression in later life. Gerontologist 42: 807–813.
13. Ossipov MH, Dussor GO, Porreca F (2010) Central modulation of pain. J Clin Invest 120: 3779–3787.
14. Millan MJ (2002) Descending control of pain. Prog Neurobiol 66: 355–474.
15. Vlaeyen JW, Linton SJ (2000) Fear-avoidance and its consequences in chronic musculoskeletal pain: a state of the art. Pain 85: 317–332.
16. Asmundson GJ, Katz J (2009) Understanding the co-occurrence of anxiety disorders and chronic pain: state-of-the-art. Depress Anxiety 26: 888–901.
17. Sareen J, Cox BJ, Clara I, Asmundson GJ (2005) The relationship between anxiety disorders and physical disorders in the U.S. National Comorbidity Survey. Depress Anxiety 21: 193–202.
18. McWilliams LA, Cox BJ, Enns MW (2003) Mood and anxiety disorders associated with chronic pain: an examination in a nationally representative sample. Pain 106: 127–133.
19. Beesdo K, Jacobi F, Hoyer J, Low NC, Hofler M, et al. (2010) Pain associated with specific anxiety and depressive disorders in a nationally representative population sample. Soc Psychiatry Psychiatr Epidemiol 45: 89–104.
20. Gerhardt A, Hartmann M, Schuller-Roma B, Blumenstiel K, Bieber C, et al. (2011) The prevalence and type of Axis-I and Axis-II mental disorders in subjects with non-specific chronic back pain: results from a population-based study. Pain Med 12: 1231–1240.
21. Gerrits MM, Vogelzangs N, van Oppen P, van Marwijk HW, van der Horst H, et al. (2012) Impact of pain on the course of depressive and anxiety disorders. Pain 153: 429–436.
22. Papakostas GI, Petersen T, Denninger J, Sonawalla SB, Mahal Y, et al. (2003) Somatic symptoms in treatment-resistant depression. Psychiatry Res 118: 39–45.
23. Teh CF, Morone NE, Karp JF, Belnap BH, Zhu F, et al. (2009) Pain interference impacts response to treatment for anxiety disorders. Depress Anxiety 26: 222–228.
24. Karp JF, Scott J, Houck P, Reynolds CF 3rd, Kupfer DJ, et al. (2005) Pain predicts longer time to remission during treatment of recurrent depression. J Clin Psychiatry 66: 591–597.
25. Gilkey DP, Keefe TJ, Peel JL, Kassab OM, Kennedy CA (2010) Risk factors associated with back pain: a cross-sectional study of 963 college students. J Manipulative Physiol Ther 33: 88–95.
26. Janwantanakul P, Sitthipornvorakul E, Paksaichol A (2012) Risk factors for the onset of nonspecific low back pain in office workers: a systematic review of prospective cohort studies. J Manipulative Physiol Ther 35: 568–577.
27. Kindler LL, Jones KD, Perrin N, Bennett RM (2010) Risk factors predicting the development of widespread pain from chronic back or neck pain. J Pain 11: 1320–1328.
28. Croft PR, Lewis M, Papageorgiou AC, Thomas E, Jayson MI, et al. (2001) Risk factors for neck pain: a longitudinal study in the general population. Pain 93: 317–325.
29. Wessely S, Nimnuan C, Sharpe M (1999) Functional somatic syndromes: one or many? Lancet 354: 936–939.
30. Nimnuan C, Hotopf M, Wessely S (2001) Medically unexplained symptoms: an epidemiological study in seven specialities. J Psychosom Res 51: 361–367.
31. Fink P, Toft T, Hansen MS, Ornbol E, Olesen F (2007) Symptoms and syndromes of bodily distress: an exploratory study of 978 internal medical, neurological, and primary care patients. Psychosom Med 69: 30–39.
32. Lucchetti G, Oliveira AB, Mercante JP, Peres MF (2012) Anxiety and fear-avoidance in musculoskeletal pain. Curr Pain Headache Rep 16: 399–406.
33. Walter SA, Jones MP, Talley NJ, Kjellstrom L, Nyhlin H, et al. (2013) Abdominal pain is associated with anxiety and depression scores in a sample of the general adult population with no signs of organic gastrointestinal disease. Neurogastroenterol Motil 25: 741–e576.
34. Shahid M, Rehmani R, Khan MM (2004) Anxiety and depression among young adults with chest pain. J Coll Physicians Surg Pak 14: 700.
35. Penninx BW, Beekman AT, Smit JH, Zitman FG, Nolen WA, et al. (2008) The Netherlands Study of Depression and Anxiety (NESDA): rationale, objectives and methods. Int J Methods Psychiatr Res 17: 121–140.
36. Wittchen HU (1994) Reliability and validity studies of the WHO–Composite International Diagnostic Interview (CIDI): a critical review. J Psychiatr Res 28: 57–84.
37. Von Korff M, Ormel J, Keefe FJ, Dworkin SF (1992) Grading the severity of chronic pain. Pain 50: 133–149.
38. Smith BH, Penny KI, Purves AM, Munro C, Wilson B, et al. (1997) The Chronic Pain Grade questionnaire: validation and reliability in postal research. Pain 71: 141–147.
39. Rush AJ, Trivedi MH, Ibrahim HM, Carmody TJ, Arnow B, et al. (2003) The 16-Item Quick Inventory of Depressive Symptomatology (QIDS), clinician rating (QIDS-C), and self-report (QIDS-SR): a psychometric evaluation in patients with chronic major depression. Biol Psychiatry 54: 573–583.
40. Rush AJ, Gullion CM, Basco MR, Jarrett RB, Trivedi MH (1996) The Inventory of Depressive Symptomatology (IDS): psychometric properties. Psychol Med 26: 477–486.
41. Beck AT, Epstein N, Brown G, Steer RA (1988) An inventory for measuring clinical anxiety: psychometric properties. J Consult Clin Psychol 56: 893–897.
42. Kabacoff RI, Segal DL, Hersen M, Van Hasselt VB (1997) Psychometric properties and diagnostic utility of the Beck Anxiety Inventory and the State-Trait Anxiety Inventory with older adult psychiatric outpatients. J Anxiety Disord 11: 33–47.
43. Bair MJ, Robinson RL, Eckert GJ, Stang PE, Croghan TW, et al. (2004) Impact of pain on depression treatment response in primary care. Psychosom Med 66: 17–22.
44. Campbell LC, Clauw DJ, Keefe FJ (2003) Persistent pain and depression: a biopsychosocial perspective. Biol Psychiatry 54: 399–409.
45. Maes M, Yirmyia R, Noraberg J, Brene S, Hibbeln J, et al. (2009) The inflammatory & neurodegenerative (I&ND) hypothesis of depression: leads for future research and new drug developments in depression. Metab Brain Dis 24: 27–53.
46. Schulz E, Zherdin A, Tiemann L, Plant C, Ploner M (2012) Decoding an individual's sensitivity to pain from the multivariate analysis of EEG data. Cereb Cortex 22: 1118–1123.
47. Mogil JS (1999) The genetic mediation of individual differences in sensitivity to pain and its inhibition. Proc Natl Acad Sci U S A 96: 7744–7751.
48. Ziv M, Tomer R, Defrin R, Hendler T (2010) Individual sensitivity to pain expectancy is related to differential activation of the hippocampus and amygdala. Hum Brain Mapp 31: 326–338.
49. Maes M, Song C, Lin A, De Jongh R, Van Gastel A, et al. (1998) The effects of psychological stress on humans: increased production of pro-inflammatory cytokines and a Th1-like response in stress-induced anxiety. Cytokine 10: 313–318.
50. Felger JC, Lotrich FE (2013) Inflammatory cytokines in depression: neurobiological mechanisms and therapeutic implications. Neuroscience 246: 199–229.
51. Sharpley CF, Agnew LL (2011) Cytokines and depression: findings, issues, and treatment implications. Rev Neurosci 22: 295–302.
52. de Oliveira CM, Sakata RK, Issy AM, Gerola LR, Salomao R (2011) Cytokines and pain. Rev Bras Anestesiol 61: 255–259, 260–255, 137–242.
53. Shubayev VI, Kato K, Myers RR (2010) Cytokines in Pain. In: Kruger L, Light AR, editors. Translational Pain Research: From Mouse to Man. Boca Raton, FL: Llc.
54. Fava M, Alpert JE, Carmin CN, Wisniewski SR, Trivedi MH, et al. (2004) Clinical correlates and symptom patterns of anxious depression among patients with major depressive disorder in STAR*D. Psychol Med 34: 1299–1308.
55. Fava M, Rush AJ, Alpert JE, Carmin CN, Balasubramani GK, et al. (2006) What clinical and symptom features and comorbid disorders characterize outpatients with anxious major depressive disorder: a replication and extension. Can J Psychiatry 51: 823–835.

56. Fava M, Rush AJ, Alpert JE, Balasubramani GK, Wisniewski SR, et al. (2008) Difference in treatment outcome in outpatients with anxious versus nonanxious depression: a STAR*D report. Am J Psychiatry 165: 342–351.
57. Scholten WD, Batelaan NM, van Balkom AJ, Wjh Penninx B, Smit JH, et al. (2013) Recurrence of anxiety disorders and its predictors. J Affect Disord 147: 180–185.
58. Pincus T, Williams A (1999) Models and measurements of depression in chronic pain. J Psychosom Res 47: 211–219.
59. Tossani E (2013) The concept of mental pain. Psychother Psychosom 82: 67–73.
60. Celano CM, Huffman JC (2011) Depression and cardiac disease: a review. Cardiol Rev 19: 130–142.
61. Roest AM, Martens EJ, de Jonge P, Denollet J (2010) Anxiety and risk of incident coronary heart disease: a meta-analysis. J Am Coll Cardiol 56: 38–46.
62. Cheng C, Wong WM, Lai KC, Wong BC, Hu WH, et al. (2003) Psychosocial factors in patients with noncardiac chest pain. Psychosom Med 65: 443–449.
63. Fraguas R Jr, Iosifescu DV, Alpert J, Wisniewski SR, Barkin JL, et al. (2007) Major depressive disorder and comorbid cardiac disease: is there a depressive subtype with greater cardiovascular morbidity? Results from the STAR*D study. Psychosomatics 48: 418–425.
64. Gladigau EL, Fazio TN, Hannam JP, Dawson LM, Jones SG (2014) Increased cardiovascular risk in patients with severe mental illness. Intern Med J 44: 65–69.
65. Nielsen TJ, Vestergaard M, Christensen B, Christensen KS, Larsen KK (2013) Mental health status and risk of new cardiovascular events or death in patients with myocardial infarction: a population-based cohort study. BMJ Open 3.
66. Kriegsman DM, Penninx BW, van Eijk JT, Boeke AJ, Deeg DJ (1996) Self-reports and general practitioner information on the presence of chronic diseases in community dwelling elderly. A study on the accuracy of patients' self-reports and on determinants of inaccuracy. J Clin Epidemiol 49: 1407–1417.
67. Leavitt F, Garron DC, D'Angelo CM, McNeill TW (1979) Low back pain in patients with and without demonstrable organic disease. Pain 6: 191–200.
68. Beck JG, Clapp JD (2011) A different kind of co-morbidity: Understanding posttraumatic stress disorder and chronic pain. Psychol Trauma 3: 101–108.
69. Roth RS, Geisser ME, Bates R (2008) The relation of post-traumatic stress symptoms to depression and pain in patients with accident-related chronic pain. J Pain 9: 588–596.

9

Suprathreshold Heat Pain Response Predicts Activity-Related Pain, but Not Rest-Related Pain, in an Exercise-Induced Injury Model

Rogelio A. Coronado[1]*, Corey B. Simon[1], Carolina Valencia[2], Jeffrey J. Parr[3], Paul A. Borsa[4], Steven Z. George[1,5]*

1 Department of Physical Therapy, University of Florida, Gainesville, Florida, United States of America, **2** Department of Applied Medicine and Rehabilitation, Indiana State University, Terra Haute, Indiana, Unites States of America, **3** Department of Sports Medicine and Nutrition, University of Pittsburgh, Pittsburgh, Pennsylvania, United States of America, **4** Department of Applied Physiology and Kinesiology, University of Florida, Gainesville, Florida, United States of America, **5** Center for Pain Research and Behavioral Health, University of Florida, Gainesville, Florida, United States of America

Abstract

Exercise-induced injury models are advantageous for studying pain since the onset of pain is controlled and both pre-injury and post-injury factors can be utilized as explanatory variables or predictors. In these studies, rest-related pain is often considered the primary dependent variable or outcome, as opposed to a measure of activity-related pain. Additionally, few studies include pain sensitivity measures as predictors. In this study, we examined the influence of pre-injury and post-injury factors, including pain sensitivity, for induced rest and activity-related pain following exercise induced muscle injury. The overall goal of this investigation was to determine if there were convergent or divergent predictors of rest and activity-related pain. One hundred forty-three participants provided demographic, psychological, and pain sensitivity information and underwent a standard fatigue trial of resistance exercise to induce injury of the dominant shoulder. Pain at rest and during active and resisted shoulder motion were measured at 48- and 96-hours post-injury. Separate hierarchical models were generated for assessing the influence of pre-injury and post-injury factors on 48- and 96-hour rest-related and activity-related pain. Overall, we did not find a universal predictor of pain across all models. However, pre-injury and post-injury suprathreshold heat pain response (SHPR), a pain sensitivity measure, was a consistent predictor of activity-related pain, even after controlling for known psychological factors. These results suggest there is differential prediction of pain. A measure of pain sensitivity such as SHPR appears more influential for activity-related pain, but not rest-related pain, and may reflect different underlying processes involved during pain appraisal.

Editor: Ruth Landau, University of Washington, United States of America

Funding: Funding for this study was received by a NIAMS/NIH grant AR055899. RAC was supported by NIH T32 Interdisciplinary Training in Rehabilitation and Neuromuscular Plasticity grant (5T32HDO43730). CBS was supported in part by the NIH/NCATS Clinical and Translational Science Awards to the University of Florida (TL1 TR000066 and UL1 TR000064). The funders had no role in study design, data collection and analysis, decision to publish, or preparation of the manuscript.

Competing Interests: The authors have declared that no competing interests exist.

* Email: rogelio.coronado@vanderbilt.edu (RAC); szgeorge@phhp.ufl.edu (SZG)

Introduction

Pain ratings are commonly queried during the assessment of individuals with musculoskeletal pain. In clinical studies, current or rest-related pain intensity is most often assessed [1], while pain ratings with specific activity (e.g., activity-related pain) are less frequently reported. A recent systematic review of post-surgical trials by Srikandarajah and Gilron [2] found that only 39% (281/726) of published trials included a measurement of activity-related pain as a clinical outcome. Failure to include a measure of activity-related pain is noteworthy as activity-related pain may have a stronger association with functional limitations, or greater sensitivity in assessing therapeutic response, than measures of rest-related pain [3,4].

Differentiating rest and activity-related pain can be difficult in clinical studies. Exercise-induced injury models may better control comparisons of rest and activity-related pain. In a study by Dannecker and Sluka [5], the authors showed that following eccentric exercise for the elbow flexors, higher pain ratings occurred with elbow extension than at rest. This study is relevant as it suggests exercise-induced injury models can induce higher levels of pain dependent on activity, and may be appropriate models for studying the prediction of rest and activity-related pain.

Predictive models have been generated to determine which factors influence pain outcomes following exercise-induced injury [6–9]. Similar to clinical studies, most exercise-induced injury studies focus on predicting rest-related pain rather than activity-related pain. Factors shown to be predictive of rest-related pain are predominantly psychological in nature, such as pain catastrophizing [9,10]. However, current limitations in the prediction of pain following exercise-induced injury are twofold. First, it is unclear whether psychological factors are predictors of activity-related pain. Second, measures of pain sensitivity have not been widely considered within predictive models for pain following exercise-induced injury [6,7]. Pain sensitivity measures are thought to reflect pain processing within the nervous system and are receiving attention as potential prognostic variables [11,12]. Pain sensitivity can potentially improve prediction models that already include psychological factors and, therefore, may allow better evaluation of different processes relevant to the perception of rest or activity-related pain. Furthermore, pain sensitivity, if found to be an important predictor, could be considered a relevant factor to include in clinical assessment, especially as it is not commonly assessed in a clinical context [13].

Thus, further investigation is needed to ascertain the influence pain sensitivity has on an individual's pain perception at rest or during activity. Specifically, we sought primarily to assess the predictive ability of 1) baseline, pre-injury pain sensitivity on post-injury rest and activity-related pain at 48 and 96-hours and 2) 48-hours post-injury pain sensitivity on post-injury rest and activity-related pain at 96-hours. We used an exercise-induced injury model in a group of healthy volunteers, as these models are standardized induced-pain methods to study the development and progression of chronic pain. In these models, the overall pain experience is shorter in duration, yet generates similar pain and impairment characteristics observed in clinical pain conditions [14–16]. Moreover, the influence of both pre-injury (e.g., pre-clinical) and post-injury (e.g., clinical) factors on the painful episode can be examined as the onset of injury is controlled within the model. We hypothesized that pain sensitivity factors would be predictive of rest and activity-related pain, even after controlling for psychological factors. We did not have a specific hypothesis on a differential influence of pain sensitivity on pain outcome.

Materials and Methods

Ethics Statement

This study was approved by the University of Florida Institutional Review Board. Prior to enrollment, all participants provided written informed consent.

Participants

Participants were recruited from the campus of the University of Florida and the surrounding community. All participants were between the ages of 18 and 85 years old and not performing strength training exercises for the upper extremity either currently or during the previous 6 weeks. Participants were not included if they 1) were currently experiencing neck or shoulder pain, 2) had neurological impairments of the upper extremity, such as loss of sensation, muscle weakness, or reflex changes, 3) were currently taking pain medication, or 4) had previous shoulder surgery.

Procedure

After providing written informed consent at the initial assessment session, all participants completed standardized questionnaires and underwent pain sensitivity testing. Testing was conducted in the same private laboratory environment controlled for room temperature and humidity, and where distractions were minimized. Next, participants performed an eccentric exercise protocol on their dominant shoulder to induce pain [8] using a Kin-Com isokinetic dynamometer (Chattanooga Group, Chattanooga, TN). Participants were seated according to manufacturer's recommendations and straps were affixed across the torso to minimize trunk motion. The dominant shoulder was placed in a standardized position within the scapular plane. After determining maximum voluntary isometric contraction (MVIC) for each individual, participants completed repetitions of isokinetic concentric/eccentric external rotation actions to induce shoulder pain. Specifically, participants performed a standard bout of 3 sets of 10 repetitions at 60°/sec with a goal of fatiguing participants so they generated 50% or less of their initial MVIC. If necessary, additional repetitions (e.g., 1 set of 8 repetitions) were performed until the standard fatigue level was reached. After completing the initial session which lasted approximately one hour, participants were then scheduled for 2 follow-up sessions. Follow-up sessions occurred at 48- and 96-hours after the initial session, where repeat measurements of psychological variables, pain sensitivity, and outcome occurred at 48-hours and outcome alone at 96-hours.

Measures

Demographics. Demographic information included age, sex, height, weight, and dominant arm. Height and weight information were used to compute body mass index (BMI) as a covariate for exercise-induced injury.

Shoulder Pain Intensity. Using a 101-point numeric pain rating scale (0 = "no pain," 100 = "worst pain imaginable"), participants verbally indicated their intensity of shoulder pain [17]. Shoulder pain intensity was asked during three states: 1) at rest (e.g., upper extremity held at side); 2) during active motion (e.g., shoulder abduction); 3) during isometric activation (e.g., resisted external rotation).

Pain Catastrophizing. Pain catastrophizing was assessed using the Pain Catastrophizing Scale (PCS) as this variable has been shown to influence pain-related outcomes [9,18,19]. The PCS is a 13-item questionnaire (score ranges from 0 to 52) that measures thoughts on various pain experiences where higher scores reflect higher levels of pain catastrophizing [20].

Fear of Movement. Fear of movement was assessed using the shortened version of the Tampa Scale of Kinesiophobia (TSK-11) and has shown to be associated with shoulder injury outcome [21,22]. The TSK-11 is a 17-item questionnaire (score ranges from 11 to 44) that measures fear of movement where higher scores reflect higher levels of fear of movement [23].

Pressure Pain Threshold. Pressure pain threshold (PPT) was measured at the tip of the acromion of the dominant shoulder using a hand-held algometer (Pain Diagnostics & Treatment, Great Neck, NY) with a 1 cm^2 diameter probe. PPT is a single stimulus threshold measure of static pain sensitivity, and is commonly used in laboratory and clinical research trials [24]. Our assessment of PPT for the shoulder undergoing exercise-induced injury is a marker of local pain sensitivity. [25,26] A trained examiner applied a standard pressure force with a target rate of approximately 1 kg/sec until the pressure sensation was first reported by the participant to be painful [25–28]. Lower PPT values were indicative of higher pain sensitivity. A total of 3 trials were obtained with rest in between each testing trial. The average of the 3 trials was used for analyses.

Suprathreshold Heat Pain Response. Suprathreshold heat pain response (SHPR) was measured at the thenar aspect of both hands using a contact thermode with 2.5 cm^2 surface area connected to a computer-controlled PATHWAY Model Contact Heat Evoked Potential Stimulator (CHEPS) (Medoc Advanced Medical Systems). SHPR is a dynamic measure of pain sensitivity and thought to be predominantly mediated by C-fiber activity [24,29]. A series of 5 consecutive heat pulses at a rate of 30°C/sec with interstimulus interval of 2.5 seconds was delivered with a peak temperature of 48°C. We used 48°C as this temperature elicits a moderate level of pain (e.g., pain ratings near 50/100 on pain rating scale) for a majority of participants [30]. Each heat pulse was rated by the participant using the same 101-point numeric pain rating scale. SHPR was identified as the pain intensity rating of the fifth heat pulse in a train of 5 heat pulses and has been used as a clinically meaningful dynamic measure of pain sensitivity [30,31]. Higher pain ratings on SHPR indicate higher pain sensitivity. The average SHPR rating of both hands was used for analyses.

Conditioned Pain Modulation. Conditioned pain modulation (CPM) was measured using the same CHEPS setup as SHPR. The CPM protocol included a measured response of a test stimulus before and after application of a conditioning stimulus [32]. The test stimulus was delivered to the thenar aspect of the non-dominant hand and involved a sequence of 5 heat pulses at a temperature that induced a moderate level of pain intensity (e.g., 50/100 on pain scale) with the same parameters as SHPR. Participants rated each heat pulse with the same 101-point numeric pain rating scale used in the SHPR protocol. The pain rating of the fifth heat pulse was used as the test stimulus response. For the conditioning stimulus, participants immersed their dominant hand into a cold water bath for up to 60 seconds. The water temperature was maintained at a constant temperature of 8°C using a refrigeration unit (NESLAB RTE 7 Digital One, Thermo Scientific Co., Massachusetts, USA) which circulated water to prevent warming. Participants were instructed to keep their hand in the cold water bath for a minimum of 30 seconds, at which time they could remove their hand, if needed. After the 60 second cold water time period, a second bout of the same test stimulus was conducted. CPM was computed as the absolute difference in SHPR before and after the conditioning stimulus [32]. Like SHPR, CPM is a dynamic measure of pain sensitivity and indicative of central sensitivity. Moreover, CPM is a behavioral correlate of endogenous pain inhibition [33]. Larger differences (e.g., larger reductions in SHPR) were indicative of greater degrees of pain modulation.

Data Analysis

We used IBM SPSS Statistics for Windows (version 21.0, SPSS, Inc., Chicago, IL) for all data analyses. Alpha was set a priori at the 0.05 level for statistical significance.

Descriptive statistics were computed for all pertinent baseline and follow-up measures. To assess whether the exercise-induced injury model induced changes in relevant factors, baseline and 48-hour psychological variables (PCS, TSK-11) and pain sensitivity (PPT, SHPR, CPM) comparisons were made using a paired samples t-test.

The primary dependent variables (e.g., outcomes) for all analyses were the exercise-induced 1) rest-related shoulder pain (pain intensity with shoulder at rest); 2) shoulder pain with motion (pain intensity during active shoulder abduction); and 3) isometric shoulder pain (pain during isometric resisted external rotation of the shoulder). The latter two dependent variables were considered measures of activity-related pain. These variables were measured at 48- and 96-hours after exercise-induced shoulder pain.

Zero-order correlation coefficients were computed for independent variables (e.g., predictors) measured at baseline (pre-injury: age, sex, BMI, PCS, TSK-11, PPT, SHPR, CPM) with dependent variables at 48- and 96-hours, and independent variables measured at 48-hours (post-injury: PCS, TSK-11, PPT, SHPR, CPM) with dependent variables at 96-hours. All variables were analyzed as continuous variables, except for sex which was a dichotomous variable (0 for female, 1 for male). These correlations coefficients express the simple relationship between each independent and dependent variable.

Subsequently, we examined the unique relationship between independent and dependent variables after controlling for other variables, using hierarchical linear regression. Hierarchical linear regression modeling allows us to account for other factors in an a-priori, theoretical fashion. Separate hierarchical linear regression models were created using 1) baseline, pre-injury independent variables for each of the three dependent variables at 48- and 96-hours and 2) baseline demographic (age, sex, BMI) and 48-hour, post-injury independent variables (PCS, TSK-11, PPT, SHPR, CPM) for each of the three dependent variables at 96-hours.

In each of the hierarchical linear regression models, demographic variables of age, sex, and BMI were entered into the first block, psychological variables of PCS and TSK-11 were entered into the second block, and pain sensitivity variables of PPT, SHPR, and CPM were entered into the third and final block. In the 96-hour prediction model, each respective independent variable outcome measured at 48-hours was entered in the first block. We built these models in this fashion to assess the unique contribution of pain sensitivity factors after accounting for relevant demographic and psychological variables.

Correlation values between independent variables were examined prior to entering into regression models in order to prevent significant inter-correlation (i.e., multicollinearity). An a-priori correlation of 0.7 or greater was used to reflect potential multicollinearity [34]. Additional multicollinearity tests were tolerance and variance inflation, which should be greater than.2 and less than 10, respectively [35]. All tests indicated a lack of multicollinearity, and therefore, confirmed the stability of our models. Overall model statistics were examined along with changes in r-squared and p-value for each model step. Relative individual predictor strength was assessed with β estimates.

Sample Size Determination

To determine the minimum acceptable sample size needed for these analyses, we used estimation criteria from Green [36], as well as the general rule of thumb of 10–15 cases per predictor, as guidelines [35,37]. Since we were interested in assessing both the overall fit of our regression modeling and testing individual predictors ($n = 8$) we used the larger of the two sample sizes needed from Green's criteria. In this case, the minimum total sample size needed was 114 participants and was approximate to the more stringent rule of thumb criteria of 120 participants (e.g., 15 cases per predictor with 8 predictors).

Results

Sample Characteristics

Descriptive data from 143 individuals who participated in this study are presented in Table 1. All enrolled participants, except for one (illness), completed study. Participants ranged in age from 18 to 58 years (mean age = 23.7 years, SD = 6.7 years) and the 59% were female (85 female, 58 male). Comparison of baseline and 48-hour values for psychological variables and pain sensitivity showed that exercise-induced shoulder pain resulted in significantly lower PPT (higher local pain sensitivity) and PCS (lower pain catastrophizing) values and higher TSK-11 values (higher fear of movement) ($p<0.05$).

Association between Predictor and Outcome Variables

Table 2 lists correlation coefficients for each pre-injury and post-injury variable and 48- and 96-hour pain outcome. For pain sensitivity predictors, pre-injury SHPR was positively associated with both measures of activity-related pain at 48- and 96-hours ($p<0.05$), but not rest-related pain at these time points ($p>0.05$). Furthermore, post-injury SHPR, along with post-injury PPT, was associated with 96-hour activity-related pain ($p<0.05$). The

Table 1. Baseline, 48-hour, and 96-hour Descriptive Data (N = 143).

	Pre-injury	Post-injury	
Variable	**Baseline**	**48-hour**	**96-hour**
Demographic			
Age (years)	23.7 (6.7)	-	-
Sex (N of females)	85	-	-
Dominant arm (N of right)	126	-	-
BMI	23.5 (4.0)		
Psychological			
PCS	9.9 (7.9)	8.0 (8.0)	-
TSK-11	18.0 (4.4)	18.8 (5.0)	-
Pain Sensitivity			
PPT (kg)	5.5 (2.0)	4.8 (1.8)	-
SHPR (x/100)	23.2 (24.4)	20.9 (22.7)	-
CPM (x/100)	−8.6 (12.8)	−7.8 (13.6)	-
Shoulder Pain Intensity (x/100)			
At Rest	-	22.2 (20.5)	7.5 (10.1)
With Active Motion	-	15.5 (16.4)	4.2 (7.4)
With Isometric Contraction	-	20.6 (18.8)	10.5 (16.3)

Values are expressed as mean (SD) unless otherwise indicated.
Abbreviations: BMI = body mass index, CPM = conditioned pain modulation, N = number, PCS = Pain Catastrophizing Scale, PPT = pressure pain threshold, SHPR = suprathreshold heat pain response, TSK-11 = Tampa Scale of Kinesiophobia.

relationship of SHPR and PPT with pain outcome was such that the more pain sensitive an individual was (e.g., higher SHPR or lower PPT), the higher the report of shoulder pain.

Prediction of Rest- and Activity-Related Pain at 48 Hours

Table 3 includes results from the hierarchical regression models predicting 48-hour rest-related shoulder pain and shoulder pain with activity using pre-injury predictors. The final regression model for 48-hour rest-related shoulder pain indicated that none of the covariate variables were predictive of outcome ($F_{8,133} = 1.145$, $p = 0.338$, $r^2 = 0.064$). In contrast, the final regression models for shoulder pain with motion ($F_{8,132} = 2.360$, $p<0.05$) and isometric shoulder pain ($F_{8,130} = 5.159$, $p<0.001$) demonstrated predictive ability explaining 12.5% and 24.1% of the variance in pain outcome, respectively. In these models, pre-injury SHPR ($\beta = 0.285$, $p<0.05$) was the strongest predictor of 48-hour shoulder pain with motion, even after accounting for psychology (PCS: $\beta = 0.209$, $p<0.05$). In addition, pre-injury SHPR ($\beta = 0.472$, $P<0.05$) was the sole predictor of 48-hour isometric shoulder pain.

Prediction of Rest- and Activity-Related Pain at 96 Hours

Table 4 includes results from the hierarchical regression models predicting 96-hour resting shoulder pain and shoulder pain with activity using pre-injury predictors. The final regression model predicting 96-hour rest-related shoulder pain was not statistically significant, and therefore, was not predictive of outcome ($F_{8,131} = 0.683$, $p = 0.706$, $r^2 = 0.040$). The final regression models for shoulder pain with motion ($F_{8,130} = 2.259$, $p = 0.027$) and isometric shoulder pain ($F_{8,128} = 3.102$, $p = 0.003$) demonstrated predictive ability, explaining 12.2% and 16.2% of the variance in pain outcome, respectively. Despite lack of significance, pre-injury SHPR ($\beta = 0.172$, $p = 0.067$) was the strongest predictor of 96-hour shoulder pain with motion. Moreover, pre-injury SHPR was a unique predictor ($\beta = 0.387$, $p<0.001$) of 96-hour isometric shoulder pain.

Table 5 includes results from the hierarchical regression models predicting 96-hour rest and activity-related pain using 48-hour post-injury predictors. The final regression model for 96-hour rest-related shoulder pain was predictive of outcome ($F_{9,129} = 4.700$, $p<0.001$), explaining 24.7% of the variance. The final regression models for shoulder pain with motion ($F_{9,128} = 9.338$, $p<0.001$) and isometric shoulder pain ($F_{9,126} = 13.266$, $p<0.001$) were also predictive, explaining 39.6% and 48.7% of the variance in pain outcome, respectively. Pain outcome measured at 48-hours was the strongest predictor across all models (i.e., rest pain at 48-hours for rest pain at 96-hours, etc.), however, post-injury PPT ($\beta = -0.164$, $p<0.05$) and post-injury SHPR ($\beta = 0.154$, $p<0.05$) also predicted 96-hour shoulder pain with motion. Furthermore, post-injury SHPR ($\beta = 0.164$, $p<0.05$) was a predictor of 96-hour isometric shoulder pain.

Discussion

We induced shoulder pain using an eccentric exercise protocol and evaluated the influence of pre-injury and post-injury factors, namely pain sensitivity, on rest and activity-related shoulder pain measured at 48- and 96-hours. We did not observe consistent predictors across both rest and activity-related pain. However, SHPR, a pain sensitivity measure, was a consistent and oft-times the sole predictor of activity-related pain. These findings suggest that rest and activity-related pain may be modulated by different underlying processes and mechanisms [10]. Specifically, the results of our study indicate that activity-related pain is more likely to be modulated by factors related to pain sensitivity. The relevance of these findings for pain research and clinical practice is further considered in subsequent sections.

Table 2. Correlation of Pre-Injury and Post-Injury Predictors with Shoulder Pain Outcome at 48 and 96-Hours.

	48-Hours			96-Hours		
		Activity-Related Pain			Activity-Related Pain	
Variable	Rest-Related Pain	Motion Pain	Isometric Pain	Rest-Related Pain	Motion Pain	Isometric Pain
Pre-injury						
Age	−0.014	0.011	−0.053	−0.123	−0.084	−0.096
Sex	−0.171*	0.066	−0.039	−0.066	0.050	0.040
BMI	−0.051	0.033	−0.062	−0.020	0.042	0.005
PCS	0.096	0.125	0.128	0.175*	0.179*	0.145
TSK-11	−0.015	−0.044	−0.003	0.073	0.073	0.091
PPT	−0.131	−0.076	−0.162*	−0.048	−0.051	−0.079
SHPR	0.045	0.251*	0.437*	0.073	0.222*	0.320*
CPM	0.091	−0.051	−0.118	−0.056	−0.197*	−0.039
Post-Injury						
48 Pain	-	-	-	0.423*	0.568*	0.670*
PCS	-	-	-	0.253*	0.176*	0.095
TSK-11	-	-	-	0.139	0.201*	0.050
PPT	-	-	-	−0.129	−0.233*	−0.203*
SHPR	-	-	-	0.162*	0.286*	0.418*
CPM	-	-	-	−0.023	−0.087	0.017

*p-value<0.05.
Values are correlation coefficients.
Abbreviations: BMI = body mass index, CPM = conditioned pain modulation, PCS = Pain Catastrophizing Scale, PPT = pressure pain threshold, SHPR = suprathreshold heat pain response, TSK = Tampa Scale of Kinesiophobia.

Relevance to Pain Research

Exercise-induced injury paradigms like the one in our study have been used to model the pain experience [5–9,11,15,16,18,19,38–42]. In general, pre-injury psychological factors have been shown to be predictive of post-injury resting pain reports [7–9,18,19]. Pain sensitivity, however, predicted activity-related pain, even after controlling for selected psychological factors. These findings are consistent with results reported by Rakel et al. [10] that examined pre-operative psychological and pain sensitivity predictors of rest and activity-related pain following total knee replacement. These authors found pre-operative pain sensitivity measures (e.g., cutaneous mechanical and thermal threshold) to be predictive of activity-related movement pain, but not rest-related pain. Additionally, PPT had limited predictive ability on either rest or activity-related pain [10], which is concordant with our PPT findings.

Our study advances current evidence by including both static (PPT) and dynamic (SHPR, CPM) pain sensitivity measures in predicting pain. In doing so, we show that a dynamic measure of pain sensitivity, SHPR, is an important predictor of clinical pain outcome in a novel pain model (e.g., exercise-induced shoulder injury model) and corroborates a previously published trial of exercise-induced pain [6,7]. Bishop et al [6] examined the influence of static and dynamic thermal pain sensitivity on exercise-induced low back pain and reported a significant association between dynamic thermal pain sensitivity (e.g., temporal summation of pain) and daily muscle pain intensity. While the authors did not specifically examine activity-related pain, measures of daily muscle pain intensity may include appraisals of activity-related pain within their metric, especially if activity-related pain coincides with moments of worst pain during the day. This may explain why we found no association between pain sensitivity and resting pain intensity, because resting pain only assesses current pain when no movement is occurring at the shoulder.

The lack of consistent predictors across rest and activity-related pain aligns with current models on the pain experience or pain perception [43,44]. Pain sensation appraisal is context-dependent and involves influence from cognitive, sensory and affective components, and is likely processed in serial, parallel, and cyclical fashion. Conceptually, individuals may appraise pain differently when at rest and during activity [45,46], and possible explanations include the following mechanisms. First, rating pain during a controlled activity (i.e., lifting arm in controlled fashion like in our study), may not be as threatening as pain during either unpredictable or uncontrollable moments (e.g., daily events or at rest when not anticipating pain). Second, evoked pain may be seen as a challenge to the sensory system and result in activity-dependent responses. Thus, pain sensitivity may be suited to reflect these underlying activity-dependent states more so than during basal states such as rest.

Relevance to Clinical Practice

While our findings are consistent with findings across pre-clinical (i.e., healthy participant) and postoperative studies [6,7,10,47–49], we used an exercise-induced injury model which is advantageous for the assessment of pre-injury influence. We are unaware of studies that assessed the association between pain sensitivity and the transition of pre-injury to post-injury states and this was one of our primary aims [47,48]. Measuring pre-injury states is difficult to conduct in clinical studies where the future development of pain is uncertain. While our findings are

Table 3. Hierarchical Regression Models Predicting 48-hour Shoulder Pain at Rest, with Motion, and with Isometric Action Using Baseline, Pre-injury Predictors.

					Activity-Related Pain							
	Rest-Related Pain				Motion Pain				Isometric Pain			
	Beta	P	Δ R^2	P	Beta	P	Δ R^2	P	Beta	P	Δ R^2	P
1			0.027	0.281			0.006	0.850			0.005	0.889
Age	0.025	0.785			<0.001	0.996			−0.027	0.771		
Sex	−0.163	0.065			0.071	0.423			−0.011	0.902		
BMI	−0.016	0.867			0.013	0.890			−0.049	0.605		
2			0.020	0.249			0.043	0.232			0.029	0.461
Age	0.061	0.512			0.054	0.564			0.013	0.893		
Sex	−0.157	0.076			0.079	0.367			−0.005	0.955		
BMI	−0.021	0.819			0.004	0.968			−0.053	0.577		
PCS	0.170	0.095			**0.247**	**0.015**			**0.202**	**0.048**		
TSK-11	−0.099	0.323			−0.149	0.135			−0.088	0.382		
3			0.017	0.338			0.076	0.021			0.207	<0.001
Age	0.071	0.449			0.054	0.552			0.011	0.899		
Sex	−0.137	0.140			0.107	0.232			0.040	0.632		
BMI	0.017	0.855			0.051	0.579			0.023	0.789		
PCS	0.170	0.100			**0.209**	**0.036**			0.133	0.149		
TSK-11	−0.074	0.466			−0.144	0.142			−0.080	0.378		
PPT	−0.057	0.533			−0.061	0.494			−0.084	0.311		
SHPR	0.083	0.384			**0.285**	**0.002**			**0.472**	**<0.001**		
CPM	0.128	0.186			0.041	0.665			0.056	0.527		

All predictor variables measured at baseline (pre-injury).
Abbreviations: BMI = body mass index, CPM = conditioned pain modulation, PCS = Pain Catastrophizing Scale, P = p-value, PPT = pressure pain threshold, SHPR = suprathreshold heat pain response, TSK = Tampa Scale of Kinesiophobia.

Table 4. Hierarchical Regression Models Predicting 96-hour Shoulder Pain at Rest, with Motion, and with Isometric Action Using Baseline, Pre-Injury Predictors.

					Activity-Related Pain							
	Rest-Related Pain				**Motion Pain**				**Isometric Pain**			
	Beta	**P**	**Δ R^2**	**P**	**Beta**	**P**	**Δ R^2**	**P**	**Beta**	**P**	**Δ R^2**	**P**
1			0.022	0.379			0.016	0.541			0.014	0.607
Age	−0.138	0.134			−0.119	0.201			−0.116	0.215		
Sex	−0.068	0.446			0.060	0.506			0.061	0.501		
BMI	0.050	0.592			0.070	0.463			0.031	0.746		
2			0.016	0.379			0.036	0.205			0.025	0.393
Age	−0.111	0.240			−0.071	0.455			−0.084	0.382		
Sex	−0.058	0.512			0.070	0.430			0.068	0.452		
BMI	0.052	0.580			0.072	0.445			0.037	0.699		
PCS	0.139	0.179			**0.204**	**0.048**			0.139	0.179		
TSK-11	−0.018	0.859			−0.012	0.900			0.038	0.702		
3			0.002	0.706			0.070	0.027			0.124	0.003
Age	−0.111	0.249			−0.087	0.348			−0.092	0.312		
Sex	−0.049	0.601			0.094	0.303			0.102	0.257		
BMI	0.059	0.541			0.121	0.193			0.088	0.340		
PCS	0.134	0.203			0.166	0.100			0.100	0.311		
TSK-11	−0.016	0.876			−0.039	0.694			0.054	0.573		
PPT	−0.024	0.794			−0.046	0.604			−0.040	0.652		
SHPR	0.033	0.736			0.172	0.067			**0.387**	**<0.001**		
CPM	0.005	0.960			−0.145	0.123			0.127	0.172		

All predictor variables measured at baseline (pre-injury).
Abbreviations: BMI = body mass index, CPM = conditioned pain modulation, PCS = Pain Catastrophizing Scale, P = p-value, PPT = pressure pain threshold, SHPR = suprathreshold heat pain response, TSK = Tampa Scale of Kinesiophobia.

Table 5. Hierarchical Regression Models Predicting 96-hour Shoulder Pain at Rest, with Motion, and with Isometric Action using 48-Hour, Post-Injury Predictors.

					Activity-Related Pain							
	Rest-Related Pain				Motion Pain				Isometric Pain			
	Beta	P	Δ R^2	P	Beta	P	Δ R^2	P	Beta	P	Δ R^2	P
1			0.216	<0.001			0.334	<0.001			0.458	<0.001
Age	−0.149	0.074			−0.111	0.150			−0.075	0.284		
Sex	0.001	0.986			0.040	0.596			0.071	0.295		
BMI	0.055	0.520			0.067	0.395			0.063	0.379		
48 Pain	**0.445**	**<0.001**			**0.563**	**<0.001**			**0.669**	**<0.001**		
2			0.018	<0.001			0.011	<0.001			0.001	<0.001
Age	−0.129	0.123			−0.103	0.190			−0.074	0.300		
Sex	0.009	0.913			0.036	0.629			0.073	0.287		
BMI	0.043	0.614			0.075	0.341			0.059	0.412		
48 Pain	**0.410**	**<0.001**			**0.566**	**<0.001**			**0.667**	**<0.001**		
PCS	0.148	0.122			−0.062	0.482			0.032	0.684		
TSK-11	−0.016	0.866			0.125	0.148			−0.034	0.665		
3			0.013	<0.001			0.052	<0.001			0.027	<0.001
Age	−0.129	0.130			−0.106	0.172			−0.086	0.232		
Sex	0.022	0.791			0.100	0.188			0.084	0.234		
BMI	0.051	0.553			0.113	0.150			0.060	0.404		
48 Pain	**0.398**	**<0.001**			**0.497**	**<0.001**			**0.594**	**<0.001**		
PCS	0.146	0.130			−0.070	0.421			0.037	0.638		
TSK-11	−0.010	0.913			0.135	0.110			−0.031	0.689		
PPT	−0.039	0.642			**−0.164**	**0.032**			−0.011	0.874		
SHPR	0.101	0.213			**0.154**	**0.041**			**0.164**	**0.035**		
CPM	0.054	0.499			<0.001	0.996			0.114	0.087		

All predictor variables except age, sex, and BMI measured at 48 hours (post-injury).
Abbreviations: 48 Pain = Pain report of each respective outcome variable at 48 hours, BMI = body mass index, CPM = conditioned pain modulation, PCS = Pain Catastrophizing Scale, P = p-value, PPT = pressure pain threshold, SHPR = suprathreshold heat pain response, TSK = Tampa Scale of Kinesiophobia.

preliminary, our results suggest that early indication of individuals at risk for persistent activity-related pain may be identified by pre-injury pain sensitivity. This has potential implications for clinical management or screening as pain sensitivity assessment may be an additional tool to predict individuals at risk for chronic pain [47]. Recommendations such as these have been made in populations including postoperative pain [50,51] and there are ongoing efforts for the identification of pain sensitivity profiles or phenotypes for improved pain management [52]. If our findings are replicated in patients with musculoskeletal pain, then current recommendations may be extended to suggest phenotypes of pain-free individuals at risk of activity-evoked pain after musculoskeletal injury.

In a well-conducted meta-analysis, Hubscher et al [53] reported a weak association between pain sensitivity responses and clinical pain intensity. Rather than reflect poor clinical validity of pain sensitivity, the apparent weak association with pain sensitivity and clinical pain potentially may suggest a more complex relationship between measures of pain sensitivity and clinical outcome. Pain sensitivity, in general, may in fact be weakly associated to resting pain ratings, but may show stronger associations when evoked pain (as occurs during movement) is considered the clinical outcome of interest. Not apparent in the review by Hubscher et al [53] is whether a distinction between rest and activity-related pain was made when assessing outcome. But, perhaps in future clinical studies the utility of pain sensitivity will not be in predicting rest-related pain, but in activity-related pain.

Furthermore, select pain sensitivity responses may yield better association or prediction than others. Hubscher et al [53] reported relatively stronger correlations between clinical pain intensity and dynamic pain sensitivity (e.g., temporal summation), as compared to static pain sensitivity. This is consistent with our current findings where SHPR showed stronger relative prediction than PPT. Interestingly, we did not find CPM to be predictive of activity-related pain and that may be because our exercise-induced injury model is a model of acute pain. Evidence suggests that a lack of inhibitory mechanisms, as inferred through CPM, is more often shown in chronic pain syndromes [54,55], so these results may be expected and future studies in clinical populations should continue to use CPM until this issue is explored further.

Study Limitations

This study has several limitations. First, we standardized the initial bout of exercise for injury induction, but allowed continued exercise performance if our fatigue criterion was not met. Thus, we did not include the dosage of exercise to induce injury into our models for those individuals requiring a larger volume to induce the same injury criterion. Second, our study results can only be generalized to a population of younger, healthy individuals with induced shoulder pain following eccentric exercise. Although similar results have been observed in experimental and clinical trials [6,7,10], further validation of these findings to older and clinical populations is warranted. Third, our results are limited to those predictive factors included in our models. Other known predictors of resting pain such as depression were not included in these analyses. Furthermore, we did not include interaction terms within our model as we did not have specific hypotheses for interactions. Our models assessed only the main effects from each of the included predictors.

Additionally, we included only select measures of pressure and heat pain sensitivity and no other modalities. Currently, there is no consensus for pain sensitivity assessment, however multiple modality testing is encouraged and we included both static and dynamic pain sensitivity [13]. We did not include assessments of pain beyond 96-hours post-injury, but it is common for resolution of pain to occur for most individuals within this timeframe. Our pain outcome assessment was limited to pain intensity as compared to unpleasantness or other pain dimension measures. We did find some discrepancy in pain outcome between our study and the study by Dannecker and Sluka [5] where our activity-related pain measures did not elicit higher pain ratings than pain at rest. This may be due to the lack of specificity in our activity. In other words, we did not selectively stress the musculoskeletal tissue that was fatigued as was done by Dannecker and Sluka [5]. Further studies should assess whether induced shoulder pain can elicit higher pain ratings with selective movements as opposed to a general active or resisted motion.

Conclusion

Our prediction models within an exercise-induced injury paradigm allowed us to assess whether pain sensitivity was related to pain outcome as a risk (pre-injury) factor or prognostic (post-injury) factor. Based on our findings, pain sensitivity and SHPR specifically is associated with activity-related pain, however further investigations are needed to validate these findings and their potential translation into clinical practice.

Supporting Information

Data S1 (XLSX)

Acknowledgments

We wish to acknowledge Dr. Kelly Larkin Kaiser for assisting with data collection.

Author Contributions

Conceived and designed the experiments: PAB SZG. Performed the experiments: RAC CBS CV JJP SZG. Analyzed the data: RAC SZG. Wrote the paper: RAC CBS CV JJP PAB SZG.

References

1. Litcher-Kelly L, Martino SA, Broderick JE, Stone AA (2007) A systematic review of measures used to assess chronic musculoskeletal pain in clinical and randomized controlled clinical trials. J Pain 8: 906–913.
2. Srikandarajah S, Gilron I (2011) Systematic review of movement-evoked pain versus pain at rest in postsurgical clinical trials and meta-analyses: a fundamental distinction requiring standardized measurement. Pain 152: 1734–1739.
3. Kehlet H, Dahl JB (2011) Assessment of postoperative pain–need for action! Pain 152: 1699–1700.
4. Wu CL, Rowlingson AJ, Partin AW, Kalish MA, Courpas GE, et al. (2005) Correlation of postoperative pain to quality of recovery in the immediate postoperative period. Reg Anesth Pain Med 30: 516–522.
5. Dannecker EA, Sluka KA (2011) Pressure and activity-related allodynia in delayed-onset muscle pain. Clin J Pain 27: 42–47.
6. Bishop MD, George SZ, Robinson ME (2012) Dynamic, but not static, pain sensitivity predicts exercise-induced muscle pain: covariation of temporal sensory summation and pain intensity. Neurosci Lett 526: 1–4.
7. Bishop MD, Horn ME, George SZ (2011) Exercise-induced pain intensity predicted by pre-exercise fear of pain and pain sensitivity. Clin J Pain 27: 398–404.
8. George SZ, Dover GC, Fillingim RB (2007) Fear of pain influences outcomes after exercise-induced delayed onset muscle soreness at the shoulder. Clin J Pain 23: 76–84.
9. George SZ, Dover GC, Wallace MR, Sack BK, Herbstman DM, et al. (2008) Biopsychosocial influence on exercise-induced delayed onset muscle soreness at the shoulder: pain catastrophizing and catechol-o-methyltransferase (COMT) diplotype predict pain ratings. Clin J Pain 24: 793–801.

10. Rakel BA, Blodgett NP, Bridget Zimmerman M, Logsden-Sackett N, Clark C, et al. (2012) Predictors of postoperative movement and resting pain following total knee replacement. Pain 153: 2192–2203.
11. Ayles S, Graven-Nielsen T, Gibson W (2011) Vibration-induced afferent activity augments delayed onset muscle allodynia. J Pain 12: 884–891.
12. Cruz-Almeida Y, Fillingim RB (2014) Can quantitative sensory testing move us closer to mechanism-based pain management? Pain Med 15: 61–72.
13. Backonja MM, Attal N, Baron R, Bouhassira D, Drangholt M, et al. (2013) Value of quantitative sensory testing in neurological and pain disorders: NeuPSIG consensus. Pain 154: 1807–1819.
14. Henriksen M, Alkjaer T, Lund H, Simonsen EB, Graven-Nielsen T, et al. (2007) Experimental quadriceps muscle pain impairs knee joint control during walking. J Appl Physiol (1985) 103: 132–139.
15. Bishop MD, Horn ME, George SZ, Robinson ME (2011) Self-reported pain and disability outcomes from an endogenous model of muscular back pain. BMC Musculoskelet Disord 12: 35.
16. Slater H, Arendt-Nielsen L, Wright A, Graven-Nielsen T (2003) Experimental deep tissue pain in wrist extensors–a model of lateral epicondylalgia. Eur J Pain 7: 277–288.
17. Price DD, McGrath PA, Rafii A, Buckingham B (1983) The validation of visual analogue scales as ratio scale measures for chronic and experimental pain. Pain 17: 45–56.
18. Parr J, Borsa P, Fillingim R, Kaiser K, Tillman MD, et al. (2014) Psychological influences predict recovery following exercise induced shoulder pain. Int J Sports Med 35: 232–237.
19. Parr JJ, Borsa PA, Fillingim RB, Tillman MD, Manini TM, et al. (2012) Pain-related fear and catastrophizing predict pain intensity and disability independently using an induced muscle injury model. J Pain 13: 370–378.
20. Sullivan MJL, Bishop SR, Pivik J (1995) The Pain Catastrophizing Scale: Development and validation. Psychological Assessment 7: 524–532.
21. Mintken PE, Cleland JA, Whitman JM, George SZ (2010) Psychometric properties of the Fear-Avoidance Beliefs Questionnaire and Tampa Scale of Kinesiophobia in patients with shoulder pain. Arch Phys Med Rehabil 91: 1128–1136.
22. Lentz TA, Barabas JA, Day T, Bishop MD, George SZ (2009) The relationship of pain intensity, physical impairment, and pain-related fear to function in patients with shoulder pathology. J Orthop Sports Phys Ther 39: 270–277.
23. Woby SR, Roach NK, Urmston M, Watson PJ (2005) Psychometric properties of the TSK-11: a shortened version of the Tampa Scale for Kinesiophobia. Pain 117: 137–144.
24. Arendt-Nielsen L, Yarnitsky D (2009) Experimental and clinical applications of quantitative sensory testing applied to skin, muscles and viscera. J Pain 10: 556–572.
25. Coronado RA, Kindler LL, Valencia C, George SZ (2011) Thermal and pressure pain sensitivity in patients with unilateral shoulder pain: comparison of involved and uninvolved sides. J Orthop Sports Phys Ther 41: 165–173.
26. Coronado RA, Simon CB, Valencia C, George SZ (2014) Experimental pain responses support peripheral and central sensitization in patients with unilateral shoulder pain. Clin J Pain 30: 143–151.
27. Chesterton LS, Sim J, Wright CC, Foster NE (2007) Interrater reliability of algometry in measuring pressure pain thresholds in healthy humans, using multiple raters. Clin J Pain 23: 760–766.
28. Persson AL, Brogardh C, Sjolund BH (2004) Tender or not tender: test-retest repeatability of pressure pain thresholds in the trapezius and deltoid muscles of healthy women. J Rehabil Med 36: 17–27.
29. Price DD, Mao J, Frenk H, Mayer DJ (1994) The N-methyl-D-aspartate receptor antagonist dextromethorphan selectively reduces temporal summation of second pain in man. Pain 59: 165–174.
30. Valencia C, Fillingim RB, George SZ (2011) Suprathreshold heat pain response is associated with clinical pain intensity for patients with shoulder pain. J Pain 12: 133–140.
31. Valencia C, Kindler LL, Fillingim RB, George SZ (2012) Investigation of central pain processing in shoulder pain: converging results from 2 musculoskeletal pain models. J Pain 13: 81–89.
32. Valencia C, Kindler LL, Fillingim RB, George SZ (2013) Stability of conditioned pain modulation in two musculoskeletal pain models: investigating the influence of shoulder pain intensity and gender. BMC Musculoskelet Disord 14: 182.
33. Kong JT, Schnyer RN, Johnson KA, Mackey S (2013) Understanding central mechanisms of acupuncture analgesia using dynamic quantitative sensory testing: a review. Evid Based Complement Alternat Med 2013: 187182.
34. Dormann CF, Elith J, Bacher S, Buchmann C, Carl G, et al. (2013) Collinearity: a review of methods to deal with it and a simulation study evaluating their performance. Ecography 36: 27–46.
35. Field AP (2009) Discovering statistics using SPSS. Los Angeles: SAGE Publications. xxxii, 821 p. p.
36. Green SB (1991) How Many Subjects Does It Take to Do a Regression-Analysis. Multivariate Behavioral Research 26: 499–510.
37. Babyak MA (2004) What you see may not be what you get: a brief, nontechnical introduction to overfitting in regression-type models. Psychosom Med 66: 411–421.
38. Dannecker EA, Hausenblas HA, Kaminski TW, Robinson ME (2005) Sex differences in delayed onset muscle pain. Clin J Pain 21: 120–126.
39. Dannecker EA, Koltyn KF, Riley JL 3rd, Robinson ME (2003) Sex differences in delayed onset muscle soreness. J Sports Med Phys Fitness 43: 78–84.
40. Frey Law LA, Evans S, Knudtson J, Nus S, Scholl K, et al. (2008) Massage reduces pain perception and hyperalgesia in experimental muscle pain: a randomized, controlled trial. J Pain 9: 714–721.
41. Slater H, Arendt-Nielsen L, Wright A, Graven-Nielsen T (2005) Sensory and motor effects of experimental muscle pain in patients with lateral epicondylalgia and controls with delayed onset muscle soreness. Pain 114: 118–130.
42. Torisu T, Wang K, Svensson P, De Laat A, Tanaka M, et al. (2010) Effects of eccentric jaw exercise on temporal summation in jaw-closing muscles of healthy subjects. Eur J Pain 14: 719–724.
43. Price DD (2002) Central neural mechanisms that interrelate sensory and affective dimensions of pain. Mol Interv 2: 392–403, 339.
44. Melzack R, Katz J (2013) Pain. Wiley Interdisciplinary Reviews-Cognitive Science 4: 1–15.
45. Parks EL, Geha PY, Baliki MN, Katz J, Schnitzer TJ, et al. (2011) Brain activity for chronic knee osteoarthritis: dissociating evoked pain from spontaneous pain. Eur J Pain 15: 843 e841–814.
46. Trost Z (2012) All pain is not created equal: differentiating between pain during movement versus pain at rest following total knee arthroplasty. Pain 153: 2161–2162.
47. Yarnitsky D, Crispel Y, Eisenberg E, Granovsky Y, Ben-Nun A, et al. (2008) Prediction of chronic post-operative pain: pre-operative DNIC testing identifies patients at risk. Pain 138: 22–28.
48. Valencia C, Fillingim RB, Bishop M, Wu SS, Wright TW, et al. (2013) Investigation of Central Pain Processing in Post-Operative Shoulder Pain and Disability. Clin J Pain.
49. Granot M, Weissman-Fogel I (2012) The effect of post-surgical neuroplasticity on the stability of systemic pain perception: a psychophysical study. Eur J Pain 16: 247–255.
50. Landau R, Kraft JC, Flint LY, Carvalho B, Richebe P, et al. (2010) An experimental paradigm for the prediction of Post-Operative Pain (PPOP). J Vis Exp.
51. Granot M (2009) Can we predict persistent postoperative pain by testing preoperative experimental pain? Curr Opin Anaesthesiol 22: 425–430.
52. Yarnitsky D, Granot M, Granovsky Y (2014) Pain modulation profile and pain therapy: between pro- and antinociception. Pain 155: 663–665.
53. Hubscher M, Moloney N, Leaver A, Rebbeck T, McAuley JH, et al. (2013) Relationship between quantitative sensory testing and pain or disability in people with spinal pain-a systematic review and meta-analysis. Pain 154: 1497–1504.
54. Lautenbacher S, Rollman GB (1997) Possible deficiencies of pain modulation in fibromyalgia. Clin J Pain 13: 189–196.
55. Pielsticker A, Haag G, Zaudig M, Lautenbacher S (2005) Impairment of pain inhibition in chronic tension-type headache. Pain 118: 215–223.

The Inhibitory Effect of Pseudolaric Acid B on Gastric Cancer and Multidrug Resistance via Cox-2/PKC-α/P-gp Pathway

Qian Sun, Yan Li*

Department of gastroenterology, Shengjing Hospital Affiliated to China Medical University, Shenyang, Liaoning, China

Abstract

Aim: To investigate the inhibitory effect of pseudolaric acid B on subcutaneous xenografts of human gastric adenocarcinoma and the underlying molecular mechanisms involved in its multidrug resistance.

Methods: Human gastric adenocarcinoma SGC7901 cells and drug-resistant SGC7901/ADR cells were injected into nude mice to establish a subcutaneous xenograft model. The effects of pseudolaric acid B with or without adriamycin treatment were compared by determining the tumor size and weight. Cyclo-oxygenase-2, protein kinaseC-α and P-glycoprotein expression levels were determined by immunohistochemistry and western blot.

Results: Pseudolaric acid B significantly suppressed the tumor growth induced by SGC7901 cells and SGC7901/ADR cells. The combination of pseudolaric acid B and the traditional chemotherapy drug adriamycin exhibited more potent inhibitory effects on the growth of gastric cancer in vivo than treatment with either pseudolaric acid B or adriamycin alone. Protein expression levels of cyclo-oxygenase-2, protein kinaseC-α and P-glycoprotein were inhibited by pseudolaric acid B alone or in combination with adriamycin in SGC7901/ADR cell xenografts.

Conclusion: Pseudolaric acid B has a significant inhibitory effect and an additive inhibitory effect in combination with adriamycin on the growth of gastric cancer in vivo, which reverses the multidrug resistance of gastric neoplasm to chemotherapy drugs by downregulating the Cox-2/PKC-α/P-gp/mdr1 signaling pathway.

Editor: Soumitro Pal, Children's Hospital Boston & Harvard Medical School, United States of America

Funding: This work was supported by Science Program Foundation of Shenyang Municipal Science and Technology Bureau (1091136-9-02). The funder had no role in study design, data collection and analysis, decision to publish, or preparation of the manuscript.

Competing Interests: The authors have declared that no competing interests exist.

* Email: yanli2955@163.com

Introduction

Gastric cancer is one of the world's most common cancers [1], and chemotherapy is an important strategy against gastric cancer [2]. Because multiple chemotherapeutic drugs of different classes are used to treat gastric cancer, the sensitivity of anticancer drugs to gastric cancer decreases gradually, and resistance to many different drugs with different chemical structures and different mechanisms of action can occur. This type of resistance is called multidrug resistance (MDR) and significantly decreases the efficiency of therapy on gastric cancer. MDR is becoming a major problem for successful cancer treatment [3]. It has been discovered that the major reason for MDR in cancer is the overexpression of P-glycoprotein (P-gp), a product of the human MDR1 gene. P-gp is an ATP-dependent efflux pump that can decrease drug accumulation in cancer cells. It is proposed that P-gp, a well-accepted biomarker of MDR, should also be considered as a molecular target in multidrug-resistant cancer [4]. Recent studies have demonstrated that in cancer cells with MDR, the expression levels of cyclo-oxygenase-2 (Cox-2) and an isoform of protein kinaseC (PKC-α) are both upregulated, and their inhibition can reverse neoplastic MDR [5–10].

Pseudolaric acid B (PAB, Figure 1), a diterpene acid isolated from the root and trunk bark of the tree *Pseudolarix kaempferi* Gordon (Pinaceae), is used in traditional Chinese medicine for its wide spectrum of biological features, such as anti-fungal effects and anti-fertility effects. In addition, its anti-angiogenic effects have also been gradually recognized in recent years [11,12]. Recent studies have demonstrated that PAB induces growth inhibition, cell cycle arrest and apoptosis. Moreover, PAB reverses the multidrug resistance of cancer cells [13,14]. PAB suppresses the growth of the gastric neoplastic AGS cell line and induces its apoptosis [15]. Our previous research demonstrated that PAB also has a dramatic inhibitory effect on human gastric cancer SGC7901 cells in vitro [16]. However, in vitro studies of the anticancer effect of PAB are rare, and neither the in vivo efficacy of this novel herbal compound against tumors nor its precise molecular mechanism against MDR has been fully investigated.

The aim of the present study is to evaluate the anti-neoplastic effect of PAB in vivo, including the reversal of MDR, using a

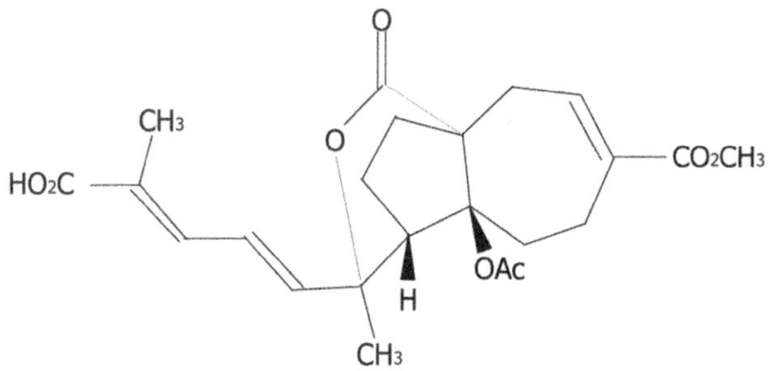

Figure 1. Chemical structure of pseudolaric acid B ($C_{23}H_{28}O_8$, MW = 432.5).

xenograft model in nude mice and explore whether PAB's underlying molecular mechanism is related to the inhibition of MDR via the Cox-2/PKC-α/P-gp pathway.

Materials and Methods

Materials

RPMI-1640 culture medium and fetal bovine serum (FBS) for cell culture were purchased from Gibco BRL, Gaithersburg, MD, USA. Rabbit anti-Cox-2 monoclonal antibody, mouse anti-PKC-α and mouse anti-P-gp monoclonal antibodies were purchased from Santa Cruz Corporation, CA, USA. Secondary antibodies against the rabbit and mouse antibodies, streptavidin-peroxidase (SP) kits, and 3,3'-diaminobenzidine (DAB) were obtained from Beijing Zhongshan Biotechnology, China. BCA protein assay kits and SDS-PAGE gel preparation kits were obtained from the Beyotime Institute of Biotechnology, Shanghai, China. PAB was purchased from the Liaoning Institute for Drug Control, China No. 201003 (the purity:>98%). Adriamycin (ADR) was obtained from Zhejiang Hisun Pharmaceutical Co., Ltd., China No. 120906. Tween80 and polyethylene glycol were purchased from Sigma Chemical, St. Louis, MO, USA.

Cell culture

Human gastric adenocarcinoma SGC7901 cells were cultured in the central laboratory of Shengjing Hospital Affiliated to China Medical University [16], and adriamycin-resistant SGC7901/ADR cells were gifted from Institute of Digestive Diseases in Xijing Hospital Affiliated to Fourth Military Medical University [17]. Human gastric adenocarcinoma SGC7901 cells and adriamycin-resistant SGC7901/ADR cells were cultured in RPMI-1640 medium supplemented with 10% FBS and antibiotics (100 U/ml penicillin and streptomycin) with 5% CO_2 in a humidified incubator at 37°C. ADR (1 μg/ml) was added to the SGC7901/ADR cell culture medium to help maintain their MDR. Cells in the logarithmic growth phase were centrifuged and diluted with RPMI-1640 medium to prepare single-cell suspensions with a concentration of 2.5×10^6/ml for seeding.

Establishment of a nude mice xenograft model

The in vivo antitumor effect of PAB was examined in a murine xenograft model. For the model, 4-6-week-old male and female immunodeficient BALB/c (nu/nu) mice, weighing 18 to 22 g, were purchased from Beijing HFK Bioscience Co., Ltd. (China) and kept in accredited facilities under standard conditions for rodents (SPF grade) in the Department of Laboratory Animal Science. Fifty mice were selected and randomly assigned into two groups (25 per group). A total of 25 mice were subcutaneously injected with 2.5×10^6/ml SGC7901 cells in 0.2 ml of RPMI-1640 medium into the left axillae, and the other 25 mice were injected with SGC7901/ADR cells into the right axillary region under germ-free conditions.

Experimental groups and medication

Seven days after cell implantation, the tumors became palpable (approximately 3 mm×3 mm in diameter), and then, the two groups injected with two different types of cells were randomly divided into five subgroups (5 mice per group): normal saline (NS) control group, TWEEN control group, ADR group, PAB group, and PAB+ADR group. For the PAB groups, PAB (25 mg/kg/d in 0.1 ml) dissolved in an aqueous solution of 6% polyethylene glycol, 3% ethanol, and 1% Tween80 was administered intraperitoneally (i.p.) daily for 20 days [13]. An identical volume of aqueous solution or NS was injected in the TWEEN control group or NS control group, respectively. For the ADR group, ADR (1.25 mg/kg in 0.1 ml) diluted in NS was administered i.p. daily for 20 days [18]. Tumor-bearing mice were administered both PAB (25 mg/kg/d) and ADR (1.25 mg/kg/day) i.p. for the same period in the PAB+ADR group. After treatment, mice from each group were sacrificed, and tumor samples of bilateral axillary regions were weighed and resected for immunohistochemical and western blot analyses. This study was performed strictly in accordance with the recommendations in the Guide for the Care and Use of Laboratory Animals of the National Institutes of Health. The protocol was approved by the Committee on the Ethics of Animal Experiments of the Shengjing Hospital Affiliated to China Medical University (Permit Number: 2013PS144K). Mice were sacrificed under 10% chloral hydrate anesthesia, and all efforts were made to minimize suffering.

Measurement and calculation of tumor volume and weight

Body weight was monitored every day, and two perpendicular diameters (length and width in millimeters) of tumors were measured every two days with calipers throughout the treatment period. Tumor volumes were estimated using two-dimensional measurements and calculated as follows: tumor volume (mm^3) = length (mm)×width^2 (mm)/2. The relative tumor volume (RTV) was calculated as follows: RTV = (mean tumor volume during therapy)/(mean tumor volume at the beginning of therapy). The antitumor effects of PAB and/or ADR were estimated with the mean inhibition rate (IR) of tumor growth using the following equation: IR (%) = [(1-mean RTV of drug-treated group/mean RTV of NS control group) ×100] [19]. The relative body weight of mice was calculated using the W_t/W_0 index, where W_t was the body weight on the day of measurement, and W_0 was the body weight at the first day of treatment. The change in body weight on days 1 and 20, representing the start and end of the experiment, respectively, was used to evaluate and analyze the effects of drugs on the body weight [20].

Immunohistochemical staining for expression of Cox-2, PKC-α and P-gp

Tumor specimens were fixed with paraformaldehyde, processed routinely by embedding in paraffin, and then sliced into 4-μm sections. Following hematoxylin and eosin (HE) staining, cells of the gastric cancer xenografts were observed under a light microscope. The expression levels of Cox-2, PKC-α and P-gp in harvested tumor cells were determined using the SP method. Briefly, after being dewaxed and rehydrated, slides were incubated in 0.3% H_2O_2 solution and dried in a microwave in citric acid buffer for 15 min to retrieve antigens. The slices were blocked with normal goat serum for 30 min at 37°C and probed with a rabbit monoclonal antibody to Cox-2 and mouse monoclonal antibodies to PKC-α and P-gp at 4°C overnight (all antibodies were diluted at 1:300). Biotinylated anti-rabbit IgG and anti-rat IgG were added and incubated at 37°C for 30 min before enzyme conjugated HRP-streptavidin was added. In addition, 3, 3'-diaminobenzidine (DAB) was used as the chromogen. Slides were counterstained with hematoxylin, dehydrated in alcohol, and mounted on neutral balsam. Controls were prepared using secondary antibodies only. Five fields of each section from every mouse in each group were selected for image collection. The results were analyzed and compared statistically using NIS-Elements Br 3.0 software, and the average optical density was obtained to quantify the expression levels of Cox-2, PKC-α and P-gp.

Western blot of Cox-2, PKC-α and P-gp in nude mice xenografts

A total of 100 mg of fresh-frozen tumor tissues from at least three mice of each group were weighed and supplemented with radio immunoprecipitation assay (RIPA) lysis buffer [containing 100 μg/ml phenylmethanesulfonyl fluoride (PMSF)]. After pulverized using scissors, extracts were homogenized using ultrasound. After centrifuging at 14000 rpm at 4°C for 30 min, a supernatant sample was frozen at −80°C for western blotting. The protein concentration of the extracts was determined using a bicinchoninic acid (BCA) protein assay kit. A total of 100 μg protein per mouse under denaturing conditions (100°C, 5 min) was electrophoresed using sodium dodecyl sulfate-polyacrylamide gel electrophoresis (SDS-PAGE) on 8% separation gel and electrotransferred onto PVDF membranes using a wet transfer system at 100 V (Cox-2, PKC-α, β-actin for 100 min, and P-gp for 3 h). After blocking with 5% nonfat dry milk in 1×TBST (Tris-buffered saline containing 0.1% Tween20) for 90 min, the membranes were then incubated with the primary antibody [rabbit monoclonal antibody to Cox-2 (1:400) or mouse monoclonal antibodies to PKC-α (1:200) and P-gp (1:200), with β-actin as an internal control for protein loading] overnight at 4°C. The antibody binding was visualized using a peroxidase-coupled secondary goat anti-rabbit antibody (1:2000) and goat anti-mouse antibody (1:2000) for 1.5 h at room temperature. Then, the membranes were visualized by enhanced chemiluminescence (ECL) reagent. The results were analyzed using Image J software.

Statistical analysis

All data are presented as the mean values±standard deviation, and multiple comparisons between any two of the treated groups were evaluated by one-way ANOVA, using SNK and LSD methods with SPSS 17.0 software. The relationship between body weight change and tumor volume were analyzed by Pearson correlation analysis. p values less than 0.05 were considered to be statistically significant.

Results

Inhibitory effect of PAB on the growth of human gastric cancer

Tumors in all treated groups formed readily after the implantation of single-cell suspensions, and the formation rate was 100%. When the xenografts became evident, there were no significant differences in the average volume of the xenografts among the different groups (Table 1), and the tumor volumes were monitored at various time points in all groups. The curves of the tumor growth of the two cell lines were graphed (Figure 2A, 2B). As shown in Table 1, for the SGC7901 cell-treated groups, no significant difference was observed between the PAB group and ADR group in the average relative volumes of the xenografts ($p > 0.05$), and the IR was 56.4% and 59.0%, respectively. The addition of ADR to PAB resulted in higher antitumor activity than that of PAB alone or ADR alone ($p < 0.05$) with an IR of 88.1%. The inhibitory effect of the PAB group was stronger compared with that of the ADR group on the xenografts of SGC7901/ADR cells, and the IR values were 64.1% and 21.9%, respectively ($p < 0.05$). Tumor growth inhibition was more evident in mice treated with PAB combined with ADR, with an IR of 85.8%. The findings of tumor weight in different groups further supported our results regarding the volume of mice xenografts. Figure 2C and 2D shows the changes of the relative body weight of the mice in the ten groups. The body weight was similar between the control groups and PAB-treated groups. However, the body weight decreased in the combination-treated groups and ADR groups, and the decrease of the ADR groups was more evident ($p < 0.05$). Moreover, Figure 3 provides a direct comparison of the tumor sizes of the SGC7901 cells and SGC7901/ADR cells in the different groups. The relationship between body weight change and tumor volume were not significant ($p > 0.05$). The dosages tested were well tolerated by the mice, and no animal lethality was observed during the experiment.

Immunohistochemical staining for the expression of Cox-2, PKC-α and P-gp

All tumors in each group, via immunohistochemical staining, displayed positive expression of the Cox-2, PKC-α and P-gp proteins. Cox-2 and PKC-α expression was defined as positive if the stained region of the tumor cells was in the cytoplasm, and P-gp staining was considered positive if staining was observed in the membrane and cytoplasm. The proteins were stained yellow or brown under optical microscope observation (Figure 4). For the SGC7901/ADR cell line, the staining of these proteins in the control groups was stronger than in the other groups ($p < 0.05$). PAB treatment reduced the intracellular staining of Cox-2, PKC-α and P-gp compared with the ADR-treated group ($p < 0.05$). After PAB and ADR treatment, the intracellular staining of these proteins was sparser and weaker compared with that of the other groups. For the xenografts of the two NS control groups, the staining of P-gp in the SGC7901 cells was significantly lower than that of the SGC7901/ADR cells ($p < 0.05$). The analysis of the staining intensity of Cox-2, PKC-α and P-gp expression revealed the same results (Table 2).

Effect of PAB on Cox-2, PKC-α, and P-gp expression in mice xenografts

To elucidate the molecular mechanism involved in the reversal effects of PAB on the SGC7901/ADR xenografts in vivo, the expression of Cox-2, PKC-α, and P-gp in tumors from different reagent-treated groups were determined by western blot analysis. As shown in Figure 5, for the NS control group, the expression levels of Cox-2, PKC-α, and P-gp in the SGC7901 cell xenografts were lower compared than those in the SGC7901/ADR cell tumors ($p < 0.05$). For the tumors of the SGC7901/ADR cells, the expression levels of the three proteins of interest in the NS control group and TWEEN control group were significantly higher compared with the other groups ($p < 0.05$), and there was no significant difference between the two groups ($p > 0.05$). The expression levels of Cox-2, PKC-α, and P-gp in the PAB-treated group were significantly lower compared with those of the ADR-treated group ($p < 0.05$). The expression of β-actin was used as an

Table 1. Antitumor effects of PAB and/or ADR on nude mice xenografts of SGC7901 cells and SGC7901/ADR cells.

	Number of animals		Body weight (g)		Volume of tumors (mm^3)		Relative tumor volume (mm^3)	Rtv/Ctv (%)	Tumor weight (g)	Inhibition rate (%)	Body weight change (%)
	Beginning	Ending	Beginning	Ending	Beginning	Ending					
SGC7901											
NS control group	5	5	21.3±2.8	21.2±2.0	13.5±2.5	596.8±109.6	44.3	100	1.05±0.09	0	−5.11±3.8
TWEEN control group	5	5	20.7±2.5	20.7±2.6	13.7±0.5	592.1±48.4	43.2	97.6	1.05±0.08	2.4	−5.13±2.9
ADR group	5	5	22.6±2.6	18.5±2.1	14.5±4.0	262.7±57.9	18.2	41.0	0.44±0.06*	59.0	−20.1±2.9
PAB group	5	5	20.7±3.5	21.0±3.7	14.4±2.1	276.8±68.6	19.3	43.6	0.49±0.1*	56.4	−0.98±6.0
PAB+ADR group	5	5	21.3±2.1	19.0±1.6	14.2±1.7	74.8±38.7	5.3	12.0	0.15±0.0*	88.1	−11.3±3.8
SGC7901/ADR											
NS control group	5	5	21.1±2.5	21.2±2.3	13.6±0.7	486.7±31.4	35.8	100	0.84±0.06	0	−3.44±2.4
TWEEN control group	5	5	20.7±2.3	21.1±2.0	13.0±1.3	486.2±71.3	37.4	104.5	0.83±0.12	−4.5	−1.90±5.2
ADR group	5	5	22.7±1.0	18.6±1.7	14.3±2.0	399.3±12.6	28.0	78.1	0.69±0.03*	21.9	−21.2±5.9
PAB group	5	5	21.1±2.5	21.0±2.2	14.1±2.0	180.8±15.6	12.8	35.9	0.32±0.03*	64.1	−1.87±2.2
PAB+ADR group	5	5	21.2±2.3	19.0±1.4	13.8±1.5	71.3±15.0	5.1	14. 2	0.13±0.04*	85.8	−10.7±3.7

Notes: * $p<0.05$ vs control group.
Rtv/Ctv (%) = (Relative tumor volume in treatment group/Relative tumor volume in NS control group) ×100.
Inhibition rate (%) = [(1-mean RTV of drug-treated group/mean RTV of NS control group) ×100].
Body weight (BW) change (%) = [(BW on day 20- tumor weight) - (BW on day 1)]/(BW on day 1) ×100.
PAB, Pseudolaric acid B; ADR, adriamycin.

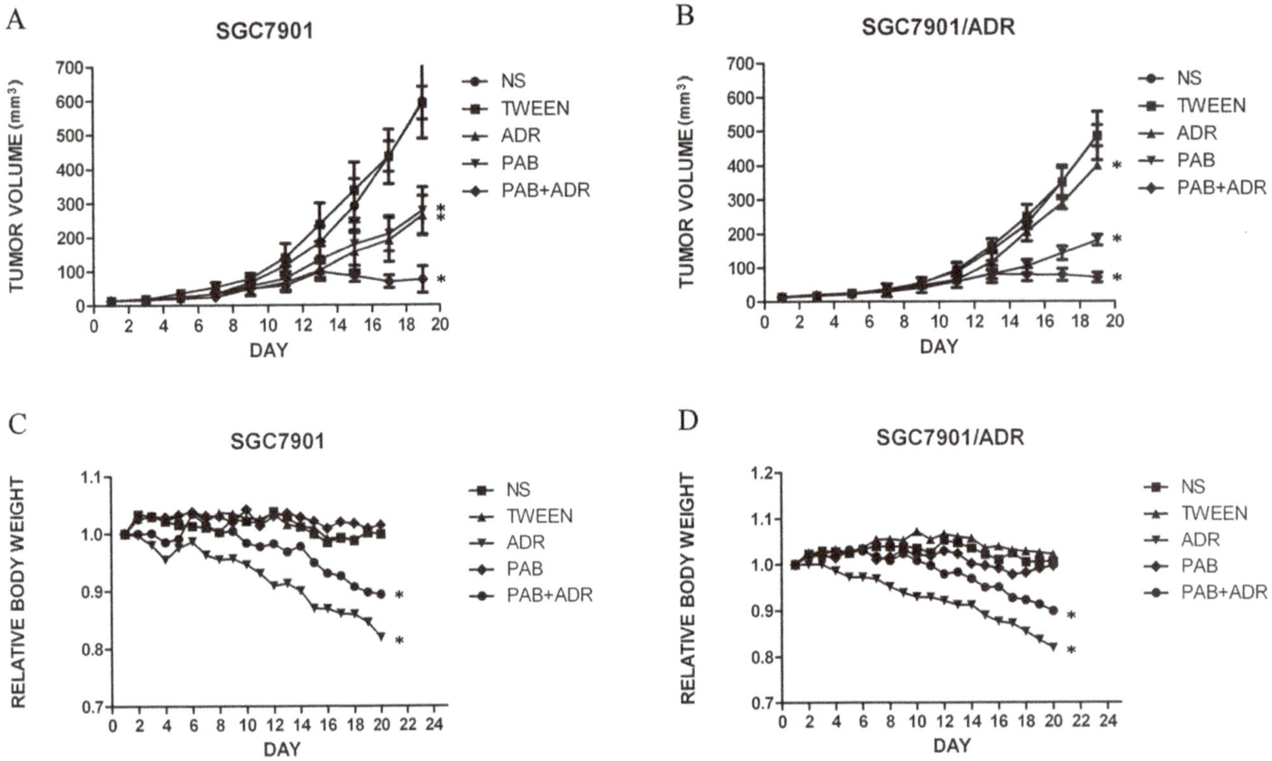

Figure 2. Inhibition of gastric tumor growth by pseudolaric acid B and mean body weight change of nude mice. A: growth curve of SGC7901 cell xenografts B: growth curve of SGC7901/ADR cell xenografts C: relative body weight change of mice with SGC7901 cell xenografts D: relative body weight change of mice with SGC7901/ADR cell xenografts. SGC7901 cells and SGC7901/ADR cells (2.5×10^6/ml) were injected subcutaneously into the axillary areas of nude mice, and when evident tumors were observed, the mice received a daily dose of 25 mg/kg pseudolaric acid B and/or 1.25 mg/kg adriamycin or normal saline (control)/tween solution (control) (n=5 per group). Tumor volumes were monitored at different time points (Day1, 3, 5, 7, 9, 11, 13, 15, 17, 19). The IR of tumor growth in the drug-treated groups were compared with that in the control groups at the end of the experiment by one-way ANOVA. *$p<0.05$ vs control group.

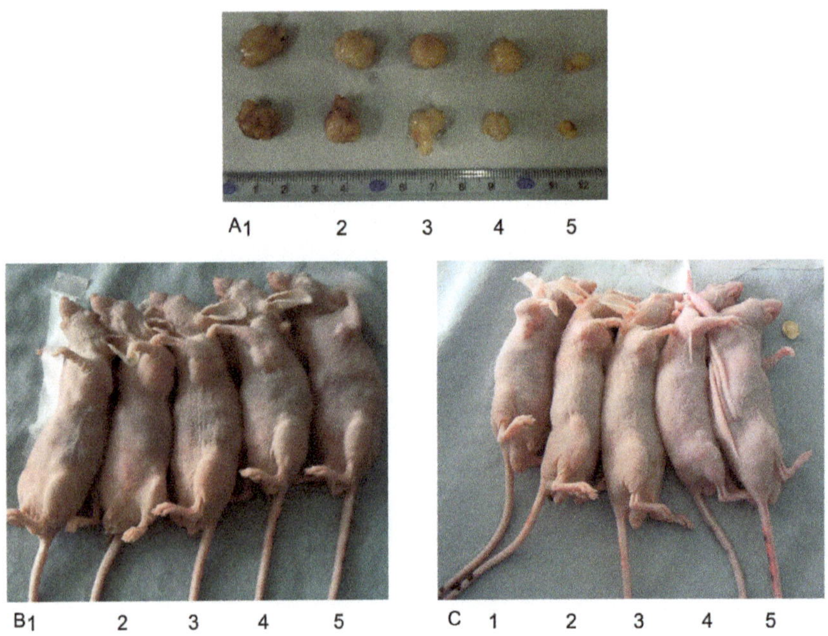

Figure 3. Subcutaneous xenografts of nude mice in different treatment groups. A: isolated tumors of SGC7901 cells (above) and SGC7901/ADR cells (below) B: subcutaneous xenografts of SGC7901 cell line in nude mice C: subcutaneous xenografts of SGC7901/ADR cell line in nude mice. (group 1): NS control group (group 2): TWEEN control group (group 3): ADR group (group 4): PAB group (group 5): PAB+ADR group.

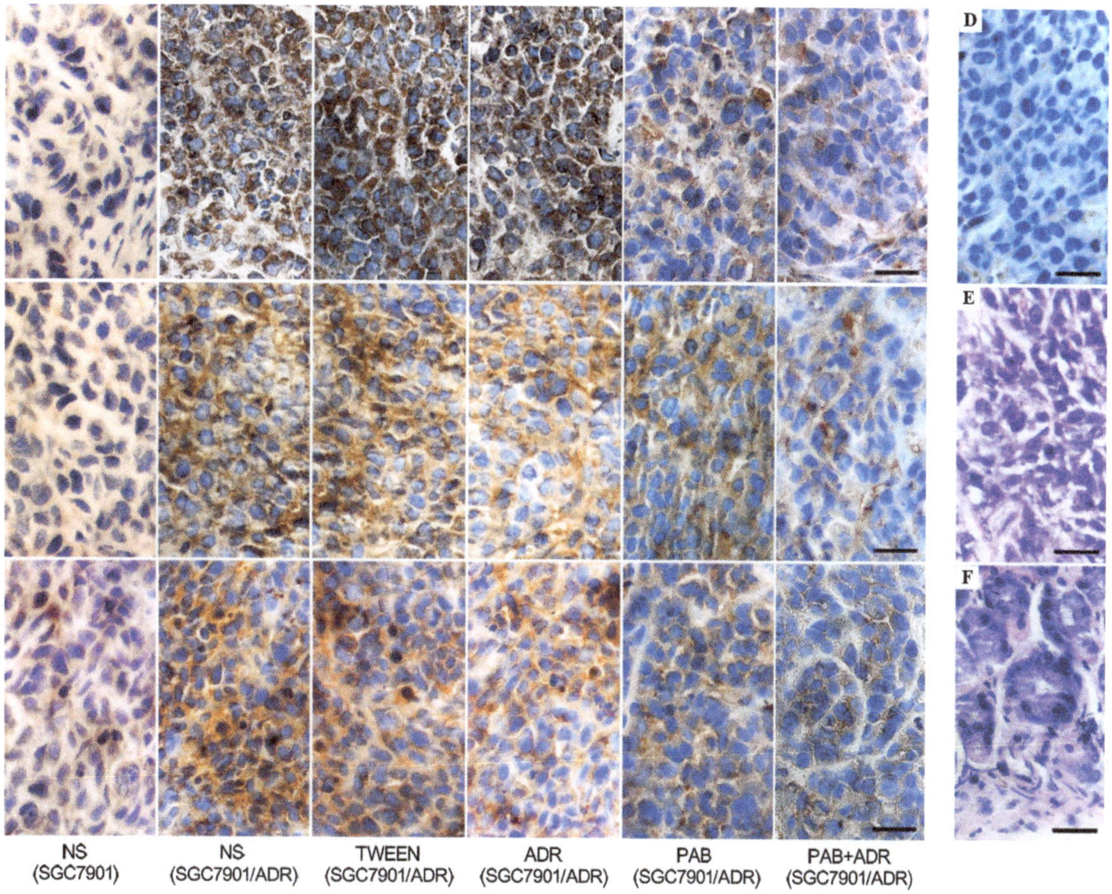

Figure 4. Cox-2, PKC-α, and P-gp expression levels of xenografts in different groups (×400). A: expression of Cox-2 in mice xenografts B: expression of PKC-α in mice xenografts C: expression of P-gp in mice xenografts D: negative control E: xenograft by HE F: normal gastric tissue by HE. Tissues were fixed, embedded, mounted and stained by the SP method or HE staining using standard procedures. Scale bar, 25 μm.

internal control, and the expression levels of Cox-2, PKC-α, and P-gp were decreased sequentially among the control groups, ADR group, PAB group and PAB+ADR group ($p<0.05$).

Discussion

PAB is one of the major biologically active components of the root bark of the medicinal plant *Pseudolarix kaempferi* and displays considerable cytotoxicity toward several cancer cell lines. In vitro studies have also demonstrated that it reverses the MDR of carcinoma by inhibiting the overexpression of P-gp without obvious side effects [13,15,20,21]. It has also been demonstrated that PAB has an antitumor effect in mice xenograft models of human colon cancer and hepatocellular carcinoma [13,20], and no known side effects of PAB on animals have been reported. Our previous study demonstrated that PAB has a potent inhibitory effect on the SGC7901 cell line in vitro and induces apoptosis of gastric cancer cells via the caspase pathway [16]. Our present in

Table 2. Average optical density of Cox-2, PKC-α and P-gp in different treatment groups (mean ± SD).

Group	n	Cox-2	PKC-α	P-gp
NS control group (SGC7901)	5	0.243±0.011*	0.192±0.012*	0.219±0.008*
NS control group (SGC7901/ADR)	5	0.302±0.004	0.285±0.006	0.292±0.008
TWEEN control group (SGC7901/ADR)	5	0.304±0.007	0.287±0.007	0.291±0.010
ADR group (SGC7901/ADR)	5	0.291±0.007*	0.252±0.002*	0.261±0.005*
PAB group (SGC7901/ADR)	5	0.255±0.004*	0.222±0.002*	0.241±0.005*
PAB+ADR group (SGC7901/ADR)	5	0.236±0.002*	0.183±0.009*	0.226±0.003*

Notes: * $p<0.05$ vs control group.
n: number of animals.
PAB, Pseudolaric acid B; ADR, adriamycin; SD, standard deviation.

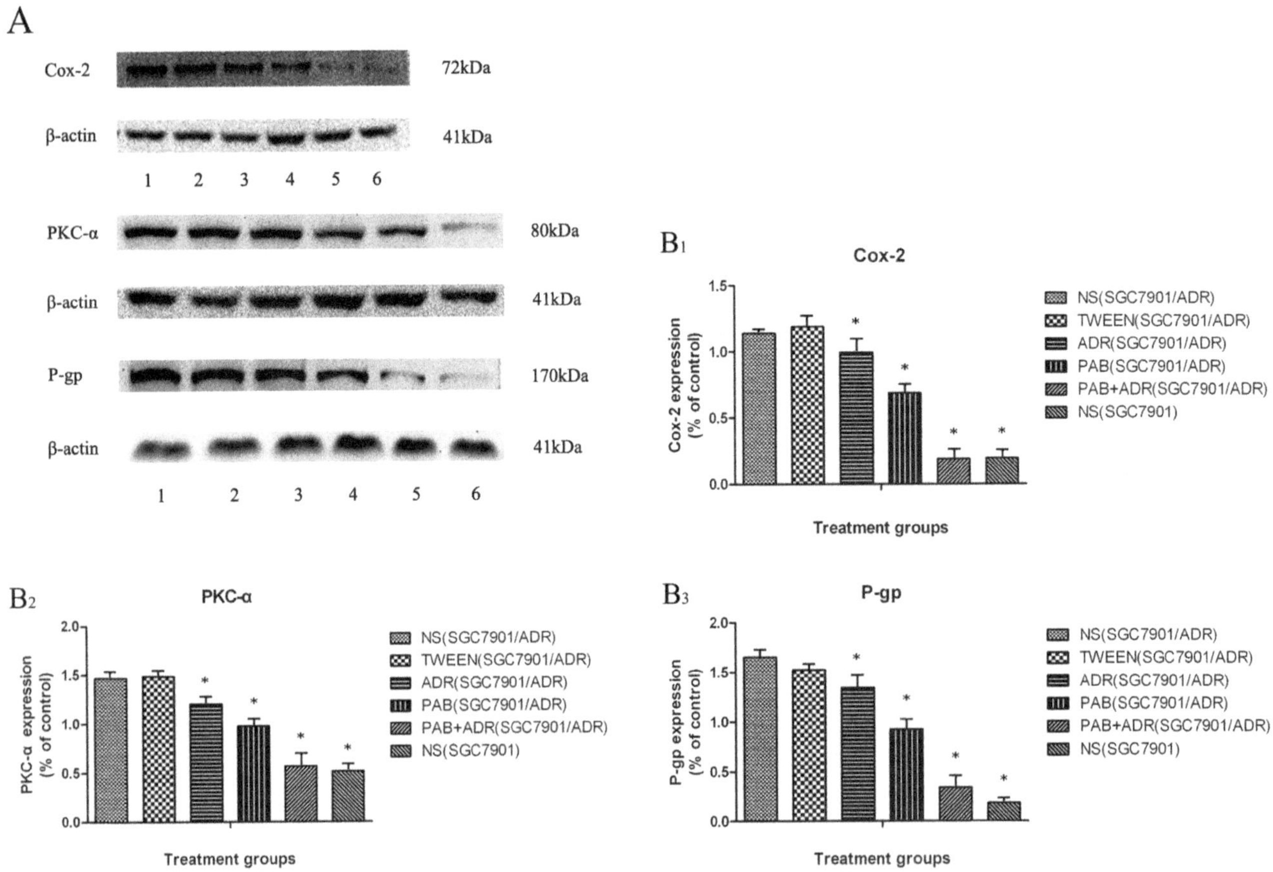

Figure 5. Inhibitory effects of PAB on expressions of Cox-2, PKC-α and P-gp in tumor tissues. A: representative immunoblots of Cox-2, PKC-α, P-gp compared with β-actin in different treatment groups. (lane 1): NS control group (SGC7901/ADR) (lane 2): TWEEN control group (SGC7901/ADR) (lane 3): ADR group (SGC7901/ADR) (lane 4): PAB group (SGC7901/ADR) (lane 5): PAB+ADR group (SGC7901/ADR) (lane 6): NS control group (SGC7901). B: relative expression levels of Cox-2 (B1), PKC-α (B2), and P-gp (B3) in different treatment groups. The tumors were isolated and homogenized to measure the protein level, and β-actin was used as an internal control. Each immunoblot was representative of three distinct experiments with similar results. *$p<0.05$ vs control group.

vivo study provides further evidence that PAB is protective against gastric tumors in murine xenograft models using SGC7901 cells and SGC7901/ADR cells. Our preliminary experiments have shown that PAB at 25 mg/kg not only inhibits the growth of gastric cancer but is also well tolerated by mice. Moreover, we included the TWEEN control group to exclude the influence of the aqueous solution that was used to dissolve PAB on tumors [13]. For sensitive cells, the anticancer effects of PAB produced no significant differences compared with ADR, a traditional chemotherapy drug. In addition, PAB is a biologically active compound that exerted its reversing effect against SGC7901/ADR cell line tumors by targeting the signaling pathway activated by P-gp overexpression in vivo.

P-gp is a 170-kDa membrane protein that acts as a drug efflux pump, resulting in a continuous defect in the intracellular accumulation of drugs [22]. The multidrug resistance phenotype is the major cause of tumor chemotherapy failure and is mainly the product of the overexpression of P-gp in the majority of cancers, including gastric neoplasms [23]. Moreover, the inhibition of this pathway might be a way to reverse the MDR of gastric cancer cells [3,24].

Cox-2, an inducible enzyme that catalyzes the conversion of arachidonic acid to prostanoids (PG) and participates in multiple physiological and pathological events, is induced by various inflammatory and mitogenic stimuli [25]. A strong association between MDR and the overexpression of Cox-2 has been reported in many different types of tumors. These previous results suggest that Cox-2 modulates the expression and activity of P-gp and is involved in the development of the MDR phenotype [26–28]. Moreover, accumulated evidence has demonstrated that Cox-2 inhibitors are able to sensitize cancer cells to the anti-proliferative effects of chemotherapeutic drugs by altering the activity of the ATP-binding cassette protein. Cox-2 inhibitors can even reverse MDR by blocking the Cox-2-mediated increase in MDR1 expression and activity in cancer, both in vitro and in vivo [6,7,29]. Therefore, we hypothesize that Cox-2 may regulate the expression of P-gp in tumor tissues and that inhibiting this pathway is of great significance to reversing the resistance of cancer to chemotherapeutic drugs.

We found that for the SGC7901/ADR cell tumors, the expression levels of Cox-2 and P-gp in the NS control group were evidently higher than those for the xenografts of SGC7901 cells. After the injection of PAB, an obvious decrease in these expression levels was observed. However, ADR was less effective for the suppression of the Cox-2 and P-gp expression levels of the SGC7901/ADR cell xenografts, and when combined with PAB, a lower level of proteins was observed. Thus, we proposed that modulation of Cox-2 expression by PAB could decrease the expression and activity of P-gp, inhibit growth and induce apoptosis, in addition to acting cooperatively with ADR in the suppression of drug-resistant tumors and even the reversal of the MDR phenotype of gastric cancer.

PKC is a serine/threonine kinase involved in the signal transduction required for cellular proliferation and differentiation [30]. Of the PKC isoforms, the overexpression and increased activity of PKC-α are most closely associated with the regulation of the MDR phenotype in human gastric cancer [31]. The results presented here support the notion that PKC-α phosphorylates P-gp, modulates P-gp efflux function, and ultimately leads to drug resistance [32]. The inhibition of PKC-α with a specific inhibitor or knocking down PKC-α with siRNA leads to reduced MDR1 expression, increased toxicity of anticancer drugs, and reversed MDR [8–10]. Therefore, we speculate that a PKC-α signal transduction system might play a role in modulating MDR1 expression in gastric cancer.

Under normal circumstances, PKC is inactive in cells, and its activation is related to upstream PGE activation. Cox-2 is coupled to membrane-associated prostaglandin E2 synthase (MPGES-1), and synthesis of PGE mediated by these proteins increases and activates the downstream PKC-α pathway [33]. It has been demonstrated that selective Cox-2 inhibition by specific inhibitors or siRNA has a therapeutic effect on inhibiting the expression of PKC-α and P-gp, while also, at the same time, reversing MDR [26,34]. A study has demonstrated that PGE2 mediates induction of MDR1 expression via the PKC pathway [35]. The results of our experiments demonstrated that PAB can inhibit PKC-α expression of xenografts of the SGC7901/ADR cell line, the effect of which was stronger than that of ADR. In addition, when PAB was combined with ADR, the PKC-α expression inhibition efficacy was even stronger. The variation tendency of PKC-α expression is consistent with that of Cox-2 and P-gp in various reagent-treated groups of drug-resistant SGC7901/ADR tumors. It has been shown that PAB induces growth arrest and apoptosis through inhibiting the Cox-2 pathway in cancer cells [20,21]. We hypothesize that PAB inhibits the expression of Cox-2 in SGC7901/ADR cell xenografts and that the coupling between Cox-2 and MPGES-1 reduces the synthesis of PGE, which reduces the activation of downstream PKC-α. As the phosphorylation of P-gp is inhibited, more drugs accumulate in the cancer cells, the toxicity of ADR is enhanced and MDR is reversed. These results provide insight into a new strategy involving the use of PAB to inhibit MDR of human gastric cancers.

One focus of our experiment is the inhibitory effect of pseudolaric acid B on subcutaneous xenografts of human gastric adenocarcinoma and the comparison of anti-tumor effects of drugs among different treatment groups. Moreover, the characteristic of SGC7901 cells and SGC7901/ADR cells are different. Through our two pre-experiment and a formal experiment, we all found the tumor volume of SGC7901/ADR cells was not larger than that of SGC7901 cells. We hypothesize the tumor volume might be associated with the cell count, growth time, characteristic of cells and other kinds of factors. Therefore, we have not compared the tumor volume between SGC7901 cell xenografts and SGC7901/ADR cell xenografts. In addition, we speculate that the body weight change of mice might be mainly related to the toxicity of drugs, and have not significant relationship to the tumor volume in our experiment.

The other focus of our experiment is the underlying molecular mechanisms involved in the multidrug resistance. Thus we have only designed NS control group of SGC7901 cell xenografts to contrast and confirm the expressions of the three kinds of protein from SGC7901/ADR cell xenografts are indeed significantly higher than that from SGC7901 cell xenografts. Besides, since the response of SGC7901 cells to anticancer drugs is rather more sensitive than SGC7901/ADR cells in both basic and clinical experiments, how to improve the sensitivity of multidrug resistance cells to anticancer drugs is our research focus. Therefore, we have not compared the expressions of Cox-2, PKC-α and P-gp for the tumors from SGC7901 and the various treatments of this group except for NS control group by western blot and immunohistochemical staining.

Our study discovered that the herbal diterpenoid PAB not only significantly suppressed gastric cancer SGC7901 cells in vivo but also displayed obvious inhibitory effects toward tumors of drug-resistant SGC7901/ADR cells. Moreover, the combination of PAB with ADR could inhibit the growth of gastric cancer and the development of xenografts in nude mice. It is worth mentioning that as a type of traditional Chinese medicine, the effect of PAB on the body weight of nude mice was quite lower than that of ADR in our experiment, which is an apparent advantage that makes PAB a more secure and tolerable drug for cancer therapy. PAB might not only be a new effective drug for the inhibition of the growth of gastric cancer and reversing its MDR, but it also can be used as an excellent adjuvant with traditional chemotherapeutics and surgical therapy following further development and research.

In the present study, we examined, for the first time, the inhibitory effect of PAB against human gastric cancer and its reversal effect on MDR in vivo via a xenograft nude mice model. We determined that its inhibition of MDR was mediated through the Cox-2/PKC-α/P-gp pathway, which provides a crucial theoretical basis concerning the molecular mechanisms of gastric cancer therapy. However, we have not studied the MDR mechanism in regards to gene expression and regulation. As the molecular mechanisms of reversing MDR are extraordinarily complicated and multiple types of proteins, genes and factors may be involved, the loop that we have proposed may be only a part of the mechanism for reversing MDR. More in-depth and concrete regulation mechanisms need to be elucidated in future studies.

In conclusion, PAB has a significant inhibitory effect on gastric cancer in vivo and can reverse the MDR of gastric cancer to chemotherapy drugs. The mechanism against MDR is mediated at least partially through the Cox-2/PKC-α/P-gp pathway. Our study provides broad prospects for future investigations of PAB in gastric cancer therapy.

Supporting Information

Checklist S1 ARRIVE Guidelines Checklist.
(DOC)

Author Contributions

Conceived and designed the experiments: YL. Performed the experiments: QS. Analyzed the data: QS. Contributed reagents/materials/analysis tools: YL QS. Wrote the paper: YL QS. Experimental guidance: YL.

References

1. Parkin DM, Pisani P, Ferlay J (1999) Estimates of the worldwide incidence of 25 major cancers in 1990. Int J Cancer 80: 827–841.
2. Ajani JA (1998) Chemotherapy for gastric carcinoma: new and old options. Oncology (*Williston Park*) 12: S44–47.

3. Borst P, Elferink RO (2002) Mammalian ABC transporters in health and disease. Annu Rev Biochem 71: 537–592.
4. Ambudkar SV, Kimchi-Sarfaty C, Sauna ZE, Gottesman MM (2003) P-glycoprotein: from genomics to mechanism. Oncogene 22: 7468–7485.
5. Nardone G, Rocco A, Vaira D, Staibano S, Budillon A, et al. (2004) Expression of COX-2, mPGE-synthase1, MDR-1 (P-gp), and Bcl-xL: a molecular pathway of H pylori-related gastric carcinogenesis. J Pathol 202: 305–312.
6. Roy KR, Reddy GV, Maitreyi L, Agarwal S, Achari C, et al. (2010) Celecoxib inhibits MDR1 expression through COX-2-dependent mechanism in human hepatocellular carcinoma (HepG2) cell line. Cancer Chemother Pharmacol 65: 903–911.
7. Vivaldi A, Ciampi R, Tacito A, Molinaro E, Agate L, et al. (2012) Celecoxib, a cyclooxygenase-2 inhibitor, potentiates the chemotherapic effect of vinorelbine in the medullary thyroid cancer TT cell line. Mol Cell Endocrinol 355: 41–48.
8. Fine RL, Chambers TC, Sachs CW (1996) P-Glycoprotein, Multidrug Resistance and Protein Kinase C. Oncologist 1: 261–268.
9. O'Brian CA, Ward NE, Stewart JR, Chu F (2001) Prospects for targeting protein kinase C isozymes in the therapy of drug-resistant cancer—an evolving story. Cancer Metastasis Rev 20: 95–100.
10. Lee SK, Shehzad A, Jung JC, Sonn JK, Lee JT, et al. (2012) Protein Kinase Cα Protects Against Multidrug Resistance in Human Colon Cancer Cells. Mol Cells 34: 61–69.
11. Yang SP, Dong L, Wang Y, Wu Y, Yue JM (2003) Antifunal diterpenoids of Pseudolarix kaempferi, and their structure-activity relationship study. Bioorg Med Chem 11: 4577–4584.
12. Tan WF, Zhang XW, Li MH, Yue JM, Chen Y, et al. (2004) Pseudolaric acid B inhibits angiogenesis by antagonizing the vascular endothelial growth factor-mediated anti-apoptotic effect. Eur J Pharmacol 499: 219–228.
13. Wong VK, Chiu P, Chung SS, Chow LM, Zhao YZ, et al. (2005) Pseudolaric acid B, a novel microtubule-destabilizing agent that circumvents multidrug resistance phenotype and exhibits antitumor activity in vivo. Clin Cancer Res 11: 6002–6011.
14. Yu JH, Cui Q, Jiang YY, Yang W, Tashiro S, et al. (2007) Pseudolaric acid B induces apoptosis, senescence, and mitotic arrest in human breast cancer MCF-7. Acta Pharmacol Sin 28: 1975–1983.
15. Li KS, Gu XF, Li P, Zhang Y, Zhao YS, et al. (2005) Effect of pseudolaric acid B on gastric cancer cells: inhibition of proliferation and induction of apoptosis. World J Gastroenterol 11: 7555–7559.
16. Xu YH, Wang XQ, Ju XH, Zhao LJ, Li Y (2008) Molecular mechanisms of pseudolaric acid B induced apoptosis in SGC7901 cells. Chinese Pharmacological Bulletin 24: 601–606.
17. Chen Y, Wei X, Yan P, Han Y, Sun S, et al. (2009) Human mitochondrial Mrs2 protein promotes multidrug resistance in gastric cancer cells by regulating p27, cyclin D1 expression and cytochrome C release. Cancer Biol Ther 8: 607–614.
18. Chen M, Huang SL, Zhang XQ, Zhang B, Zhu H, et al. (2012) Reversal effects of pantoprazole on multidrug resistance in human gastric adenocarcinoma cells by down-regulating the V-ATPases/mTOR/HIF-1α/P-gp and MRP1 signaling pathway in vitro and in vivo. J Cell Biochem 113: 2474–2487.
19. Kobunai T, Watanabe T, Fukusato T (2011) Antitumour activity of S-1 in combination with cetuximab on human gastric cancer cell lines in vivo. Anticancer Res 31: 3691–3696.
20. Hou L, Xu B, Guo W, Ran FX, Liu JT, et al. (2012) Pseudolaric acid B inhibits inducible cyclooxygenase-2 expression via downregulation of the NF-κB pathway in HT-29 cells. J Cancer Res Clin Oncol.
21. Ko JK, Leung WC, Ho WK, Chiu P (2007) Herbal diterpenoids induce growth arrest and apoptosis in colon cancer cells with increased expression of the nonsteroidal anti-inflammatory drug-activated gene. Eur J Pharmacol 559: 1–13.
22. Gottesman MM, Ling V (2006) The molecular basis of multidrug resistance in cancer: the early years of P-glycoprotein research. FEBS Lett 580: 998–1009.
23. Breier A, Barancík M, Sulová Z, Uhrík B (2005) P-glycoprotein—implications of metabolism of neoplastic cells and cancer therapy. Curr Cancer Drug Targets 5: 457–468.
24. Longley DB, Johnston PG (2005) Molecular mechanisms of drug resistance. J Pathol 205: 275–292.
25. Méric JB, Rottey S, Olaussen K, Soria JC, Khayat D, et al. (2006) Cyclooxygenase-2 as a target for anticancer drug development. Crit Rev Oncol Hematol 59: 51–64.
26. Ratnasinghe D, Daschner PJ, Anver MR, Kasprzak BH, Taylor PR, et al. (2001) Cyclooxygenase-2, P-glycoprotein-170 and drug resistance; is chemoprevention against multidrug resistance possible?. Anticancer Res 21: 2141–2147.
27. Sorokin A (2004) Cyclooxygenase-2: potential role in regulation of drug efflux and multidrug resistance phenotype. Curr Pharm Des 10: 647–657.
28. Yu L, Wu WK, Li ZJ, Liu QC, Li HT, et al. (2009) Enhancement of doxorubicin cytotoxicity on human esophageal squamous cell carcinoma cells by indomethacin and 4-[5-(4-chlorophenyl)-3-(trifluoromethyl)-1H-pyrazol-1-yl]-benzenesulfonamide (SC236) via inhibiting P-glycoprotein activity. Mol Pharmacol 75: 1364–1373.
29. Fantappiè O, Solazzo M, Lasagna N, Platini F, Tessitore L, et al. (2007) P-glycoprotein mediates celecoxib-induced apoptosis in multiple drug-resistant cell lines. Cancer Res 67: 4915–4923.
30. Clemens MJ, Trayner I, Menaya J (1992) The role of protein kinase C isoenzymes in the regulation of cell proliferation and differentiation. J Cell Sci 103: 881–887.
31. Han Y, Han ZY, Zhou XM, Shi R, Zheng Y, et al. (2002) Expression and function of classical proteinkinase C is oenzymes in gastric cancer cell line and its drug-resistant sublines. World J Gastroenterol 8: 441–445.
32. Ahmad S, Glazer RI (1993) Expression of the antisense cDNA for protein kinase C alpha attenuates resistance in doxorubicin-resistant MCF-7 breast carcinoma cells. Mol Pharmacol 43: 858–862.
33. Murakami M, Naraba H, Tanioka T, Semmyo N, Nakatani Y, et al. (2000) Regulation of prostaglandin E2 biosynthesis by inducible membrane-associated prostaglandin E2 synthase that acts in cyclooxygenase-2. J Biol Chem 275: 32783–32792.
34. Kalle AM, Sachchidanand S, Pallu R (2010) Bcr-Abl-independent mechanism of resistance to imatinib in K562 cells: Induction of cyclooxygenase-2 (COX-2) by histone deacetylases (HDACs). Leuk Res 34: 1132–1138.
35. Puhlmann U, Ziemann C, Ruedell G, Vorwerk H, Schaefer D, et al. (2005) Impact of the cyclooxygenase system on doxorubicin-induced functional multidrug resistance 1 overexpression and doxorubicin sensitivity in acute myeloid leukemic hl-60 cells. J Pharmacol Exp Ther 312: 346–354.

11

Assessment of Activity Limitations with the Health Assessment Questionnaire Predicts the Need for Support Measures in Patients with Rheumatoid Arthritis: A Multicenter Observational Study

Xavier Janssens[1]*, Saskia Decuman[1,2], Filip De Keyser[1], and the Belgian Rheumatoid Arthritis Disability Assessment study group

1 Department of Rheumatology, Ghent University Hospital, Ghent, Belgium, 2 Department of Internal Medicine, Ghent University, Ghent, Belgium

Abstract

Objective: This study investigated whether the Health Assessment Questionnaire (HAQ) can be used as an instrument to assess the need for social support measures that address activity limitations and participation issues in patients with rheumatoid arthritis (RA).

Methods: This multicenter observational study included patients with RA and disease duration of at least one year, consulting their rheumatologist for routine evaluation of disease activity. In the single study visit data on demographics, disease history and current treatment were collected. DAS28 values were collected to evaluate current RA disease activity. Patients were asked to fill out the HAQ and SF-36 questionnaires. Receiver Operator Characteristics (ROC) curves were constructed to evaluate the performance of the HAQ, SF-36 and DAS28 in predicting the need for nine supporting measures available for chronically ill patients in the Belgian social security system. The expert opinion of the treating rheumatologist was used as a reference.

Results: The study included 316 patients with a mean age of 59.8±12.6 years, disease duration of 11.4±9.3 years, mean DAS28 values of 2.83±1.17. Mean HAQ score was 0.95±0.73, mean SF-36 score 56.5±21.3. HAQ scores >1 were observed in 39.4% of patients. The area under the HAQ ROC curve was consistently >0.7 and higher for the HAQ than for SF-36 or DAS28 for all support measures. Rheumatologists on average recommended 3.67 support measures.

Conclusion: The HAQ score was found to be a good predictor of the need for social support measures in patients with RA.

Editor: Arvind Chopra, Center for Rheumatic Diseases, India

Funding: This work was supported by an unrestricted educational grant from Roche, by the 'Fonds de la Recherche de l'Association Polyarthrite-FRAP' and by the 'Fonds voor Wetenschappelijk Reuma Onderzoek/Fonds pour la Recherche Scientifique en Rhumatologie'. The funders had no role in study design, data collection and analysis,decision to publish, or preparation of the manuscript.

Competing Interests: F. De Keyser received research support from Roche, UCB, Actelion; served as consultant for MSD/Schering Plough, Abbott, UCB, Roche, GSK. Funding from Roche was received for this specific study. X. Janssens and S. Decuman declare that they have no conflicts of interest. There are no patents, products in development or marketed products to declare. This does not alter the authors' adherence to all the PLOS ONE policies on sharing data and materials, as detailed online in the guide for authors.

* Email: janssens.reuma@skynet.be

Introduction

As a chronic inflammatory disease, rheumatoid arthritis (RA) can lead to impairment of physical functioning and mobility, loss of productivity, and difficulties in performing normal daily activities. Patients with RA are confronted with extra costs to compensate for these difficulties, as well as with extra health care costs, often in combination with loss of income [1,2].

To limit the impact of RA on functioning and quality of life, support measures addressing activity limitations and participation issues are an important complement to the medical treatment. In order to promote equitable allocation of supporting measures and determine the level and type of supporting measures needed, objective and reliable evaluation of the level and area of activity limitations in patients is essential.

The Health Assessment Questionnaire (HAQ) was developed three decades ago at Stanford University by Fries and colleagues as a patient-reported outcome instrument designed to measure health status and health-related quality of life. It is a 20-item questionnaire covering activities of daily living in 8 domains. Respondents indicate for every item whether they can do the activity 'without any difficulty', with 'some' or 'much difficulty' or are 'unable to do' the activity. The HAQ yields a disability index (HAQ-DI) score between 0 and 3, where 0 means no disability and 3 represents total dependence on others [3–5]. HAQ scores >1 are considered to indicate the presence of disability.

The HAQ is one of the most important patient-reported outcome measures in RA clinical trials, but is also commonly used by rheumatologists in daily practice [6,7], to assess the functional status of their patients. The HAQ has been translated in many languages [8] and has proven validity and reliability in patients with RA [9,10].

In the Belgian social security system, nine different social support measures are currently available for persons with chronic daily activity limitations and loss of autonomy, to promote their reintegration and participation. These support measures comprise financial benefits, disease cost reduction measures, tax benefits and social benefits (see Table 1). There is no validated score for allocation of these benefits.

In this study, we investigated whether the HAQ can predict the need for such social support measures in patients with RA, with the expert opinion of the treating rheumatologist as a reference and compared the performance of HAQ, DAS28 and SF-36.

Patients and Methods

Ethics Statement

All patients gave written informed consent and the study was approved by the Ethics Committee of the University Hospital Ghent (ref. 2010-094) and the ethical committees of the participating clinical centers.

Study Design

Patients eligible for inclusion in this multicenter observational study were at least 18 years of age, met the American College of Rheumatology (ACR) classification criteria for RA [11], had a disease duration of at least one year and consulted their rheumatologist for routine half-yearly outpatient evaluation (according to nomenclature number 478030 of the Belgian social security system). No specific exclusion criteria were defined.

To obtain a representative population of patients with RA, participating rheumatologists asked the first eligible patient in every consultation time block to participate in the study. Patients who gave their written informed consent were included in the study and proceeded with the study data collection in the same visit.

Data collected comprised patient demographics, disease history, current treatment, DAS28, HAQ and SF-36 questionnaires. The treating rheumatologists scored the need for each of 9 different supporting measures (Table 1) available for chronically ill patients in the Belgian social security system on a four item categorical scale as: certainly needed, probably needed, probably not needed or certainly not needed. HAQ and SF-36 questionnaires were filled out independently by the patient; the rheumatologists were unaware of the SF-36 or HAQ scores, which were only calculated during data analysis.

Data analysis and statistics

Data are presented as mean ± standard deviation for normally distributed variables, as median (range) for variables not following a normal distribution or as percentages. Statistical analysis was performed with SPSS version 20 software (IBM Corporation, Armonk, New York, USA). A p-value <0.05 was considered statistically significant.

The Kolmogorov-Smirnov test was used to assess the normal distribution of variables. To compare age groups <65 y versus ≥ 65 y, unpaired t-test or Mann-Whitney U-test was used for continuous variables, and chi-square test for categorical variables.

To evaluate the performance of the HAQ, SF-36 and DAS28 as tests to predict the need for social support measures by patients with RA, Receiver Operator Characteristics (ROC) curves were constructed and the area under the ROC curve (AUC) was calculated [12], with the recommendation of the treating rheumatologist for all nine support measures (Table 1) as the reference. To this end, the scores 'certainly needed' and 'probably needed' were considered as a positive recommendation for a particular support measure, unless otherwise stated. For the purpose of constructing the ROC-curve with sensitivity and specificity for the outcome that at least one support measure is considered necessary by the treating rheumatologist, only the score 'certainly needed' was considered as a positive score. The relevance of such exercise is that a cut-off for this criterium could define a subpopulation of RA patients who would certainly need at least one support measure and a complimentary subpopulation in which no essential support measures apply.

The AUCs of the ROC curves for HAQ, SF-36 and DAS28 were compared using ANOVA.

Table 1. Social support measures for chronically ill patients in Belgium.

Support measure	Type	Description
Integration allowance	Financial benefit (<65 years)	To compensate extra costs due to diminished autonomy and to enhance social participation of person with special needs.
Allowance for help to the aged	Financial benefit (>65 years)	For seniors with chronic health disorders confronted with supplementary costs due to loss of autonomy, in order to enhance their social participation.
Tax reduction	Tax benefit	Income tax exemption for families with one or more disabled persons.
Parking card	Promotion of mobility	For persons with mobility restrictions. Allows parking in parking places reserved for disabled persons and parking without time limit in areas of time restricted parking.
Vehicle tax waiver	Tax benefit	Exemption of car tax for disabled persons
Free public transportation for attendant	Promotion of mobility	Free public transportation access for companions of people with mobility restrictions who can't travel alone
Social telephone rate	Cost reduction	Reduced telephone connection rate, subscription fee and call charges for people with functional limitations.
Social rate utility services	Cost reduction	Exemption of regular allowance and free delivery of a fixed amount of gas and electricity for disabled persons.
Allowance for chronic illness	Financial benefit (<65 years)	Premium for persons with a chronic disease confronted with high medical costs.

Table 2. Population characteristics.

Population characteristics		Overall	<65 y	≥65 y
Nr of patients		316	200	116
% of patients		100	63.3	36.7
Age (y)		59.8±12.6	52.6±9.9	72.31±5.4
Gender ratio (% female)		69.9	73.5	63.8
RA characteristics				
Disease duration (y)		11.4±9.3	10.8±8.98	12.2±9.8
RF (% positive)		72.9	71.5	75.2
Anti-CCP (% positive)		58.7	60.5	55.6
Erosions (% positive)		65.5	65.3	66.0
DAS 28		2.83±1.17	2.89±1.16	2.71±1.18
HAQ		0.95±0.73	0.91±0.68	1.01±0.81
	% HAQ >1	39.4	37.0	42.2
SF-36	Total	56.5±21.3	54.0±20.8	60.9±21.6
	MCS	60.6±21.6	58.2±21.4	64.7±21.2
	PCS	49.4±21.4	47.02±20.9	53.6±21.6
Treatment (% of patients)				
DMARDs		86.4	86.0	87.1
DMARDs - no biologicals		51.6	45.5	62.1
Biologicals		45.9	52.5	34.5
Corticosteroids		44.6	56.5	46.6
NSAIDs		42.2	44.5	38.4

Data are expressed as mean ± standard error or as percentages. *Abbreviations: CRP: C-reactive protein, DAS28: disease activity score using 28 joint counts, DMARDs: Disease-modifying anti-rheumatic drugs, HAQ: Health Assessment Questionnaire, MCS: mental component summary, NSAIDs: non-steroidal anti-inflammatory drugs, PCS: physical component summary, SF-36: Short Form-36.*

The Youden index (sensitivity + specificity − 1) was used to provide a single statistic to capture the performance of the predictive tests [13].

Results

Population characteristics

Table 2 summarizes the study population characteristics. The study included 316 patients with RA. Patients were on average 59.8±12.6 years old, with 36.7% (n = 116) of patients aged 65 or older, 69.9% were female. Mean disease duration was 11.4±9.3 years, rheumatoid factor was present in 72.9% of patients and anti-CCP in 58.7%. DAS28 values were 2.83±1.17, HAQ scores were 0.95±0.73 and 39.4% of patients had a HAQ score >1. SF-36 scores were 56.5±21.3, with lower scores on the physical than on the mental subscale, suggesting a larger impact of RA on physical than on mental functioning. HAQ scores and DAS28 values did not differ significantly between patients below 65 years of age and older patients, but patients aged 65 or older had significantly higher SF-36 scores (Figure 1A).

Current RA treatment included DMARDs in 86.4% of patients, 45.9% of patients were on biologicals. Corticosteroids were used by 44.6% and NSAIDs by 42.2% of patients.

Assessment of the need for social support measures by the rheumatologist

The need for the social support measures listed in Table 1 was scored for every patient by the rheumatologist as certainly or probably needed or certainly or probably not needed. Rheumatologists on average recommended 3.67 support measures per patient.

The most frequently recommended support measures were the allowance for chronic illness (62.2%), tax reduction (51.5%) and social telephone rate (49.5%). Integration allowance was recommended for 43.6% of patients <65 years of age, allowance for help to the aged was recommended for 48.6% of patients older than 65. Rheumatologists recommended the social rate for utility services in 42.2% of patients. Vehicle tax waiver, parking card and free public transportation for an attendant were recommended for respectively 45.6%, 37.8% and 26.9% of patients. (Figure 2).

Predicting the need for social support measures

The number of benefits recommended by the rheumatologist clearly increased with increasing HAQ scores, but not with increasing DAS28 values. Likewise, the number of benefits recommended did not increase with decreasing SF-36 scores (Figure 1B).

In order to assess whether measures of disease activity or functioning can predict the need for social support measures, ROC curve analysis was performed with HAQ, SF-36 and DAS28 for each of the social support measures, with the recommendation of the rheumatologist as reference or gold standard.

The AUC of these ROC curves are presented in Table 3. For all support measures, AUCs were significantly higher for the HAQ than for either SF-36 or DAS28, with AUC values for HAQ of at least 0.7 for all measures (ANOVA, $p = 0.001$), indicating that the HAQ score is a valuable predictor of the need for social support measures in patients with RA and is superior in that function to

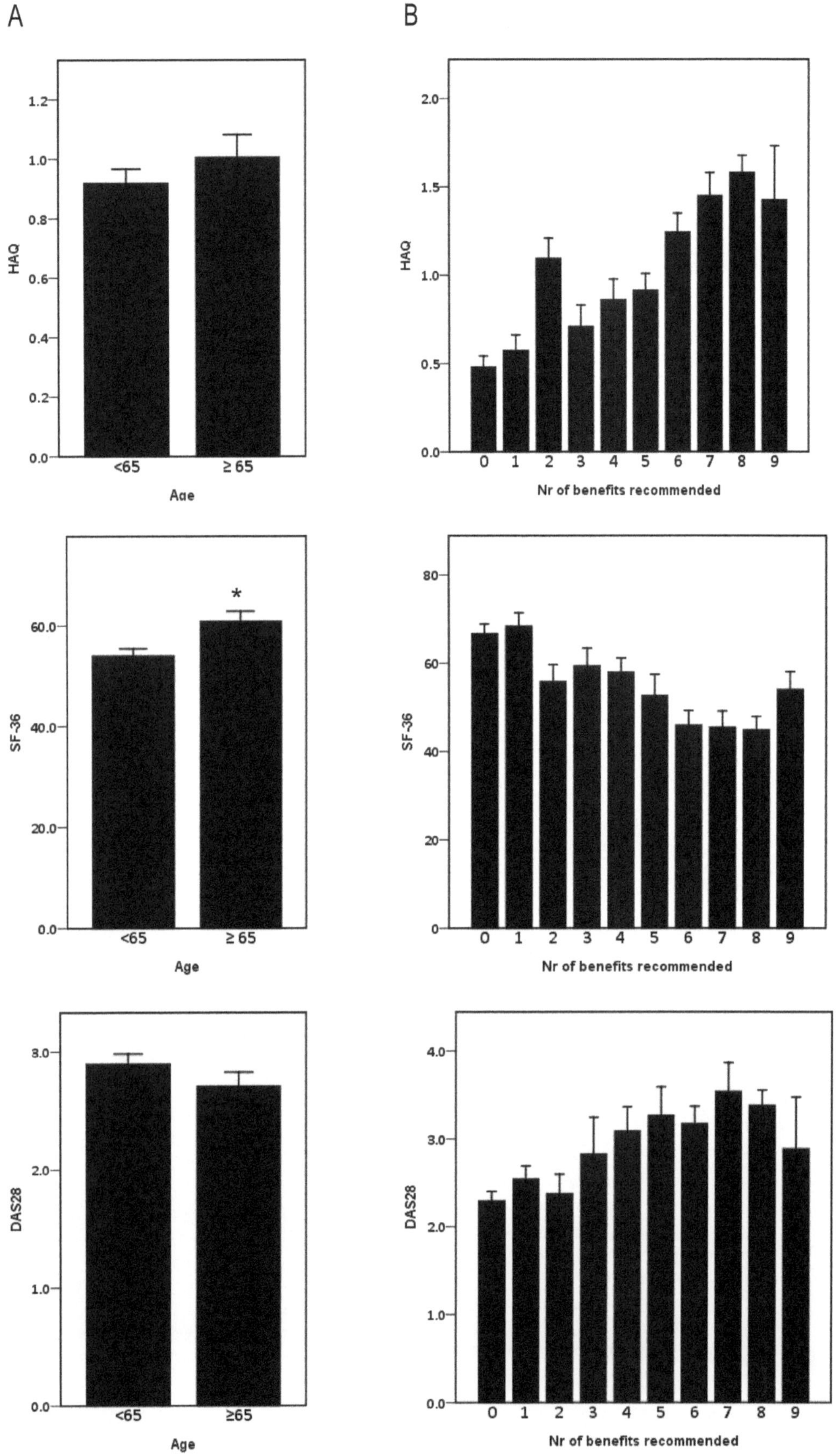

Figure 1. HAQ, SF-36 and DAS 28. A. In function of patient age category. Means for HAQ and DAS28 did not differ between patients below 65 y of age and patients of 65 or older, but patients in the latter age category had significantly higher SF-36 scores *: $p<0.05$ (t-test, error bars represent standard error of the mean). B. In function of number of benefits recommended by the rheumatologist. (Error bars represent standard error of the mean).

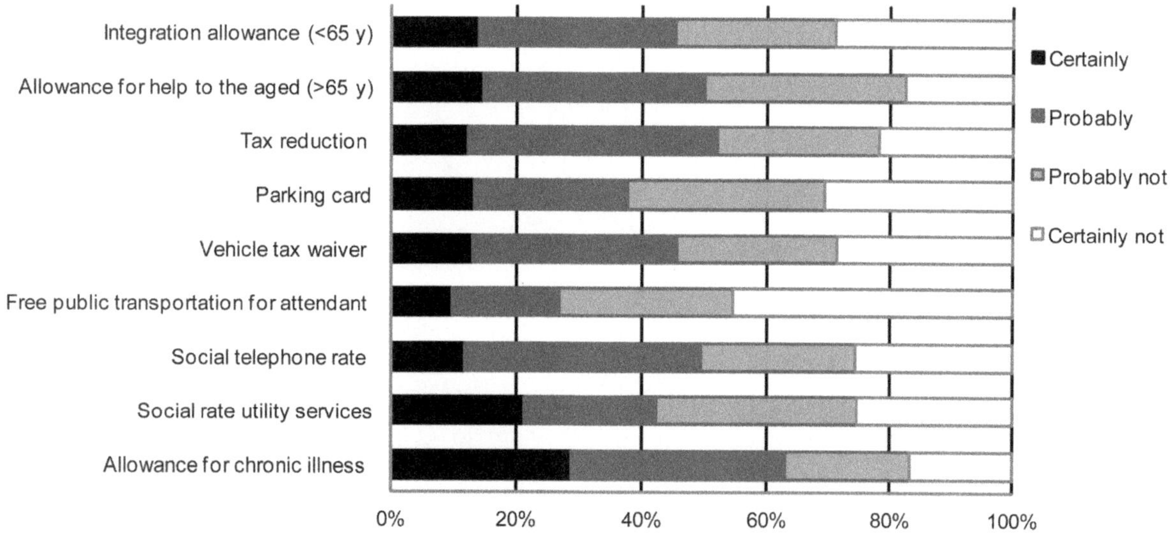

Figure 2. Assessment of need for social support measures by the rheumatologist. Data are expressed as percentage of patients. For support measures with age limits, the patient percentage refers only to the patients in the age category eligible to receive the benefit.

DAS28 and SF-36. Figure 3 shows the ROC curves of the HAQ as predictor for the need for support measures. See File S1 for the raw data for these ROC curves.

An additional purpose was to create a ROC-curve with sensitivity and specificity for the outcome that at least one support measure is considered certainly necessary by the treating rheumatologist. In this way, one can propose a cut-off to define a subpopulation of RA patients who would certainly need at least one support measure and a complimentary subpopulation in which no essential support measures apply. Thus, in the latter subpopulation with a score beneath such cut-off, one would not miss any essential support measure. The AUC for such ROC-curve with HAQ, SF-36 and DAS28 was respectively 0.750, 0.698 and 0.656. For the HAQ, the Youden Index for this analysis reached a maximum of 0.391 for a HAQ cut-off of 0.69 (sensitivity 80.8% and specificity 58.3%). In our study population, 133 patients (42.1%) had a HAQ score below 0.69.

No support measures were recommended by the rheumatologist in 24.4% of patients overall and in 43.3% of patients with a HAQ score below 0.69.

Discussion

Optimal care for patients with RA needs to include support measures to compensate for difficulties in performing daily activities and participation issues. Together, they may alleviate the substantial impact this disease may have.

In this study we evaluated whether disease activity parameters such as DAS28, indicators of functioning such as HAQ, or a measure of health status like SF-36 can predict the need for social support measures, since equitable allocation of benefits requires a reliable measure to evaluate activity limitation.

In this representative, unselected population of patients with longstanding RA, the HAQ score was found to be the best predictor for the need of social support measures, with AUC of the ROC curve of at least 0.7 for all support measures investigated.

Table 3. AUC of ROC- curves for HAQ, SF-36 and DAS28.

	HAQ	SF-36	SF-36 PCS	DAS28
Integration allowance (<65 y)	0.806	0.725	0.779	0.695
Allowance for help to the aged (>65 y)	0.798	0.798	0.776	0.785
Tax reduction	0.766	0.727	0.748	0.713
Parking card	0.831	0.728	0.750	0.703
Vehicle tax waiver	0.778	0.710	0.715	0.632
Free public transportation for attendant	0.700	0.642	0.650	0.660
Social telephone rate	0.775	0.708	0.721	0.665
Social rate utility services	0.755	0.735	0.748	0.647
Allowance for chronic illness	0.707	0.639	0.657	0.641

Areas under the curve (AUC) of the ROC curve analysis performed with HAQ, SF-36, SF-36 physical component score (PCS) and DAS28 for the social support measures available in Belgium in order to assess whether these instruments can be used to predict the need for social support measures in patients with RA. The recommendation of the rheumatologist was used as reference.

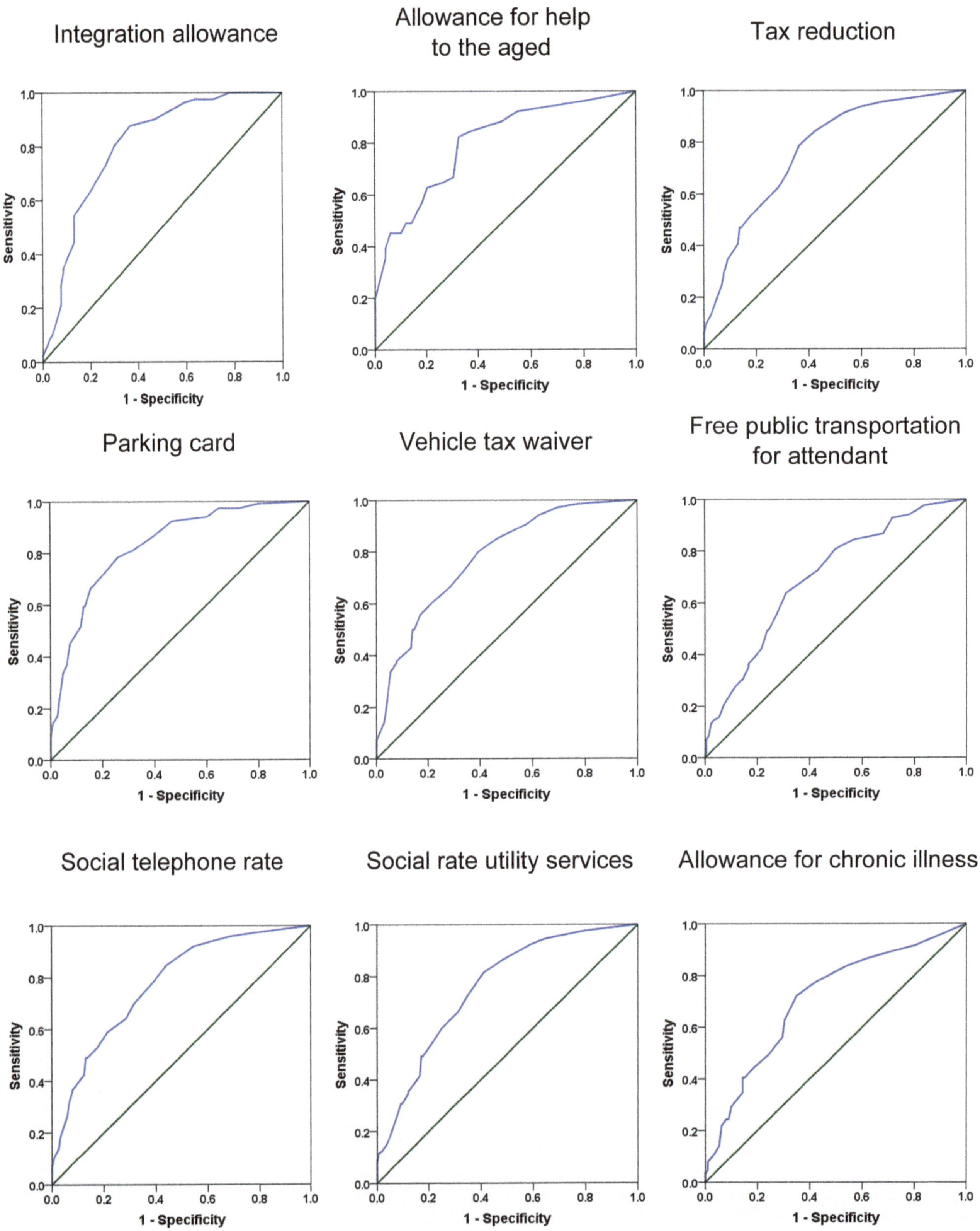

Figure 3. ROC curves for HAQ predicting the need for different social support measures. Receiver operator characteristic analysis (ROC) demonstrates that the Health Assessment Questionnaire (HAQ) performs well as a tool to predict the need for social support measures in patients with RA. The recommendation by the treating rheumatologist was used as reference.

Previous studies in the United Kingdom (UK) showed that the HAQ can be used to predict successful application for access to benefits and financial support [14–16]. In the UK, 69% of the patients with RA or osteoarthritis of hip or knee and a HAQ score >1.5 who applied were awarded the benefit [15].

In our study, no data were collected on actual applications to receive the social support measures studied, nor on actual allocation of these benefits, so that the results of our study solely represent the expert opinion of the treating rheumatologists on their patients' needs. We did not attempt to calculate HAQ cut-off values for the different support measures investigated, but instead chose to include the raw data of the ROC curves as supplementary data (File S1). Consequently, the data from this study can be used to calculate HAQ cut-offs to suit the sensitivity or specificity limits one wishes to use or to fit the budget available for these benefits.

Based upon our analysis, we propose a HAQ cut-off value of 0.69 to define two RA subpopulations according to whether or not these patients absolutely require at least one of the described support measures. The relevance of this cut-off could be that in case the HAQ score is lower than this cut-off, one could justify not pursuing further efforts for allocation of support measures.

Functioning may be further impaired by factors such as age and comorbidity. It is an important strength of the HAQ to provide a comprehensive assessment of a patient's functioning, not only determined by RA, but also by old age or limitations as a consequence of superimposed comorbidity. The need of support measures will increase with this global loss of functioning and not just with the functional limitations of RA.

We did not collect socioeconomic parameters or educational status in this study. The impact of these parameters on functioning are still controversial: a Swedish cross sectional study reported no influence of socioeconomic factors and education on disability in RA patients [17] but a number of studies have found RA disease activity and severity to be more pronounced in patients with lower socio-economic status [18,19].

Our findings indicate that it would be feasible to expand the scope of application of the HAQ to include its use as an instrument for allocating access to financial or social support measures or to tax benefits for patients with RA. Such an approach would have the added benefit of reducing the administrative burden involved with benefit allocation by using the results of a test that is widely used and accepted for clinical monitoring of patients with RA.

Additional research is needed to investigate whether the use of HAQ score to determine the need of support can be generalized to other regions, with other types of support measures available, and to determine what the impact would be of using the HAQ for the actual allocation of social support measures. A follow-up study investigating which domains of the HAQ determine best the need for which kind of support measures is currently ongoing.

In summary, the HAQ score was found to be a good predictor (better than DAS28 and SF-36) for the need for social support measures in patients with RA, as assessed by the rheumatologist.

Supporting Information

File S1 ROC curve data tables for the HAQ. Tables with coordinates of the ROC curve analysis investigating the performance of the Health Assessment Questionnaire (HAQ) as an instrument to evaluate the need for social support measures in patients with RA. The expert opinion of the treating rheumatologist on the need for social support measures was used as a reference.
(DOCX)

Acknowledgments

The Belgian Rheumatoid Arthritis Disability Assessment study group: Ackerman C (Lead author, AZ St Lucas, Gent, christine.ackerman@azstlucas.be), André B (CHU Sart Tilman Liège), Brasseur J-P (Clinique Saint-Pierre, Ottignies), Cremer D (Hôpital Saint-Joseph, Liège), De Brabanter G (AZ St-Lucas, Brugge), De Keyser F (AZ Alma, Sijsele), Durez P (Cliniques Universitaires Saint-Luc, Bruxelles), Fontaine M-A (Hôpital Saint-Joseph, Liège), Gyselbrecht L (ASZ, Aalst), Houssiau F (Cliniques Universitaires Saint-Luc, Bruxelles), Lauwerys B (Cliniques Universitaires Saint-Luc, Bruxelles), Maeyaert B (AZ St-Lucas, Brugge), Stubbe M (ULB, Erasme), Vandenberghe M (ASZ, Aalst), Vanden Berghe M (GHDC Hôpital Saint-Joseph, Gilly), Van Mullem X (GHDC Hôpital Saint-Joseph, Gilly), Verschueren P (UZ Gasthuisberg, Leuven), Westhovens R (UZ Gasthuisberg, Leuven).

The authors acknowledge the contribution of Veerle Persy, MD, PhD as an independent medical writer on behalf of Hugin Mugin Research.

Author Contributions

Conceived and designed the experiments: XJ FDK. Performed the experiments: XJ SD FDK. Analyzed the data: XJ SD FDK. Contributed reagents/materials/analysis tools: FDK. Wrote the paper: XJ.

References

1. Yelin E, Wanke L (1999) An assessment of the annual and long-term direct costs of rheumatoid arthritis: the impact of poor function and functional decline. Arthritis Rheum 42: 1209–1218. doi:10.1002/1529-0131(199906)42:6<1209::AID-ANR18>3.0.CO;2-M.
2. Huscher D, Merkesdal S, Thiele K, Zeidler H, Schneider M, et al. (2006) Cost of illness in rheumatoid arthritis, ankylosing spondylitis, psoriatic arthritis and systemic lupus erythematosus in Germany. Ann Rheum Dis 65: 1175–1183. doi:10.1136/ard.2005.046367.
3. Bruce B, Fries JF (2003) The Stanford Health Assessment Questionnaire: a review of its history, issues, progress, and documentation. J Rheumatol 30: 167–178.
4. Bruce B, Fries JF (2003) The Stanford Health Assessment Questionnaire: dimensions and practical applications. Health Qual Life Outcomes 1: 20. doi:10.1186/1477-7525-1-20.
5. Bruce B, Fries JF (2005) The Health Assessment Questionnaire (HAQ). Clin Exp Rheumatol 23: S14–8.
6. Wolfe F, Kleinheksel SM, Cathey MA, Hawley DJ, Spitz PW, et al. (1988) The clinical value of the Stanford Health Assessment Questionnaire Functional Disability Index in patients with rheumatoid arthritis. J Rheumatol 15: 1480–1488.
7. Pincus T (2006) The DAS is the most specific measure, but a patient questionnaire is the most informative measure to assess rheumatoid arthritis. J Rheumatol 33: 834–837.
8. Zandbelt MM, Welsing PM, van Gestel a M, van Riel PL (2001) Health Assessment Questionnaire modifications: is standardisation needed? Ann Rheum Dis 60: 841–845.
9. Linde L, Sørensen J, Ostergaard M, Hørslev-Petersen K, Hetland ML (2008) Health-related quality of life: validity, reliability, and responsiveness of SF-36, 15D, EQ-5D [corrected] RAQoL, and HAQ in patients with rheumatoid arthritis. J Rheumatol 35: 1528–1537.
10. Sokka T, Kautiainen H, Hannonen P, Pincus T (2006) Changes in Health Assessment Questionnaire disability scores over five years in patients with rheumatoid arthritis compared with the general population. Arthritis Rheum 54: 3113–3118. doi:10.1002/art.22130.
11. Arnett FC, Edworthy SM, Bloch DA, McShane DJ, Fries JF, et al. (1988) The American Rheumatism Association 1987 revised criteria for the classification of rheumatoid arthritis. Arthritis Rheum 31: 315–324.
12. Bewick V, Cheek L, Ball J (2004) Statistics review 13: receiver operating characteristic curves. Crit Care 8: 508–512. doi:10.1186/cc3000.
13. Youden WJ (1950) Index for rating diagnostic tests. Cancer 3: 32–35.
14. Memel DS, Kirwan JR, Langley C, Hewlett S, Hehir M (2002) Prediction of successful application for disability benefits for people with arthritis using the Health Assessment Questionnaire. Rheumatology (Oxford) 41: 100–102.
15. Langley C, Memel DS, Kirwan JR, Pollock J, Hewlett S, et al. (2004) Using the Health Assessment Questionnaire and welfare benefits advice to help people disabled through arthritis to access financial support. Rheumatology (Oxford) 43: 863–868. doi:10.1093/rheumatology/keh184.

16. Fruin C, Pitt PI (2008) Welfare benefit promotion within a district general hospital rheumatology centre: a joint project with the local Citizens Advice Bureau. Musculoskeletal Care 6: 211–219. doi:10.1002/msc.133.
17. Bendtsen P, Bjurulf P, Trell E, Lindström F, Larsson JE (n.d.) Cross-sectional assessment and subgroup comparison of functional disability in patients with rheumatoid arthritis in a Swedish health-care district. Disabil Rehabil 17: 94–99.
18. Harrison MJ, Farragher TM, Clarke AM, Manning SC, Bunn DK, et al. (2009) Association of functional outcome with both personal- and area-level socioeconomic inequalities in patients with inflammatory polyarthritis. Arthritis Rheum 61: 1297–1304. doi:10.1002/art.24830.
19. Massardo L, Pons-Estel BA, Wojdyla D, Cardiel MH, Galarza-Maldonado CM, et al. (2012) Early rheumatoid arthritis in Latin America: low socioeconomic status related to high disease activity at baseline. Arthritis Care Res (Hoboken) 64: 1135–1143. doi:10.1002/acr.21680.

12

Pyrroloquinoline Quinone (PQQ) Inhibits Lipopolysaccharide Induced Inflammation in Part via Downregulated NF-κB and p38/JNK Activation in Microglial and Attenuates Microglia Activation in Lipopolysaccharide Treatment Mice

Chongfei Yang[1], Lifeng Yu[1], Lingbo Kong[2], Rui Ma[3], Juliang Zhang[1], Qingsheng Zhu[1], Jinyu Zhu[1]*, Dingjun Hao[2]*

1 Institute of Orthopaedic Surgery, Xijing Hospital, Fourth Military Medical University, Xi'an, China, **2** Hong-Hui Hospital, Xi'an Jiaotong University College of Medicine, Xi'an, China, **3** Department of Anesthesiology, Xijing Hospital, Fourth Military Medical University, Xi'an, China

Abstract

Therapeutic strategies designed to inhibit the activation of microglia may lead to significant advancement in the treatment of most neurodegenerative diseases. Pyrroloquinoline quinone (PQQ) is a naturally occurring redox cofactor that acts as an essential nutrient, antioxidant, and has been reported to exert potent immunosuppressive effects. In the present study, the anti-inflammatory effects of PQQ was investigated in LPS treated primary microglia cells. Our observations showed that pretreatment with PQQ significantly inhibited the production of NO and PGE2 and suppressed the expression of pro-inflammatory mediators such as iNOS, COX-2, TNF-a, IL-1b, IL-6, MCP-1 and MIP-1a in LPS treated primary microglia cells. The nuclear translocation of NF-κB and the phosphorylation level of p65, p38 and JNK MAP kinase pathways were also inhibited by PQQ in LPS stimulated primary microglia cells. Further a systemic LPS treatment acute inflammation murine brain model was used to study the suppressive effects of PQQ against neuroinflammation *in vivo*. Mice treated with PQQ demonstrated marked attenuation of neuroinflammation based on Western blotting and immunohistochemistry analysis of Iba1-against antibody in the brain tissue. Indicated that PQQ protected primary cortical neurons against microglia-mediated neurotoxicity. These results collectively suggested that PQQ might be a promising therapeutic agent for alleviating the progress of neurodegenerative diseases associated with microglia activation.

Editor: Karin E. Peterson, National Institute of Allergy and Infectious Diseases - Rocky Mountain Laboratories, United States of America

Funding: This research was supported by the National Natural Science Foundation of China (Grant No. 81301541). The funders had no role in study design, data collection and analysis, decision to publish, or preparation of the manuscript.

Competing Interests: The authors have declared that no competing interests exist.

* Email: jinyuzhu@outlook.com (JZ); dhao.honghui@outlook.com (DH)

These authors contributed equally to this work.

Introduction

Neuroinflammation characterized by the activation of glia has been closely associated with the pathogenesis of a number of neurodegenerative diseases (NDDs), including Alzheimer's disease (AD), Parkinson's disease (PD), amyotrophic lateral sclerosis (ALS) [1]. Microglia, the resident immune cells of the central nervous system, become activated and induce significant and highly detrimental neurotoxic effects by excessively producing a large array of cytotoxic and pro-inflammatory mediators, including inflammatory enzymes such as: inducible Nitric Oxide Synthase (iNOS) and Cyclooxygenase-2 (COX-2); pro-inflammatory cytokines such as: Interleukin-1β (IL-1β) and Tumor Necrosis Factor-α (TNF-α); chemokines such as: Monocyte Chemoattractant Protein (MCP-1), and transcription factors such as: Nuclear Factor-κB (NF-κB) [2–4]. Therefore, anti-inflammatory treatment *via* inhibition of microglial activation is regarded as a promising strategy for preventing NDDs in the clinic.

Pyrroloquinoline quinone (PQQ) is an anionic, water soluble compound that is a redox cycling planar orthoquinone (Fig. 1) [5], which also has free radical scavenging properties [6,7]. Only one prior report by Jensen et al. [8] showed that PQQ given intraperitoneally at 30 min prior to hypoxia reduces infarct size without causing measurable neurobehavioral side effects in an *in vivo* cerebral hypoxia/ischemia model in 7-day-old rat pups. Recently PQQ has been reported to depress N-methyl-Dasparate (NMDA)-induced electrical responses and is neuroprotective *in vitro* against NMDA-mediated neurotoxic injury [9]. Further, combined with other previous studies we have shown that PQQ regulate several intracellular signaling pathways, including Ras-related ERK1/2 activation, CREB dependent mitochondriogenesis, and JAK/STAT activation [10–12]. However, little information is available about the effects of PQQ on neuroinflammation by using the *in vitro* and *in vivo* study. Therefore, in this study, we aimed to investigate the anti-inflammatory effects of PQQ involved in LPS stimulated mice primary microglia cells activation, and its therapeutic effects on the early stage of neuroinflammation induced by systemic LPS treatment in mice.

Materials and Methods

Pyrroloquinoline quinine (PQQ) disodium salt was purchased from Wako (Wako Pure Chemical Industries, Ltd. Osaka, Japan). Dulbecco's Eagle's Medium (DMEM), fetal bovine serum (FBS), penicillin and streptomycin, and trypsin/EDTA were purchased from Gibco. LPS from *E.coli* serotype O55:B5 was from Sigma–Aldrich (St. Louis, USA). Antibodies against p38, JNK, phospho-p38, phospho-JNK and NF-κB were purchased from Cell Signaling Biotechnology (Hertfordshire, England). Antibodies against iNOS and COX-2 were from BD Biosciences (Laguna Hills, CA, U.S.A.). Antibody against β-actin and the secondary antibodies were obtained from Santa Cruz Biotechnology (Santa Cruz, CA, U.S.A.). FITC labeled goat anti-rabbit IgG and goat anti-mouse IgG were purchased from Invitrogen (Frederick, MD, USA). Enhanced Chemilumincescence (ECL) kit was from Millipore (Amersham Pharmacia Biotech, Piscataway, NJ). PCR primers were synthesized at Invitrogen (Frederick, MD, USA). The total nitrate assay kit was obtained from Beyotime (Nanjing, China)

Cell culture

Mice primary microglia cells were prepared from 1 day old C57BL/6J mice as previously described [13]. Briefly, the cerebral cortex was gently dissociated and digested in 0.25% trypsin for 10 min at 37°C. The cells were passed through a 70 μm pore filter and the primary mixed glial cells were resuspended in DMEM supplemented with 10% FBS, 100 U/ml penicillin and 100 mg/ml streptomycin. Cells were seeded in 75 cm^2 flasks for 10–12 days. Primary microglia cells were separated from the mixed glial cells by shaking the flasks for 3 h at 260 r.p.m. in a rotary shaker at 37°C. Detached cells were cultured in the complete medium and seeded into 24-well plates at a density of 5×10^5 cells/well for 2–3 days. The purity of the primary microglia cells were more than 95% as determined by Iba-1 staining.

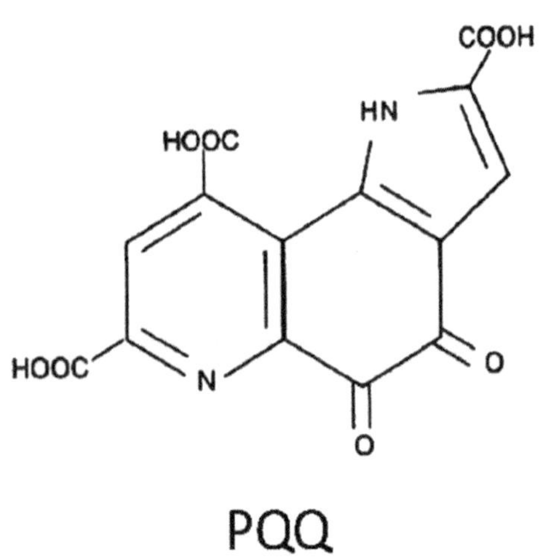

Figure 1. Structure of pyrroloquinoline quinone (PQQ).

Cytotoxicity assay for PQQ

Primary microglia seeded in 96-well plates at a density of 5×10^3 cells/well were treated with PQQ in the presence and absence of LPS for 24 h. Subsequently, MTT solution was added and incubated at 37°C in 5% CO_2 for 4 h. The dark blue formazan crystals were dissolved in DMSO and the absorbance at 540 nm was determined with a microplate reader. Results were expressed as the percentages of live cells over control cells.

Measurement of nitrite and PGE2

Primary microglia were seeded at 1.0×10^5 cells/well in 24-well culture plates, treated with or without PQQ for 1 h followed by LPS treatment (1 μg/ml) for 24 h. Cultured supernatants were collected. Accumulated nitrite was assessed using the Griess reaction. The absorbance was obtained at 570 nm and the results were expressed as mean change fold change of the control. Potassium nitrite was performed as a standard curve. The concentration of PGE2 was measured by a competitive enzyme immunoassay kit (R&D systems, Shanghai, China) following the manufacturer's instructions.

RNA isolation and real-time quantitative PCR

Total RNA was extracted using Trizol reagent according to the manufacturer's instructions and subsequently reversed transcribed to cDNA using a PrimeScript RT reagent kit. Quantitative PCR was performed using SYBR Premix Ex Taq on an ABI 7500 PCR instrument (Applied Biosystems, USA) as previously described [14]. Relative gene expression was analyzed by the $2^{-(\Delta\Delta Ct)}$ method with normalization to the expression of the internal control, glyceraldehyde-3-phosphate dehydrogenase (GAPDH). The primers used are as previously described [14].

Western blot analysis

Equal amounts of protein were separated by a 10% SDS–polyacrylamide gel and transferred to polyvinylidene difluoride (PVDF) membrane. The membrane was blocked with 5% skim milk in TBST for 1 h at room temperature and incubated with primary antibodies against *COX-2* (1:500), *iNOS* (1:100), *p38* (1:1000), *p-p38* (1:1000), *JNK* (1:1000), *p-JNK* (1:1000) over night, then followed by appropriate horseradish peroxidase (HRP)-conjugated secondary antibody (1:5000), and visualized with the ECL detection kit. The optical density of targeted bands was quantified with densitometry. *β-actin* (1:5000) was used as a loading control.

Immunofluorescence analysis

Primary microglia were seeded on cover slips in 24-well culture plates and exposed to LPS (1 μg/ml) for 2 h with or without 1 h PQQ pretreatment. Briefly, cells were washed twice with PBS and fixed in cold 4% parafomaldehyde for 25 min at room temperature. After washing twice in PBS PH 7.4 containing 0.25% Triton X-100, cells were blocked in 3% BSA in PBS for 1 h at room temperature. Subsequently, the cells were incubated overnight with anti-NF-κB p65 in 0.25% PBST and then incubated with FITC-conjugated goat anti-mouse IgG at room temperature for 2 h. DAPI counterstaining was performed to locate the nuclei. Finally, the cover slips were mounted and images were viewed by Olympus BX51 microscope.

Animal Experiments

Forty-eight healthy female 8-wk-old C57BL/6J mice with a mean weight of 19.9±1.9 g were used in this study. All animal protocols were approved by the Ethics Committee for the Care and Use of Laboratory Animals at the Fourth Military Medical University. The animals were housed in plastic cages at a constant temperature (22±2°C) and humidity (55±10%) with 12 h–12 h light–dark conditions. The animals were allowed free access to food and water before the experiment. A peripheral injection of LPS was administered to evoke neuroinflammation in mice as previously described [15]. Briefly, experimental Groups Mice were randomly divided into four groups. In the sham control group (Normal) mice were injected intraperitoneally (i.p.) with saline (3 mg/kg) was allowed free access to food and water without any treatment. The control group (LPS) was intraperitoneally (i.p.) injected with a single dose of saline (3 mg/kg) and vehicle (normal saline) 1 h before the 1.0 mg/kg LPS (*E.coli*, serotype 055:B5, Sigma) injection. The PQQ treatment groups: LPS+PQQ3 and LPS+PQQ10 were administered two doses of PQQ (3 or 10 mg/kg) once 1 h prior to LPS injection respectively. Their body weights were monitored daily; in a subset of animals, core body temperature was also monitored (DC temperature controller, World Precision Instrument).

Immunohistochemistry

Microglia activation in the brain tissue was observed with immunohistochemistry. At 4 h after the LPS injection, the mice were deeply anesthetized and perfused transcardially with 0.05 M phosphate-buffered saline (PBS) containing 4% paraformaldehyde. The brain was removed and was post-fixed in the same perfusing solution overnight at 4°C. Coronal sections of 30 μm thickness were made using a freezing microtome (Leica, 2800N, Germany). The brain sections were stained by a free-floating DAB reaction. The sections were rinsed with 0.05 M PBS and then incubated for 15 min in 1% hydrogen peroxide PBS at room temperature. The sections were incubated overnight at 4°C with primary antibodies against Iba-1 (Wako, Japan), as a microglia marker. The sections were then incubated with biotinylated anti-mouse secondary antibody (Vector Laboratories, USA) for 1 h at room temperature, after which the avidinbiotin complex (Vector Laboratories, USA) method was carried out with peroxidase coupling in a mixture containing 0.05% DAB (Sigma-Aldrich, USA) and 0.03% H_2O_2 for 2–5 min.

Count of Iba-1 Immuno-positive Cells

Immunohistochemistry stained sections were used for analysis of the number of the immunopositive cells. The count of Iba-1 immunopositive microglia was analyzed by using ImageJ software (Ver. 1.44p, NIH, U.S.A.). Four sections and four fields per section were chosen for analysis in each rat. Data were normalized with the same area (10^5 μm^2) and the mean values for the four sections in each rat were used for statistical analysis.

Statistical Analysis

Data were expressed as the mean ± S.E.M. of three to five independent experiments. Significant differences were evaluated by ANOVA test followed by *Bonferroni post hoc* multiple comparison test using the SPSS software 18.0. *p-values*<0.05 were considered as statistically significant.

Results

Cytotoxicity of PQQ in Primary Microglia

To test the cytotoxicity of PQQ, various concentrations of PQQ were applied alone or together with LPS (1 μg/ml) to primary microglia for 24 h. Cell viability was determined by MTT assay. Normal untreated primary microglia were considered as control. MTT results demonstrated that either treatment of PQQ alone or with LPS had no effect on the cell viability of primary microglia in the performed concentrations. Based on these findings, concentrations of PQQ used in the present study were ranged from 1 to 15 μM.

PQQ Attenuated LPS-induced NO Production and iNOS Expression in Primary Microglia

To examine the effects of PQQ on NO production in LPS-induced primary microglia, cells were treated with LPS in the presence or absence of PQQ (1, 15 μM) for 24 h and NO levels in the cell culture supernatants were measured. PQQ pretreatment for 1 h effectively decreased LPS-stimulated NO production in a dose-dependent manner in primary microglia cells (Fig. 2A). Subsequently, we further determined the iNOS mRNA and protein levels by real-time PCR and western blot in primary microglia cells respectively. Consistent with the down-regulation of NO production, PQQ pretreatment significantly attenuated LPS-induced iNOS mRNA (Fig. 2B) and protein levels (Fig. 2E) at 15 μM in primary microglia cells.

PQQ Suppressed LPS-induced PGE2 Production and COX-2 Expression in Primary Microglia

To examine the effect of PQQ on PGE2 production in LPS-induced primary microglia, cells were treated with or without PQQ following the treatment of LPS for 24 h. Concentrations of PGE2 in the culture supernatants were measured by ELISA. As shown in Fig. 2C, LPS-stimulated PGE2 production was markedly decreased by PQQ pretreatment in a dose-dependent manner in primary microglia. To further examine whether the down-regulation of COX-2 contributed to the decrease in PGE2 production, real-time PCR and western blot analysis were performed to analyze the expression of COX-2. Treatment with PQQ 1 h prior to LPS stimulation significantly suppressed both LPS-induced COX-2 mRNA (Fig. 2D) and protein levels (Fig. 2E) at 15 μM. Results demonstrated that inhibition of COX-2 expression by PQQ pretreatment was probably associated with the reduction of PGE2 production in LPS-induced microglia.

PQQ downregulated LPS-induced mRNA levels of pro-inflammatory Mediators in Primary Microglia

To examine the effect of PQQ on LPS-induced mRNA overexpression of pro-inflammatory cytokines and chemokines, primary microglia cells were treated with PQQ (1 μM, 15 μM) for 1 h prior to stimulation with LPS for 6 h. Results of real-time PCR show the mRNA expression of pro-inflammatory factors in primary microglia cells was all dramatically increased in response to LPS stimuli compared to the control. However, the production of these pro-inflammatory factors was significantly reduced in a dose-dependent manner by pretreatment with PQQ. These results indicated that LPS-induced excessive mRNA expression of TNF-α, IL-1β, IL-6, MCP-1 and MIP-1α were effectively down-regulated by PQQ pretreatment (Fig. 3).

PQQ Inhibited LPS-induced Activation of NF-κB in Primary Microglia

NF-κB is an important regulator of gene expression of pro-inflammatory mediators such as COX-2, iNOS, TNF-α and IL-6 in LPS-induced microglia. Therefore, we identified the effects of PQQ on NF-κB activity using immunofluoresence microscopy. As shown in Fig. 4A, LPS exposure induced significant nuclear translocation of NF-κB p65 subunit in primary microglia. In contrast, PQQ pretreatment strongly inhibited this response.

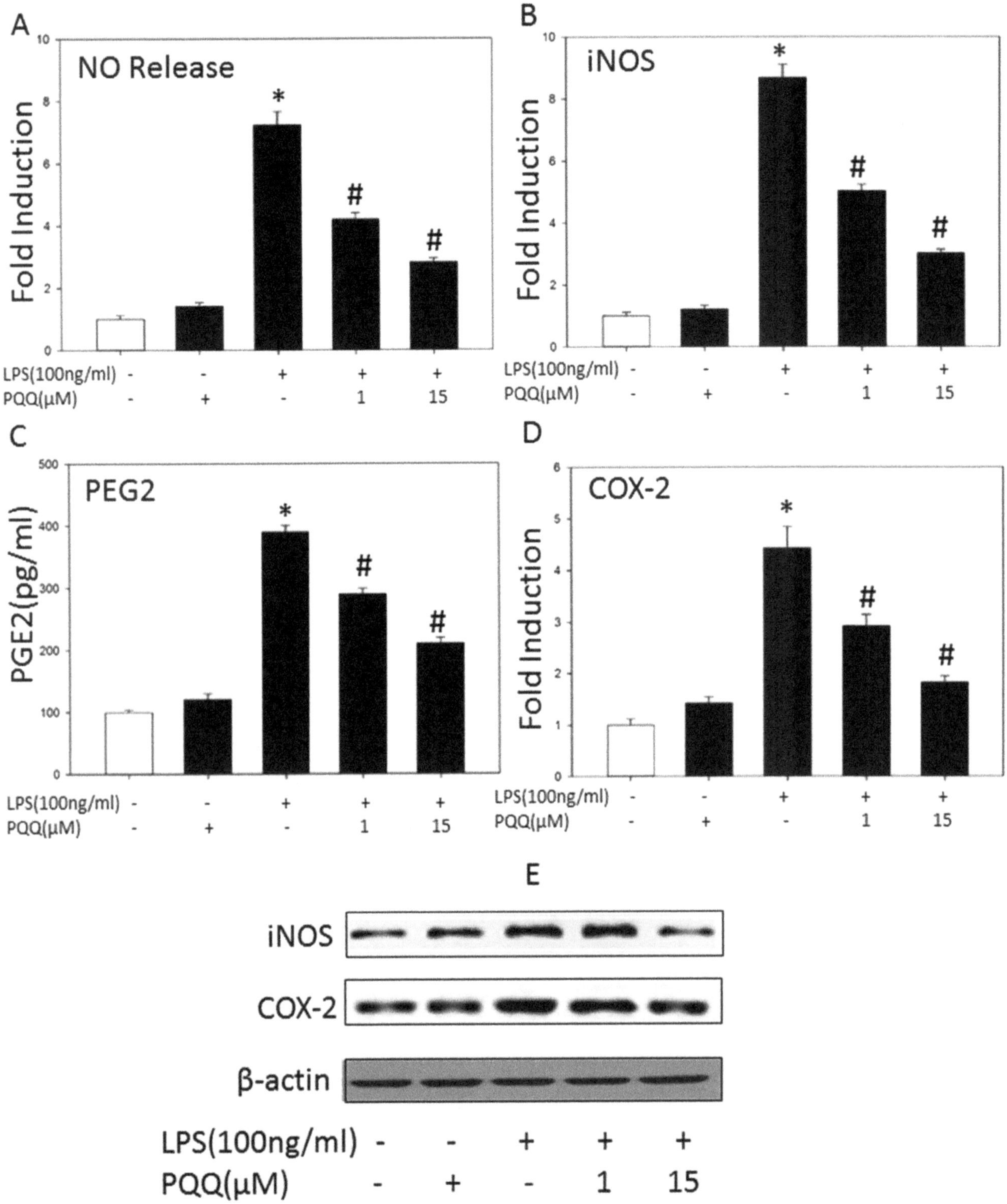

Figure 2. Effects of PQQ on LPS-induced NO, PGE2 production and iNOS, COX-2 expression in microglia cells. Primary microglia were pretreated with or without PQQ for 1 h followed by LPS (100 ng/ml) treatment for indicated durations. Culture supernatants were collected 24 h later, the released NO in primary microglia (A) was determined by the Griess assay, total mRNA was harvested 6 h later, and the mRNA level of iNOS (B) and COX-2 (D) was measured by real-time PCR. (C) Concentrations of PGE2 in the culture supernatants of primary microglia were determined by ELISA. (E) 24 h later, the protein level of iNOS and COX-2 were detected by western blot analysis in primary microglia cells. The results presented as mean ± S.E.M. of at least three independent experiments, **p<0.05 vs. control group, #p<0.05 vs. only LPS group.*

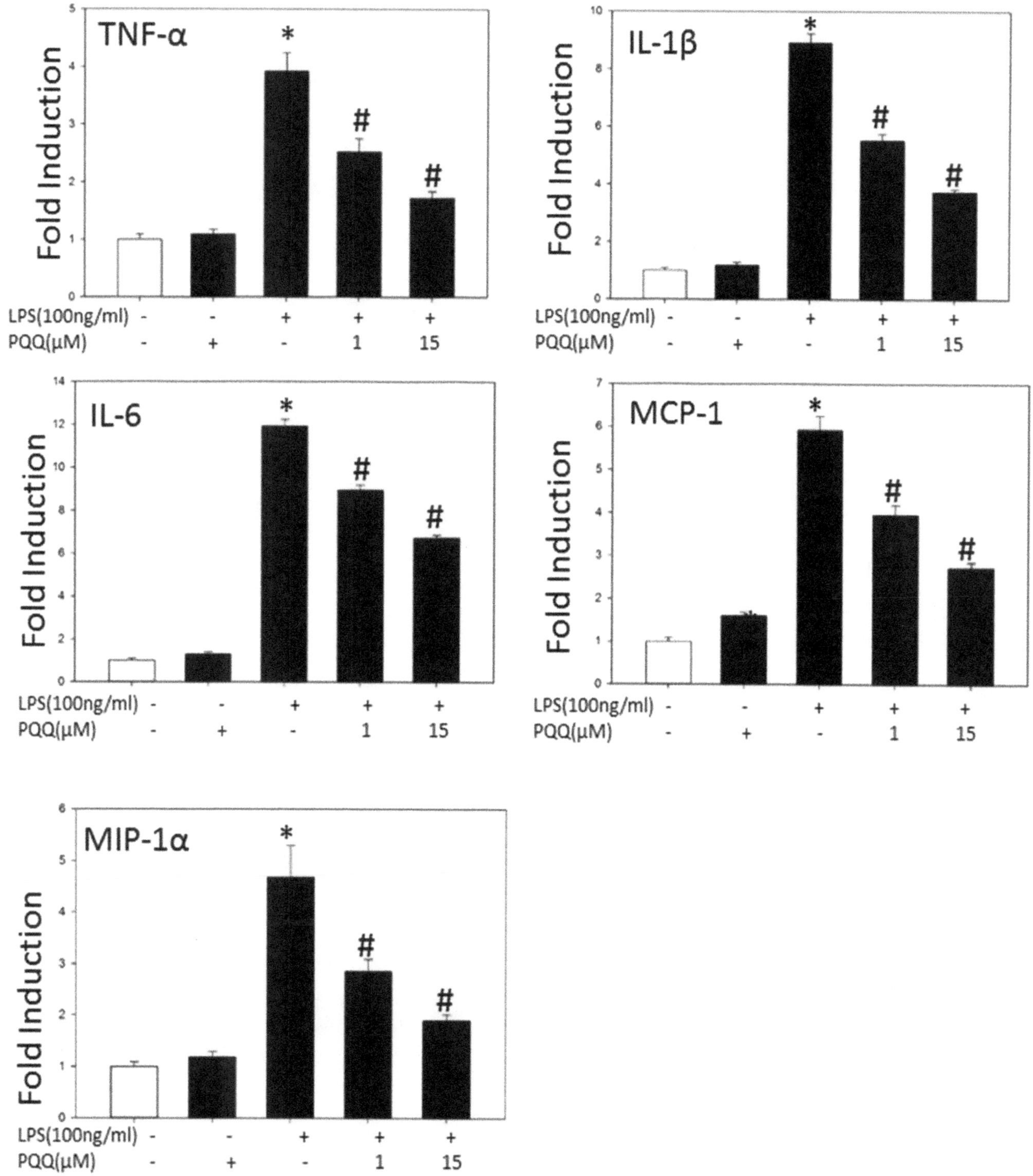

Figure 3. Effects of PQQ on LPS-stimulated expression of pro-inflammatory mediators in microglial cells. Cells were treated with the indicated concentrations of PQQ 1 h prior to 6 h co-treatment of LPS (100 ng/ml). Primary microglia were harvested and total RNA was prepared. The mRNA expression of pro-inflammatory mediators: TNF-a, IL-1β, IL-6, COX-2, MCP-1 and MIP-1α was measured by real-time PCR. GAPDH was used as an internal control. The results shown are mean ± S.E.M. of three independent experiments. **p<0.05 vs. control group, #p<0.05 vs. only LPS group.*

These results indicated that PQQ may attenuate NF-κB activation through inhibiton of NF-κB p65 nuclear translocation.

PQQ Attenuated the Phosphorylation Levels of p38 and JNK in LPS-treated Primary Microglia

MAP kinases signaling is one of the most important pathway in modulating inflammatory activation in microglia [16]. Therefore,

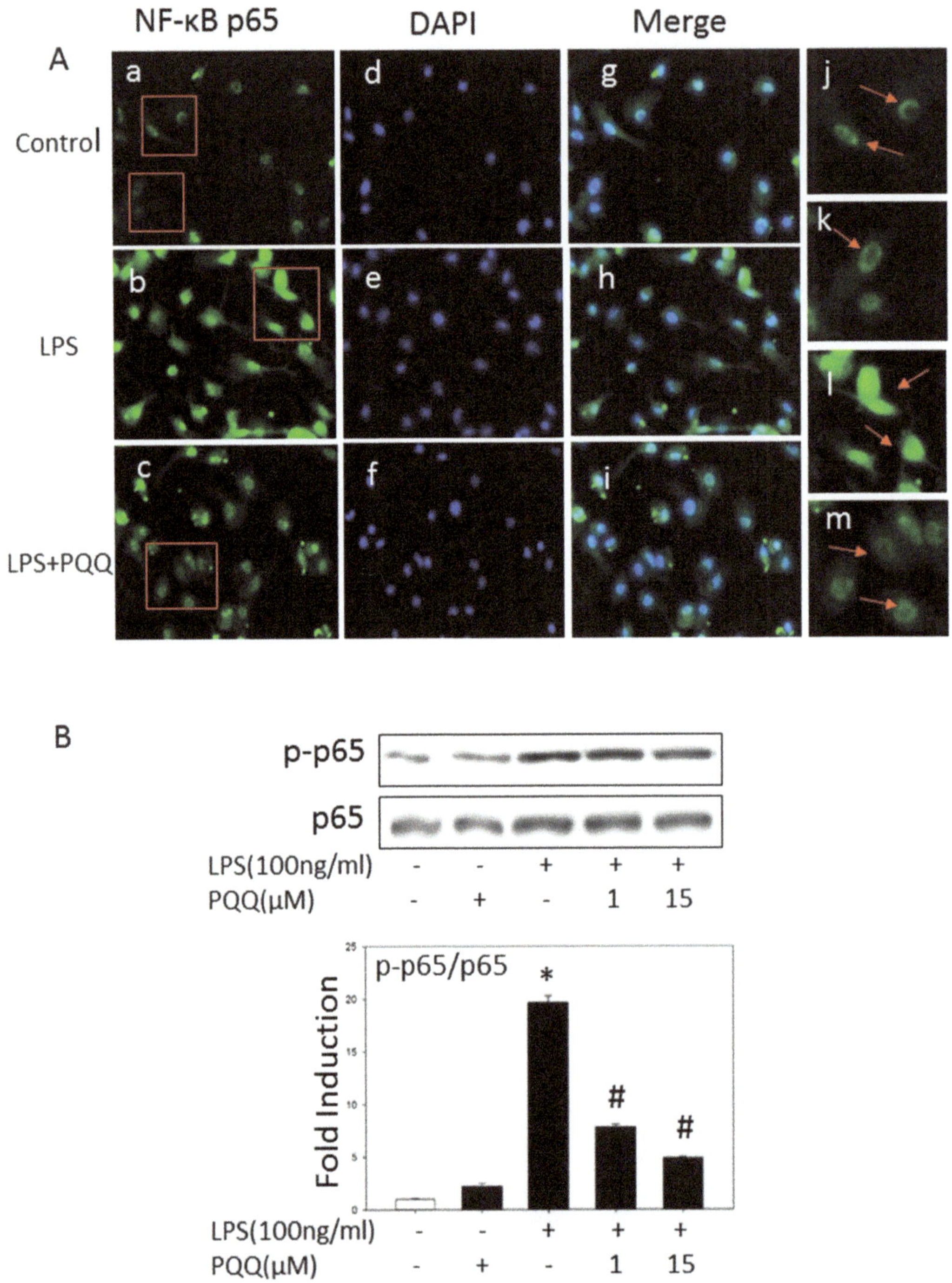

Figure 4. Effects of PQQ on LPS-induced p65 and NF-κB activity in microglial cells. (A) Representative images of NF-κB p65 in microglial cells of each group. Cells were pretreated with or without PQQ for 1 h followed by 100 ng/ml LPS treatment for 2 h. Microglial cells were incubated with NF-κB p65 antibody and immunofluorescence microscopy was used to visualize the localization of NF-κB p65 (Green; a-c), boxed regions in (a-c) are also shown at×200 (j-m). Nuclei were visualized using DAPI counterstaining (Blue; d-f). (B) Cells were treated with 100 ng/m LPS for indicated time. p65 protein level was measured by western blot analysis. Non-phosphorylated p65 was used as loading control, and the expression of p-p65 was normalized to control and quantified by densitometric analysis. The results shown are mean ± S.E.M. of three independent experiments. **p<0.05 vs. control group, #p<0.05 vs. only LPS group.*

we also studied the role of PQQ in LPS-induced activation of MAP kinases pathways in primary microglia. As shown in Fig.5, LPS stimulation led to rapid activation of p38 and JNK, then cells were treated with or without PQQ for 4 h. Western blot analysis showed that PQQ pretreatment significantly inhibited LPS-stimulated phosphorylation of p38 and JNK while no changes were observed in the expression of non-phosphorylated p38 and JNK. These results indicated that inhibition of pro-inflammatory mediators by PQQ in LPS-induced primary microglia was partly associated with down-regulation of the activity of p38 and JNK.

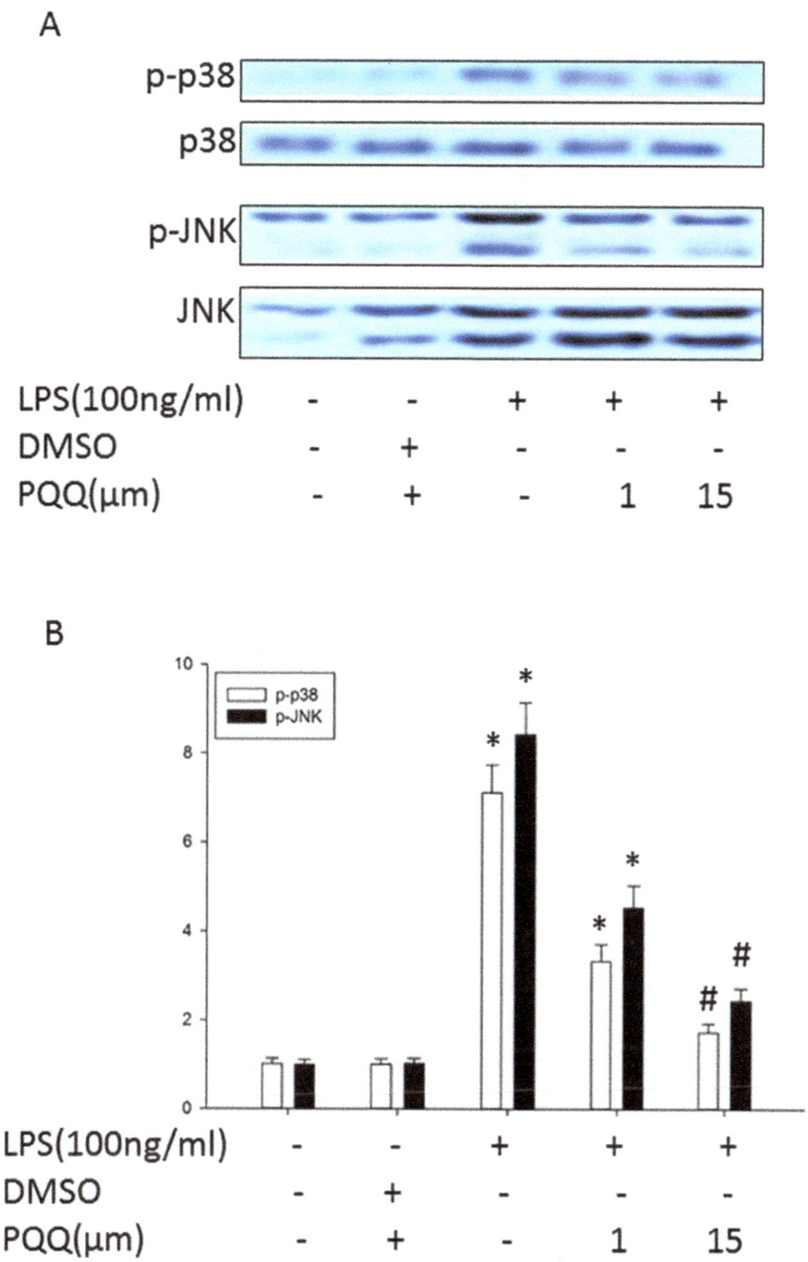

Figure 5. Effects of PQQ on LPS-induced MAP kinases activity in microglial cells. (A) Microglial cells were treated with or without PQQ 1 h prior to 4 h co-treatment with LPS. The protein expression of p-p38 and p-JNK was determined by western blot analysis. Non-phosphorylated form of each targeted protein was used as loading control. (B) Bar graph represents the average levels of p-p38 and p-JNK compared to the control. The results shown are mean ± S.E.M. of three independent experiments. **p<0.05 vs. control group, #p<0.05 vs. only LPS group.*

PQQ Attenuates Microglia Activation in the Brain Tissue of LPS-Treated Mice

The effects of PQQ on microglia activation following systemic LPS injection were tested by quantification of Iba-1 protein with Western blotting and immunohistochemistry against Iba-1 antibody in the brain tissue at 4 h after LPS injection. LPS increased the % increase of Iba-1 expression in brain tissue (169.20±11.97%). PQQ treatment attenuated, significantly and dose dependently, the % increase of Iba-1 expression in the brain tissue at doses of 3 and 10 mg/kg (139.91±9.29%, $p<0.05$; 119.37±3.93%, $p<0.05$; respectively) as compared to the LPS group (Fig.6).

The LPS injection activated microglia, as displayed by an increase in cell size, irregular shape, thickened and shortened processes and intensified Iba-1 immunostaining density in the cerebral cortex and dentate gyrus (DG) of hippocampus (Fig. 7A). However, compared with the LPS group, PQQ treatment dramatically attenuated the morphological changes to activated-form of microglia. To examine the effect of PQQ on microglia activation, the number of Iba-1 immunostained microglia was counted and normalized with the same area (10^5 μm^2). In the cerebral cortex area, the LPS group was 78.7±7.9 cells/10^5 μm^2. However, the PQQ treatment groups were 58.9±6.9 cells/10^5 μm^2 ($p<0.05$) and 41.3±3.9 cells/10^5 μm^2 ($p<0.05$) respec-

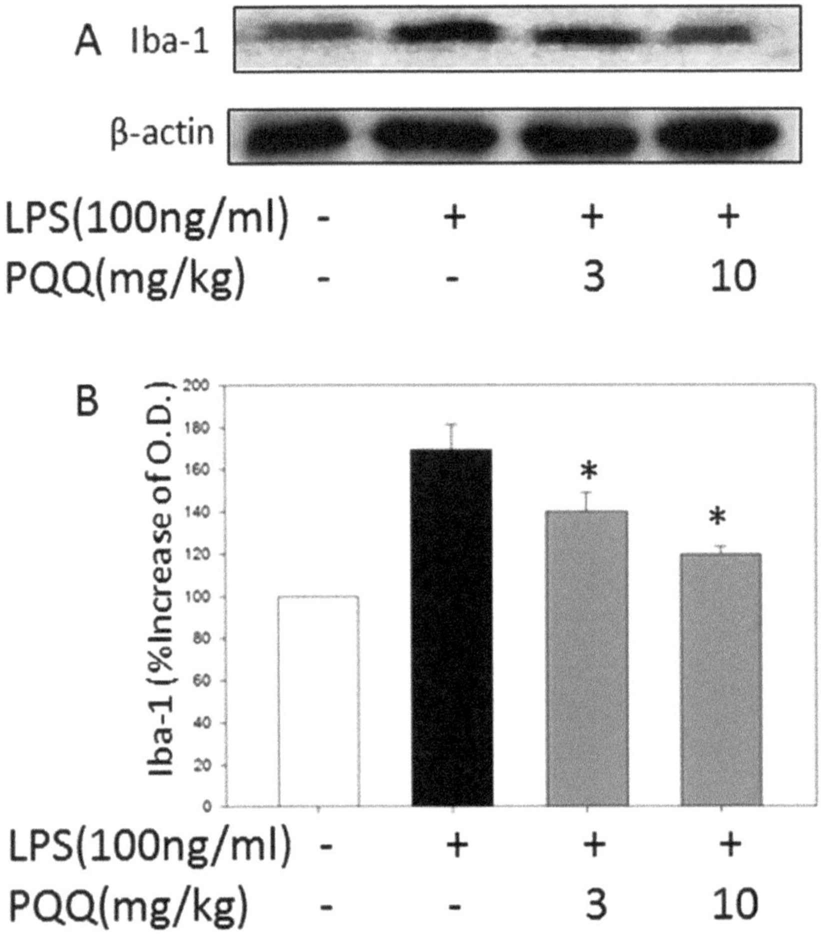

Figure 6. Effect of PQQ on Iba-1 Expression in the Brain. Representative Western blots illustrate differences in the bands of Iba-1 (A). LPS up-regulates Iba-1 expression in brain tissue, while PQQ treatment attenuates up-regulation of Iba-1 expression at doses of 3 and 10 mg/kg administration (B). The results shown are mean ± S.E.M. (*n* = 6 in each group) of three independent experiments. **p<0.05 vs. control group, #p<0.05 vs. only LPS group.*

tively (Fig. 7B). In the dentate gyrus (DG) area, the LPS group was 64.1±6.19 cells/10^5 μm^2. However, the PQQ treatment groups were 36.3±3.3 cells/10^5 μm^2 ($p<0.05$) and 27.7±2.9 cells/ 10^5 μm^2 ($p<0.05$) respectively (Fig. 7B). Those results indicate that PQQ attenuated microglia activation in the brain induced by systemic LPS injection.

Discussion

The present study demonstrated for the first time that PQQ attenuated the synthesis of NO and PGE2, suppressed the expression of iNOS and COX-2 at the mRNA and proteins levels and inhibited the mRNA levels of TNF-α, IL-1β, IL-6, MCP-1 and MIP-1α in LPS-stimulated primary microglia cells. The nuclear translocation of NF-κB and the activation of p38 MAP kinase and JNK were also suppressed by PQQ *in vitro*. Moreover, PQQ exhibits suppressive effects against neuroinflammation induced by systemic LPS treatment *in vivo*. These data suggested that PQQ would be a potential therapeutic agent for alleviating neuroinflammation desease accompanied by activated microglia.

Microglia-mediated neurotoxicity is a hallmark of the pathogenesis of various neurodegenerative diseases [17]. High levels of pro-inflammatory cytokines and chemokines released by activated microglia are implicated in the process of neuronal injury [18]. Many recent studies have reported that agents exert their neuroprotective effects through inhibition of production of pro-inflammatory mediators [19–22]. Moreover, excessive activation of microglia characterized by robust production and secretion of a variety of pro-inflammatory substances has been implicated in the pathogenesis of a number of neurodegenerative diseases, such as AD and PD [23]. Accumulation of these pro-inflammatory molecules leads to neurodegeneration and eventually neurological diseases [24]. Thus, therapeutic approaches targeting activated microglia may be a promising treatment of these diseases. Despite major roles of microglia on inflammatory responses in the brain, there were no reports to demonstrate effects of PQQ on microglia activation *in vitro* or *in vivo*.

COX-2 is upregulated in response to various inflammatory stimuli including overproduction of PGE2. Up-regulation of COX-2 contributes to the development of many chronic inflammatory diseases [25,26]. Moreover, NO also is an important regulatory mediator involved in cell survival and death exerts a number of pro-inflammatory effects during several physiological and pathological processes. Prolonged activation of microglial cells leads to excessive release of NO by iNOS in the brain [27]. Under conditions in neurodegenerative diseases, increased production of

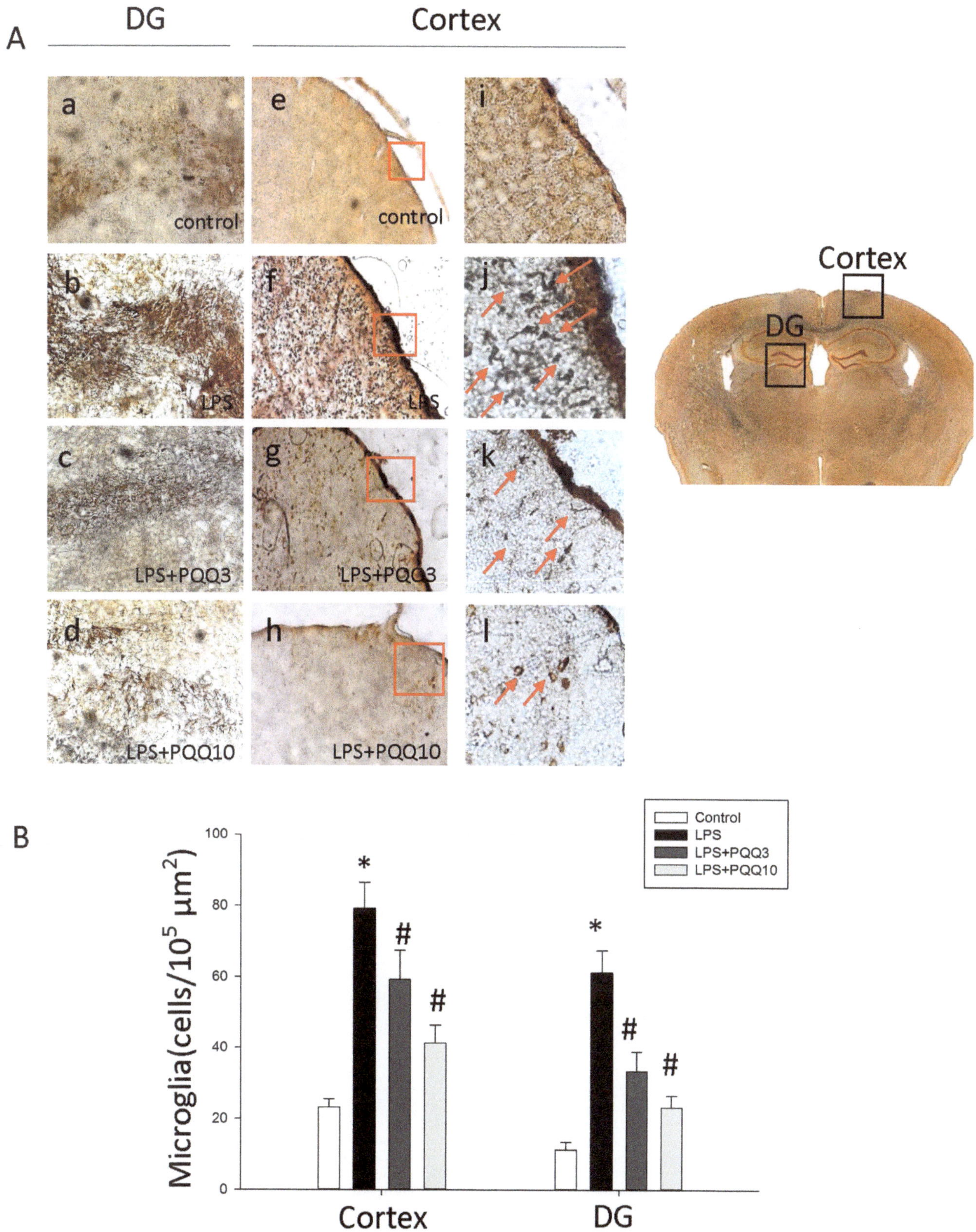

Figure 7. Effect of PQQ on Microglia Activation in the Brain. Representative photographs show Iba-1 immuno-stained microglia of the mouse brain (A). LPS group shows mostly an activated-form of microglia which display an increased size, irregular shape, thickened and shortened processes and intensified Iba-1 immunostaining density, in the dentate gyrus of hippocampus (DG) and cerebral cortex (Cortex) compared to the normal group. Moreover, both PQQ treated groups show a decrease of morphological activation of microglia in all brain regions with respect to LPS group. Representative DG (a–d) and Cortex (e–h) immunostained slices are presented at ×40. High power images of Iba-1-expressed microglia in the boxed

regions in (f), (g) and (h) are also shown at×200 (i–l). Arrow indicates the Iba-1-expressed microglia. The number of microglia was counted and normalized in the corresponding same area (B). LPS increases the number of Iba-1-expressed microglia in the brain. PQQ treatment significantly reduces the number of Iba-1-expressed microglia both in the cerebral cortex and DG. The results shown are mean ± S.E.M. ($n = 6$ in each group) of three independent experiments. *$^*p<0.05$ vs. control group, $\#p<0.05$ vs. only LPS group.*

NO mainly results from the up-regulated expression of iNOS in activated astrocytes and microglia cells [28]. Therefore, agents that inhibit the release of NO and attenuate iNOS and COX-2 expression could be beneficial for preventing and delaying the progression of neuroinflammatory disease. In the present study, PQQ treatment to primary microglia stimulated by LPS effectively decreased iNOS and COX-2 levels and the release of their respective end-products, NO and PGE2. This inhibition exhibited by PQQ may be attributed to suppression of iNOS and COX-2 mRNA transcription and a subsequent reduction in protein expression.

The transcription factor NF-κB is a pleiotropic regulator of diverse genes involved in regulating the expression of various pro-inflammatory mediators and has been found to be a promising target for inflammatory diseases [29]. NF-κB activates several cellular signal transduction pathways that are involved in the production of iNOS, COX-2, and various cytokines [30–32]. As the expression of these pro-inflammatory mediators is modulated by NF-κB, blocking NF-κB transcriptional activity may be an important target for treating inflammatory diseases. Therefore in this study, we investigated the inhibition effects of PQQ on NF-κB activity. We found that PQQ pretreatment markedly suppressed LPS-induced nuclear translocation of NF-κB p65, suggesting that inhibition of pro-inflammatory factors by PQQ was at least partially mediated through blockade of NF-κB activation.

MAP kinases are also crucial in regulating the pro-inflammatroy substances such as TNF-α, IL-6, iNOS and COX-2 expression in LPS-stimulated microglia cells [33,34]. One of the important MAPK families, p38, is positively related to LPS signaling in microglial cells, which respond to pro-inflammatory cytokines [16]. Moreover, p38 MAPK is a key mediator of cellular stressors such as inflammation and apoptosis. Both *in vitro* and *in vivo* studies have shown that p38 MAPK regulates the production of the pro-inflammatory cytokines, NO, and PGE2 by increasing cytokine release or messenger RNA transcription [35,36]. Thus, we further determined whether the anti-inflammatory effects of PQQ in LPS-stimulated primary microglia was due to suppression of MAP kinases. Results from our study shown that exposure of primary microglia to LPS resulted in strongly increased expression of phosphorylated p38 and JNK, indicating that p38 and JNK are additional pathways by which PQQ inhibited LPS-induced inflammatory activation of primary microglia.

At the *in vivo* experiment, we used the systemic LPS treatment acute inflammation murine brain model to study the suppressive effects of PQQ against neuroinflammation. Microglia are activated in response to brain injuries and immunological stimuli to undergo dramatic alterations in morphology, changing from resting, ramified microglia into activated, amoeboid microglia, which is believed to favor phagocytosis and mobility [37]. In our present *in vivo* study, according immunohistochemical analyses, we found PQQ lessened the microglia morphological changes to an activated-form which can manifest as increased cell size, irregular shape, thickened and shortened processes in all brain regions. Moreover, PQQ significantly reduced Iba-1 protein expression in the brain compared to that of LPS group. Iba-1, which is highly and specifically expressed in microglia and macrophage [36], and is involved in RacGTPase-dependent membrane ruffling and phagocytosis [38]. By immunohistochemical analyses, anti-Iba-1 antibody was found to specifically recognize ramified microglia in normal rat brain, and Iba-1 protein was strongly upregulated in activated microglia. Therefore, Iba-1 may play significant roles in the regulation of some immunological and pathophysiological functions of microglia, and serve as a novel marker of detecting the activation of microglia. However, this study is the first time to show that PQQ plays a modulatory role in microglia activation using an *in vivo* animal study.

In conclusion, PQQ showed significant anti-neuroinflammatory actions in microglial cells regulating *via* NF-κB and p38 MAPK signaling pathways *in vitro*. Further, the *in vivo* efficacy of PQQ was confirmed with an animal model of systemic LPS treatment acute inflammation murine brain model. Given that microglial activation and the consequent release of various inflammatory components contributes to neurodegeneration, PQQ may potentially protect against microglia-mediated neurodegenerative diseases. Further in-depth and long term research is required to confirm these findings.

Author Contributions

Conceived and designed the experiments: J. Zhu DH CY LY LK. Performed the experiments: CY LK LY RM J. Zhu QZ. Analyzed the data: J. Zhang RM CY LY. Contributed reagents/materials/analysis tools: LK CY LY DH. Wrote the paper: CY LY LK J. Zhu QZ J. Zhang RM.

References

1. Jha MK, Jeon S, Suk K (2012) Glia as a Link between Neuroinflammation and Neuropathic Pain. Immune Netw 12(2): 41–47.
2. Block ML, Zecca L, Hong JS (2007) Microglia-mediated neurotoxicity: uncovering the molecular mechanisms. Nat Rev Neurosci. 8(1), 57–69.
3. McGeer PL, McGeer EG (1995) The inflammatory response system of brain: implications for therapy of Alzheimer and other neurodegenerative diseases. Brain Res Brain Res Rev. 21(2):195–218.
4. Block ML, Hong JS (2005) Microglia and inflammation-mediated neurodegeneration: multiple triggers with a common mechanism. Prog. Neurobiol. 76(2):77–98.
5. Zhang Y, Feustel PJ, Kimelberg HK (2006) Neuroprotection by pyrroloquinoline quinone (PQQ) in reversible middle cerebral artery occlusion in the adult rat. Brain Res 13;1094(1):200–6.
6. Gallop PM, Henson E, Paz MA, Greenspan SL, Flückiger R (1989) Acid-promoted tautomeric lactonization and oxidation reduction of pyrroloquinoline quinone (PQQ). Biochem.Biophys. Res. Commun. 163(2): 755–63.
7. Gallop PM, Paz MA, Flückiger R, Henson E (1993) Is the antioxidant, anti-inflammatory putative new vitamin, PQQ, involved with nitric oxide in bone metabolism? Connect Tissue Res. 29(2):153–61.
8. Jensen FE, Gardner GJ, Williams AP, Gallop PM, Aizenman E, et al (1994) The putative essential nutrient pyrroloquinoline quinone is neuroprotective in a rodent model of hypoxic/ischemic brain injury. Neuroscience. 62(2): 399–406.
9. Alexandrova ML, Bochev PG (2005) Oxidative stress during the chronic phase after stroke. Free Radic Biol Med. 39(3):297–316.
10. Kumazawa T, Hiwasa T, Takiguchi M, Suzuki O, Sato K (2007) Activation of Ras signaling pathways by pyrroloquinoline quinone in NIH3T3 mouse fibroblasts. Int J Mol Med 19(5):765–770.
11. Chowanadisai W, Bauerly KA, Tchaparian E, Wong A, Cortopassi GA, et al. (2010) Pyrroloquinoline quinone stimulates mitochondrial biogenesis through cAMP response element-binding protein phosphorylation and increased PGC-1a expression. J Biol Chem 285(1):142–52.
12. Kong L, Yang C, Yu L, Smith W, Zhu S, et al. (2013) Pyrroloquinoline Quinine Inhibits RANKL-Mediated Expression of NFATc1 in Part via Suppression of c-

Fos in Mouse Bone Marrow Cells and Inhibits Wear Particle-Induced Osteolysis in Mice. PLoS ONE 8(4): e61013.
13. Kitayama M, Ueno M, Itakura T, Yamashita T (2011) Activated microglia inhibit axonal growth through RGMa. PLoS One. 6(9):e25234.
14. Chen ZB, Huang DQ, Niu FN, Zhang X, Li EG, et al. (2010) Human urinary kallidinogenase suppresses cerebral inflammation in experimental stroke and downregulates nuclear factor-kappaB. J Cereb Blood Flow Metab. 30(7):1356–1365.
15. Qin L, Wu X, Block ML, Liu Y, Breese GR, et al. (2007) Systemic LPS causes chronic neuroinflammation and progressive neurodegeneration. Glia. 55(5):453–62.
16. Han L, Yin K, Zhang S, Wu Z, Wang C, et al. (2013) Dalesconols B inhibits lipopolysaccharide induced inflammation and suppresses NF-κB and p38/JNK activation in microglial cells. Neurochem Int. 62(7):913–21.
17. Blinzinger K, Kreutzberg G (1968) Displacement of synaptic terminals from regenerating motoneurons by microglial cells. Z. Zellforsch. Mikrosk. Anat. 85(2):145–57.
18. Magrone T, Marzulli G, Jirillo E (2012) Immunopathogenesis of neurodegenerative diseases: current therapeutic models of neuroprotection with special reference to natural products. Curr Pharm Des 18(1):34–42.
19. Haga S, Akai K, Ishii T (1989) Demonstration of microglial cells in and around senile (neuritic) plaques in the Alzheimer brain. An immunohistochemical study using a novel monoclonal antibody. Acta Neuropathol. 77(6):569–75.
20. Cagnin A, Brooks D J, Kennedy AM, Gunn RN, Myers R, et al. (2001) In-vivo measurement of activated microglia in dementia. Lancet 358(9280), 461–7.
21. Cameron B, Landreth GE (2010) Inflammation, microglia, and Alzheimer's disease. Neurobiol Dis. 37(3):503–9.
22. Beumer W, Gibney SM, Drexhage RC, Pont-Lezica L, Doorduin J, et al. (2012) The immune theory of psychiatric diseases: a key role for activated microglia and circulating monocytes. J Leukoc Biol. 92(5):959–75.
23. Block ML, Hong JS (2005) Microglia and inflammation-mediated neurodegeneration: multiple triggers with a common mechanism. Prog Neurobiol 76(2):77–98.
24. Block ML, Zecca L, Hong JS (2007) Microglia-mediated neurotoxicity: uncovering the molecular mechanisms. Nat Rev Neurosci. 8(1):57–69.
25. Sheng W, Zong Y, Mohammad A, Ajit D, Cui J (2011) Pro-inflammatory cytokines and lipopolysaccharide induce changes in cell morphology, and upregulation of ERK1/2, iNOS and $sPLA_2$-IIA expression in astrocytes and microglia. J Neuroinflammation. 8: 121.
26. Li P, Lu J, Kaur C, Sivakumar V, Tan KL, et al. (2009) Expression of cyclooxygenase-1/-2, microsomal prostaglandin-E synthase-1 and E-prostanoid receptor 2 and regulation of inflammatory mediators by PGE2in the amoeboid microglia in hypoxic postnatal rats and murine BV-2 cells. Neuroscience.164(3):948–62.
27. Possel H, Noack H, Putzke J, Wolf G, Sies H (2000) Selective upregulation of inducible nitric oxide synthase (iNOS) by lipopolysaccharide (LPS) and cytokines in microglia: in vitro and in vivo studies. Glia. 32(1):51–9.
28. Boje KM, Arora PK (1992) Microglial-produced nitric oxide and reactive nitrogen oxides mediate neuronal cell death. Brain Res. 587(2):250–6.
29. Karin M, Yamamoto Y, Wang QM (2004) The IKK NF-kappa B system: a treasure trove for drug development. Nat Rev Drug Discov. 3(1):17–26.
30. Pascual O, Achour SB, Rostaing P, Triller A, Bessis A (2012) Microglia activation triggers astrocyte-mediated modulation of excitatory neurotransmission. Proc Natl Acad Sci USA. 109(4):E197–205.
31. Peça J, Feng G (2012) Cellular and synaptic network defects in autism. Curr Opin Neurobiol. 22(5):866–72.
32. Perry VH, Cunningham C, Holmes C (2007) Systemic infections and inflammation affect chronic neurodegeneration. Nat Rev Immunol. 7(2):161–7.
33. Bhat NR, Zhang P, Lee JC, Hogan EL (1998) Extracellular signal-regulated kinase and p38 subgroups of mitogen-activated protein kinases regulate inducible nitric oxide synthase and tumor necrosis factor-alpha gene expression in endotoxin-stimulated primary glial cultures. J Neurosci. 18(5):1633–41.
34. Waetzig V, Czeloth K, Hidding U, Mielke K, Kanzow M, et al. (2005) C-Jun N-terminal kinases (JNKs) mediate pro-inflammatory actions of microglia. Glia. 50(3):235–46.
35. Streit WJ, Walter SA, Pennell NA (1999) Reactive microgliosis. Prog Neurobiol. 57(6):563–81.
36. Ito D, Tanaka K, Suzuki S, Dembo T, Fukuuchi Y (2001) Enhanced expression of Iba1, ionized calcium-binding adapter molecule 1, after transient focal cerebral ischemia in rat brain. Stroke. 32(5):1208–15.
37. Park SM, Choi MS, Sohn NW, Shin JW (2012) Ginsenoside Rg3 Attenuates Microglia Activation Following Systemic Lipopolysaccharide Treatment in Mice. Biol Pharm Bull. 35(9):1546–52.
38. Kanazawa H, Ohsawa K, Sasaki Y, Kohsaka S, Imai Y (2002) Macrophage/microglia-specific protein Iba1 enhances membrane ruffling and Rac activation via phospholipase C-gamma-dependent pathway. J Biol Chem. 277(22):20026–32.

13

Butanol Isomers Exert Distinct Effects on Voltage-Gated Calcium Channel Currents and Thus Catecholamine Secretion in Adrenal Chromaffin Cells

Sarah McDavid[1]§, Mary Beth Bauer[1]§, Rebecca L. Brindley[1], Mark L. Jewell[2], Kevin P. M. Currie[3]*

1 Department of Anesthesiology, Vanderbilt University School of Medicine, Nashville, Tennessee, United States of America, **2** Department of Pharmacology, Vanderbilt University School of Medicine, Nashville, Tennessee, United States of America, **3** Department of Anesthesiology, Department of Pharmacology, and Vanderbilt Brain Institute, Vanderbilt University School of Medicine, Nashville, Tennessee, United States of America

Abstract

Butanol ($C_4H_{10}OH$) has been used both to dissect the molecular targets of alcohols/general anesthetics and to implicate phospholipase D (PLD) signaling in a variety of cellular functions including neurotransmitter and hormone exocytosis. Like other primary alcohols, 1-butanol is a substrate for PLD and thereby disrupts formation of the intracellular signaling lipid phosphatidic acid. Because secondary and tertiary butanols do not undergo this transphosphatidylation, they have been used as controls for 1-butanol to implicate PLD signaling. Recently, selective pharmacological inhibitors of PLD have been developed and, in some cases, fail to block cellular functions previously ascribed to PLD using primary alcohols. For example, exocytosis of insulin and degranulation of mast cells are blocked by primary alcohols, but not by the PLD inhibitor FIPI. In this study we show that 1-butanol reduces catecholamine secretion from adrenal chromaffin cells to a much greater extent than tert-butanol, and that the PLD inhibitor VU0155056 has no effect. Using fluorescent imaging we show the effect of these drugs on depolarization-evoked calcium entry parallel those on secretion. Patch-clamp electrophysiology confirmed the peak amplitude of voltage-gated calcium channel currents (I_{Ca}) is inhibited by 1-butanol, with little or no block by secondary or tert-butanol. Detailed comparison shows for the first time that the different butanol isomers exert distinct, and sometimes opposing, effects on the voltage-dependence and gating kinetics of I_{Ca}. We discuss these data with regard to PLD signaling in cellular physiology and the molecular targets of general anesthetics.

Editor: J. David Spafford, University of Waterloo, Canada

Funding: This work was supported in part by a pilot and feasibility grant from the Vanderbilt Diabetes Research and Training Center to KC [Grant P30 DK20593], and by the National Institutes of Health [Grant R01 NS052446] to KC. The funders had no role in study design, data collection and analysis, decision to publish, or preparation of the manuscript.

Competing Interests: Kevin Currie currently serves as an academic editor for PLOS ONE. This does not alter the authors' adherence to PLOS ONE policies on sharing data and materials.

* Email: kevin.currie@vanderbilt.edu

§ These authors contributed equally to this work.

Introduction

Butanol ($C_4H_{10}OH$) exists as multiple isomers; primary (1-butanol) and secondary butanol (2-butanol) have a straight carbon chain with the hydroxyl group located at the terminal or second carbon, respectively. The four-carbon chain can also be branched with the hydroxyl group located at a terminal carbon (isobutanol; also called 2-methyl-1-propanol) or at the internal carbon (tert-butanol; also called 2-methyl-2-propanol). Like other primary alcohols, 1-butanol serves as a substrate for phospholipase D (PLD) [1]. In the absence of alcohols, PLD catalyzes the hydrolysis of phosphatidylcholine to produce choline and phosphatidic acid, with the latter acting directly or indirectly through intracellular signaling cascades to control a diverse array of cellular functions [2–11]. However, in the presence of 1-butanol, PLD produces phosphatidylbutanol rather than phosphatidic acid [1]. Neither secondary nor tertiary butanols undergo this transphosphatidylation, so these alcohols are commonly used as controls for 1-butanol to implicate phosphatidic acid/PLD signaling. Recently, several selective pharmacological inhibitors of PLD have been developed [12–14], and some reports have noted a disparity between the effects of these and 1-butanol on cellular function. For example, 1-butanol inhibits insulin secretion, but the PLD inhibitor FIPI has no effect [12]. Similarly, 1-butanol inhibits membrane ruffling, blebbing, and degranulation (exocytosis) in mast cells, but FIPI does not [15]. The implication from these studies is that acute application of 1-butanol blocks exocytosis by a mechanism(s) distinct from PLD signaling.

This raises the question by which other target(s) might butanol inhibit exocytosis? It is known that primary alcohols induce anesthesia and act in a manner similar to inhalational anesthetics [16]. Potential molecular targets for alcohols/general anesthetics include ligand-gated, voltage-gated, and other ion channels [17–23]. Although much attention has focused on post-synaptic ligand-gated ion channels, there is also evidence for presynaptic effects of alcohols/anesthetics [23–25]. The critical roles of voltage-gated channels make them an attractive potential target for disruption of stimulus-secretion coupling by butanol (and other alcohols/

anesthetics). Voltage-gated sodium and potassium channels control electrical excitability, while calcium entry through voltage-gated calcium channels controls a multitude of cellular functions including vesicular trafficking and neurotransmitter/hormone secretion. Indeed, primary alcohols have been shown to modulate voltage-gated channels: 1-butanol inhibits voltage-gated sodium channel currents [26], voltage-gated potassium channel currents [27–29], and voltage-gated calcium channel currents (I_{Ca}) [30–32]. However, it is not known if butanol isomers differ in their modulation of voltage-gated ion channel function.

In this study we investigated the effects of butanol isomers on catecholamine secretion and I_{Ca} in adrenal chromaffin cells, an important neuroendocrine component of the sympathetic nervous system and a well-characterized neurosecretory model [33]. Both PLD1 and PLD2 are expressed in chromaffin cells, and PLD1 has been implicated in controlling catecholamine secretion [11,34]. However, to our knowledge the effects of newer PLD inhibitors have not been reported prior to this study. We show that 1-butanol reduces catecholamine secretion to a much greater extent than tert-butanol, but VU0155056, a newly developed cell membrane permeable inhibitor of both PLD1 and PLD2 [13,14], has no effect. Fluorescent imaging approaches reveal parallel effects on depolarization-evoked calcium entry. With patch-clamp electrophysiology we demonstrate concentration-dependent inhibition of I_{Ca} by 1-butanol with little or no block by secondary or tert-butanol. Detailed comparison shows for the first time that different butanol isomers exert distinct, and sometimes opposing, effects on the gating and kinetics of I_{Ca}. We discuss these data with regard to PLD signaling in cellular physiology and the molecular targets of general anesthetics.

Materials and Methods

Cell culture

Bovine adrenal glands were obtained from a local slaughterhouse (C & F Meat Co. Inc., College Grove, TN), and chromaffin cells were prepared by digestion with collagenase followed by density gradient centrifugation as described previously [35]. The cells were plated onto coverslips coated with collagen (at a density of 0.3–0.4×10^6 cells/mL for $[Ca^{2+}]_i$ measurements or ~0.2×10^6 cell/mL for patch clamp recordings). For secretion studies, cells were plated in 24-well tissue culture plates at a density of ~0.3×10^6 cells per well. Fibroblasts were effectively suppressed with cytosine arabinoside (10 μM) (Sigma-Aldrich; St Louis MO), leaving relatively pure chromaffin cell cultures. The culture medium consisted of Dulbecco's modified Eagle medium \ F12 (1:1) supplemented with fetal bovine serum (10%), glutamine (2 mM), penicillin/streptomycin (100 unit mL^{-1}/100 μg mL^{-1}), cytosine arabinoside (10 μM) and 5-fluorodeoxyuridine (10 μM). Tissue culture reagents were from Life Technologies (Grand Island, NY). The culture medium was replaced the day after isolation and experiments were performed 2–5 days following cell isolation.

$[Ca^{2+}]_i$ Measurements

Free cytosolic Ca^{2+} concentration ($[Ca^{2+}]_i$) was measured using an InCyt IM2 fluorescence imaging system (Intracellular Imaging Inc., Cincinnati, OH) and a Nikon TE2000 fluorescence microscope (Nikon Instruments Inc., Melville, NY) [35]. Cells were washed twice with HEPES-buffered Hanks Balanced Salt Solution and incubated in the dark for 30–45 minutes with 3-5 μM FURA2-AM or FURA4F-AM at 37°C. Cells were then washed (in the dark) in FURA-free solution for 30–60 minutes before recording. The coverslip was transferred to a recording bath (volume ~300–400 μL) and continually perfused with fresh solution at a flow rate of ~4 ml/min from gravity-fed reservoirs. Cells were excited at 340 nm and 380 nm and emission at 510 nm detected using a Pixelfly digital camera. The ratio of fluorescence emission at 340 nm/380 nm excitation was collected every 1–2 s throughout the experiment and converted to $[Ca^{2+}]_i$ using an *in vitro* calibration curve. Data were transferred to OriginPro software (Originlab Corporation, Northampton, MA) for analyses.

Catecholamine secretion experiments

Cells in 24-well plates were washed twice with extracellular solution and equilibrated in this solution for 30 mins at ~37°C. This was next replaced with fresh solution to determine basal release or with solution containing 30 mM KCl to stimulate secretion. After a five-minute stimulation period at ~37°C the cells were placed on ice, and the solution was removed and added to an equal volume of ice-cold 0.4 M perchloric acid. The cells were lyzed by addition of perchloric acid and scraping to extract the non-secreted catecholamines. The catecholamine content of the samples was determined by a specific high performance liquid chromatography (HPLC) assay utilizing an Antec Decade (oxidation potential: 0.7 V) electrochemical detector in the Neurochemistry Core of the Vanderbilt Brain Institute as described previously [35]. The amount of catecholamine secreted during the 5-minute stimulation period was expressed as a percentage of the total catecholamine content for that dish of cells. For each experiment, duplicate wells for each condition (control and drug treated) were averaged (to yield n = 1). 1-butanol (0.4% v/v; ~44 mM), tert-butanol (0.4% v/v; ~42 mM), the PLD inhibitor VU0155056 (1 μM), or DMSO (0.01%) (vehicle for VU0155056) was added to the cells for 10 minutes during the preincubation period and throughout the stimulation with KCl. Statistical analyses were performed using Prism5 software (GraphPad Software Inc., La Jolla, CA).

Patch-clamp electrophysiology

Patch pipette electrodes were pulled from borosilicate glass capillary tubes (World Precision Instruments, Sarasota, FL) using a Sutter P-97 pipette puller (Sutter Intrument, Novato, CA), coated with dental wax (Electron Microscopy Sciences, Hatfield, PA) and fire-polished to a final resistance of ~2 MΩ when filled with a CsCl-based internal solution. Cells were voltage-clamped in the conventional whole-cell configuration using either an Axopatch 200B amplifier, Digidata 1400A interface, and PClamp10 (Clampex) acquisition software (Molecular Devices, Sunnyvale, CA) or a HEKA EPC10 amplifier and PatchMaster acquisition software (HEKA instruments). Analog data were filtered at 2–3 kHz and digitized at 50 kHz. Series resistance was partially compensated (~50–80%) and data for I_{Ca} were subjected to linear capacitance and leak subtraction using P/N protocols (P/-4 or P/-8) with the leak pulses applied following the test pulses. The recording bath (volume ~300 μL) was continually perfused with fresh solution at a flow rate of ~4 ml/min from gravity-fed reservoirs. The exception was when ω-conotoxin GVIA (CgTx) was used to block the N-type I_{Ca}. For these experiments the CgTx was added as a 50 μL bolus of 2 μM CgTx into a static bath. The estimated final concentration of CgTx was ~0.5–1 μM. Blockade of the channels by CgTx is irreversible over the time course of these experiments. Following plateau of the current inhibition by CgTx (approximately 4–5 minutes), the bath flow was restarted and butanol applied. Raw data were analyzed using PClamp10 (Clampfit) or HEKA FitMaster software. Graphing and statistical analyses were performed using Origin or Prism.

Solutions, drugs and reagents

The extracellular solution for calcium imaging and secretion studies comprised (in mM): 136 NaCl, 2 KCl, 1 MgCl, 10 glucose, 10 HEPES, 2 CaCl, pH 7.3 osmolarity ~305 mOsm. The extracellular solution for patch-clamp recording was (in mM): 136 NaCl, 2 KCl, 1 MgCl, 10 glucose, 10 HEPES, 5 CaCl, pH 7.3 osmolarity ~310 mOsm. Tetrodotoxin (TTX) (0.5–1 μM) was added to block voltage-gated sodium channels. The intracellular (patch pipette) solution consisted of (in mM): CsCl 110, $MgCl_2$ 4, HEPES 20, EGTA 10, GTP 0.35, adenosine triphosphate 4, creatine phosphate 14, pH 7.3, osmolarity ~310–315 mOsm.

The AM-ester of FURA was prepared as 1 mM stock in dimethyl sulfoxide (DMSO) and aliquots frozen until use. The pentapotassium salt used for in vitro calibration curves was prepared as an aqueous stock and stored at 4°C. Butanol was added to the extracellular solutions at the indicated concentrations on the day of each experiment. VU0155056 was kindly provided by Dr. Alex Brown (Vanderbilt University) (also available from Avanti Polar Lipids Inc., Alabaster, Alabama). Stock solutions were prepared in DMSO (10 mM) and diluted into extracellular solution (1 μM final concentration) on the day of use. Tetrodotoxin (R&D systems, Minneapolis, MN) was prepared as a 1 mM aqueous stock and aliquots frozen until use (final concentration when diluted into extracellular solution was ~0.5 μM). ω-conotoxin GVIA (R&D systems, Minneapolis, MN) was prepared as a 100–300 μM aqueous stock and stored as frozen aliquots until use. On the day of the use, the aliquot was diluted to 2 μM in extracellular solution and a 50 μL bolus of this solution was added to the static recording bath (300–400 μL).

Results

Differential inhibition of calcium entry and catecholamine secretion by butanol isomers and the PLD inhibitor VU0155056

Dishes of chromaffin cells were stimulated with 30 mM KCl for 5 minutes to evoke membrane depolarization, calcium entry through voltage-gated calcium channels, and thus catecholamine secretion. Pre-incubation of the cells with 1-butanol (0.4%; ~44 mM) dramatically reduced epinephrine secretion measured using HPLC (Fig 1A). Tert-butanol (0.4%; ~42 mM) also reduced catecholamine secretion but to a significantly lesser extent than 1-butanol (Fig 1A). In contrast, 1 μM VU0155056, a newly developed cell membrane permeable inhibitor of both PLD1 and PLD2 [13], had no effect on secretion compared to DMSO controls (Fig 1B). These results suggest that 1-butanol exerts the bulk of its inhibitory effect on exocytosis at a site(s) other than PLD.

Because calcium entry through voltage-gated calcium channels plays a pivotal role in catecholamine secretion [36–39], we used ratiometric imaging of FURA2-loaded cells to determine if 1-butanol altered KCl-evoked calcium entry. Cells were stimulated with three successive applications of 30 mM KCl (Fig 1C). 1-butanol (0.4%; ~44 mM) reversibly reduced the peak calcium transient by 52±3% (n = 51 cells: $p<0.001$, Tukey's post-test following repeated measures ANOVA). In contrast, only slight reductions in calcium entry were produced by tert-butanol (9±2%) or VU-155056 (12±3%), and these did not reverse upon washout of the drugs. In other experiments, we used longer preincubations with butanol or VU0155056 (10 - 15 minute preincubation) and measured the peak intracellular calcium transient evoked by a single application of KCl. The peak calcium transient in control cells was 1319±65 nM (n = 43) and was significantly smaller in cells treated with 0.4% 1-butanol

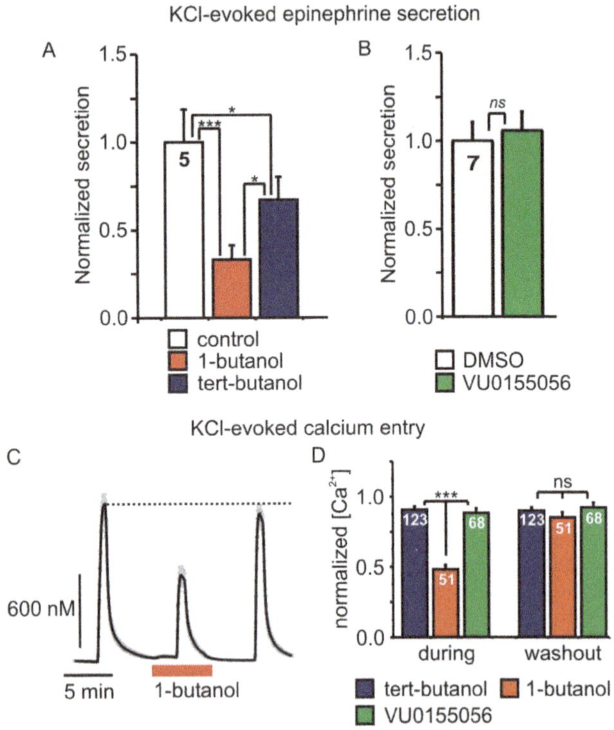

Figure 1. 1-butanol but not the phospholipase D inhibitor VU0155056 inhibits catecholamine secretion and calcium entry. A) Secretion was evoked by application of 30 mM KCl for five-minutes. Epinephrine secretion from cells treated with 1-butanol (0.4%; ~44 mM) or tert-butanol (0.4%; ~42 mM) was normalized to that from controls. Secretion was significantly inhibited by 1-butanol and to a lesser extent by tert-butanol (one-way ANOVA, $F = 20.98$, $p = 0.0007$: * $p<0.05$, *** $p<0.001$ for pairwise comparisons using Tukey's post-hoc test). **B)** KCl-evoked epinephrine secretion was not altered by the phospholipase D inhibitor VU0155056 (1 μM) ($p = 0.49$, paired t-test). **C)** A representative experiment showing the intracellular calcium transients evoked by 30 mM KCl (60 s applications) applied before, during, and after washout of 0.4% 1-butanol. **D)** Mean data from several experiments like that shown in panel C. The peak increase in intracellular $[Ca^{2+}]$ evoked by KCl in the presence (during) of 1-butanol (0.4%; ~42 mM), tert-butanol (0.4%; ~42 mM), or VU0155056 (1 μM) was normalized to the first control response in each cell. 1-butanol significantly inhibited Ca^{2+} entry compared to both tert-butanol and VU0155056 (one-way ANOVA, $F = 54.8$, $p<0.0001$: *** $p<0.001$ for pairwise comparisons using Tukey's post-hoc test). After washout of the drugs (washout) Ca^{2+} entry was not significantly different in any of the three treatment groups (one-way ANOVA, $F = 1.03$, $p = 0.36$).

(797±38 nM; n = 62; $p<0.001$ ANOVA with Tukey's post-test). In contrast, neither tert-butanol (1153±29 nM, n = 99) nor VU0155056 (1112±84 nM; n = 71) significantly reduced the peak calcium transient compared to controls (ANOVA followed by pair-wise comparison with Tukey's post-test).

Differential effects of butanol isomers on voltage-gated calcium channel currents (I_{Ca})

Based on the calcium imaging data (Fig 1), we compared the effects of butanol isomers on I_{Ca} using patch clamp electrophysiology. Cells were voltage-clamped in the standard whole-cell recording configuration and I_{Ca} activated by short (10–20 ms) steps from −80 mV to +10 mV every 20 s (Fig 2A). Acute application of 1-butanol (0.4%; ~44 mM) rapidly and reversibly inhibited the peak amplitude of I_{Ca}. The inhibition of I_{Ca} was concentration-dependent with an estimated EC_{50} of 52 mM (~0.48%) (Fig 2B). We then compared the ability of 1-butanol, 2-butanol, and tert-butanol (all at 0.4%) to inhibit the peak amplitude of I_{Ca}. 1-butanol inhibited I_{Ca} from 640±88 pA to 399±57 pA (n = 17, p<0.0001 paired t-test); 2-butanol inhibited I_{Ca} from 652±81 pA to 547±81 pA (n = 5; p<0.001 paired t-test); tert-butanol only slightly reduced the amplitude of I_{Ca} from 632±83 pA to 583±78 pA (n = 18, p = 0.06 paired t-test). The percent inhibition by 1-butanol was significantly greater than either 2-butanol or tert-butanol (Fig 2C).

1-butanol inhibits N-type and P/Q-type I_{Ca} to the same extent

The whole cell I_{Ca} in bovine chromaffin cells has been well characterized and is comprised of ~10% L-type current (blocked by dihydropyridine antagonists) with the remaining current carried by N-type and P/Q-type I_{Ca} in roughly equal proportions [37,40,41]. To determine if the N- and P/Q-type channels were differentially inhibited by 1-butanol, we pharmacologically isolated the two current components. Cells were voltage-clamped at −70 mV and nitrendipine (3 μM) was present throughout the experiment to block the L-type current. Cells were stimulated every 20 s with a 20 ms step to +10 mV. The inhibition of I_{Ca} produced by 1-butanol was determined twice, once before and once after application of ω-conotoxin GVIA (CgTx) to block the N-type channels (Fig 2D). Consistent with previous reports, CgTx blocked 48±7% (n = 5) of the current [37,42,43]. We have previously shown that the remaining CgTx resistant component of I_{Ca} is almost fully comprised of P/Q-type channels, as it is blocked by ω-Agatoxin IVA [42]. Calculating the "difference current" (i.e. subtracting the data recorded after CgTx from that recorded before CgTx) yields the CgTx-sensitive N-type I_{Ca}. Using this pharmacological dissection, we found that 1-butanol inhibited N-type I_{Ca} by 46±5% and P/Q-type I_{Ca} by 49±3.7% (n = 5) (Fig 2D).

Differential effects of primary and tert-butanol on channel activation

To assess the inhibition of I_{Ca} in more detail, current-voltage relationships were determined. 1-butanol inhibited the amplitude of I_{Ca} across a range of voltages with no obvious shift in the I-V curve (Fig 3A). In contrast, 2-butanol had much smaller effects (Fig 3B) and especially for tert-butanol there was an obvious hyperpolarizing shift in the I-V curve (Fig 3C). Indeed, the amplitude of I_{Ca} elicited by a step to −10 mV was significantly *increased* by tert-butanol (p<0.01, repeated measures ANOVA with pairwise comparison using Bonferroni post-test).

Given that tert-butanol produced a prominent shift in the I-V curve, we assessed the voltage-dependence of I_{Ca} activation by measuring the tail current amplitude following a series of depolarizing steps (Fig 4A). Figures 4B and 4C show the effects of 1-butanol and tert-butanol on the activation curves. The V_{50}

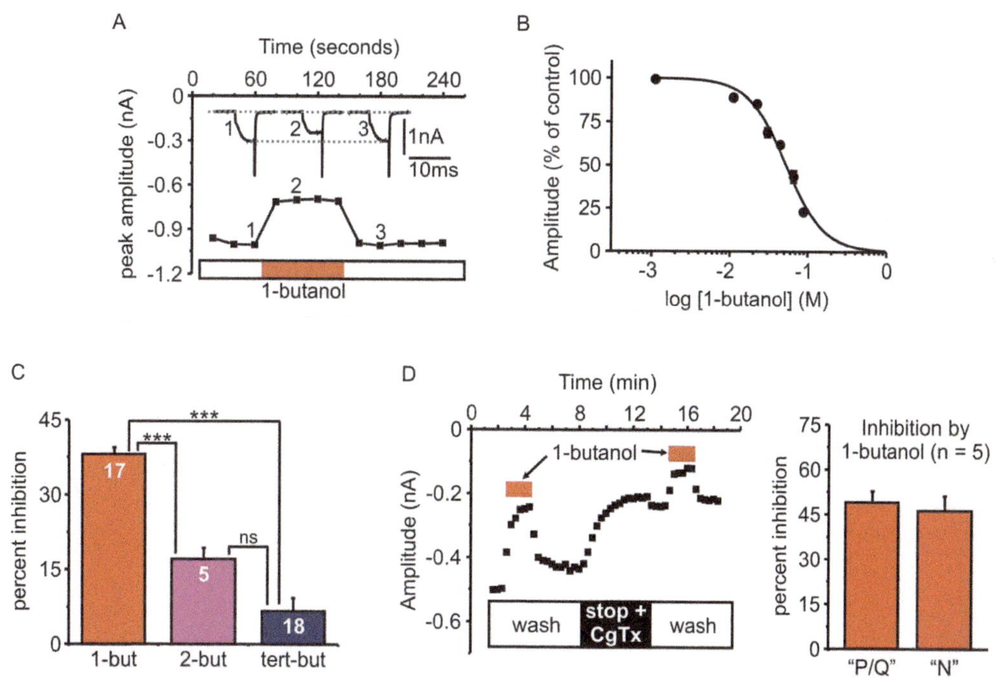

Figure 2. Concentration-dependent inhibition of I_{Ca} by 1-butanol. A) Representative time-course showing reversible inhibition of peak I_{Ca} amplitude by 1-butanol (0.4%; ~44 mM). Currents were evoked by 10 ms duration steps from −90 mV to +10 mV. **B)** Concentration-response curve showing the percent inhibition of I_{Ca} amplitude by 1-butanol. Points are mean ± s.e.m. of 4–17 cells (error bars are within the data points in some cases). The solid line shows the fit to a standard dose-response relationship which yielded an estimated EC_{50} of 52 mM and Hill slope of −1.73. **C)** Percent inhibition of peak I_{Ca} amplitude (elicited by a step from −90 mV to +10 mV) by 1-butanol (n = 17), 2-butanol (n = 5), or tert-butanol (n = 18) (all butanol isomers at 0.4%) (one-way ANOVA, F = 60.7, p<0.0001: *** p<0.001, ns = "not significant" for pairwise comparisons using Tukey's post-hoc test). **D)** *Left panel*: Representative experiment showing peak I_{Ca} amplitude plotted against time (elicited by a step from −70 mV to +10 mV). Nitrendipine (3 μM) was present throughout the experiment to block any L-type calcium channels. The bath was continually perfused with fresh solution (wash) and 1-butanol applied as indicated by the red bars. At the time indicated by the black bar, the solution flow was stopped and a bolus of ω-conotoxin GVIA was added to the bath (stop + CgTx) to irreversibly block N-type calcium channels. *Right panel*: The percent inhibition of pharmacologically isolated P/Q-type and N-type I_{Ca} by 1-butanol. "P/Q-type" I_{Ca} was defined as the CgTx resistant current (i.e. the current remaining after washout of CgTx). "N-type" I_{Ca} was defined as the CgTx sensitive component (i.e. the data after Cgtx subtracted from data before CgTx).

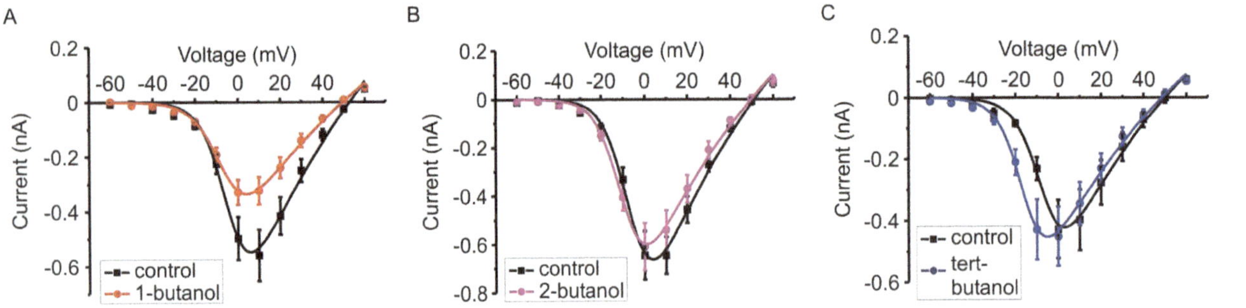

Figure 3. Differential effects of butanol isomers on the current-voltage relationship of I_{Ca}. Cells were stimulated by a series of steps, from a holding potential of −90 mV to test potentials ranging from −60 mV to +60 mV, first in control conditions and then in the presence of either 0.4% (~44 mM) 1-butanol (panel A, n = 6), 2-butanol (panel B, n = 5), or tert-butanol (panel C, n = 5). The mean current amplitude elicited by each step is plotted. Tert-butanol elicited a clear hyperpolarizing shift in the I-V relationship.

(potential at which half maximal activation is achieved) was determined by fitting a Boltzmann curve to the data. 1-butanol did not significantly shift the V_{50} for activation (0.6±0.4 mV in control conditions compared to −0.1±0.9 mV in the presence of 1-butanol, n = 6; p = 0.35, paired t-test). However, tert-butanol hyperpolarized the activation curve (Fig 4C) and significantly shifted the V_{50} from −2.7±1.4 mV to −11.4±0.8 (n = 6; p = 0.0018, paired t-test). The slope of the activation curve was significantly reduced by 1-butanol (Fig 4B) but not by tert-butanol (Fig 4C). Thus, the different butanol isomers exert distinct effects on channel activation which is opposed by 1-butanol but favored by tert-butanol.

Opposite effects of primary and tert-butanol on the deactivation kinetics of I_{Ca}

Figure 5A shows examples of tail currents following steps to + 40 mV to maximally activate I_{Ca}. The mean tail current amplitude was significantly reduced by 1-butanol (from 1.81±0.33 nA to 0.92±0.15 nA; n = 6; p = 0.006, paired t-test) but not by tert-butanol (1.17±0.22 nA to 1.01±0.15 nA; n = 6; p = 0.14, paired t-test). The decay of the tail currents reflects channel deactivation (i.e. the open to closed transition upon membrane hyperpolarization) and is well fit with a single exponential. 1-butanol significantly accelerated the decay (Fig 5B, C), decreasing the time constant of the exponential fit from 300±13 µS to 217±7 µS (n = 6, p = 0.004, paired t-test) (Fig 5C). In contrast, tert-butanol significantly slowed the decay of the tail currents, increasing the time constant of the exponential fit from 340±33 µS to 514±68 µS (n = 6, p = 0.03, paired t-test) (Fig 5B, C).

Primary and tert-butanol both promote voltage-dependent inactivation of I_{Ca}

The voltage-dependence of steady-state inactivation was determined by incrementally increasing the holding potential from − 90 mV to −20 mV for durations of 30 s (Fig 6A). Following recovery at −90 mV the cell was then exposed to either 1-butanol (0.4%; ~44 mM) or tert-butanol (0.4%; ~42 mM) and the

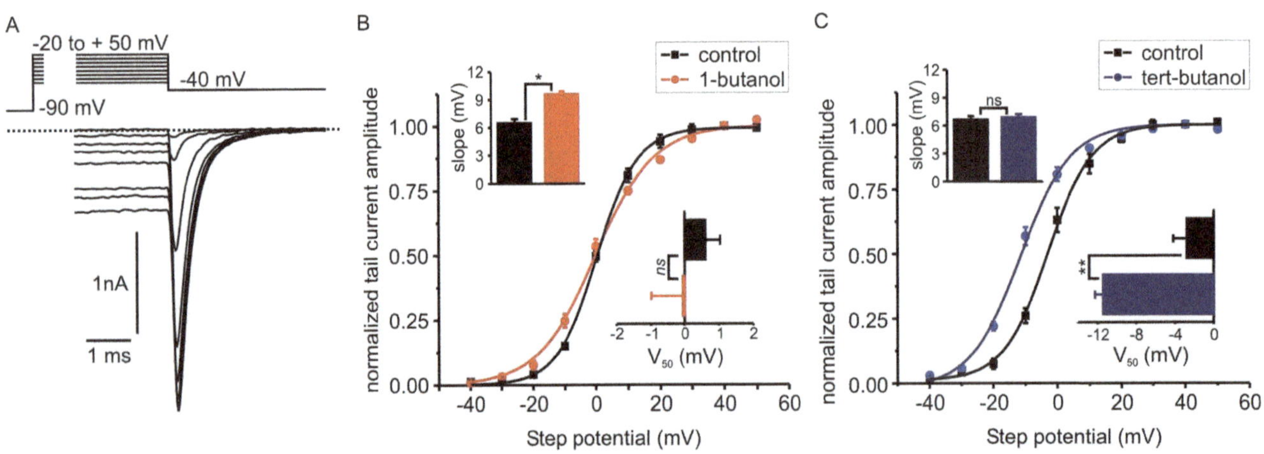

Figure 4. Butanol isomers differentially modulate the voltage-dependence of I_{Ca} activation. A) The upper panel shows the voltage command protocol and the lower panel shows a family of representative I_{Ca} tail current recordings. Cells were stimulated with depolarizing steps from a holding potential of −90 mV to test potentials ranging from −20 to +50 mV and tail currents were recorded upon repolarization to −40 mV. **B, C)** In each cell, tail currents were recorded first under control conditions and then in the presence of either 1-butanol (panel B, n = 6) or tert-butanol (panel C, n = 6). Tail current amplitude was normalized to that evoked by the +40 mV step and plotted against the potential of the step depolarization (mean ± s.e.m.). The solid line shows the fit with a Boltzmann curve. The inset bar graphs show the mean slope and V_{50} (potential at half maximal activation) derived from the Boltzmann fits to individual cells. 1-butanol had no effect on V_{50} but the slope of the curve was significantly shallower. In contrast, tert-butanol had no effect on the slope, but produced a strong hyperpolarizing shift in the V_{50} (* $p<0.05$; ** $P<0.01$; ns = not significant; paired t-test).

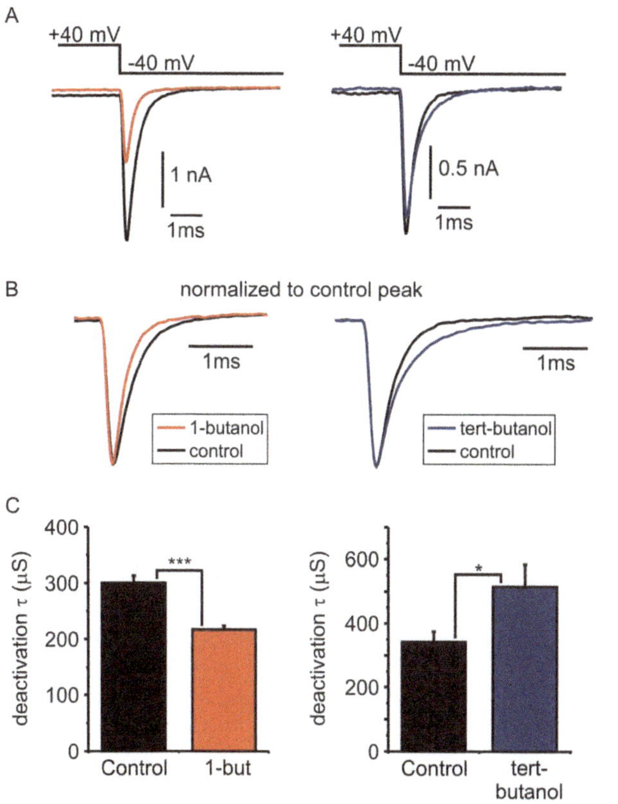

Figure 5. Differential effects of butanol isomers on the deactivation kinetics of I_{Ca}. **A)** Representative tail currents activated by a step depolarization from −90 mV to +40 mV. In each cell, tail currents were recorded first in control conditions and then in the presence of either 1-butanol (left) or tert-butanol (right). **B)** The same traces as in panel A, but the time-base was expanded and the currents in the presence of butanol were scaled to the same amplitude as control to more clearly illustrate changes in the decay kinetics. **C)** The decay of the tail currents was fit with a single exponential function. Bar charts plot the mean time constant of the fit (τ) in control conditions and in the presence of 1-butanol (n = 6) or tert-butanol (n = 6). (* $p < 0.05$; *** $p < 0.001$ compared to matched controls; paired t-test).

inactivation protocol was repeated. Both butanol isomers produced a similar hyperpolarizing shift in the inactivation curves (Fig 6B, C). 1-butanol significantly shifted the V_{50} (potential at half maximal inactivation) from −37.4±3.6 mV to -54.3±5.1 mV (n = 5, p = 0.0016, paired t-test). Similarly, tert-butanol shifted the V_{50} from -37.8±2.4 mV to −55.1±4.2 mV (n = 6, p = 0.0006, paired t-test).

The effect of butanol on voltage-dependent inactivation during a sustained depolarizing step was also determined (Fig 7A, B). EGTA (10 mM) was present in the patch-pipette solution to block Ca^{2+}-dependent inactivation. Cells were stimulated by a voltage step to +10 mV lasting 500 ms before and during application of either 1-butanol (0.4%; ~44 mM) or tert-butanol (0.4%; ~42 mM). Both butanol isomers significantly increased inactivation during the 500 ms step (Fig 7B). Accelerated inactivation will reduce calcium entry into cells during sustained or repetitive stimulation. To quantify this we calculated the charge (i.e. the integral) of I_{Ca} evoked by a 500 ms step depolarization. 1-butanol significantly inhibited the charge of I_{Ca} from 328±35 pC to 116±14 pC (n = 9; $p<0.0001$, paired t-test). Even though tert-butanol has little effect on the peak amplitude, it significantly reduced the charge of I_{Ca} from 297±48 pC to 184±40 pC (n = 7; $p<0.001$, paired t-test). Reflecting the dual actions of 1-butanol on both peak amplitude and inactivation, the integral of I_{Ca} was inhibited to a greater extent by 1-butanol (65±3%, n = 9) than by tert-butanol (41±4%, n = 7; $p<0.001$, independent t-test).

Discussion

In this study we investigated the effects of butanol isomers on calcium signaling and catecholamine secretion from adrenal chromaffin cells, an important component of the sympathetic nervous system and powerful model for investigating neurosecretory mechanisms. The rationale for the current investigation arose from two general uses of butanol in cellular physiology: implication of phosphatidic acid/PLD signaling in cellular functions, and investigating the molecular targets of general anesthetics. In spite of these two uses, there is little data comparing the effects of butanol isomers on pertinent cellular targets including voltage-gated ion channels.

Our data show that 1-butanol inhibited secretion to a much greater extent than tert-butanol, but the PLD inhibitor VU0155056 had no effect (Fig 1). We used VU0155056 at 1 μM, a concentration well above the reported cellular IC_{50} for PLD1 (20 nM) and PLD2 (380 nM) [13,14]. Our data parallel a previous report showing that 1-butanol inhibits insulin secretion but the PLD inhibitor FIPI has no effect [12]. Similarly, 1-butanol but not FIPI blocks degranulation (exocytosis) of mast cells [15]. Together, our data and these previous studies imply that acute application of 1-butanol blocks exocytosis by a PLD-independent mechanism(s). Our data demonstrate that disrupted calcium signaling is a likely mechanism by which 1-butanol acts. Using cellular imaging, we show that the calcium transient evoked by KCl-mediated depolarization was significantly reduced by 1-butanol, while tert-butanol and VU0155056 had negligible effects (Fig 1). Furthermore, we used patch clamp electrophysiology to confirm that 1-butanol rapidly and reversibly inhibited the peak amplitude of I_{Ca} while secondary and tert-butanol had minimal effects (Fig 2).

Ten genes encode for the pore-forming α_1 subunit of voltage-gated calcium channels, and these are sub-divided into three major families based on sequence homology (Ca_V1, Ca_V2, Ca_V3) [44,45]. Chromaffin cells from adult animals typically express Ca_V1 and Ca_V2 channels with the relative expression level depending on the species [37,39–41]. Low threshold T-type channels (Ca_V3) are typically not functionally expressed under normal conditions, but can be recruited by various signaling pathways or hypoxia [46–49]. In bovine cells, we have previously demonstrated that the whole cell I_{Ca} is comprised of ~10% L-type current and ~90% N + P/Q-type current in a roughly 1:1 ratio [42,50]. The concentration response relationship to 1-butanol (Fig 2B) shows that higher concentrations almost fully blocked I_{Ca}, suggesting that all the calcium channel subtypes present in these cells were targeted. To confirm this, we pharmacological dissected I_{Ca} using ω-conotoxin GVIA (a selective blocker of N-type channels) and found that the N-type and P/Q-type I_{Ca} were equally blocked by 1-butanol (Fig 2D). We speculate that L-type channels will be modulated in a similar manner, but due to the small amplitude of the L-type current in bovine chromaffin cells we did not determine this. In rodent chromaffin cells L-type channels ($Ca_V1.2$ and $Ca_V1.3$) comprise ~40% of the whole cell calcium current, and have been implicated in controlling action potential firing at rest or during sustained depolarization [51]. It is interesting to speculate that the butanol isomers will differentially modulate these aspects of rodent chromaffin cell function, but further experiments are needed to confirm this.

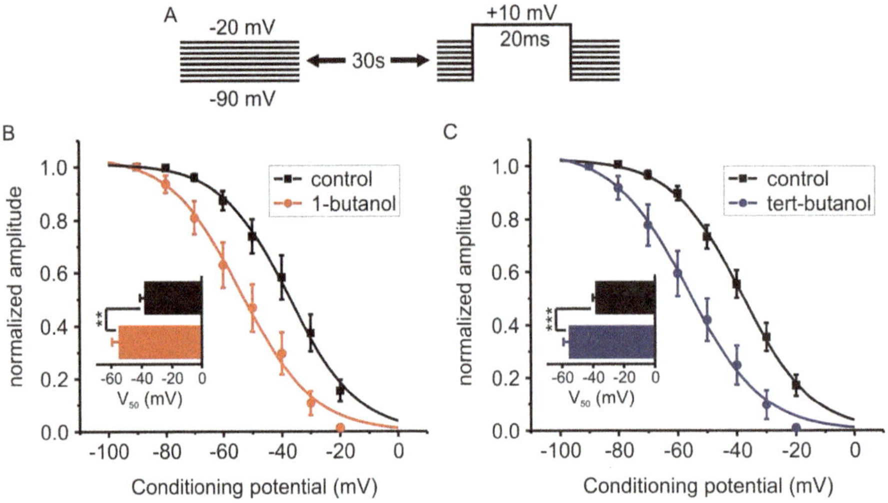

Figure 6. 1-butanol and tert-butanol produce a similar hyperpolarization of closed-state inactivation. A) Schematic depiction of the voltage-stimulus protocol. I_{Ca} were elicited by steps to +10 mV. The holding potential was increased in 10 mV increments from −90 mV to −20 mV and maintained at each potential for 30 s. In each cell this was done first in control conditions and then in the presence of either 1-butanol (panel B; n = 5) or tert-butanol (panel C; n = 6). **B, C**) I_{Ca} amplitude was normalized to that evoked from a holding potential of −90 mV and plotted against the holding potential. The graphs show the mean data fit using a Boltzmann function with three free parameters (upper plateau, slope, and V_{50}) and the lower plateau was constrained to ≥0. The inset bar graphs show the hyperpolarizing shift in mean V_{50} (voltage at half maximal inactivation) derived from the Boltzmann fits to individual cells (** p<0.01; *** p<0.001 compared to matched controls; paired t-test).

Our data showing isomer-specific block of I_{Ca} by butanol suggests the need to reassess at least some cellular functions previously attributed to PLD signaling using primary alcohols, especially those in which calcium signaling plays a prominent role. There is a body of work supporting a role for PLD in calcium-dependent exocytosis from chromaffin or PC12 cells [9,11,34],

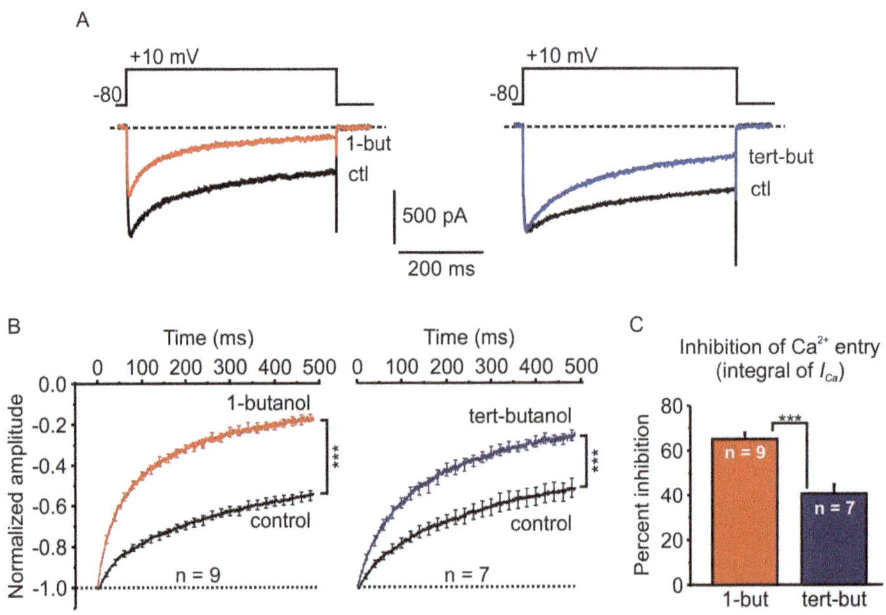

Figure 7. Butanol accelerates voltage-dependent inactivation and reduces total calcium entry during sustained depolarization. A) Representative recordings of I_{Ca} elicited by a 500 ms step depolarization under control conditions (ctl) and in the presence of either 0.4% (~44 mM) 1-butanol (1-but) or 0.4% (~42 mM) tert-butanol (tert-but). The patch pipette solution contained 10 mM EGTA to block calcium-dependent inactivation. Thus, the decay in I_{Ca} is due to voltage-dependent inactivation. 1-butanol inhibited the peak amplitude and accelerated the the inactivation of I_{Ca}. Tert-butanol also accelerated inactivation, but had minimal effects of the peak amplitude of I_{Ca}. **B**) Pooled data (mean ± sem) from multiple experiments like that shown in panel A. To facilitate comparison of inactivation, the amplitude of I_{Ca} in the presence of butanol was normalized to control conditions. For clarity, the displayed traces begin at the peak amplitude and error bars are only shown for some data points. 1-butanol and tert-butanol both significantly increased the extent of inactivation. (*** p<0.001 for the extent of inactivation at 490 ms in the presence of butanol compared to control conditions; paired t-test). **C**) The charge (integral) of I_{Ca} is directly proportional to the amount of calcium entry during the depolarizing step. 1-butanol produced a significantly greater inhibition than tert-butanol (*** p<0.001; paired t-test).

although some other studies have found no such link [52–54]. While the precise mechanism remains unclear, it has been proposed that generation of phosphatidic acid at vesicle release sites induces membrane curvature and thereby promotes the final stages of vesicle fusion with the plasma membrane [11]. Phosphatidic acid has also been shown to interact directly with SNARE proteins [55], or could lead to changes in other signaling lipids such as diacylglycerol or PiP2 [10]. Several approaches including RNAi-mediated knockdown of PLD and overexpression of wild-type or dominant negative mutants have been used to implicate PLD, and in particular PLD1, in exocytosis (for reviews see [9,11]). However, acute interventions have typically involved the use of primary alcohols, and to our knowledge the effects of newer PLD inhibitors have not been reported prior to this study. The main focus of the current investigation was not to dissect the role of PLD in catecholamine secretion *per se*, but our data suggest that acute block of PLD does not have a dramatic impact. Subtle effects on secretion are still possible as these would not be resolved in the assays used in this study, and we did not assess the impact of longer term block of PLD signaling. Further investigations will be required to address these issues and the precise role of PLD in neurotransmitter/hormone secretion.

This paper also provides the first detailed comparison of how butanol isomers modulate the function of voltage-gated channels. We used a concentration of 0.4% (~44 mM), typical for experiments probing PLD signaling and close to the EC_{50} for block of peak I_{Ca} amplitude by 1-butanol (Fig 2B). Although tert-butanol had minimal effects on peak I_{Ca} amplitude, it was not simply inert with respect to channel function. Tert-butanol accelerated inactivation of I_{Ca} during sustained depolarization and produced a pronounced (approximately −20 mV) shift in the steady state inactivation curve (Figs 6, 7). Distinct, even opposing effects of the butanol isomers were seen on other channel gating parameters, including the voltage-dependence of activation. 1-butanol produced no shift in the V_{50} and a modest reduction in the slope of the activation curve (Fig 4B). In contrast, tert-butanol hyperpolarized the V_{50} by ~−9 mV, with no change in the slope (Fig 4C). This likely will not increase the small "window current" (overlap of activation and inactivation curves (Figs 4 and 6)) because the much larger shift in steady-state inactivation will dominate. However, the hyperpolarizing shift in activation was apparent in the I-V relationship, and resulted in tert-butanol significantly *potentiating* the amplitude of I_{Ca} evoked by steps to −10 mV (Fig 3). The two isomers also had opposing effects on the kinetics of deactivation (tail current decay), which was accelerated by 1-butanol and slowed by tert-butanol (Fig 5). Again, as with the effects on activation gating, this would favor a potentiation of I_{Ca} by tert-butanol and inhibition by 1-butanol.

Perhaps the complex effects of butanol on I_{Ca} reflect multiple binding sites on the channel, some of which discern between the structurally distinct primary and tert-butanol isomers. 1-butanol has been used to map a binding site for general anesthetics/alcohols near the activation gate of Shaw-2 voltage-gated potassium channels [28,29]. The effects we observe on activation and deactivation gating are consistent with there being a similar binding site for butanol on the voltage-gated calcium channels, although this remains to be determined. Another recent study has reported multiple binding sites for general anesthetics on the bacterial sodium channel NaChBac [56]. It is also interesting to note that in virtually all cases reported to date, alcohols/general anesthetics *inhibit* voltage-gated channels. However, sevoflurane can potentiate voltage-gated potassium channels [57] and NaChBac [56]. It will be of interest in future to determine if sevoflurane also potentiates Ca_V channels, and conversely if tert-butanol potentiates potassium and sodium channels.

Although much progress has been made, the molecular targets and mechanisms of general anesthetics/alcohols are not completely understood. There is general consensus that post-synaptic ligand gated ion channels (e.g GABA, ACh) are important targets, but some evidence also points to presynaptic effects, perhaps on voltage-gated channels or the exocytotic machinery itself including SNARE proteins and munc18 [58–61]. In this study the estimated EC_{50} for 1-butanol block of peak I_{Ca} amplitude was ~52 mM (Fig 2B), which is somewhat higher than that producing anesthesia in vivo (10–20 mM) [62–64]. Moreover, even though secondary and tert-butanol also produce anesthesia, they had minimal effects on I_{Ca} amplitude (Fig 2,3). This would argue against Ca_V2 voltage-gated calcium channels being a primary target for the anesthetic actions. However, even relatively small changes in I_{Ca} can have a significant impact on neurotransmitter release, and as already discussed the effects of butanol are complex and extend well beyond the simple block of peak current amplitude. Further, investigations will be required to determine if these channels contribute to some of the anesthetic actions and/or side effects of alcohols/inhalational anesthetics.

In conclusion, we show for the first time that butanol isomers have distinct effects on the amplitude and gating properties of Ca_V2 voltage-gated calcium channel currents. This adds to existing literature demonstrating complex modulation of voltage-gated channels by alcohols and anesthetic agents. Our data also suggest the need to reassess at least some cellular functions previously attributed to PLD signaling by using primary alcohols as a tool, especially those in which calcium signaling plays a prominent role.

Supporting Information

Data S1 This file is provided as part of the PLOS ONE data availability policy. For figures in the manuscript that present averaged data (e.g. mean ± sem), the underlying raw data used to calculate those averages are provided. Refer to the main text of the manuscript or figure legends for further explanation of experimental design, protocols, etc.
(PDF)

Acknowledgments

We would like to thank: Ray Johnson, Manager of the Vanderbilt Brain Institute Neurochemistry Core, for assistance with high performance liquid chromatography analyses of catecholamines and Dr. Alex Brown, Dept. of Pharmacology, Vanderbilt University, for generously providing samples of the PLD inhibitor.

Author Contributions

Conceived and designed the experiments: KC. Performed the experiments: SM MB RB MJ. Analyzed the data: SM MB RB KC. Wrote the paper: SM MB RB MJ KC.

References

1. Brown HA, Henage LG, Preininger AM, Xiang Y, Exton JH (2007) Biochemical analysis of phospholipase D. Methods Enzymol 434: 49–87.
2. Cockcroft S (2001) Signalling roles of mammalian phospholipase D1 and D2. Cell Mol Life Sci 58: 1674–1687.
3. Exton JH (2000) Phospholipase D. Ann N Y Acad Sci 905: 61–68.

4. Selvy PE, Lavieri RR, Lindsley CW, Brown HA (2011) Phospholipase D: enzymology, functionality, and chemical modulation. Chem Rev 111: 6064–6119.
5. Peng X, Frohman MA (2012) Mammalian phospholipase D physiological and pathological roles. Acta Physiol (Oxf) 204: 219–226.
6. Rudge SA, Wakelam MJ (2009) Inter-regulatory dynamics of phospholipase D and the actin cytoskeleton. Biochim Biophys Acta 1791: 856–861.
7. Gomez-Cambronero J (2010) New concepts in phospholipase D signaling in inflammation and cancer. ScientificWorldJournal 10: 1356–1369.
8. Stace CL, Ktistakis NT (2006) Phosphatidic acid- and phosphatidylserine-binding proteins. Biochim Biophys Acta 1761: 913–926.
9. Bader MF, Vitale N (2009) Phospholipase D in calcium-regulated exocytosis: lessons from chromaffin cells. Biochim Biophys Acta 1791: 936–941.
10. Jenkins GM, Frohman MA (2005) Phospholipase D: a lipid centric review. Cell Mol Life Sci 62: 2305–2316.
11. Vitale N (2010) Synthesis of fusogenic lipids through activation of phospholipase D1 by GTPases and the kinase RSK2 is required for calcium-regulated exocytosis in neuroendocrine cells. Biochem Soc Trans 38: 167–171.
12. Su W, Yeku O, Olepu S, Genna A, Park JS, et al. (2009) 5-Fluoro-2-indolyl des-chlorohalopemide (FIPI), a phospholipase D pharmacological inhibitor that alters cell spreading and inhibits chemotaxis. Mol Pharmacol 75: 437–446.
13. Scott SA, Selvy PE, Buck JR, Cho HP, Criswell TL, et al. (2009) Design of isoform-selective phospholipase D inhibitors that modulate cancer cell invasiveness. Nat Chem Biol 5: 108–117.
14. Scott SA, Mathews TP, Ivanova PT, Lindsley CW, Brown HA (2014) Chemical modulation of glycerolipid signaling and metabolic pathways. Biochim Biophys Acta.
15. Yanase Y, Carvou N, Frohman MA, Cockcroft S (2010) Reversible bleb formation in mast cells stimulated with antigen is Ca2+/calmodulin-dependent and bleb size is regulated by ARF6. Biochem J 425: 179–193.
16. Fang Z, Ionescu P, Chortkoff BS, Kandel L, Sonner J, et al. (1997) Anesthetic potencies of n-alkanols: results of additivity and solubility studies suggest a mechanism of action similar to that for conventional inhaled anesthetics. Anesth Analg 84: 1042–1048.
17. Howard RJ, Trudell JR, Harris RA (2014) Seeking structural specificity: direct modulation of pentameric ligand-gated ion channels by alcohols and general anesthetics. Pharmacol Rev 66: 396–412.
18. Garcia PS, Kolesky SE, Jenkins A (2010) General anesthetic actions on GABA(A) receptors. Curr Neuropharmacol 8: 2–9.
19. Dopico AM, Lovinger DM (2009) Acute alcohol action and desensitization of ligand-gated ion channels. Pharmacol Rev 61: 98–114.
20. Franks NP (2006) Molecular targets underlying general anaesthesia. Br J Pharmacol 147 Suppl 1: S72–81.
21. Orestes P, Todorovic SM (2010) Are neuronal voltage-gated calcium channels valid cellular targets for general anesthetics? Channels (Austin) 4: 518–522.
22. Hemmings HC, Jr. (2009) Sodium channels and the synaptic mechanisms of inhaled anaesthetics. Br J Anaesth 103: 61–69.
23. Herold KF, Hemmings HC, Jr. (2012) Sodium channels as targets for volatile anesthetics. Front Pharmacol 3: 50.
24. Barclay JW, Graham ME, Edwards MR, Johnson JR, Morgan A, et al. (2010) Presynaptic targets for acute ethanol sensitivity. Biochem Soc Trans 38: 172–176.
25. Siggins GR, Roberto M, Nie Z (2005) The tipsy terminal: presynaptic effects of ethanol. Pharmacol Ther 107: 80–98.
26. Horishita T, Harris RA (2008) n-Alcohols inhibit voltage-gated Na+ channels expressed in Xenopus oocytes. J Pharmacol Exp Ther 326: 270–277.
27. Covarrubias M, Vyas TB, Escobar L, Wei A (1995) Alcohols inhibit a cloned potassium channel at a discrete saturable site. Insights into the molecular basis of general anesthesia. J Biol Chem 270: 19408–19416.
28. Bhattacharji A, Klett N, Go RC, Covarrubias M (2010) Inhalational anaesthetics and n-alcohols share a site of action in the neuronal Shaw2 Kv channel. Br J Pharmacol 159: 1475–1485.
29. Barber AF, Liang Q, Amaral C, Treptow W, Covarrubias M (2011) Molecular mapping of general anesthetic sites in a voltage-gated ion channel. Biophys J 101: 1613–1622.
30. Oyama Y, Akaike N, Nishi K (1986) Effects of n-alkanols on the calcium current of intracellularly perfused neurons of Helix aspersa. Brain Res 376: 280–284.
31. Hawthorn MH, Ferrante JN, Kwon YW, Rutledge A, Luchowski E, et al. (1992) Effect of an homologous series of aliphatic alcohols on neuronal and smooth muscle voltage-dependent Ca2+ channels. Eur J Pharmacol 229: 143–148.
32. Oz M, Tchugunova YB, Dunn SM (2001) Direct inhibition of voltage-dependent Ca(2+) fluxes by ethanol and higher alcohols in rabbit T-tubule membranes. Eur J Pharmacol 418: 169–176.
33. Jewell ML, Currie KPM (2013) Control of CaV2 calcium channels and neurosecretion by heterotrimeric G protein coupled receptors. In: Stephens GJ, Mochida S, editors. Modulation of presynaptic calcium channels: Springer Publishing. pp. 101–130.
34. Vitale N, Caumont AS, Chasserot-Golaz S, Du G, Wu S, et al. (2001) Phospholipase D1: a key factor for the exocytotic machinery in neuroendocrine cells. Embo J 20: 2424–2434.
35. Todd RD, McDavid SM, Brindley RL, Jewell ML, Currie KP (2012) Gabapentin inhibits catecholamine release from adrenal chromaffin cells. Anesthesiology 116: 1013–1024.
36. Douglas WW (1968) Stimulus-secretion coupling: the concept and clues from chromaffin and other cells. Br J Pharmacol 34: 451–469.
37. Garcia AG, Garcia-De-Diego AM, Gandia L, Borges R, Garcia-Sancho J (2006) Calcium signaling and exocytosis in adrenal chromaffin cells. Physiol Rev 86: 1093–1131.
38. Currie KP (2010) Inhibition of Ca2+ channels and adrenal catecholamine release by G protein coupled receptors. Cell Mol Neurobiol 30: 1201–1208.
39. Mahapatra S, Calorio C, Vandael DH, Marcantoni A, Carabelli V, et al. (2012) Calcium channel types contributing to chromaffin cell excitability, exocytosis and endocytosis. Cell Calcium 51: 321–330.
40. Marcantoni A, Carabelli V, Comunanza V, Hoddah H, Carbone E (2008) Calcium channels in chromaffin cells: focus on L and T types. Acta Physiol (Oxf) 192: 233–246.
41. Fox AP, Cahill AL, Currie KP, Grabner C, Harkins AB, et al. (2008) N- and P/Q-type Ca2+ channels in adrenal chromaffin cells. Acta Physiol (Oxf) 192: 247–261.
42. Currie KPM, Fox AP (1997) Comparison of N- and P/Q-type voltage-gated calcium channel current inhibition. J Neurosci 17: 4570–4579.
43. McDavid S, Currie KP (2006) G-proteins modulate cumulative inactivation of N-type (Cav2.2) calcium channels. J Neurosci 26: 13373–13383.
44. Ertel EA, Campbell KP, Harpold MM, Hofmann F, Mori Y, et al. (2000) Nomenclature of voltage-gated calcium channels. Neuron 25: 533–535.
45. Catterall WA, Perez-Reyes E, Snutch TP, Striessnig J (2005) International Union of Pharmacology. XLVIII. Nomenclature and structure-function relationships of voltage-gated calcium channels. Pharmacol Rev 57: 411–425.
46. Novara M, Baldelli P, Cavallari D, Carabelli V, Giancippoli A, et al. (2004) Exposure to cAMP and beta-adrenergic stimulation recruits Ca(V)3 T-type channels in rat chromaffin cells through Epac cAMP-receptor proteins. J Physiol 558: 433–449.
47. Carabelli V, Marcantoni A, Comunanza V, de Luca A, Diaz J, et al. (2007) Chronic hypoxia up-regulates alpha1H T-type channels and low-threshold catecholamine secretion in rat chromaffin cells. J Physiol 584: 149–165.
48. Souvannakitti D, Nanduri J, Yuan G, Kumar GK, Fox AP, et al. (2010) NADPH oxidase-dependent regulation of T-type Ca2+ channels and ryanodine receptors mediate the augmented exocytosis of catecholamines from intermittent hypoxia-treated neonatal rat chromaffin cells. J Neurosci 30: 10763–10772.
49. Hill J, Chan SA, Kuri B, Smith C (2011) Pituitary adenylate cyclase-activating peptide (PACAP) recruits low voltage-activated T-type calcium influx under acute sympathetic stimulation in mouse adrenal chromaffin cells. J Biol Chem 286: 42459–42469.
50. Currie KPM, Fox AP (1996) ATP serves as a negative feedback inhibitor of voltage-gated Ca2+ channel currents in cultured bovine adrenal chromaffin cells. Neuron 16: 1027–1036.
51. Marcantoni A, Vandael DH, Mahapatra S, Carabelli V, Sinnegger-Brauns MJ, et al. (2010) Loss of Cav1.3 channels reveals the critical role of L-type and BK channel coupling in pacemaking mouse adrenal chromaffin cells. J Neurosci 30: 491–504.
52. Glenn DE, Thomas GM, O'Sullivan AJ, Burgoyne RD (1998) Examination of the role of ADP-ribosylation factor and phospholipase D activation in regulated exocytosis in chromaffin and PC12 cells. J Neurochem 71: 2023–2033.
53. Purkiss J, Murrin RA, Owen PJ, Boarder MR (1991) Lack of phospholipase D activity in chromaffin cells: bradykinin-stimulated phosphatidic acid formation involves phospholipase C in chromaffin cells but phospholipase D in PC12 cells. J Neurochem 57: 1084–1087.
54. Coorssen JR (1996) Phospholipase activation and secretion: evidence that PLA2, PLC, and PLD are not essential to exocytosis. Am J Physiol 270: C1153–1163.
55. Lam AD, Tryoen-Toth P, Tsai B, Vitale N, Stuenkel EL (2008) SNARE-catalyzed fusion events are regulated by Syntaxin1A-lipid interactions. Mol Biol Cell 19: 485–497.
56. Barber AF, Carnevale V, Klein ML, Eckenhoff RG, Covarrubias M (2014) Modulation of a voltage-gated Na+ channel by sevoflurane involves multiple sites and distinct mechanisms. Proc Natl Acad Sci U S A 111: 6726–6731.
57. Barber AF, Liang Q, Covarrubias M (2012) Novel activation of voltage-gated K(+) channels by sevoflurane. J Biol Chem 287: 40425–40432.
58. Nagele P, Mendel JB, Placzek WJ, Scott BA, D'Avignon DA, et al. (2005) Volatile anesthetics bind rat synaptic snare proteins. Anesthesiology 103: 768–778.
59. Herring BE, Xie Z, Marks J, Fox AP (2009) Isoflurane inhibits the neurotransmitter release machinery. J Neurophysiol 102: 1265–1273.
60. Xie Z, McMillan K, Pike CM, Cahill AL, Herring BE, et al. (2013) Interaction of anesthetics with neurotransmitter release machinery proteins. J Neurophysiol 109: 758–767.
61. Graham ME, Edwards MR, Holden-Dye L, Morgan A, Burgoyne RD, et al. (2009) UNC-18 modulates ethanol sensitivity in Caenorhabditis elegans. Mol Biol Cell 20: 43–55.
62. Krasowski MD, Harrison NL (2000) The actions of ether, alcohol and alkane general anaesthetics on GABAA and glycine receptors and the effects of TM2 and TM3 mutations. Br J Pharmacol 129: 731–743.
63. Alifimoff JK, Firestone LL, Miller KW (1989) Anaesthetic potencies of primary alkanols: implications for the molecular dimensions of the anaesthetic site. Br J Pharmacol 96: 9–16.
64. Firestone S, Firestone LL (1995) Staurosporine, a protein kinase inhibitor, increases the intoxicating potencies of ethanol and other n-alkanols in Rana pipiens tadpoles. Alcohol Clin Exp Res 19: 416–419.

14

Involvement of Trigeminal Transition Zone and Laminated Subnucleus Caudalis in Masseter Muscle Hypersensitivity Associated with Tooth Inflammation

Kohei Shimizu[1,3]*, Kunihito Matsumoto[2,3], Noboru Noma[4,5], Shingo Matsuura[1], Kinuyo Ohara[1], Hiroki Komiya[1], Tetsuro Watase[1], Bunnai Ogiso[1,3], Yoshiyuki Tsuboi[6,7], Masamichi Shinoda[6,7], Keisuke Hatori[1,3], Yuka Nakaya[4], Koichi Iwata[6,7,8]

1 Department of Endodontics, Nihon University School of Dentistry, Tokyo, Japan, **2** Department of Radiology, Nihon University School of Dentistry, Tokyo, Japan, **3** Divisions of Advanced Dental Treatment, Dental Research Center, Nihon University School of Dentistry, Tokyo, Japan, **4** Department of Oral Diagnosis, Nihon University School of Dentistry, Tokyo, Japan, **5** Divisions of Clinical Research, Dental Research Center, Nihon University School of Dentistry, Tokyo, Japan, **6** Department of Physiology, Nihon University School of Dentistry, Tokyo, Japan, **7** Division of Functional Morphology, Dental Research Center, Nihon University School of Dentistry, Tokyo, Japan, **8** Division of Applied System Neuroscience Advanced Medical Research Center, Nihon University Graduate School of Medical Science, Tokyo, Japan

Abstract

A rat model of pulpitis/periapical periodontitis was used to study mechanisms underlying extraterritorial enhancement of masseter response associated with tooth inflammation. Periapical bone loss gradually increased and peaked at 6 weeks after complete Freund's adjuvant (CFA) application to the upper molar tooth pulp (M1). On day 3, the number of Fos-immunoreactive (IR) cells was significantly larger in M1 CFA rats compared with M1 vehicle (veh) rats in the trigeminal subnucleus interpolaris/caudalis transition zone (Vi/Vc). The number of Fos-IR cells was significantly larger in M1 CFA and masseter (Mass) capsaicin applied (M1 CFA/Mass cap) rats compared with M1 veh/Mass veh rats in the contralateral Vc and Vi/Vc. The number of phosphorylated extracellular signal-regulated kinase (pERK)-IR cells was significantly larger in M1 CFA/Mass cap and M1 veh/Mass cap rats compared to Mass-vehicle applied rats with M1 vehicle or CFA in the Vi/Vc. Pulpal CFA application caused significant increase in the number of Fos-IR cells in the Vi/Vc but not Vc on week 6. The number of pERK-IR cells was significantly lager in the rats with capsaicin application to the Mass compared to Mass-vehicle treated rats after pulpal CFA- or vehicle-application. However, capsaicin application to the Mass did not further affect the number of Fos-IR cells in the Vi/Vc in pulpal CFA-applied rats. The digastric electromyographic (d-EMG) activity after Mass-capsaicin application was significantly increased on day 3 and lasted longer at 6 weeks after pulpal CFA application, and these increase and duration were significantly attenuated by i.t. PD98059, a MEK1 inhibitor. These findings suggest that Vi/Vc and Vc neuronal excitation is involved in the facilitation of extraterritorial hyperalgesia for Mass primed with periapical periodontitis or acute pulpal-inflammation. Furthermore, phosphorylation of ERK in the Vi/Vc and Vc play pivotal roles in masseter hyperalgesia after pulpitis or periapical periodontitis.

Editor: Theodore J. Price, University of Texas at Dallas, United States of America

Funding: This study was supported in part by Research grants from Sato and Uemura Funds from Nihon University School of Dentistry, and Grant from Dental Research Center, Nihon University School of Dentistry; Nihon University multidisciplinary research grant and Individual Research Grant; a Grant from the Ministry of Education, Culture, Sports, Science and Technology to promote multi-disciplinary research Projects (KAKENHI (Grant-in-Aid for Young Scientist (B)) # 21791868 and # 23792192 to KS, # 22792021 to MS, KAKENHI (Challenging Exploratory Research) #24659832 to KI); grants from the Ministry of Education, Culture, Sports, Science, Technology to promote multidisciplinary research projects "Brain Mechanisms for Cognition, Memory and Behavior" and "Translational Research Network on Orofacial Neurological Disorders" at Nihon University. The funders had no role in study design, data collection and analysis, decision to publish, or preparation of the manuscript.

Competing Interests: The authors have declared that no competing interests exist.

* Email: shimizu.kouhei01@nihon-u.ac.jp

Introduction

Orofacial persistent pain following trigeminal nerve injury or orofacial inflammation is known to cause various motor as well as sensory disorders in the orofacial regions such as mastication or swallowing dysfunction [1]. Orofacial dysesthesia is known as the secondary hyperalgesia often associated with pulpitis and/or periapical periodontitis [2], suggesting that oral and craniofacial organs are target regions for ectopic pain following intraoral inflammation. Furthermore, it has been reported that the chronic orofacial pain associated with pulpitis and/or periapical periodontitis is one of the most frequent referred pain in the orofacial region, and pulpitis or periapical periodontitis is also known to be involved in the referred pain in various intraoral structures [3,4]. Referred pain in non-inflamed orofacial areas associated with pulpitis or periapical periodontitis is often accounted for misdiagnosis or inappropriate clinical treatment. Thus, it is very important to understand the mechanisms underlying orofacial-referred pain associated with pulpitis or periapical periodontitis to develop appropriate diagnosis and treatment of these patients.

The spinal trigeminal subnucleus caudalis (Vc) has been known as a key nucleus to relay tooth pulp afferent inputs to the higher central nervous system, and a large number of nociceptive neurons in the Vc are activated by orofacial noxious stimulation as well as tooth pulp stimulation [5,6]. Electrical stimulation of the tooth pulp produces Fos protein expression in many neurons in the transition zone between the subnucleus interpolaris (Vi) and Vc (Vi/Vc) and the caudal Vc and upper cervical cord [5]. These two areas are thought to play differential roles in processing noxious information from the tooth pulp as well as orofacial skin or muscles [7,8]. It has been reported that Vi/Vc and Vc have a role to process masseter muscle pain [9]. Furthermore, many neurons in these two areas are also known to receive noxious as well as non-noxious inputs from the orofacial regions [7,10]. Therefore, it is highly possible that nociceptive neurons in the Vi/Vc and Vc enhance their firings following pulpitis or periapical periodontitis and play a role in orofacial cutaneous and/or Mass nociception as well as processing tooth pulp or periapical inputs. We hypothesized therefore that Vi/Vc and Vc neurons are involved in masseter muscle hypersensitivity associated with tooth pulp and periapical inflammation.

Extracellular signal-regulated protein kinase (ERK) is a member of mitogen-activated protein kinase family that can be activated by calcium influx within 10 min after noxious stimulation [11]. Phosphorylated ERK-immunoreactive (pERK-IR) cells are known to be distributed in Vc with somatotopic organization, and the number of pERK-IR cells increased in an intensity-dependent manner in the Vc [12]. Previous studies indicated that C-fiber but not A-fiber stimulation accelerates ERK phosphorylation in dorsal root ganglion and spinal dorsal horn (SDH) neurons [13]. These findings indicate that ERK phosphorylation in Vc neurons could be a reliable indicator of neuronal activation following noxious stimulation of the orofacial regions.

Fos-IR cells have been widely used as a marker of neuronal activation in the SDH following noxious stimulation [14]. Fos expression could be detected 0.5–1 hour after noxious stimulation and lasts for 2–3 hours after stimulation. Recently, we have also reported that many pERK-IR cells show Fos-IR in Vc neurons following noxious mechanical stimulation of the periodontal tissues [15], suggesting that ERK phosphorylation is followed by Fos protein expression after noxious stimulation.

To clarify the central mechanisms underlying Mass hypersensitivity associated with pulpitis or periapical periodontitis following CFA application to the tooth pulp, we studied ERK phosphorylation and Fos expression in Vi/Vc and Vc neurons in tooth pulp- or periapical inflamed rats.

Materials and Methods

This study was approved by the Animal Experimentation Committee at the Nihon University (Animal protocol AP10D001). All surgery and animal care were conducted in accordance with the National Institutes of Health Guide for the Care and Use of Laboratory Animals and the guidelines for Institutional Animal Care, and the guidelines of the International Association for the Study of Pain [16]. Male Sprague-Dawley rats (n = 152) weighing 250–450 g were used in this study. The rats were housed under 12 h light/dark cycle conditions and had free access to food and water except during the test period. To minimize animal suffering, the number of animals used was based on the minimum required for statistically valid results. Immunohistochemical and Electrophysiological analysis were carried out in a blind manner.

Pulpal or periapical inflammation

Rats were lightly anesthetized with 2% isoflurane (Mylan, Canonsburg, PA), then deeply anesthetized with intraperitoneal (i.p.) application of sodium pentobarbital (50 mg/kg; Schering Plough, Whitehouse Station, NJ), and placed on a warm mat (37°C) in a dorsal recumbent position. To allow for application of CFA (n = 4, Sigma-Aldrich, 50% CFA was diluted in saline) or vehicle (n = 4, isotonic physiological saline) to the right maxillary first molar (M1) tooth pulp, the rats' mouth was gently opened and the dental pulp was exposed by means of low-speed dental drill with a round tungsten carbide bur (No. 1-4: JOTA, Tokyo) under water cooling. CFA or vehicle was applied to the tooth pulp by a small piece of dental paper point (diameter, 0.15 mm; length, 1.5 mm; PIERCE ABSORBENT POINTS, #15) soaked with CFA or vehicle. After CFA or vehicle application with dental points, the cavity was tightly sealed with dental cement (GC Fuji I, Tokyo). The bone loss around the tooth apex was evaluated using in vivo Micro X-ray CT System R_mCT (R_mCT, Rigaku, Tokyo). There were no any abnormal animal behaviors such as grooming, locomotion and feeding. The rats did not lose weight during experimental period.

The sagittal CT images for tooth apex were obtained at 300 μm intervals, and then the bone loss around tooth apex was drawn using Neurolucida (Micro-Brightfield Inc., Colchester, VT). The drawn images were integrated and 3D image of the periapical bone loss was constructed. The change in the volume was calculated by the Neuroexplore software (Micro-Brightfield Inc., Colchester, VT). Furthermore, on day 3 or week 6 after CFA application to upper molar tooth pulp, rats were anesthetized with sodium pentobarbital (80 mg/kg, i.p.) and perfused with 4% paraformaldehyde. Maxillar bone and M1 were removed and decalcified overnight and 15 mm serial sections were cut. Then sections were stained with hematoxylin and eosin and coverslipped.

pERK and Fos immunohistochemistries

For double immunofluorescence histochemistry for pERK and NeuN, sections were rinsed in PBS, 10% normal goat serum in PBS for 1 h, and then incubated in rabbit antiphospho-p44/42 MAP Kinase Antibody (1:200, Cell Signaling Technology) for 72 h at room temperature. Then the sections were incubated in mouse anti-neuronal nuclei monoclonal Antibody (1:500, Chemicon, Temicula, CA) for 2 h at room temperature. Next, the sections were incubated in Alexa Fluor 488 anti-rabbit IgG (1:200 in 0.01 M PBS; Invitrogen, Paisley) and in Alexa Fluor 568 anti-mouse IgG (1:200 in 0.01 M PBS; Invitrogen) for 2 h at room temperature. After rinsing with 0.01 M PBS, sections were coverslipped in mounting medium (Thermo Fisher Scientific, Fremont, CA) and examined under a fluorescence microscope and analyzed using a BZ-9000 system (Keyence, Osaka).

At 3 days and 6 weeks after CFA or vehicle application to M1 (n = 6 each), rats were deeply anesthetized with 2% isoflurane, and a 26 G needle with a Hamilton syringe was inserted into the ipsilateral Mass. After 30 min rest period, capsaicin was applied to the ipsilateral Mass, and at 5 minutes after capsaicin application, rats were transcardially perfused with isotonic saline followed by a fixative containing 4% paraformaldehyde in 0.1 M phosphate buffer (pH 7.4). The whole brain including medulla and upper cervical cord was removed and post-fixed in the same fixative for 3 days at 4°C. The tissues were then transferred to 20% sucrose (w/v) in 0.01 M phosphate-buffered saline (PBS) for several days for cryoprotection. Thirty-micron-thick sections were cut with a freezing microtome, and every fourth section was collected in PBS. Free-floating tissue sections were washed in PBS and rinsed in 1% hydrogen peroxide with 0.75% Triton X-100 (Sigma, St. Louis, MO) in PBS for 1 hour. After washing in PBS, the sections were incubated in 10% normal goat serum in PBS, and then incubated in polyclonal rabbit anti-Fos antibody (c-Fos ab-5, 1:5,000 dilution; Oncogene, Cambridge, MA) for overnight at 4°C. Next, the sections were incubated in biotinylated goat anti-rabbit IgG (1:600; Vector Labs, Burlingame, CA) for 2 h at room temperature. After washing in PBS, the sections were incubated in peroxidase-conjugated avidin-biotin complex (1:100; ABC, Vector Labs) for 2 h at room temperature. After washing in 0.05 M Tris Buffer (TB), the sections were incubated in 0.035% 3,3-diaminobenzidine-tetra HCl (DAB, Sigma, St. Louis, MO), 0.2% nickel ammonium sulfate and 0.05% peroxide in 0.05 M TB (pH 7.4). After washing in PBS and incubated in 10% normal horse serum in PBS, the sections reacted with Fos antibody were incubated in mouse anti-phospho-p44/42 MAP Kinase Antibody (pERK, 1 1000, Cell Signaling Technology) for 72 h at 4°C. The following immunohistochemical procedures were similar to those of c-Fos immunohistochemistry. The reaction products of biotinylated horse anti-mouse antiserum and avidin-conjugated horseradish peroxidase were visualized with 0.035% DAB and 0.05% hydrogen peroxide without nickel.

The sections were washed in PBS, serially mounted on gelatin-coated slides, dehydrated in alcohols and cover slipped. The pERK-IR, Fos protein-IR and double-labeled neurons were drawn under the light microscope using Neurolucida drawing tube. The neurons stained with DAB as brown in the nuclei and cytoplasm were determined as pERK-IR cells. The neurons stained with DAB as black in the nuclei were determined as Fos-IR cells. The number of pERK-IR, Fos protein-IR neurons was counted from every 8th section. The total number of IR neurons from 3 of every 8th section was calculated, and the mean number of those cells (3 sections/rat) was obtained from each animal.

Digastric electromyographic recording after capsaicin application into the Mass

On day 3 or week 6 after CFA or vehicle application to the M1 tooth pulp (n = 6 each), rats were anesthetized with 2% isoflurane and a pair of bipolar wire electrodes (enamel-coated stainless steel wire, inter-polar distance: 5 mm) was inserted into the digastric muscle on the side ipsilateral to the tooth. After that, a 26G needle connected with a Hamilton syringe was gently inserted into the ipsilateral Mass.

The digastric electromyographic (d-EMG) activity was continuously monitored before, during and after the application of capsaicin, dissolved in 100% ethanol and 7% Tween 80 in saline (3 μM, 100 μl), into the Mass. Before capsaicin application, baseline of d-EMG activity was monitored for 20 min, and d-EMG activity was continuously monitored for an additional 20 min. Then, the d-EMG activity was amplified, rectified and integrated, and the area under the curve of d-EMG activity was calculated by the Spike 2 software (CED, Cambridge). The area under the curve of d-EMG activity was measured for every 1 min before and after capsaicin application, and mean d-EMG activity was calculated in each time period. The calculated d-EMG value more than 2 standard deviation of the baseline after capsaicin application was selected and evaluated.

PD98059 administration

Rats were anesthetized with 2% isoflurane and placed in a stereotaxic apparatus. After a midline skin incision, an opening was made in the caudal part of the skull with a dental drill to insert intrathecally (i.t.) a soft polyethylene tube (PE45, ID, 0.58 mm; OD, 0.96 mm; Natsume, Tokyo, Japan) [17]. The tube was connected to a mini-osmotic pump (Alzet model 2001, Alzet, Cupertino, CA, USA; total volume, 200 μL) filled with the drug and embedded subcutaneously in the dorsal portion of the body. Thus, the MEK1 inhibitor PD98059 was intrathecally applied for 7 days (1.0 μL/h). The dosage and duration of the drug (0.1 μg/μL) for pump infusion was chosen primarily based on previous reports [18–21]. For the rats with periapical periodontitis, CFA was applied into the M1 at 35 days before PD98059 or saline administration, and then capsaicin was applied to the Mass on 7 days after PD98059 administration. For the rats with pulpitis, CFA was applied into the M1 at 4 days after PD98059 or saline administration, and then capsaicin was applied into the Mass at 3 days after CFA application. The d-EMG activity was continuously monitored before and after capsaicin application (n = 6 each).

For pERK and Fos immunohistochemistries, capsaicin was applied into the Mass in CFA-treated rats on day 7 after PD98059 or saline administration (n = 6 each). At 5 minutes after capsaicin application, the rats were perfused, and the pERK and Fos immunohistochemistries were performed.

All subsequent d-EMG recording and staining steps and counting analysis were the same as described above. All d-EMG recording and immunohistochemical experiments were conducted on animals without any obvious neurological deficits. Also, the Alzet pump was removed at the end of each experiment, and the amount of the drug remaining in the pump was checked. If there was still residual drug in the pump, the data from that rat were excluded from the final analysis.

Statistical analysis

Data were expressed as mean ± SEM. Statistical analyses were performed by Student's t-test, one-way or two-way repeated-measures analysis of variance (ANOVA) followed by Turkey or Dunnet test appropriately. A value of $p<0.05$ was considered as significant.

Results

1. The effect of CFA on tooth and periapical tissues

The application of CFA to the M1 tooth pulp induced inflammation in the tooth pulp on day 3 and in the periapical tissues on week 6 (Fig. 1). The detail tooth structures of M1 were indicated in Fig. 1A–C. In naive rats or the rats with CFA application to the M1 tooth pulp on day 3, periapical bone loss was not observed (Fig. 1A, B), indicating that the CFA-induced inflammation is limited within the pulp or at the apex region of the tooth. The periapical bone loss was clearly detected at 3 weeks after CFA application to the pulp, as shown by formation of granuloma in the periapical periodontitis (Fig. 1C–I). The bone loss was gradually increased and peaked at 6 weeks after CFA application (Fig. 1J). The volume of bone loss measured by 3D micro-CT imaging analysis software was significantly greater in CFA-treated rats compared with vehicle-treated rats from 3 weeks after CFA application ($p<0.05$, Fig. 1J).

2. Change in d-EMG activities following tooth pulp or periapical inflammation

We observed significant increase in the d-EMG activity within 1 min after capsaicin application into the Mass in pulpal CFA-applied rats ($p<0.01$, Fig. 2A, B). On the other hand, the duration of d-EMG activities after pulpal-CFA or pulpal-vehicle application was about 2 minutes, and no significant difference was observed between CFA and vehicle groups (Fig. 2C).

The d-EMG activities elicited by capsaicin application into the Mass at 6 weeks after pulpal-CFA application were shown in Fig. 2D. Compared with the pulpal-vehicle applied rats, the d-EMG activity was significantly increased (Fig. 2E) and the duration of the d-EMG activity was significantly lasted (Fig. 2F)

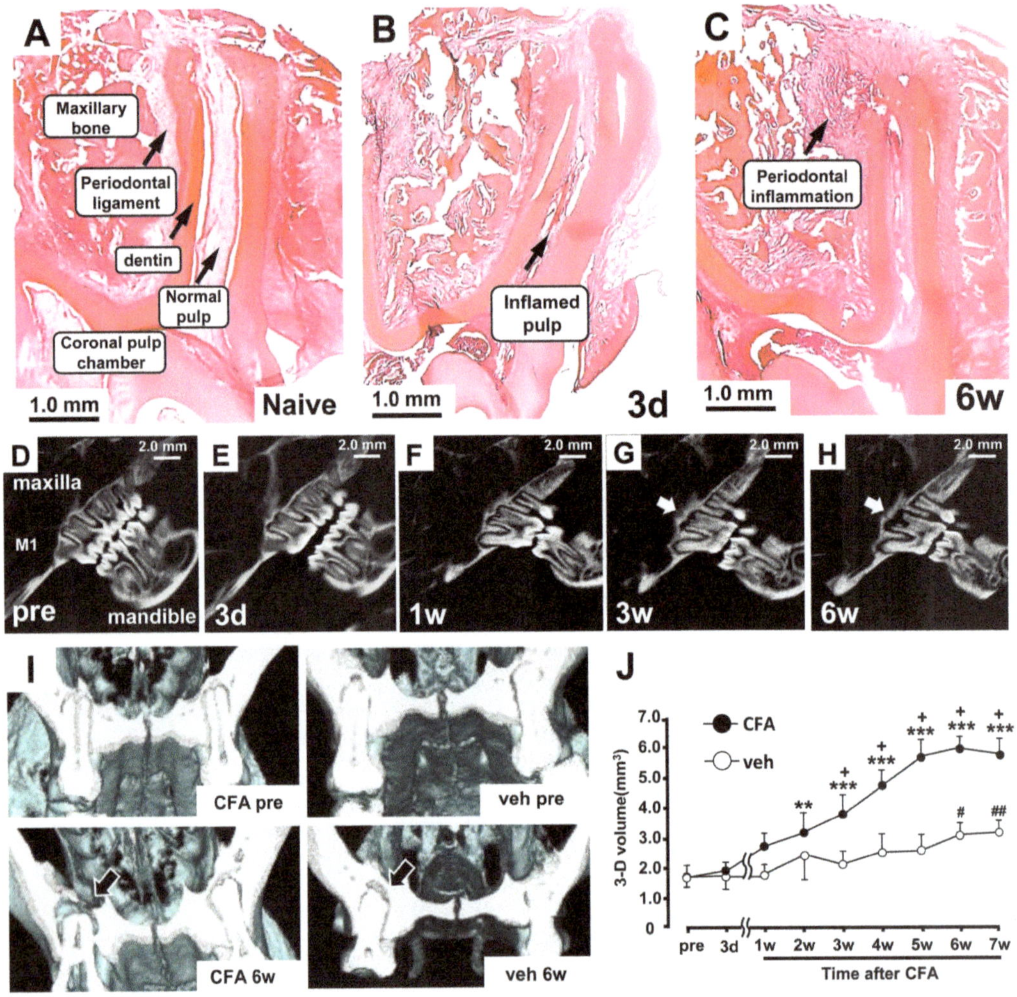

Figure 1. The change in the apical periapical tissues after CFA application to M1 tooth pulp. A, B and C: Photomicrographs of periapical tissues of the naive rats (A) and the rats on day 3 (B) and week 6 (C) after CFA application to the pulp. D–H: Lateral views of 3D X-lay photographs of periapical tissues of pre-CFA application (D), on day 3 (E), on 1 week (F), 3 week (G) and 6 week (H) after CFA application. I: Sagittal views of X-lay micro-CT images of the periapical tissues before and at 6 week after CFA or vehicle application to the pulp. J: Time course change in the size of the bone loss at the periapical tissues after CFA application to the M1 pulp (n = 4 each). Solid arrows in A-C indicate detail tooth and periapical structures. White arrows in G and H, and black arrow in I indicate periapical bone loss. veh: vehicle in this and following figures. *: Pre vs. post (CFA), #: Pre vs. post (veh), +: CFA vs. veh, +, #: $p<0.05$, ##, **: $p<0.01$, ***: $p<0.001$.

after capsaicin application into the Mass at 6 weeks after pulpal CFA application.

3. pERK-IR and Fos-IR cells and Rostral-caudal distribution in Vi/Vc or Vc

To examine the effect of M1 pulpitis or periapical periodontitis on the neuronal excitability, the ERK phosphorylation and Fos expression were studied in Vi/Vc and Vc neurons following unilateral capsaicin application into the Mass. A number of pERK-IR cells in the Vi/Vc and Vc induced by capsaicin at 3 days or 6 weeks after pulpal CFA application were double-stained with NeuN, a neuronal marker (Fig. 3A–C). However, some of the pERK-positive cells lacked NeuN staining. These results suggest that ERK phosphorylation occurs in grail cells as well as neurons. A large number of pERK-IR and Fos-IR cells were observed in the ventral portion of the Vi/Vc and in the dorsal portion of the Vc after capsaicin application into the Mass on day 3 or week 6 after CFA application into the M1 tooth pulp (Fig. 3G and 4A). Though we observed a few cells double-stained (Fig. 3F) with Fos (Fig. 3D) and pERK (Fig. 3E) antibodies, there are no double-stained cells in the Vi/Vc and Vc.

Rostral-caudal distribution of pERK-IR and Fos-IR cells in the medulla and upper cervical spinal cord were shown in Fig. 3G, H and Fig. 4A and B. A large number of pERK-IR and Fos-IR cells were observed in the Vi/Vc and Vc following capsaicin application into the ipsilateral Mass on day 3 or week 6 after pulpal CFA application (Fig. 3H and 4B). The total number of cells in Vc and Vi/Vc region indicated by red squares in Fig. 3H and 4B were calculated and the results of statistical analysis were shown in Fig. 3I and Fig. 4C, respectively. Blank indicate a lack of significant difference. The total number of pERK- or Fos-IR cells in the Vi/Vc or Vc in each group was compared respectively (Fig. 3I and Fig. 4C).

On day 3 (Fig. 3I), the number of Fos-IR cells was significantly larger in M1 CFA/Mass veh and M1 CFA/Mass cap rats compared to M1 veh/Mass cap rats in the ipsilateral Vi/Vc. The number of Fos-IR cells was significantly larger in M1 CFA/Mass

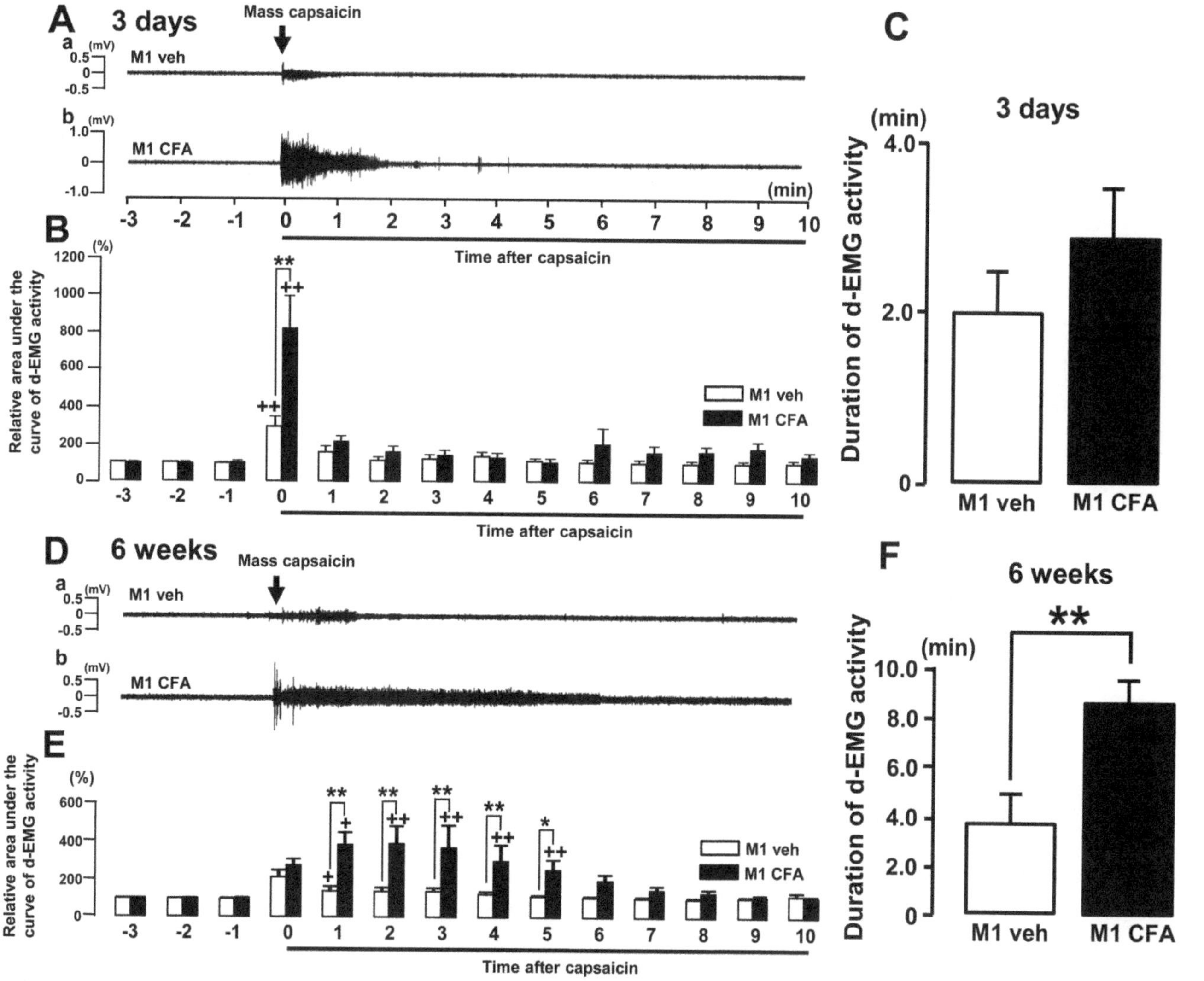

Figure 2. The d-EMG activities after tooth pulp or periapical inflammation. The capsaicin was applied into the Mass in the rats with CFA or vehicle application to the tooth pulp on day 3 and week 6. A: The d-EMG activity following capsaicin application into the Mass in the rats with pulpal-vehicle or pulpal-CFA application on day 3. B: Relative d-EMG activity following capsaicin application into the Mass in the rats with pulpal-vehicle or pulpal-CFA application. C: Mean duration of d-EMG activity following capsaicin application into the Mass in the rats with pulpal-vehicle or pulpal-CFA application. D: The d-EMG activity following capsaicin application into the Mass in the rats with pulpal-vehicle or pulpal-CFA application on week 6. E: Relative d-EMG activity following capsaicin application into the Mass in the rats with pulpal-vehicle or pulpal-CFA application. F: Mean duration of d-EMG activity following capsaicin application into the Mass in the rats with pulpal-vehicle or pulpal-CFA application. +: vs. −1 min, *: veh vs. CFA, +, *: $p<0.05$, ++, **: $p<0.01$.

capsaicin rats compared to M1 veh/Mass veh rats in the contralateral Vi/Vc and Vc.

Furthermore, the numbers of pERK-IR cells was significantly larger in M1 veh/Mass cap and M1 CFA/Mass cap rats compared to M1 veh/Mass veh rats and M1 CFA/Mass veh in the ipsilateral Vi/Vc or Vc, respectively. In the contralateral side to injections, the number of pERK-IR cells was significantly larger in M1 veh/Mass cap compared to M1 CFA/Mass veh in the Vi/Vc.

On week 6 (Fig. 4C), the number of Fos-IR cells was significantly larger in M1 CFA/Mass veh or M1 CFA/Mass cap rats compared to M1 veh/Mass cap rats in the ipsilateral Vi/Vc, respectively. The number of pERK-IR cells was also significantly larger in M1 CFA/Mass cap rats compared to M1 veh/Mass veh, M1 veh/Mass cap or M1 CFA/Mass veh rats in the ipsilateral Vi/Vc. Furthermore, the number of pERK-IR cells was significantly larger in M1 veh/Mass cap or M1 CFA/Mass cap rats compared to M1 CFA/Mass veh rats in the ipsilateral Vc. In the contralateral side to M1 injections, the number of pERK-IR cells was significantly larger in M1 CFA/Mass cap compared to M1 CFA/Mass veh in the Vi/Vc.

4. Comparison of pERK-IR and Fos-IR cells on day 3 and week 6

To examine the difference for the expression of pERK-IR and Fos-IR cells on day 3 and week 6, the ERK phosphorylation and Fos expression were studied in Vi/Vc and Vc neurons following unilateral saline or capsaicin application into the Mass.

In the rats with saline application into the Mass, the number of Fos-IR cells was significantly larger in M1 veh/Mass veh rats in the ipsilateral Vi/Vc or in M1 CFA/Mass veh rats in the ipsi- and

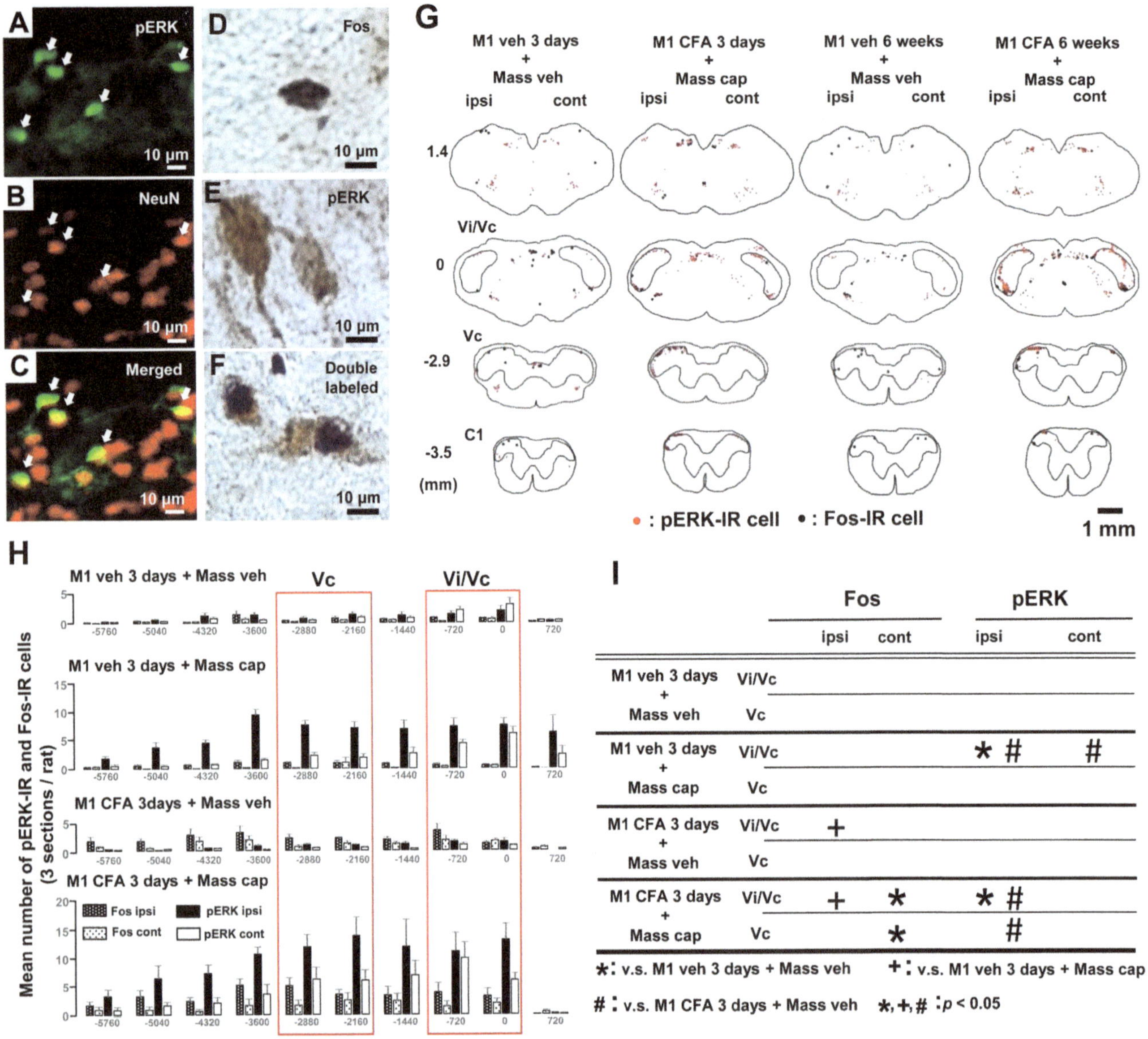

Figure 3. Photomicrographs and Rostral-caudal distribution for pERK-IR cells and Fos-IR cells after tooth pulp inflammation in Vi/Vc and Vc. A: pERK-IR cells. B: NeuN-IR cells. C: A merged with B. D: Fos-IR cell stained with nickel-conjugated DAB. E: pERK-IR cell stained with DAB. F: double stained cells (black: Fos-IR, brown: pERK-IR). G: Neurolucida drawings of pERK-IR (red and triangle dots) and Fos-IR cells (black and round dots) in the Vi/Vc and Vc. H: Rostral-caudal distribution of pERK-IR and Fos-IR cells in the Vi/Vc and Vc. I: *, + and # signs indicate significant expression of pERK-IR or Fos-IR cells compared to each region in M1 veh/Mass veh, M1 veh/Mass cap and M1 CFA/Mass veh on day 3, respectively. Arrows in A indicate pERK-IR cells, those in B indicate NeuN-IR cells and those in C are pERK-IR cells merged with NeuN-IR cells. The negative numbers on the left in G indicate the distance caudal to the obex (0 mm). cap: capsaicin, veh: vehicle, ipsi: ipsilateral, cont: contralateral.

contralateral Vi/Vc and ipsilateral Vc on week 6 compared to those in M1 veh/Mass veh rats on day 3 ($p<0.05$). The number of pERK-IR cells was also significantly larger in M1 CFA/Mass veh rats on week 6 compared to M1 veh/Mass veh on day 3, M1 veh/Mass veh on week 6 or M1 CFA/Mass veh rats on day 3 in the ipsilateral Vi/Vc ($p<0.05$).

In the rats with capsaicin application into the Mass, the number of Fos-IR cells was significantly larger in M1 CFA/Mass cap rats on week 6 compared to M1 veh/Mass cap rats on day 3 or M1 veh/Mass cap rats on week 6 in the ipsilateral Vi/Vc ($p<0.05$).

5. The effect of PD98059 in the Vi/Vc and Vc neurons

We further examined the effect of MEK1 inhibitor PD98059-pretreatment for the Mass hypersensitivity in the rats with M1 pulpitis or periapical periodontitis. We observed significant decrease in the d-EMG activity within 1 minute after capsaicin application into the Mass in the PD98059 i.t.-pretreated rats compared with saline i.t.-pretreated rats on day 3 after M1 CFA application ($p<0.01$, Fig. 5A, B).

On the other hand, the durations of d-EMG activities after capsaicin application were about 2 minutes, and no significant difference was observed between PD98059- or saline-pretreated rats on day 3 after M1 CFA application (Fig. 5C).

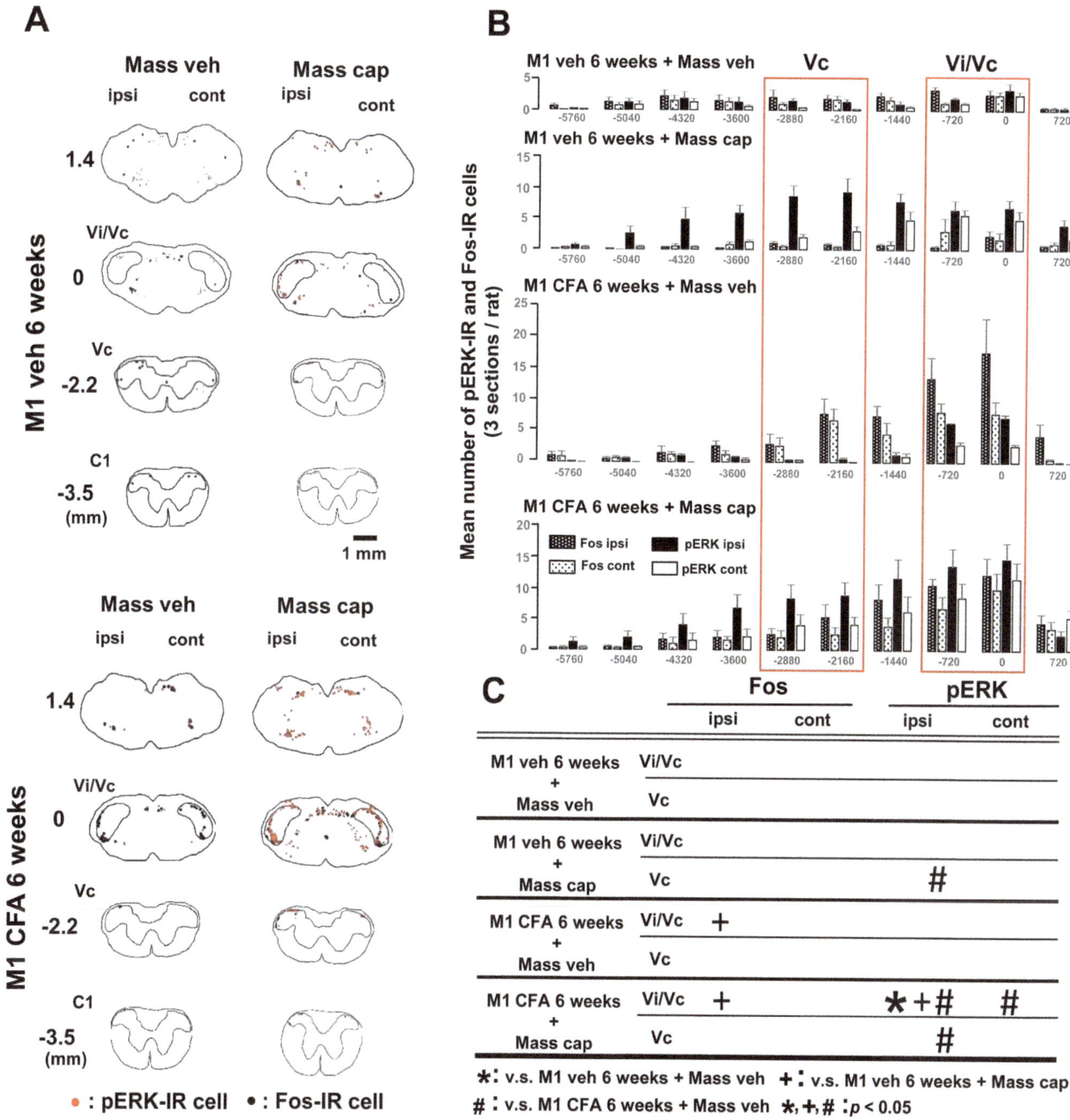

Figure 4. Rostral-caudal distribution for pERK-IR cells and Fos-IR cells after periapical inflammation in Vi/Vc and Vc. The capsaicin was applied into the Mass in the rats with CFA or vehicle application to the tooth pulp on week 6. A and B: Neurolucida drawings (A) and Rostral-caudal distribution (B) of pERK-IR and Fos-IR cells in the Vi/Vc and Vc. C: *, + and # signs indicate significant expression of pERK-IR or Fos-IR cells compared to each region in M1 veh/Mass veh, M1 veh/Mass cap and M1 CFA/Mass veh on day 3, respectively.

We observed significant attenuation in the d-EMG activity with in 2 minute after capsaicin application into the Mass in the PD98059 i.t.-pretreated rats compared with saline i.t.-pretreated rats on week 6 after M1 CFA application ($p<0.01$, Fig. 5D, E).

Furthermore, the mean duration of d-EMG activities after capsaicin application was significantly decreased in the PD98059-pretreated rats compared with saline-pretreated rats on 6 week after M1 CFA application ($p<0.01$, Fig. 5F).

To examine the effect of PD98059 on ERK phosphorylation caused by M1 pulpitis or periapical periodontitis, the change in the number of ERK-IR cells following pretreatment with PD98059 was studied in Vi/Vc and Vc following capsaicin application into the Mass (Fig. 6A and B).

On day 3 and week 6, the number of pERK-IR cells after Mass-capsaicin application was significantly decreased following PD98059 i.t. administration compared to saline i.t. administration in the ipsilateral Vi/Vc and Vc of the M1 CFA rats. Furthermore, the number of Fos-IR cells was not altered after the pretreatment of PD98059 or saline on day 3 or week 6 in the rats with M1 CFA/Mass cap (Fig. 6C).

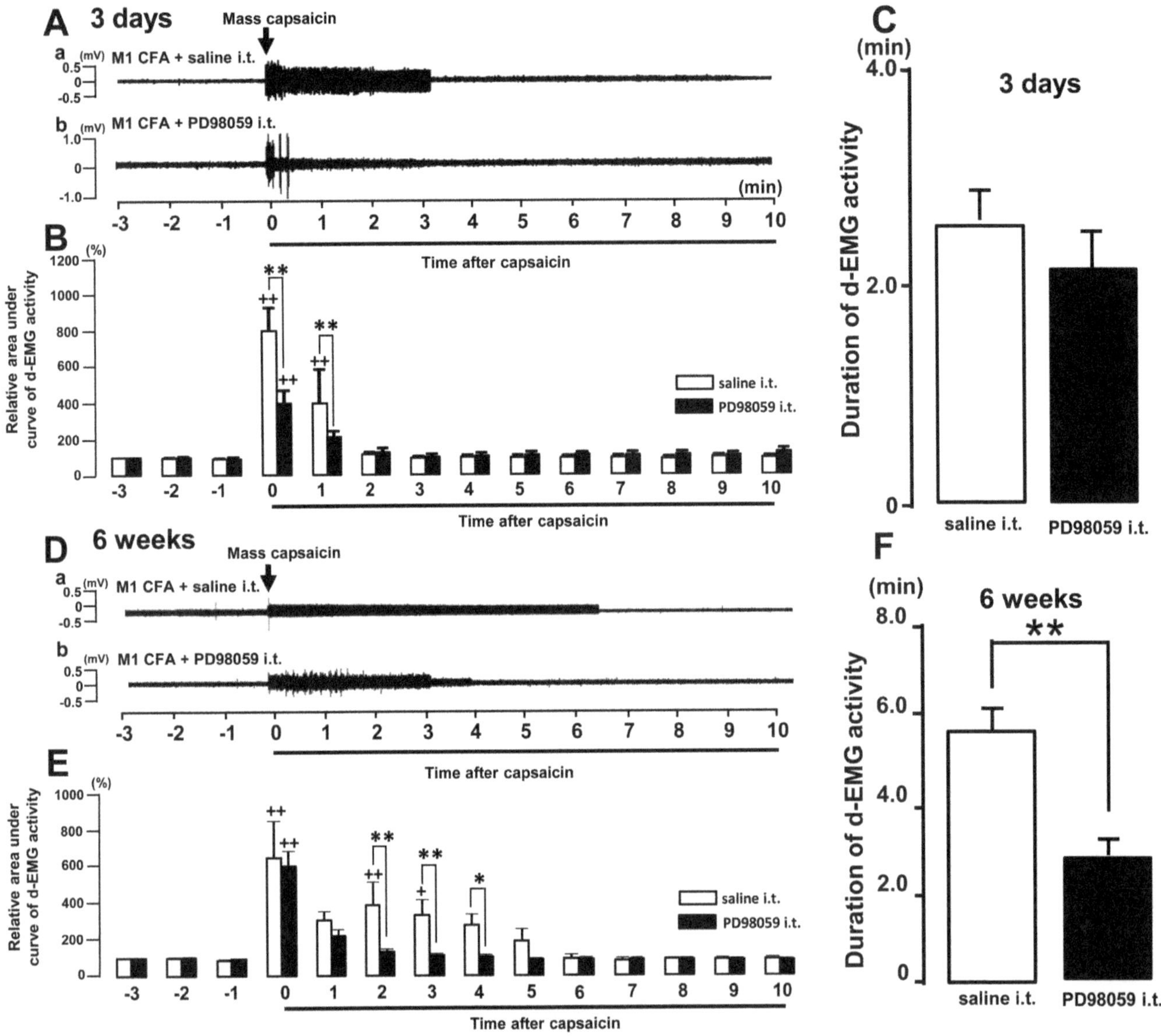

Figure 5. The effect of PD98059 on the d-EMG activities after tooth pulp or periapical inflammation. The capsaicin was applied into the Mass after pretreatment of PD98059 in the rats with M1 CFA application on day 3 and week 6. A: The d-EMG activity following capsaicin application into the Mass after pretreatment of PD98059 or saline in the rats with M1 CFA application on day 3. B: Relative d-EMG activity following capsaicin application into the Mass after pretreatment with PD98059 or saline in the rats with M1 CFA application. C: Mean duration of d-EMG activity following capsaicin application into the Mass after pretreatment with PD98059 or saline in the rats with M1 CFA application. D: The d-EMG activity following capsaicin application into the Mass after pretreatment of PD98059 or saline in the rats with M1 CFA application on week 6. E: Relative d-EMG activity following capsaicin application into the Mass after pretreatment with PD98059 or saline in the rats with M1 CFA application. C: Mean duration of d-EMG activity following capsaicin application into the Mass after pretreatment of PD98059 or saline in the rats with M1 CFA application. +: vs. −1 min, *: saline i.t. vs. PD98059 i.t., +,*: $p<0.05$., ++, **: $p<0.01$.

Discussion

Periapical inflammation frequently causes referred pain in the orofacial cutaneous tissue and/or muscle as well as tooth pulp [22]. It is well known that inflammation within the tooth pulp often extends into the periapical tissues after pulpal inflammation, resulting in pulpal necrosis and periapical inflammation. At the early stage of periapical inflammation, severe persistent pain occurs in the apex region of the tooth [23]. Eventually, periapical pain could change its' quality from an acute to a chronic state. Chronic periapical pain is dull and persistent, lasts for a long period, and also causes referred pain in the orofacial skin and/or muscles. The orofacial referred pain originated from the periapical inflammation is difficult to diagnose and treat [3]. Despite increasing necessity of the clarification of the pathogenesis for the odontogenic referred pain in the orofacial region, it is still unclear on the mechanisms underlying extraterritorial orofacial persistent pain associated with periapical inflammation. In the present study, therefore, we examined the excitability of the Vi/Vc and Vc neurons in a rat model of experimental pulpitis/periodontitis and its' involvement in the enhancement of d-EMG activity.

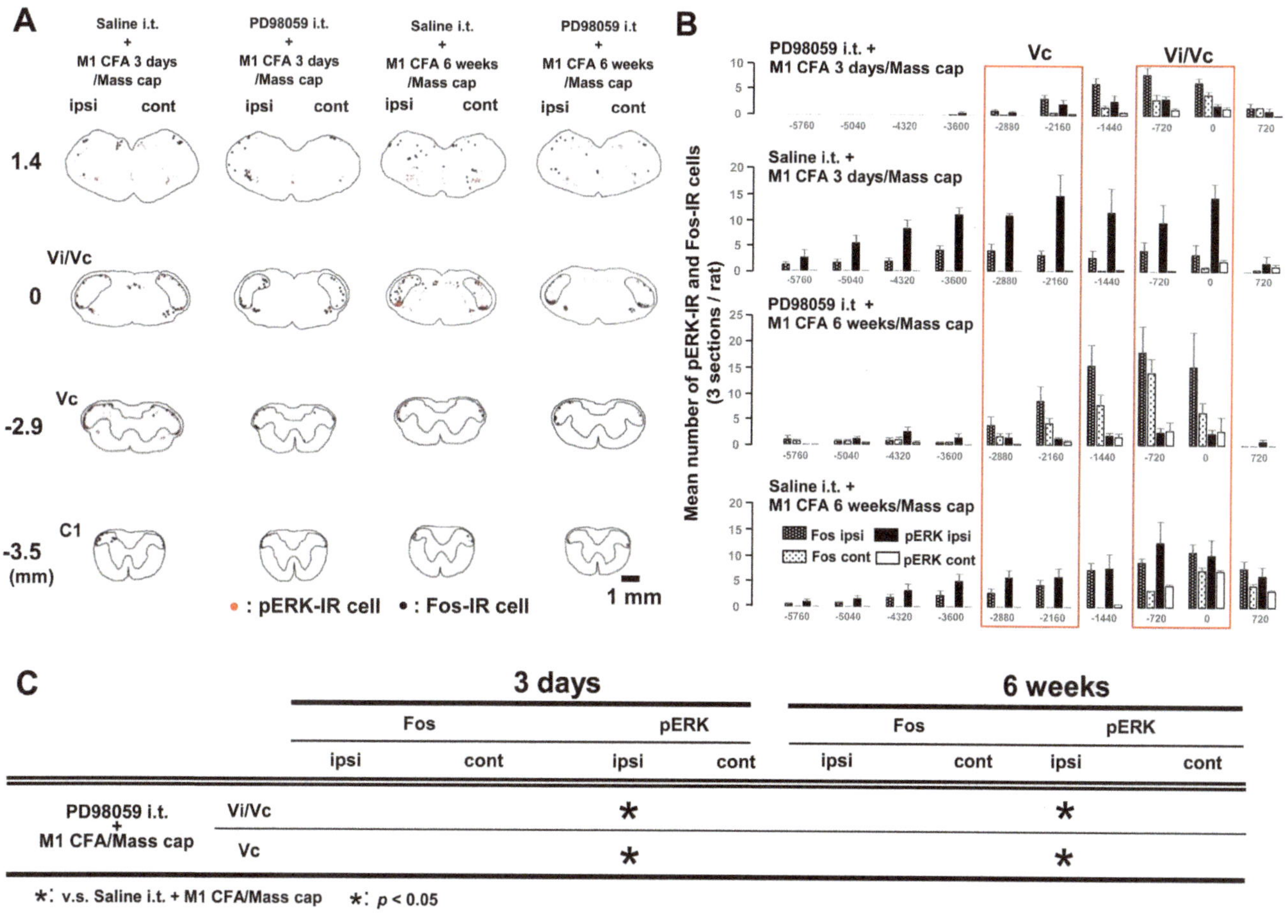

Figure 6. The effect of PD98059 on ERK phosphorylation in Vi/Vc and Vc neurons after tooth pulp or periapical inflammation. The capsaicin was applied into the Mass after PD98059 i.t. administration in the rats with M1 CFA on day 3 or week 6. A and B: Neurolucida drawings (A) and Rostral-caudal distribution (B) of pERK-IR and Fos-IR cells in the Vi/Vc and Vc. C: * indicates significant decrease in the number of pERK-IR or Fos-IR cells. Each region in each model was compared with M1 CFA/Mass cap rats with saline i.t. on day 3 or week 6, respectively.

1. Rat model of periapical inflammation

It is well known that periapical bone loss is observed during development of the periapical inflammation, suggesting that the periapical bone loss could be one of the reliable indicators for the periapical inflammation [24]. Thus, we analyzed the time-course change in the bone loss using X-ray micro-CT imaging to quantify the periapical inflammation. The advantage of this technique is that the size of bone loss can be measured in same rats throughout the experimental period. Periapical bone loss was detected at 3 weeks after pulpal application of CFA, and the largest bone loss was observed at 6 weeks after CFA application to the pulp, indicating that chronic phase characterized by lesion stabilization was commenced from 6 weeks after CFA application. The time-course of bone loss we observed in this study is similar to that of previous study [24], suggesting that this model can be used as a reliable animal model with experimental periodontitis following long lasting pulpal inflammation.

2. Changes in the Vi/Vc and Vc neuronal activities following pulpal or periapical inflammation

The d-EMG activity elicited by noxious stimulation is known as a good indicator of the noxious responses in the trigeminal system [25]. We observed significant increase in the d-EMG activity after capsaicin application into the Mass on day 3 and week 6 after pulpal-CFA or pulpal-vehicle application. Furthermore, the d-EMG activity elicited by Mass-capsaicin application was significantly higher in M1 CFA-applied rats compared with M1-vehicle applied rats. The number of Fos-IR cells in the Vi/Vc was significantly larger in M1 CFA applied rats compared with M1 vehicle-applied rats on day 3 and week 6. On the other hand, ERK phosphorylation in the Vi/Vc and/or Vc neurons significantly increased in Mass-capsaicin applied rats compared with Mass-vehicle applied rats both in pulpal CFA- or vehicle applied rats. These indicate that noxious stimulus to the Mass induces the enhancement of noxious responses in the orofacial region following pulpal or periapical inflammation. It is strongly suggested that the increase in d-EMG activities and pERK expression in Vi/Vc and Vc neurons are the result of enhancement of Vi/Vc and/or Vc neuronal activities following pulpal or periapical inflammation. Taken together, the EMG activities and pERK expression were significantly enhanced after capsaicin application into the Mass on day 3 and week 6 after pulpal CFA application, suggesting that pathogenesis of pulpal or periapical inflammation might induce pain hypersensitivity in remote organs or tissues in the orofacial region.

We also observed that the duration of EMG activity was significantly longer at 6 weeks after pulpal CFA application compared with that of pulpal vehicle application. The enhancement of EMG activity and the increased duration were significantly reversed following i.t. administration of PD98059. These results indicate that periapical inflammation may induce and maintain pain hypersensitivity in the remote organs or tissues in orofacial region, whereas pulpal inflammation may only induce pain hypersensitivity. Furthermore, the ERK phosphorylation in Vi/Vc and Vc neurons has a pivotal role in the maintenance and/ or modulation of pain processing in remote regions after tooth pulp or periapical inflammation.

3. Involvement of the Vi/Vc and Vc neurons in Mass hypersensitivity

Fos protein expression in SDH neurons following noxious stimulation of the peripheral structures is known to be caused 1–2 hours and lasted 24 hours after noxious stimulation [26], and therefore Fos protein expression in SDH neurons is thought to be a good marker of the excitation of nociceptive neurons [27]. The ventral portion of the Vi/Vc is known to have a various functions in trigeminal nociception [28]. Many Vi/Vc neurons are known to express Fos-IR products following CFA application into the Mass or noxious stimulation of the cornea [29,30]. Many of them were also observed on both sides of the Vi/Vc following unilateral noxious stimulation.

It has been reported that the number of pERK-IR cells increases unilaterally in the Vc following increase in noxious stimulus intensity [31]. In the trigeminal system, ERK can be phosphorylated in a large number of dorsal horn neurons in the Vc and C1-C2 within 5 min after noxious stimulation to various orofacial regions; these pERK-IR neurons are somatotopically organized in Vc and C1-C2, and the number of pERK-IR neurons increases following increases in the noxious stimulus intensity [12,20], indicating that ERK phosphorylation in Vc and C1-C2 neurons is a reliable marker of excitable neurons following orofacial noxious stimulation.

We observed that pERK expression was significantly enhanced after capsaicin application into the Mass both in M1 CFA- and vehicle-applied rats compared with Mass-vehicle applied rats in both Vi/Vc and Vc on day 3 and week 6. Furthermore, on day 3 after pulpal application, we observed a large number of Fos-IR cells in the bilateral Vi/Vc in pulpal CFA-applied rats. Meanwhile, on week 6 after pulpal-CFA application, we observed a large number of Fos-IR cells just in the ipsilateral Vi/Vc in pulpal CFA-applied rats, and the number of them was also significantly larger in CFA-applied rats compared with vehicle-applied rats. These findings suggest that nociceptive neurons in the Vi/Vc and Vc may have important roles for orofacial pain hypersensitivity associated with tooth pulp inflammation and periapical inflammation.

Furthermore, we could not observe significant change in the number of Fos-IR cells in these two areas between Mass-capsaicin and vehicle applied rats, suggesting that Fos expression may be mainly due to the CFA application to the tooth pulp but not Mass-capsaicin application.

Conclusions

The present findings revealed that the Vi/Vc and Vc neurons was involved in the enhancement of Mass nociception under acute pulpal-inflamed state as well as chronic periapical inflammation, suggesting that nociceptive neurons in these areas are involved in pain hypersensitivity for orofacial muscle associated with acute pulpal and chronic periapical inflammation.

Author Contributions

Conceived and designed the experiments: KS. Performed the experiments: KS KM NN SM KO KH KD TW HK YT. Analyzed the data: KS KM NN SM KO YN YT. Contributed reagents/materials/analysis tools: BO. Wrote the paper: KS KI. Contributed to discussion and reviewed/edited the manuscript: MS KI BO.

References

1. Ertekin C, Secil Y, Yuceyar N, Aydogdu I (2004) Oropharyngeal dysphagia in polymyositis/dermatomyositis. Clin Neurol Neurosurg 107: 32–37.
2. Grushka M, Sessle BJ (1984) Applicability of the McGill Pain Questionnaire to the differentiation of 'toothache' pain. Pain 19: 49–57.
3. Bender IB (2000) Pulpal pain diagnosis–a review. J Endod 26: 175–179.
4. Wright EF (2008) Pulpalgia contributing to temporomandibular disorder-like pain: a literature review and case report. J Am Dent Assoc 139: 436–440.
5. Iwata K, Takahashi O, Tsuboi Y, Ochiai H, Hibiya J, et al. (1998) Fos protein induction in the medullary dorsal horn and first segment of the spinal cord by tooth-pulp stimulation in cats. Pain 75: 27–36.
6. Sessle BJ (1987) The neurobiology of facial and dental pain: present knowledge, future directions. J Dent Res 66: 962–981.
7. Sessle BJ, Hu JW, Amano N, Zhong G (1986) Convergence of cutaneous, tooth pulp, visceral, neck and muscle afferents onto nociceptive and non-nociceptive neurones in trigeminal subnucleus caudalis (medullary dorsal horn) and its implications for referred pain. Pain 27: 219–235.
8. Shimizu K, Asano M, Kitagawa J, Ogiso B, Ren K, et al. (2006) Phosphorylation of Extracellular Signal-Regulated Kinase in medullary and upper cervical cord neurons following noxious tooth pulp stimulation. Brain Res 1072: 99–109.
9. Wang H, Wei F, Dubner R, Ren K (2006) Selective distribution and function of primary afferent nociceptive inputs from deep muscle tissue to the brainstem trigeminal transition zone. J Comp Neurol 498: 390–402.
10. Amano N, Hu JW, Sessle BJ (1986) Responses of neurons in feline trigeminal subnucleus caudalis (medullary dorsal horn) to cutaneous, intraoral, and muscle afferent stimuli. J Neurophysiol 55: 227–243.
11. Shoda E, Kitagawa J, Suzuki I, Nitta-Kubota I, Miyamoto M, et al. (2009) Increased phosphorylation of extracellular signal-regulated kinase in trigeminal nociceptive neurons following propofol administration in rats. J Pain 10: 573–585.
12. Noma N, Tsuboi Y, Kondo M, Matsumoto M, Sessle BJ, et al. (2008) Organization of pERK-immunoreactive cells in trigeminal spinal nucleus caudalis and upper cervical cord following capsaicin injection into oral and craniofacial regions in rats. J Comp Neurol 507: 1428–1440.
13. Dai Y, Iwata K, Fukuoka T, Kondo E, Tokunaga A, et al. (2002) Phosphorylation of extracellular signal-regulated kinase in primary afferent neurons by noxious stimuli and its involvement in peripheral sensitization. J Neurosci 22: 7737–7745.
14. Harris JA (1998) Using c-fos as a neural marker of pain. Brain Res Bull 45: 1–8.
15. Hasegawa M, Kondo M, Suzuki I, Shimizu N, Sessle BJ, et al. (2012) ERK is involved in tooth-pressure-induced Fos expression in Vc neurons. J Dent Res 91: 1141–1146.
16. Zimmermann M (1983) Ethical guidelines for investigations of experimental pain in conscious animals. Pain 16: 109–110.
17. Terayama R, Omura S, Fujisawa N, Yamaai T, Ichikawa H, et al. (2008) Activation of microglia and p38 mitogen-activated protein kinase in the dorsal column nucleus contributes to tactile allodynia following peripheral nerve injury. Neuroscience 153: 1245–1255.
18. Gasparini F, Lingenhohl K, Stoehr N, Flor PJ, Heinrich M, et al. (1999) 2-Methyl-6-(phenylethynyl)-pyridine (MPEP), a potent, selective and systemically active mGlu5 receptor antagonist. Neuropharmacology 38: 1493–1503.
19. Honda K, Kitagawa J, Sessle BJ, Kondo M, Tsuboi Y, et al. (2008) Mechanisms involved in an increment of multimodal excitability of medullary and upper cervical dorsal horn neurons following cutaneous capsaicin treatment. Mol Pain 4: 59.
20. Honda K, Noma N, Shinoda M, Miyamoto M, Katagiri A, et al. (2011) Involvement of peripheral ionotropic glutamate receptors in orofacial thermal hyperalgesia in rats. Mol Pain 7: 75.
21. Kobayashi A, Shinoda M, Sessle BJ, Honda K, Imamura Y, et al. (2011) Mechanisms involved in extraterritorial facial pain following cervical spinal nerve injury in rats. Mol Pain 7: 12.
22. Sessle BJ (1978) Oral-facial pain: old puzzles, new postulates. Int Dent J 28: 28–42.
23. Morse DR (1977) Immunologic aspects of pulpal-periapical diseases. A review. Oral Surg Oral Med Oral Pathol 43: 436–451.
24. Stashenko P, Yu SM, Wang CY (1992) Kinetics of immune cell and bone resorptive responses to endodontic infections. J Endod 18: 422–426.

25. Sunakawa M, Chiang CY, Sessle BJ, Hu JW (1999) Jaw electromyographic activity induced by the application of algesic chemicals to the rat tooth pulp. Pain 80: 493–501.
26. Hunt SP, Pini A, Evan G (1987) Induction of c-fos-like protein in spinal cord neurons following sensory stimulation. Nature 328: 632–634.
27. Williams S, Evan GI, Hunt SP (1990) Changing patterns of c-fos induction in spinal neurons following thermal cutaneous stimulation in the rat. Neuroscience 36: 73–81.
28. Ren K, Dubner R (2011) The role of trigeminal interpolaris-caudalis transition zone in persistent orofacial pain. Int Rev Neurobiol 97: 207–225.
29. Bereiter DA, Hathaway CB, Benetti AP (1994) Caudal portions of the spinal trigeminal complex are necessary for autonomic responses and display Fos-like immunoreactivity after corneal stimulation in the cat. Brain Res 657: 73–82.
30. Imbe H, Dubner R, Ren K (1999) Masseteric inflammation-induced Fos protein expression in the trigeminal interpolaris/caudalis transition zone: contribution of somatosensory-vagal-adrenal integration. Brain Res 845: 165–175.
31. Ji RR, Baba H, Brenner GJ, Woolf CJ (1999) Nociceptive-specific activation of ERK in spinal neurons contributes to pain hypersensitivity. Nat Neurosci 2: 1114–1119.

15

Decreased Peripheral and Central Responses to Acupuncture Stimulation following Modification of Body Ownership

Younbyoung Chae[1,2*], In-Seon Lee[2], Won-Mo Jung[1], Dong-Seon Chang[3], Vitaly Napadow[4,5], Hyejung Lee[2], Hi-Joon Park[2], Christian Wallraven[1*]

1 Department of Brain and Cognitive Engineering, Korea University, Seoul, Korea, **2** Acupuncture and Meridian Science Research Center, College of Korean Medicine, Kyung Hee University, Seoul, Korea, **3** Department of Human Perception, Cognition and Action, Max Planck Institute for Biological Cybernetics, Tübingen, Germany, **4** Martinos Center for Biomedical Imaging, Massachusetts General Hospital, Harvard Medical School, Charlestown, Massachusetts, United States of America, **5** Department of Biomedical Engineering, Kyunghee University, Yongin, Korea

Abstract

Acupuncture stimulation increases local blood flow around the site of stimulation and induces signal changes in brain regions related to the body matrix. The rubber hand illusion (RHI) is an experimental paradigm that manipulates important aspects of bodily self-awareness. The present study aimed to investigate how modifications of body ownership using the RHI affect local blood flow and cerebral responses during acupuncture needle stimulation. During the RHI, acupuncture needle stimulation was applied to the real left hand while measuring blood microcirculation with a LASER Doppler imager (Experiment 1, $N = 28$) and concurrent brain signal changes using functional magnetic resonance imaging (fMRI; Experiment 2, $N = 17$). When the body ownership of participants was altered by the RHI, acupuncture stimulation resulted in a significantly lower increase in local blood flow (Experiment 1), and significantly less brain activation was detected in the right insula (Experiment 2). This study found changes in both local blood flow and brain responses during acupuncture needle stimulation following modification of body ownership. These findings suggest that physiological responses during acupuncture stimulation can be influenced by the modification of body ownership.

Editor: Marcello Costantini, University G. d'Annunzio, Italy

Funding: This research was supported by the Basic Science Research Program through the National Research Foundation of Korea (NRF) funded by the Ministry of Education, Science and Technology (No. 2011-0009913 & 2014K2A3A1000166). VN was supported by the following NIH grants from the USA: NCCAM: P01-AT006663, R01-AT005280, R01-AT007550; NIAMS: R01-AR064367. The funders had no role in study design, data collection and analysis, decision to publish, or preparation of the manuscript.

Competing Interests: The authors have declared that no competing interests exist.

* Email: ybchae@khu.ac.kr (YC); wallraven@korea.ac.kr (CW)

Introduction

The importance of an accurate representation of the body by the brain has been documented in many different studies involving both healthy participants and clinical patients [1,2]. Body ownership specifically, which refers to the sense that a part of one's body belongs to oneself, has been studied as a fundamental aspect of bodily self-consciousness [3,4]. Moreover, body ownership and aspects of bodily self-awareness influence clinical outcomes because they can modulate the regulation of one's physical self [5,6,7].

The rubber hand illusion (RHI) is an experimental paradigm that manipulates body ownership of the hand and is widely used to investigate the processes that underlie various aspects of bodily self-awareness [6,8]. When participants watch a rubber hand being stroked by a paintbrush in synchrony with strokes applied to their own corresponding hand, they typically experience a change in body ownership such that the rubber hand "feels like one's own hand" [9]. This illusory feeling of body ownership is thought to be associated with the multimodal integration of visual, tactile, and proprioceptive information in the brain [10]. When participants take ownership of the artificial counterpart, the real hand exhibits a decrease in skin temperature, slower processing of tactile information, and enhanced histamine reactivity, which suggests that a cortical body matrix integrates the perceptual and homeostatic regulation of the body [2,6,11]. The experience of the RHI is associated with in a distributed network in the brain [7]. The ventral premotor cortex has been suggested as a key brain structure for the multisensory representation of one's own body during the RHI [12]. When the rubber hand is fully incorporated into the body, artificial limbs were able to evoke a similar level of activity in the insula and the anterior cingulate cortex, indicating that the bodily ownership of the rubber hand is associated with changes in the interoceptive system [13]. The experience of body ownership of the rubber hand as measured by the effect of multisensory integration and recalibration of hand position was positively correlated with activity in the right posterior insula [14].

Acupuncture, an ancient East Asian therapeutic technique, uses needles to stimulate a particular part of the body for the purpose of inducing beneficial effects during clinical treatment [15]. Acupuncture stimulation affects microcirculatory blood flow near the inserted needle as well as regional blood flow in various organs [16,17]. Neuroimaging studies investigating acupuncture have observed overlapping brain responses in a number of cortical and subcortical brain regions. For example, activation has been observed in cortical sensorimotor and salient networks such as the insula, thalamus, anterior cingulate cortex, as well as primary and secondary somatosensory cortices, whereas deactivation has been identified in the limbic-paralimbic neocortical network in areas such as the medial prefrontal cortex, caudate, amygdala, posterior cingulate cortex, and parahippocampus [18,19]. Accordingly, recent reviews of functional magnetic resonance imaging (fMRI) studies revealed common brain activations in the sensorimotor cortical network and common deactivations in the limbic-paralimbic-neocortical network following acupuncture needle stimulation [20,21]. A number of convergent results and promising new data provide some pointers for understanding the neural mechanisms of acupuncture therapy in the context of the modern medical mainstream [20,21]. Despite recent progress, however, some questions still remain controversial and a) Are specific traditional acupuncture points related to their specifically claimed functions? (Question of Point-specificity) [19,22,23], b) How is the acupuncture-specific sensation, called *DeQi* sensation, located functionally in the brain? [24,25,26], c) Are pain-related areas desensitized in the brain during or after acupuncture treatment, explaining the phenomenon of acupuncture analgesia? [27,28,29,30], d) Can the specific (physiological) effects be distinguished with non-specific (psychological or placebo) effects of acupuncture? [15,31,32,33]. e) What is the role of the interceptive attention system, such as somato-spatial attention, body awareness, and anticipation of stimulation in the physiological responses to acupuncture? [34,35] The answers to these questions have been somewhat contradictory, and left mostly controversial.

From the perspective of cognitive neuroscience, acupuncture is not only seen as a 'simple needling' but also as a complex treatment comprised of multimodal sensory stimulation that interacts with various factors, including bodily self-awareness [36,37]. The role of psychosocial and contextual factors, including body image and body schema, are thought to exert an important influence on the clinical effects of acupuncture [38]. Neuroimaging studies have suggested that the insula, which is known to modulate the interoceptive system, plays an important role in the effects of acupuncture [35,39]. The insula was activated to a greater extent during real acupuncture than during the placebo intervention in patients with osteoarthritis [39]. Considering a salient component of acupuncture analgesia, focused attention and accentuated bodily awareness on the specific body part with acupuncture-induced sensation could contribute to the top-down modulation of nociceptive afference and the central pain matrix [35]. Conversely, we can assume that acupuncture might not properly exert its influence under reduced bodily awareness. Thus, it is conceived that components of this bodily self-awareness can be involved in the modulation of physiological responses to acupuncture stimulation. In the current study, we hypothesized that modification of body ownership can reduce the neurophysiological responses to acupuncture stimulation, especially through the disruption of the interoceptive system in the brain.

The present study aimed to investigate whether modifications of body ownership would result in measurable physiological changes in response to acupuncture stimulation using LASER Doppler and fMRI, respectively.

Methods and Materials

Procedures for measuring changes in local blood flow (Experiment 1)

Participants. Advertisements were used to recruit a total of 28 right-handed participants (age: 22.8±0.5 years; 15 males and 13 females) for this study from the general population of students, staff, and visitors to Kyung Hee University in Seoul, Republic of Korea. Participants with no history of neurological, psychiatric, or visual disorders were included in this study. Handedness was self-reported by the participants in a screening questionnaire prior to the experiment, and participants were prohibited from drinking alcohol or caffeine or taking any drugs or medications on the day of the experiment. Each participant received a detailed explanation of the study, and written informed consent was obtained prior to participation. All experiments in this study were conducted in accordance with the guidelines issued by the human subjects committee and approved by the Institutional Review Board of Korea University in Seoul, Republic of Korea.

Experimental design. The setup followed standard procedure and was designed and executed almost identically to a previous study [9], placing a rubber hand in front of each participant while their left hand was hidden from sight. The experiments followed a within-subjects cross-over design in which the independent variable was a synchronous versus an asynchronous brush touch on the hand to measure illusory body ownership. In both the synchronous and asynchronous sessions, participants received 180 seconds of acupuncture needle stimulation on the hidden (real) left hand immediately after the RHI (Fig. 1A). The order was randomized such that participants were randomly assigned to one of two groups (i.e., they received either the synchronous or the asynchronous session first). The interval between the two sessions was approximately 2 days.

Tactile stimulation for the induction of the rubber hand illusion. Participants were told to fixate on the rubber hand (Korean Prosthetic Limbs Research Institute; Seoul, Korea), to not look elsewhere, and to not move any of their fingers during the experiment. Two small paintbrushes were used to stroke both the rubber hand and the participant's hidden real left hand (strokes were approximately 2 cm in length) at a frequency of 1 Hz for 180 sec. This was done synchronously under one condition (synchronous condition) and asynchronously under the other condition (asynchronous condition).

Acupuncture stimulation. First, participants were informed that physiological data, including LASER Doppler measurements, would be recorded while they received acupuncture stimulation. Then, each participant was led to the experimental room and seated with their left and right arms on a table in the same manner as in a standard RHI experiment [9]. At the beginning of the session, an acupuncture needle was inserted at acupoint LI4 on the dorsum of the left hand radial to the midpoint of the second metacarpal bone. The needles were 0.20 mm in diameter and 40 mm long (Seirin Acupuncture, Inc.; Kasei, Japan). Participants were instructed to look at the rubber hand during the acupuncture stimulation.

After the tactile stimulation on the rubber hand and the real hand, standard acupuncture needle stimulation (the same as in clinical acupuncture treatments) was applied by a licensed and experienced Doctor of Korean Medicine, which consisted of rotating the needle at a frequency of 1 Hz for the duration of 10 seconds every 1 minute. Therefore, the total duration of acupuncture insertion was 3 minutes, including a total of 30 seconds (3×10 seconds) of acupuncture needle manipulation.

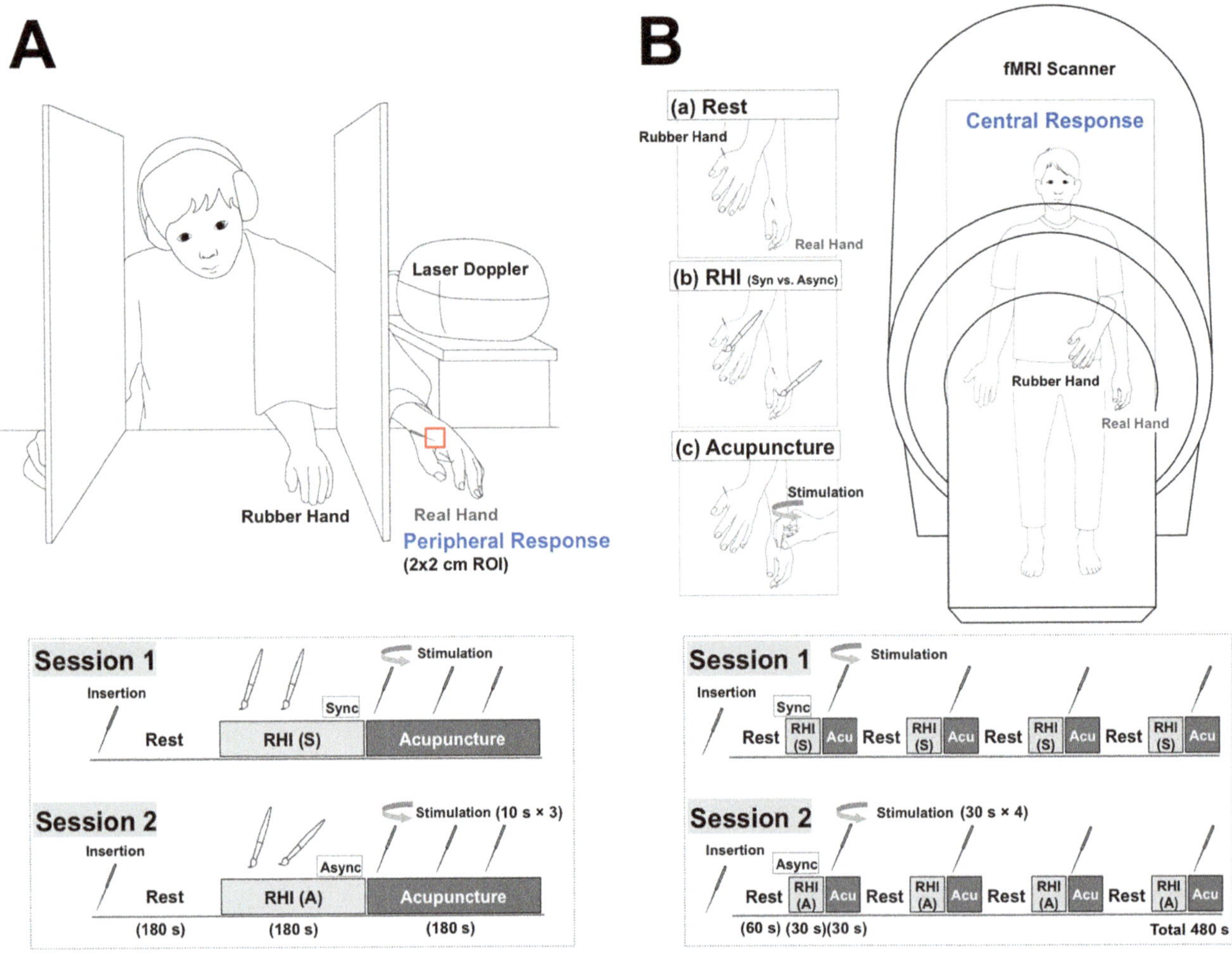

Figure 1. Experimental procedures. A: Procedures for peripheral responses (Experiment 1). Two small paintbrushes stroked the rubber hand (strokes were approximately 2 cm in length) and the hidden real left hand of the participant at a frequency of 1 Hz for 180 seconds as synchronously as possible under one condition (synchronous condition: S) and asynchronously under the other condition (asynchronous condition: A); RHI: Rubber hand illusion induction. Participants received acupuncture needle stimulation at a frequency of 1 Hz for 10 seconds every 1 minute during the 3-minute acupuncture stimulation period on the hidden (real) left hand immediately after commencing the RHI under the synchronous or asynchronous condition (Acu: Acupuncture stimulation). B: Procedures for brain responses (Experiment 2). There were two randomized sessions: a synchronous condition (S) and an asynchronous condition (A). The acupuncture needle was stimulated at the LI4 acupoint in the left hand out of sight of the participant according to the beats of a 1-Hz metronome transmitted via earphones (Acu: Acupuncture stimulation). One session included a four-block tactile-stimulation condition (30 seconds) for the RHI and a four-block acupuncture stimulation (30 seconds); these were performed successively. Tactile stimulation was synchronously or asynchronously applied with short strokes from two brushes (approximately 2 cm in length) at a frequency of 1 Hz during the tactile-stimulation block; RHI: Rubber hand illusion induction.

To confirm that the synchronous and the asynchronous sessions did not differ in terms of manual acupuncture stimulation, Acusensor2 force sensors (Stromatec Inc, Burlington, VT, USA) were attached to the needle handle to measure the degree of stimulation (rotation frequency) and the biomechanical force (torque amplitude: rotation force) [40]. The rotation frequency and torque amplitude were calculated over a period of 10 seconds based on raw data. During needle rotation, the rotation frequency was calculated using fast Fourier analyses of the raw data by Data Viewer software (Stromatec Inc.), and the torque amplitude of peaks was calculated manually as the mean value.

LASER Doppler measurement. Measurements of skin blood perfusion around the site of acupuncture stimulation (acupoint LI4) were performed using a LASER Doppler perfusion imager (LDPR; PeriScan PIM III system; Perimed AB, Sweden). Before the tactile stimulation for the induction of the RHI, the real hand (left hand) of participants was immobilized with a cylindrical object to ensure positioning, and measurements were carried out every 5 seconds for a total duration of 180 seconds. The temperature in the laboratory room was kept consistent and controlled (24–26°C) throughout the experiment. The LASER Doppler scanning was conducted on the participants' real hand out of sight without any sound and did not produce any sensation. Peripheral blood flow (PBF; symbolized as $R_{i,\ [i\,=\,1,\,2,\,3,\,\ldots,\,36]}$) was defined as the mean blood flux in each scan (5 seconds) around the LI4 acupoint (2×2 cm), and the change in PBF was calculated using the following formula: $(R_i\text{-}R_1)/R_1$. For assessing the responses during and after acupuncture stimulation, each 5 sec was subtracted from a 10 s baseline prior to the initial acupuncture stimulation (onset) and averaged across the 180 s of each session, resulting in change in scores that reflected increases from the baseline.

Rubber hand illusion and self-reported DeQi sensation rating. Right after the completion of tactile stimulation on the rubber hand and real hand (synchronous and asynchronous), participants reported their perception of the RHI by answering the most relevant question (Q3) on the RHI Perception Scale: "I felt as if the rubber hand were my hand" [9]. Acupuncture is generally accompanied by the perception of a complex set of sensations, called "*DeQi*" including aching, dull, heavy, numb, radiating, spreading and tingling [41]. It is considered to be associated with acupuncture treatment outcomes [42]. After each acupuncture stimulation session, participants evaluated their acupuncture-induced *DeQi* sensation, including heaviness, soreness, and numbness, using a 100-mm visual analogue scale [43].

Data analysis. All values are expressed as means ± standard errors. RHI ratings, subjective pain ratings, and PBF changes under the synchronous brush-stroking (induction of illusory body ownership) and the asynchronous brush-stroking (control) sessions were compared using paired *t*-tests. The level of significance was set at 0.05 for all analyses. Statistical analyses were performed using the Statistical Package for Social Sciences for Windows 20.0 (SPSS Inc.; Chicago, IL, USA).

Procedures for measuring brain responses with fMRI (Experiment 2)

Participants. A total of 17 right-handed participants (age: 23.0±0.8 years; 10 males and 7 females) were recruited by advertisement from the general population of students, staff, and visitors to Kyung Hee University in Seoul, Republic of Korea for participation in this study. Participants with no history of neurological, psychiatric, or visual disorders were included in this study. Handedness was self-reported by the participants in a screening questionnaire prior to the experiment, and participants were prohibited from drinking alcohol or caffeine or taking any drugs or medications on the day of the experiment. Each participant received a detailed explanation of the study and written informed consent was obtained prior to participation. All experiments in this study were conducted in accordance with the guidelines issued by the human subjects committee and approved by the Institutional Review Board of Korea University in Seoul, Republic of Korea.

Experimental design. During the brain scans, participants lay in a supine position on the MRI table, and their left hand was comfortably placed on the MRI table while the rubber hand was placed 15 cm above their left hand so that their real hand was hidden under the rubber hand. The rubber hand was orientated in an anatomically plausible position, pointing slightly right toward the midline of the body (20°–30°). The right hand was also comfortably placed on the MRI table. A mirror attached to the head coil enabled participants to look at the rubber hand; the position of the rubber hand and/or the head-coil mirror was adjusted to ensure a clear view of the rubber hand. Before the start of scanning, the acupuncture needle was inserted at the LI4 acupoint (on the dorsum of radial to the midpoint of the second metacarpal bone) both in the left rubber hand and left real hand out of sight of the participant. Prior to scanning, we ensured that none of the participants was able to see their own hand. The two sessions (synchronous and asynchronous conditions) were conducted in a random order. Each session included four blocks of tactile stimulation (30 seconds) to invoke the RHI and four subsequent blocks of acupuncture stimulation (30 seconds) immediately after. A total of 240 volumes were acquired during each session for 480 seconds (Fig. 1B).

Induction of the rubber hand illusion and acupuncture stimulation. The participants were told to look at the rubber hand (Korean Prosthetic Limbs Research Institute), to not look elsewhere, and to not move any of their fingers during the experiment. Two small paintbrushes (approximately 2 cm in length) were used to stroke the rubber hand and the hidden real left hand of the participant at a frequency of 1 Hz for 180 seconds. This was done synchronously under one condition (synchronous condition) and asynchronously under the other condition (asynchronous condition).

Acupuncture stimulation was always applied at acupoint LI4 on the left hand by a licensed and experienced Doctor of Korean Medicine using non-magnetic titanium sterile acupuncture needles that were 40 mm long and 0.20 mm in diameter (DongBang Acupuncture Inc.; Boryeoung, Republic of Korea). All stimulations were administered according to the beat of a 1-Hz metronome transmitted via earphones. Following each trial, subjects were asked about their experience of the illusion via headphones in the scanner.

fMRI data acquisition. The fMRI scans were acquired with a MAGNETOM Trio 3 T scanner (Siemens, Erlangen, Germany) using echo planar imaging (EPI) with a 64×64 matrix (TE = 30 ms, TR = 2000 ms) across 37 slices with a thickness of 4 mm. To minimize movement artifacts, the head of each participant was fixed using a head holder. All scans were acquired by a well-trained professional operator. Each scan session contained 210 volumes of the whole brain in a 37 axial slice acquisition (TR = 2000 ms, TE = 30 ms, flip angle = 90°, field of view = 240×240 mm^2 , voxel size = 3.8×3.8×4.0 mm^3). As an anatomical reference, a 3-dimensional T1-weighted magnetization-prepared rapid gradient echo (MPRAGE) image data set was acquired using the following parameters: TR = 2000 ms, TE = 2.37 ms, flip angle = 9°, field of view = 240×240 mm^2 , voxel size = 0.9×0.9×1.0 mm^3 , 192 slices.

fMRI data analysis. Analysis of the fMRI data was performed using Statistical Parametric Mapping software (SPM8; Wellcome Institute of Imaging Neuroscience; London, UK) implemented in Matlab 7.1 (Mathworks Inc.; Natick, MA). The data were realigned and co-registered on a mean image, normalized to a template, and smoothed with an 8-mm full-width-at-half-maximum (FWHM) Gaussian kernel. The model was estimated by applying individual movement regressors.

The first four volumes of each session were discarded to allow for T1 equilibration. All the remaining functional images were corrected for slice acquisition timing and head motion. For each participant, the functional images were realigned to the first task-relevant image to correct for head motion and were co-registered to the structural T_1-weighted anatomical images. To decrease spatial noise, the images were spatially normalized using the Montreal Neurological Institute (MNI) template, resampled with an isotropic 2 mm×2 mm×2 mm voxel size, and smoothed with an 8-mm FWHM isotropic Gaussian kernel.

Each acupuncture stimulation was modeled as a boxcar function convolved with a canonical hemodynamic response function that began at the onset of each stimulation. Contrast maps were generated for brain reactivity to acupuncture stimulation, and the individual contrast images in each session were then included in a second-level random-effects analysis. Brain responses to acupuncture stimulation were recorded under both synchronous and asynchronous conditions. For statistical inference, a threshold of $P<0.05$ was used following a correction for multiple comparisons (family-wise error corrections, FWE). To plot the regions of brain activation associated with acupuncture stimulation, the neuronal activity in specific brain areas was correlated over time by extracting the averaged percent signal change in regions of interests (ROIs) separately in the common brain areas (i.e. insula and secondary somatosensory cortex (SII)). The anatomical ROIs for insula and SII were obtained using the Wake-Forest University PickAtlas tool box version 2.4 (WFU PickAtlas; [44]. Signal changes were extracted using the MarsBaR ROI toolbox for SPM8 (http://marsbar.sourceforge.net/).

A multiple regression analysis was conducted to evaluate the association of the contrast images to acupuncture stimulation between asynchronous and synchronous session with individual ratings as two separate covariate vectors (1) the differences of RHI score (synchronous – asynchronous session) and (2) the differences of *DeQi* score (asynchronous – synchronous session). For the regression analysis, activation was considered significant at $p < 0.001$ (uncorrected) with a minimum cluster extent threshold of 10 contiguous voxels.

Rubber hand illusion and self-reported DeQi sensation ratings. After finishing each session (synchronous and asynchronous), participants reported their perception of the RHI by answering question 3 on the RHI Perception Scale: "I felt as if the rubber hand were my hand" [9]. The participants also filled out the acupuncture-induced *DeQi* sensation questionnaire using a seven-point Likert scale ranging from "strongly disagree" (−3) to "strongly agree" (+3).

Data analysis. All values are expressed as means ± standard errors. RHI ratings, subjective *DeQi* ratings, and BOLD signal changes were compared between the synchronous and asynchronous sessions using paired *t*-tests. The level of significance was set at 0.05 for all analyses. Statistical analyses were performed using the Statistical Package for Social Sciences for Windows 20.0 (SPSS Inc.).

Results

Experiment 1

Changes in local blood flow following acupuncture stimulation during the RHI. Local blood flow measurements are presented as the mean PBF change over time. A significant difference was observed in the increase in local blood-flow change following acupuncture stimulation when the asynchronous and synchronous brush-stroking sessions were compared (18.6±3.3 vs. 9.3±2.8%, $t = 2.544$, $P < 0.05$; Fig. 2). No significant differences were observed between the asynchronous and synchronous brush-stroke sessions in rotation frequency (degree of stimulation) or torque amplitude (biomechanical force) (frequency: 1.3±0.1 vs. 1.3±0.1 Hz, $t = -0.414$, $P > 0.684$; torque: 15.4±5.0 vs. 13.8±4.2 μNm, $t = -0.295$ $P > 0.771$, respectively).

Perception of the rubber hand illusion and self-reported DeQi sensation rating. We found a significant difference between the asynchronous and synchronous brush-stroke sessions in the self-reported perception of the RHI (−1.0±0.3 vs. 1.5±0.2, $t = 8.520$, $P < 0.001$). No significant differences were observed in self-reported *DeQi* sensations when the asynchronous and synchronous brush-stroking sessions were compared (heaviness: 3.6±0.6 vs. 3.1±0.5, $t = 0.769$ $P > 0.449$; soreness: 3.4±0.5 vs. 3.7±0.6, $t = 0.403$ $P > 0.690$; numbness: 3.8±0.6 vs. 3.6±0.6, $t = 0.256$ $P > 0.800$).

Experiment 2

Brain responses to acupuncture stimulation during the rubber hand illusion. Brain activations following acupuncture stimulation were observed in the contralateral secondary somatosensory cortex (SII) and insula under both the asynchronous (right SII: 44, −26, 26; $t = 11.52$; $Z = 5.9$; right insula: 44, 2, 8; $t = 9.78$; $Z = 5.5$) and synchronous (right SII: 50, −20, 20; $t = 9.33$; $Z = 5.39$; right insula: 56, 20, 0; $t = 8.9$; $Z = 5.27$) sessions (Table 1). All peaks are $p < 0.05$, corrected, and all coordinates are in MNI space (Fig. 3A).

Comparison of asynchronous and synchronous sessions revealed that the brain responses following acupuncture stimulation were significantly altered in the insula during the RHI. Differences in signal change (less brain activation during the synchronous sessions) were significant in the right insula (0.32±0.04 vs. 0.23±0.05%, $t = 2.517$, $P < 0.05$) but not in SII (0.34±0.05 versus 0.29±0.05%, $t = 1.413$, $P > 0.177$; Fig. 3B).

Perception of the rubber hand illusion and self-reported DeQi sensation rating. In Experiment 2, a significant difference between the asynchronous and synchronous brush-stroking sessions was observed in the self-reported perception of the RHI (−0.6±0.4 vs. 0.9±0.3, $t = 4.622$, $P < 0.001$). No significant differences were observed in self-reported *DeQi* sensation when comparing the asynchronous and synchronous brush-stroke sessions (1.6±0.4 vs. 2.2±0.2, $t = 1.830$, $P > 0.086$).

Individual differences in rubber hand illusion score and *DeQi* score co-varied with brain activations to acupuncture stimulation during rubber hand illusion. We determined whether individual differences in RHI score (synchronous vs. asynchronous session) co-varied with functional brain activity responses to acupuncture stimulation (asynchronous vs. synchronous session). Higher RHI scores demonstrated significant co-variation with activities in the right ventral premotor cortex ($x = 52$, $y = 16$, $z = 26$, $Z = 3.34$, $r = 0.571$, $p < 0.05$, Fig. 4A).

We also determined whether individual differences in *DeQi* score (asynchronous vs. synchronous session) co-varied with functional brain activity responses to acupuncture stimulation (asynchronous vs. synchronous session). Higher *DeQi* scores demonstrated significant co-variation with activities in the right posterior insula ($x = 46$, $y = -8$, $z = -10$, $Z = 4.38$, $r = 0.752$, $p < 0.001$, Fig. 4B).

Discussion

The current study demonstrated that a disrupted sense of body ownership induces significant changes in both local PBF and brain BOLD responses during acupuncture needle stimulation. Experiment 1 used LASER Doppler technology and found that the degree of increased blood flow around the site of acupuncture manipulation was significantly decreased when disembodiment (disrupted sense of body ownership) was induced in the same hand receiving the acupuncture stimulation. Experiment 2 used fMRI and found that brain activations following acupuncture stimulation were significantly reduced in the right insula when disembodiment was induced in the hand receiving the acupuncture stimulation. These findings suggest that body ownership is a crucial factor that influences physiological responses during acupuncture stimulation.

In Experiment 1, when body ownership and bodily self-awareness were preserved in a normal way (asynchronous session), an increase in PBF was observed during acupuncture stimulation (Fig. 2). These findings are consistent with previous studies that reported enhanced microcirculatory blood flow near the acupoints following acupuncture stimulation [16,17]. In contrast, when body ownership was disrupted (synchronous sessions), a significant decrease in peripheral microcirculation was observed around acupoint LI4 relative to asynchronous session. These findings indicate that the peripheral physiological responses following acupuncture stimulation are influenced by modifications of body ownership, at least around the site of acupuncture stimulation (left hand). To assure that the differences in PBF following acupuncture stimulation were not derived from discrepancies in acupuncture

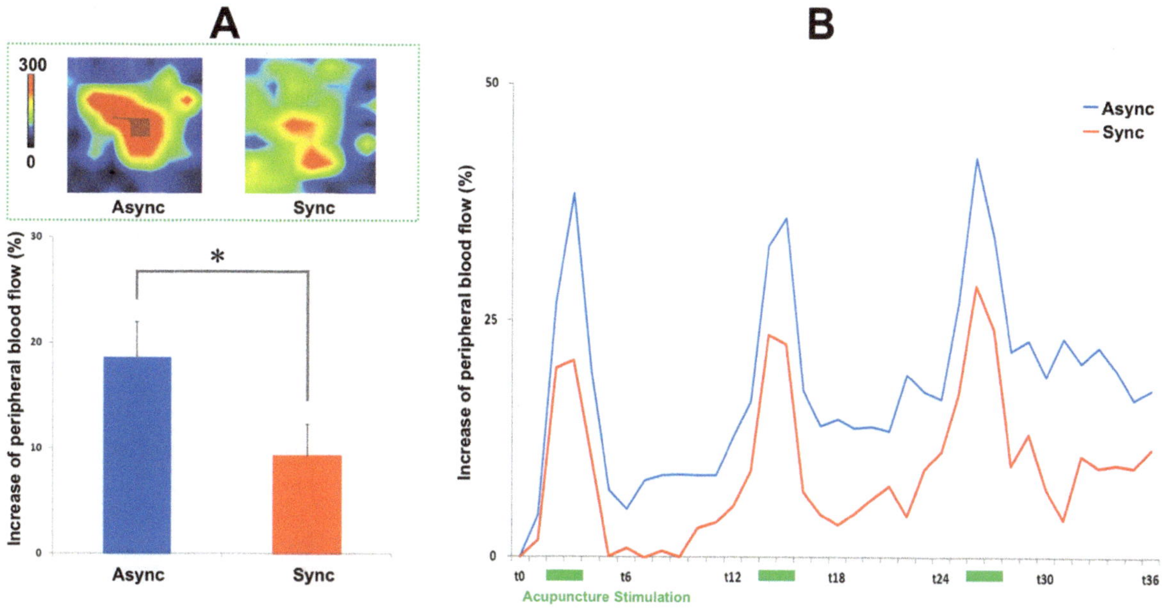

Figure 2. Peripheral responses to acupuncture stimulation during the RHI. A representative example of the peripheral responses to acupuncture stimulation around the LI4 acupoint (2×2 cm) is shown in upper column A. The increase in peripheral responses to acupuncture stimulation was significantly different between the synchronous and asynchronous brush-stroke sessions, as seen in lower column A (18.6±3.3 vs. 9.3±2.8%, $t = 2.544$, $P < 0.05$). Peripheral responses to acupuncture stimulation are presented as the mean peripheral blood-flow change over time. Values are means ± standard errors.

manipulations, the degree of and the biomechanical force behind the acupuncture manipulation were controlled for with force sensors. In our experiment, an experimenter conducted acupuncture manipulation immediately after he stroke both the rubber hand and the hidden real hand. In order to minimize a possible confounding factor in which a non-blinded acupuncturist could be biased to conduct acupuncture differently between the synchronous and the asynchronous sessions, we tried to make the acupuncturists conduct the manipulation using similar rotation frequencies, torques, and amplitudes during the acupuncture manipulation. The sensor measurements confirmed that there was no significant difference of the degree of stimulation (rotation frequency) and the biomechanical force (torque amplitude: rotation force) between the two sessions. Although unlikely given the professional training of the acupuncturist, we cannot exclude other possible bias to the outcome, such as tone of voice.

In Experiment 2, brain activations in the right insula and SII were observed in all sessions in which acupuncture stimulation was applied, whereas significant differences in BOLD signal change were observed only in the right insula when comparing synchronous and asynchronous brush-stroke sessions (Fig. 3). The common brain activations in the insula and SII in the both asynchronous and synchronous session were generally consistent with previous studies, which found that acupuncture stimulation leads to enhanced sensorimotor cortical network [20]. The observation of less activity in the right insula following acupuncture stimulation during the induction of the RHI (synchronous sessions) is noteworthy. The insula is known to generally modulate awareness of pain, temperature, sensual touch, and other bodily feelings using cutaneous mechanoreceptive stimuli [45]. It has often been suggested that the insular cortex is a unique neural substrate that instantiates subjective feelings from the body and feelings of emotion in the immediate present, which is highlighted by the central role of this area in "interoception" and "awareness of bodily signals" [46].

Table 1. Activated brain regions to acupuncture stimulation in asynchronous session and synchronous session (n = 17).

Activated regions	MNI Coordinates			Peak *t*	*p* value (FWE corrected)	Cluster size
	X	Y				
Async						
(R) Insula	44	2	8	9.78	<0.05	106
(R) SII	44	−26	26	11.52	<0.05	200
Sync						
(R) Insula	56	20	0	8.9	<0.05	36
(R) SII	50	−20	20	9.33	<0.05	59

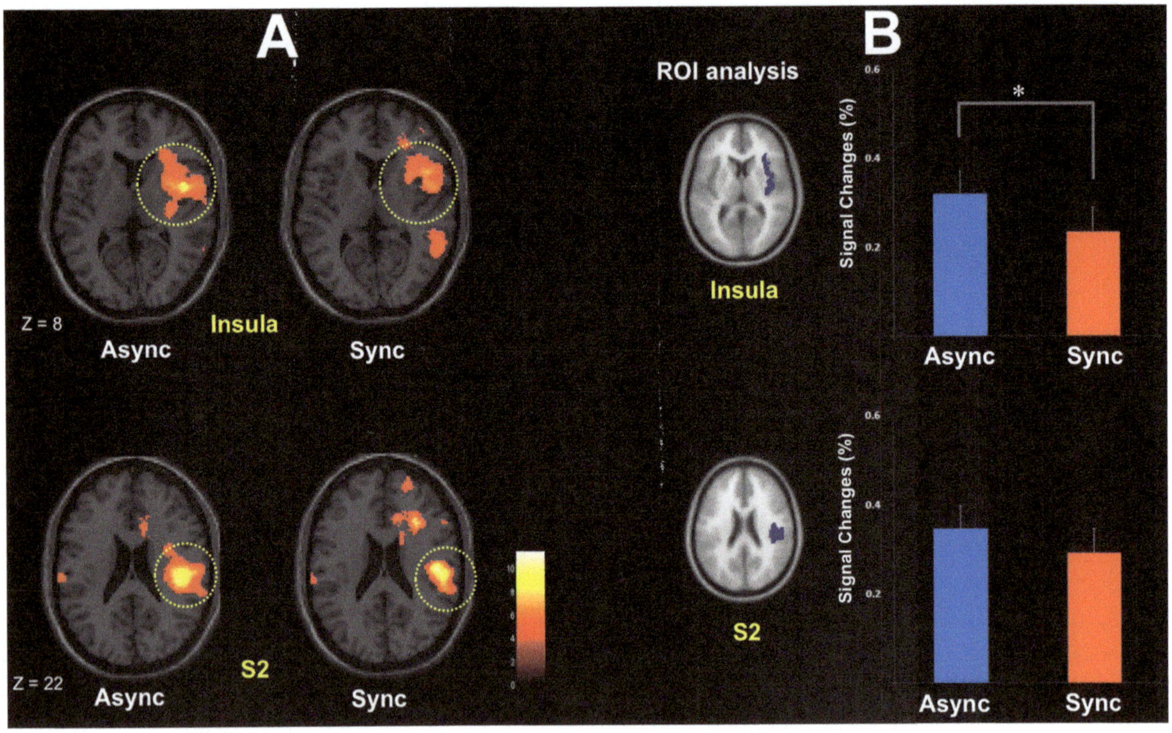

Figure 3. Brain activations in response to acupuncture stimulation. A: Brain activations in response to acupuncture stimulations were observed in the contralateral secondary somatosensory cortex (SII) and insula under both the asynchronous (right SII: 44, −26, 26; $t = 11.52$; $Z = 5.9$; right insula: 44, 2, 8; $t = 9.78$; $Z = 5.5$) and synchronous (right SII: 50, −20, 20; $t = 9.33$; $Z = 5.39$; right insula: 56, 20, 0; $t = 8.9$; $Z = 5.27$) conditions. All two peaks were $p < 0.05$, corrected, and all coordinates are in MNI space. B: To plot the regions of brain activation involved in acupuncture stimulation, the averaged percent signal change in anatomical regions of interests (ROIs), including the right insula and SII, were extracted. When the acupuncture stimulation occurred, BOLD responses in the right insula (0.32±0.04 vs. 0.23±0.05%, $t = 2.517$, $P < 0.05$; A) but not the SII (0.34±0.05 vs. 0.29±0.05%, $t = 1.413$, $P > 0.177$; B) differed significantly under the asynchronous and synchronous sessions.

With the multiple regression analyses, we demonstrated differences in neural substrates for subjective ratings from the RHI and the *DeQi* sensation. Firstly, the RHI scores significantly correlated with the brain activations to acupuncture stimulation (asynchronous vs. synchronous session) in the ventral premotor cortex (Fig. 4A). Ventral premotor cortex has been shown to play a crucial role in multisensory integration in the context of the RHI [12,47]. Previous studies have demonstrated that neural activity in the premotor cortex was correlated with the strength of illusory perceptions during the RHI [12], and damages in fibers connecting the ventral premotor cortex with other brain regions impaired the occurrence of RHI sensations [47]. It is therefore likely that the different brain responses in premotor cortex responding to the acupuncture stimulation between asynchronous and synchronous condition were much more associated with the degrees of the RHI across the subjects. Secondly, the difference of *DeQi* sensation significantly correlated with the brain activations to acupuncture stimulation (asynchronous vs. synchronous session) in the posterior insula in the current study (Fig. 4B). The insula, as a key structure of the interoceptive system, has been studied in relation to acupuncture treatment under some conditions [35,39]. It is assumed that the differential brain responses in the posterior insula in response to acupuncture stimulation between the two sessions were reflected in the substantial variability between subjects in the change of *DeQi* sensation.

The phenomenal incorporation of the rubber hand is also reflected by brain activation in the insula, which can be explained by its association with the basic processes of self-consciousness [14]. Previous fMRI and positron emission tomography (PET) studies have observed brain activations in the insula when comparing BOLD responses during real acupuncture and sham (placebo) acupuncture stimulation. This suggests that enhanced bodily attention following acupuncture may operate as a therapeutic mechanism under some conditions [35,39]. Taken together, these findings indicate that bodily self-awareness plays a central role during acupuncture treatment and that modifications of body ownership may disturb the function of acupuncture as a somatosensory-guided mind-body therapy via modulation of the interoceptive system that is represented by the insula. Further studies using sham-acupuncture are needed to address this issue in detail.

Our results suggest important implications for acupuncture research. In East Asian cultures, acupuncture stimulation is frequently employed for various clinical treatments, and the concept of *Qi* is often used to describe a distinct kind of bodily perception that explains how people feel, control, and experience their own sense of self. Achievement of appropriate *DeQi* sensation is considered to be vital for acupuncture treatment. It is thought that such perceived needling-induced sensations not only direct patients' attention to the specific points on the body, but that they also modulate cognitive and affective aspects [20,38]. In fact, certain components ascribed to the *DeQi* sensation, or perceived *Qi* during acupuncture treatment, may share the characteristics of particular aspects of "bodily self-awareness" because feeling and the perception of oneself are crucial components of both. Recently, aspects of "bodily awareness" have been increasingly attracting the interest of researchers in many disciplines [48]. Studies in the fields of neuroscience and neurology have shown

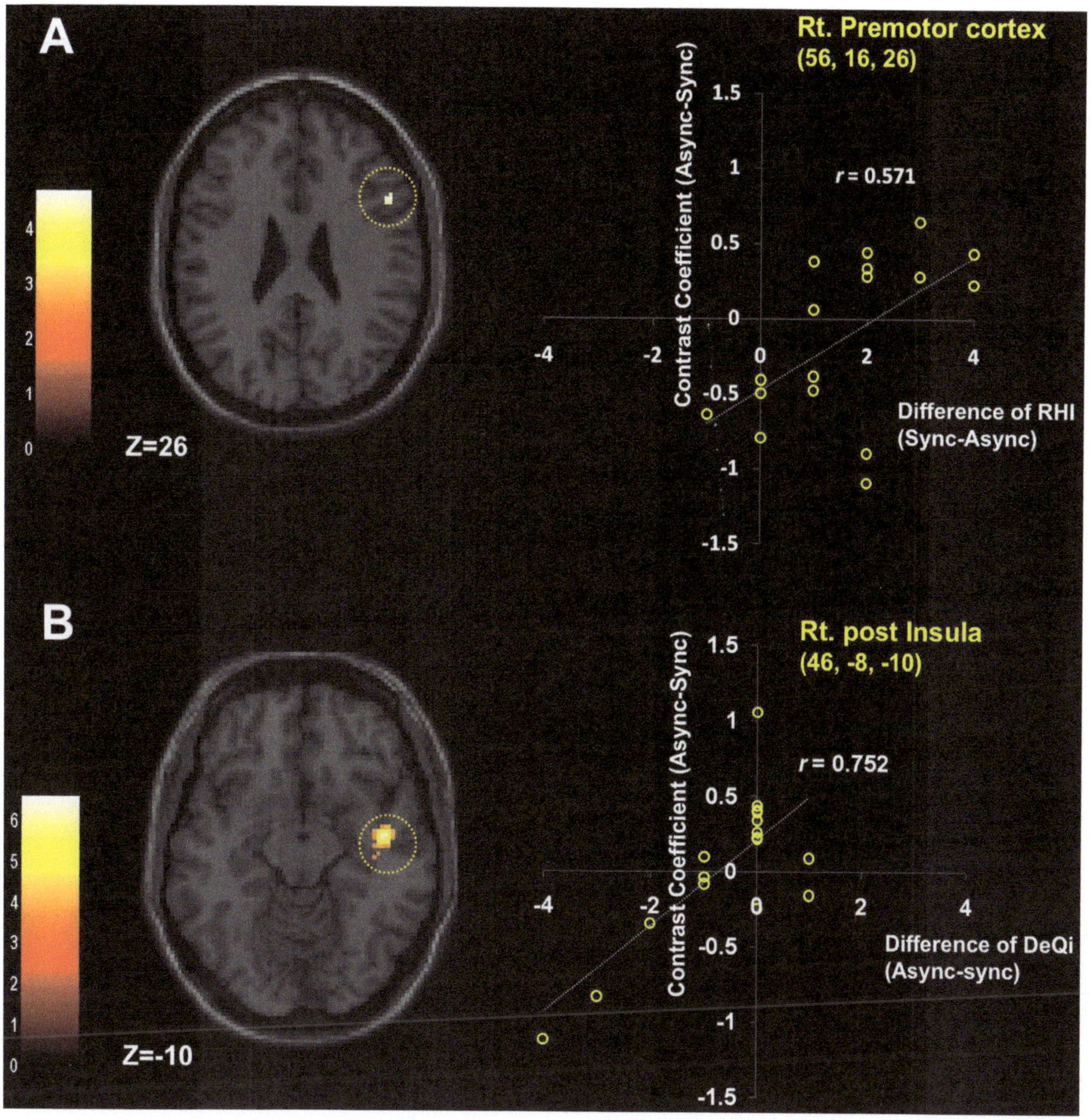

Figure 4. Individual differences in brain activations to acupuncture stimulation. A: Correlation between rubber hand illusion score and brain activations to acupuncture stimulation during reduced body ownership. Normalized SPM T-maps overlaid on the corresponding axial T1-weighted images showing statistically significant ($p<0.001$, uncorrected with 10 continuous voxels) brain activation correlations between the rubber hand illusion (synchronous vs. asynchronous session) and brain responses to acupuncture stimulation in asynchronous condition compared to synchronous condition. Brain activation was observed in the right ventral premotor cortex ($x=52$, $y=16$, $z=26$, $Z=3.34$, $r=0.571$, $p<0.05$). B: Correlation between *DeQi* score and brain activations to acupuncture stimulation during reduced body ownership. Brain activation related to *DeQi* score (asynchronous vs. synchronous session) was observed in the right posterior insula ($x=46$, $y=-8$, $z=-10$, $Z=4.38$, $r=0.752$, $p<0.001$).

that the conscious sense of one's physical self is closely linked to the physiological regulation of one's physical self [3,7]. It has also been shown that any disruption in the awareness of one's physical self can have an important impact on the physiological regulation of the self [6]. It has been suggested that a body matrix, or a multi-sensory representation of peri-personal space and the space directly around the body, serves to maintain the integrity of the body at both the homeostatic and psychological levels and allows for the adaptation of our body structure and orientation to changes in the environment [2]. Findings demonstrating that components of this bodily self-awareness are also involved in the modulation of the clinical effects of acupuncture may have important implications for acupuncture research. Mohan et al. have failed to demonstrate that the RHI modulate pain threshold or pain evoked by individually calibrated high and low painful stimuli delivered on the real arm [49]. Our previous study also found no significant differences in self-reported pain rating to acupuncture stimulation between the asynchronous and the synchronous session [36]. In the current study, we found no significant differences of subjective *DeQi* ratings between the two sessions. Even though there were two different characteristics of acupuncture sensations, such as the pain domain and *DeQi* domain [41], our findings are partially supporting the previous findings that there were no differences of pain ratings during the

RHI [36,49]. Although we did not find significant differences of subjective *DeQi* ratings between the two sessions, differences of brain activations to acupuncture stimulation in the posterior insula was associated with the difference of *DeQi* sensation *between the two sessions* in the current study. It is believed that the insula plays a crucial role in the enhanced body awareness on the specific body site by acupuncture evoked-*DeQi* sensation. Further studies are needed to determine whether reduced embodiment around the acupuncture points during RHI can affect the *DeQi* sensation and/or clinical outcome.

Still, our study possesses several limitations. First, as we did not implement a 2×2 (Body ownership×Intervention) factorial design using a tactile control (such as a non-penetrating placebo needle), we cannot claim that bodily self-awareness is a crucial factor influencing physiological responses that is restricted only to acupuncture stimulation. The rationale for not conducting such a control lies in the difficulty of providing non-penetrating sham acupuncture. Such needles are commonly used as a placebo control for acupuncture experiments [50]. In our previous study, we demonstrated specific patterns of brain activations related to genuine acupuncture compared to sham acupuncture, i.e. non-penetrating placebo needles [15,31]. As such a needle relies on the visual impression that a real needle is being inserted to the skin, however, researchers have claimed that its validity is limited when using such placebo acupuncture out of sight of the participant [51]. Given that participants in the present study can only see the rubber hand in front of them and are not able to see their own hand, a non-penetrating placebo needle would not work well as a placebo control stimulation. Further studies are necessary in order to explore the role of body ownership specific to acupuncture stimulation when compared to other types of tactile stimulation. Second, the acupuncture needle was inserted into only the real hand in experiment 1. In order to minimize visual differences between the rubber hand and the real hand, on the other hand, we performed experiment 2 with the acupuncture needle inserted into the real hand as well as in the rubber hand. In our previous study, the sympathetic activations to acupuncture stimulation in the real hand were markedly higher during the synchronous session compared to that of the asynchronous session only when a visual expectation of the acupuncture needle stimulation existed in the rubber hand [36]. In this case, it is assumed that the participants seemed to have already allowed the incorporation of the artificial body part into their self-representation, and can experience an additional "visual capture" of the acupuncture needling. Future research will be needed to investigate the role of the visual factor of the acupuncture needle in the rubber hand during reduced body ownership. Last but not at least, we did not include a control condition in which a rubber hand was not displayed. It is well established that some participants can still feel a sense of embodiment or ownership towards the rubber hand even without any touch. In order to minimize other confounding factor, such as touch, we were trying to compare the physiological changes of acupuncture between asynchronous and synchronous session in this study. As we did not examine the physiological responses to acupuncture in a third condition without the rubber hand, however, we cannot explicitly analyze the role of the visual factor provided by the artificial hand in our experiments.

The current study demonstrates that both local blood flow changes and brain responses following acupuncture needle stimulation are altered by modifications of body ownership. When body ownership was disrupted by the RHI during acupuncture treatment, local blood flow to the site of acupuncture stimulation was reduced and brain activations during acupuncture stimulation were significantly decreased in the insula, a key region involved in the interoceptive system. Acupuncture can be regarded as a complex treatment comprised of multimodal sensory stimulation that interacts with various factors, including bodily self-awareness [36,37]. These findings suggest that physiological responses during acupuncture stimulation can be influenced by the modification of body ownership. Further research is necessary to ascertain whether the clinical effects of acupuncture are associated with enhanced bodily self-awareness and, if so, how strongly.

Author Contributions

Conceived and designed the experiments: YC CW. Performed the experiments: YC ISL WMJ. Analyzed the data: ISL YC. Contributed reagents/materials/analysis tools: HL HJP. Contributed to the writing of the manuscript: VN DSC YC.

References

1. Lopez C, Halje P, Blanke O (2008) Body ownership and embodiment: vestibular and multisensory mechanisms. Neurophysiol Clin 38: 149–161.
2. Moseley GL, Gallace A, Spence C (2012) Bodily illusions in health and disease: physiological and clinical perspectives and the concept of a cortical body matrix'. Neurosci Biobehav Rev 36: 34–46.
3. Gallagher II (2000) Philosophical conceptions of the self: implications for cognitive science. Trends Cogn Sci 4: 14–21.
4. Newport R, Pearce R, Preston C (2010) Fake hands in action: embodiment and control of supernumerary limbs. Exp Brain Res 204: 385–395.
5. Herbert BM, Pollatos O (2012) The body in the mind: on the relationship between interoception and embodiment. Top Cogn Sci 4: 692–704.
6. Moseley GL, Olthof N, Venema A, Don S, Wijers M, et al. (2008) Psychologically induced cooling of a specific body part caused by the illusory ownership of an artificial counterpart. Proc Natl Acad Sci U S A 105: 13169–13173.
7. Tsakiris M (2010) My body in the brain: a neurocognitive model of body-ownership. Neuropsychologia 48: 703–712.
8. Folegatti A, de Vignemont F, Pavani F, Rossetti Y, Farne A (2009) Losing one's hand: visual-proprioceptive conflict affects touch perception. PLoS One 4: e6920.
9. Botvinick M, Cohen J (1998) Rubber hands feel' touch that eyes see. Nature 391: 756.
10. Makin TR, Holmes NP, Ehrsson HH (2008) On the other hand: dummy hands and peripersonal space. Behav Brain Res 191: 1–10.
11. Barnsley N, McAuley JH, Mohan R, Dey A, Thomas P, et al. (2011) The rubber hand illusion increases histamine reactivity in the real arm. Curr Biol 21: R945–946.
12. Ehrsson HH, Spence C, Passingham RE (2004) That's my hand! Activity in premotor cortex reflects feeling of ownership of a limb. Science 305: 875–877.
13. Ehrsson HH, Wiech K, Weiskopf N, Dolan RJ, Passingham RE (2007) Threatening a rubber hand that you feel is yours elicits a cortical anxiety response. Proc Natl Acad Sci U S A 104: 9828–9833.
14. Tsakiris M, Hesse MD, Boy C, Haggard P, Fink GR (2007) Neural signatures of body ownership: a sensory network for bodily self-consciousness. Cereb Cortex 17: 2235–2244.
15. Chae Y, Lee H, Kim H, Sohn H, Park JH, et al. (2009) The neural substrates of verum acupuncture compared to non-penetrating placebo needle: an fMRI study. Neurosci Lett 450: 80–84.
16. Hsiu H, Hsu WC, Hsu CL, Huang SM (2011) Assessing the effects of acupuncture by comparing needling the hegu acupoint and needling nearby nonacupoints by spectral analysis of microcirculatory laser Doppler signals. Evid Based Complement Alternat Med 2011: 435928.
17. Uchida S, Hotta H (2008) Acupuncture affects regional blood flow in various organs. Evid Based Complement Alternat Med 5: 145–151.
18. Dhond RP, Kettner N, Napadow V (2007) Neuroimaging acupuncture effects in the human brain. J Altern Complement Med 13: 603–616.
19. Fang J, Jin Z, Wang Y, Li K, Kong J, et al. (2009) The salient characteristics of the central effects of acupuncture needling: limbic-paralimbic-neocortical network modulation. Hum Brain Mapp 30: 1196–1206.
20. Chae Y, Chang DS, Lee SH, Jung WM, Lee IS, et al. (2013) Inserting needles into the body: a meta-analysis of brain activity associated with acupuncture needle stimulation. J Pain 14: 215–222.
21. Huang W, Pach D, Napadow V, Park K, Long X, et al. (2012) Characterizing acupuncture stimuli using brain imaging with FMRI–a systematic review and meta-analysis of the literature. PLoS One 7: e32960.

22. Kong J, Kaptchuk TJ, Webb JM, Kong JT, Sasaki Y, et al. (2009) Functional neuroanatomical investigation of vision-related acupuncture point specificity-a multisession fMRI study. Hum Brain Mapp 30: 38–46.
23. Liu H, Xu JY, Li L, Shan BC, Nie BB, et al. (2013) FMRI evidence of acupoints specificity in two adjacent acupoints. Evid Based Complement Alternat Med 2013: 932581.
24. Asghar AU, Green G, Lythgoe MF, Lewith G, MacPherson H (2009) Acupuncture needling sensation: the neural correlates of deqi using fMRI. Brain Res 1315: 111–118.
25. Hui KK, Marina O, Liu J, Rosen BR, Kwong KK (2010) Acupuncture, the limbic system, and the anticorrelated networks of the brain. Auton Neurosci 157: 81–90.
26. Hui KK, Nixon EE, Vangel MG, Liu J, Marina O, et al. (2007) Characterization of the "deqi" response in acupuncture. BMC Complement Altern Med 7: 33.
27. Dougherty DD, Kong J, Webb M, Bonab AA, Fischman AJ, et al. (2008) A combined [11C]diprenorphine PET study and fMRI study of acupuncture analgesia. Behav Brain Res 193: 63–68.
28. Harris RE, Zubieta JK, Scott DJ, Napadow V, Gracely RH, et al. (2009) Traditional Chinese acupuncture and placebo (sham) acupuncture are differentiated by their effects on mu-opioid receptors (MORs). Neuroimage 47: 1077–1085.
29. Napadow V, LaCount L, Park K, As-Sanie S, Clauw DJ, et al. (2010) Intrinsic brain connectivity in fibromyalgia is associated with chronic pain intensity. Arthritis Rheum 62: 2545–2555.
30. Zhang WT, Jin Z, Huang J, Zhang L, Zeng YW, et al. (2003) Modulation of cold pain in human brain by electric acupoint stimulation: evidence from fMRI. Neuroreport 14: 1591–1596.
31. Chae Y, Lee H, Kim H, Kim CH, Chang DI, et al. (2009) Parsing brain activity associated with acupuncture treatment in Parkinson's diseases. Mov Disord 24: 1794–1802.
32. Kong J, Kaptchuk TJ, Polich G, Kirsch I, Vangel M, et al. (2009) Expectancy and treatment interactions: a dissociation between acupuncture analgesia and expectancy evoked placebo analgesia. Neuroimage 45: 940–949.
33. Kong J, Kaptchuk TJ, Polich G, Kirsch I, Vangel M, et al. (2009) An fMRI study on the interaction and dissociation between expectation of pain relief and acupuncture treatment. Neuroimage 47: 1066–1076.
34. Lee J, Napadow V, Kim J, Lee S, Choi W, et al. (2014) Phantom acupuncture: dissociating somatosensory and cognitive/affective components of acupuncture stimulation with a novel form of placebo acupuncture. PLoS One 9: e104582.
35. Napadow V, Dhond RP, Kim J, LaCount L, Vangel M, et al. (2009) Brain encoding of acupuncture sensation-coupling on-line rating with fMRI. Neuroimage 47: 1055–1065.
36. Chang DS, Kim YJ, Lee SH, Lee H, Lee IS, et al. (2013) Modifying Bodily Self-Awareness during Acupuncture Needle Stimulation Using the Rubber Hand Illusion. Evid Based Complement Alternat Med 2013: 849602.
37. Langevin HM, Wayne PM, Macpherson H, Schnyer R, Milley RM, et al. (2011) Paradoxes in acupuncture research: strategies for moving forward. Evid Based Complement Alternat Med 2011: 180805.
38. Liu T (2009) Acupuncture: what underlies needle administration? Evid Based Complement Alternat Med 6: 185–193.
39. Pariente J, White P, Frackowiak RS, Lewith G (2005) Expectancy and belief modulate the neuronal substrates of pain treated by acupuncture. Neuroimage 25: 1161–1167.
40. Davis RT, Churchill DL, Badger GJ, Dunn J, Langevin HM (2012) A new method for quantifying the needling component of acupuncture treatments. Acupunct Med 30: 113–119.
41. Park H, Park J, Lee H (2002) Does Deqi (needle sensation) exist? Am J Chin Med 30: 45–50.
42. Choi YJ, Lee JE, Moon WK, Cho SH (2013) Does the effect of acupuncture depend on needling sensation and manipulation? Complement Ther Med 21: 207–214.
43. Kang OS, Chang DS, Lee MH, Lee H, Park HJ, et al. (2011) Autonomic and subjective responses to real and sham acupuncture stimulation. Auton Neurosci 159: 127–130.
44. Maldjian JA, Laurienti PJ, Kraft RA, Burdette JH (2003) An automated method for neuroanatomic and cytoarchitectonic atlas-based interrogation of fMRI data sets. Neuroimage 19: 1233–1239.
45. Craig AD (2003) Interoception: the sense of the physiological condition of the body. Curr Opin Neurobiol 13: 500–505.
46. Craig AD (2009) How do you feel–now? The anterior insula and human awareness. Nat Rev Neurosci 10: 59–70.
47. Zeller D, Gross C, Bartsch A, Johansen-Berg H, Classen J (2011) Ventral premotor cortex may be required for dynamic changes in the feeling of limb ownership: a lesion study. J Neurosci 31: 4852–4857.
48. Mehling WE, Gopisetty V, Daubenmier J, Price CJ, Hecht FM, et al. (2009) Body awareness: construct and self-report measures. PLoS One 4: e5614.
49. Mohan R, Jensen KB, Petkova VI, Dey A, Barnsley N, et al. (2012) No pain relief with the rubber hand illusion. PLoS One 7: e52400.
50. Dincer F, Linde K (2003) Sham interventions in randomized clinical trials of acupuncture-a review. Complement Ther Med 11: 235–242.
51. Tsukayama H, Yamashita H, Kimura T, Otsuki K (2006) Factors that influence the applicability of sham needle in acupuncture trials: two randomized, single-blind, crossover trials with acupuncture-experienced subjects. Clin J Pain 22: 346–349.

16

Oridonin Attenuates $A\beta_{1-42}$-Induced Neuroinflammation and Inhibits NF-κB Pathway

Sulei Wang[1]☯, Hui Yang[1]☯, Linjie Yu[2], Jiali Jin[2], Lai Qian[2], Hui Zhao[2], Yun Xu[1,2]*, Xiaolei Zhu[2]*

1 Department of Neurology, Nanjing Drum Tower Hospital Clinical College of Traditional Chinese and Western Medicine, Nanjing University of Chinese Medicine, Nanjing, P. R. China, 2 Department of Neurology, Affiliated Drum Tower Hospital of Nanjing University Medical School, Nanjing, P. R. China

Abstract

Neuroinflammation induced by beta-amyloid (Aβ) plays a critical role in the pathogenesis of Alzheimer's disease (AD), and inhibiting Aβ-induced neuroinflammation serves as a potential strategy for the treatment of AD. Oridonin (Ori), a compound of Rabdosia rubescens, has been shown to exert anti-inflammatory effects. In this study, we demonstrated that Ori inhibited glial activation and decreased the release of inflammatory cytokines in the hippocampus of $A\beta_{1-42}$-induced AD mice. In addition, Ori inhibited the NF-κB pathway and $A\beta_{1-42}$-induced apoptosis. Furthermore, Ori could attenuate memory deficits in $A\beta_{1-42}$-induced AD mice. In conclusion, our study demonstrated that Ori inhibited the neuroinflammation and attenuated memory deficits induced by $A\beta_{1-42}$, suggesting that Ori might be a promising candidate for AD treatment.

Editor: Zhongcong Xie, Massachusetts General Hospital, United States of America

Funding: This study was supported by the National Nature Science Foundation of China (81200839, 81230026, and 81171085), the Natural Science Foundation (BL2012013) and the Bureau of Health (LJ201101) of the Jiangsu Province of China. The funders had no role in study design, data collection and analysis, decision to publish, or preparation of the manuscript.

Competing Interests: The authors have declared that no competing interests exist.

* Email: xuyun20042001@aliyun.com (YX); zhuquelee@126.com (XZ)

☯ These authors contributed equally to this work.

Introduction

Alzheimer's disease (AD), as the major cause of dementia, is an irreversible neurodegenerative disorder with progressive cognitive dysfunction, memory impairment and behavioral damage. According to the World Alzheimer Report 2012, there are 36 million people suffering from dementia worldwide in 2010 [1]. The pathological features of AD compose of beta-amyloid (Aβ) plaques (accumulation of extracellular Aβ) and neurofibrillary tangles (NFTs, deposition of intracellular hyperphosphorylated tau protein) [2,3]. Although the exact mechanism of AD still remains unclear, evidence from experimental models and human brain studies indicates that Aβ-mediated neuroinflammation is associated with the development of AD [4,5]. The clinical trials also demonstrate that the levels of pro-inflammatory cytokines are significantly increased in the cerebrospinal fluid (CSF) of AD patients [6], and anti-inflammatory drugs including nonsteroidals have shown great benefits in the treatment of AD [7].

Emerging evidence suggests that Aβ plays important roles in the induction of neuroinflammation in AD [8]. The depositions of Aβ activates the astrocytes and microglia [9], which would release a series of proinflammatory and cytotoxic factors, such as inducible nitric oxide synthase (iNOS), interleukin-1β (IL-1β), cyclooxygenase-2 (COX-2) and tumor necrosis factor alpha (TNF-α) [10]. These cytokines contribute to neuronal damage and eventually cellular death [11]. Nuclear factor-κB (NF-κB) regulates the process of inflammation by targeting the downstream genes, such as TNF-α, IL-1β, iNOS, and COX-2 [12]. Reports have indicated that activation of NF-κB pathway, which subsequently results in the secretion of proinflammatory cytokines, is involved in the degeneration of neurons in AD patients [13,14]. Inhibition of NF-κB signaling can ameliorate neurodegeneration and memory impairment [15]. These results indicate that suppression of neuroinflammation and NF-κB pathway may be a beneficial therapy for AD.

Oridonin (Ori), a diterpenoid originated from Chinese herb of Rabdosia rubescens, exhibits a diverse of biological activities, such as anti-inflammation, anti-tumor and anti-oxidation [16–18]. Recent studies have demonstrated that Ori inhibits the release of proinflammatory mediators through modulating the functions of microglia [19]. In addition, Ori inhibits the NF-κB activity in TNF-α-induced HepG2 cells [20]. In the current study, we investigated whether Ori could inhibit $A\beta_{1-42}$–induced inflammation and attenuate memory deficits in $A\beta_{1-42}$ induced AD mice.

Materials and Methods

$A\beta_{1-42}$ induced AD mice model and Ori treatment

The $A\beta_{1-42}$ (Millipore, CA, USA) was dissolved in 1% $NH_3 \cdot H_2O$ at a concentration of 1 μg/μl and incubated at 37°C for 5 days to allow for fibril formation. Ori (Chengdu Must Bio-Technology Co., Ltd, Sichuan, China, purity more than 98% measured by reverse phase high-performance liquid chromatography) was dissolved in DMSO at a concentration of 20 mg/ml and diluted to the desired concentration in saline. $A\beta_{1-42}$ (4 μg) was injected into the bilateral hippocampus of male C57BL/6 (B6) mice by infusion cannulae as described previously [21]. Mice were divided into three groups: the control mice with saline, $A\beta_{1-42}$-induced AD mice with saline, and $A\beta_{1-42}$-induced AD mice with Ori (10 mg/kg/day, i.p. for 15 days). Our preliminary data has shown that Ori did not attenuate the memory impairment in $A\beta_{1-42}$-induced AD mice at higher dose (20–50 mg/kg/day) (data not shown). After Ori treatment, the mice were trained and tested in Morris water maze for 6 days, and then sacrificed for the following experiments. All experimental procedures were approved by Animal Care Committee of Nanjing University.

Real-time PCR

As described previously [22], total RNA of the hippocampus was isolated using Trizol (Invitrogen, USA) and reversed transcribed to cDNA using a reverse transcriptase kit (Takara, Dalian, China). Quantitative PCR was performed using ABI 7500 system (Applied Biosystems, USA) by a SYBR green kit (Takara, Dalian, China). The primers (Invitrogen, USA) are as follows:

IL-1β: F: AAGCCTCGTGCTGTCGGACC, R: TGAGGCCCAAGGCCACAGGT;

IL-6: F: GCTGGTGACAACCACGGCCT, R: AGCCTCCGACTTGTGAAGTGGT;

IL-10: F: GGCATGAGGATCAGCAGGGGC, R: TGGCTGAAGGCAGTCCGCAG;

iNOS: F: CAGCTGGGCTGTACAAACCTT, R: CATTGGAAGTGAAGCGTTTCG;

COX-2: F: GATGACTGCCCAACTCCC, R: AACCCAGGTCCTCGCTTA;

TNF-α: F: CAAGGGACAAGGCTGCCCCG, R: GCAGGGGCTCTTGACGGCAG;

MCP-1: F: CCAGCACCAGCACCAGCCAA, R: TGGATGCTCCAGCCGGCAAC;

GAPDH: F: GCCAAGGCTGTGGGCAAGGT, R: TCTCCAGGCGGCACGTCAGA.

Western blotting

Western blotting analysis was performed as previously [23]. Briefly, cytoplasmic and nuclear proteins of the hippocampus were collected using cytoplasmic and nuclear protein extraction kit (Thermo, USA) according to the manufacturer's instruction. The proteins were separated by SDS-PAGE and electrophoretically transferred onto polyvinylidene fluoride membranes. Membranes were blocked with 5% skimmed milk for 1 h and incubated overnight at 4°C with anti-COX-2 (1:1000, Santa Cruz, USA), anti-iNOS (1:500, Bioworld, USA), anti-NF-κB p65 (1:1000, Cell Signaling, USA), anti-IκBα (1:1000, Cell Signaling, USA), anti-p-IκBα (1:1000, Cell Signaling, USA), anti-Bcl-2 (1:2000, Bioworld, USA), anti-Bax (1:1000, Cell Signaling, USA), anti-cytochrome c (1:500, Abcam, USA), anti-VDAC1 (1:500, Bioworld, USA), anti-Histone (1:1000, Epitomics, USA) or anti-β-actin (1:5000, Bioworld, USA). β-actin was used as a loading control. Subsequently, the membranes were incubated with the corresponding secondary antibodies and the reaction was visualized with chemiluminescence reagents provided with an ECL kit (Bioworld) and exposed to a film. The intensity of the blots was quantified with densitometry.

Immunostaining

Mice were anesthetized and transcardially perfused with 0.9% saline, then perfused with paraformaldehyde. The brains were removed and cut into consecutive frozen sections and then incubated overnight with anti-ionized calcium-binding adaptor molecule 1 (Iba1) (1:400, Abcam, USA) and anti-glial fibrillary acidic protein (GFAP) (1:100, BD, USA) at 4°C. The secondary antibody (1:200, Invitrogen) was applied to the sections for 1 h at room temperature. The images were performed by a fluorescent microscope (Olympus, Japan). All images were analyzed by Image J for counting of automatically recognized cells. The means were calculated from 5 randomly selected fields in the hippocampus and 5 consecutive sections were analyzed for each brain. All counting procedures were conducted in a randomized and blinded manner.

Morris water maze text

The Morris water maze text was prepared as previously described [21]. Briefly, mice were trained to find a platform in an open circular pool 2 cm under the water surface in the middle of one quadrant. Four training trials per day were conducted for five consecutive days. In each trial, the latency to escape onto the platform was recorded up to 1 min. If a mouse could found the platform, it was allowed to remain on the platform for 5 s, and then returned to the home cage. If the mouse failed to find the platform within 1 min, it was picked up and placed on the platform for 10 s, and the latency was recorded for 1 min. On the 6th day, a probe trial was given for memory retention by removing the platform from the pool, and each mouse was allowed to swim freely for 1 min, the numbers of crossings of the platform were recorded. All data were collected using a computerized video system.

Statistical analysis

The results were expressed as means ± SEM. The data were subjected to statistical analysis using SPSS version 13.0 (SPSS, Chicago, IL, USA). Group differences in the escape latency and swimming distance during the MWM test were analyzed by two-way analysis of variance (ANOVA) with repeated measures followed by Bonferroni multiple comparison test with day and treatment as the sources of variation. All other data were analyzed with a one-way ANOVA followed by Bonferroni's post hoc. $P < 0.05$ were considered statistically significant.

Results

Ori Inhibits the Release of Pro-inflammatory Factors in the Hippocampus of $A\beta_{1-42}$-induced AD Mice

To examine the effects of Ori on $A\beta_{1-42}$-induced inflammation *in vivo*, the relative mRNA levels of IL-1β, IL-6, IL-10, COX-2, iNOS, TNF-α, and MCP-1, and the relative protein levels of iNOS and COX-2 in the hippocampus of mice were tested. The results showed that $A\beta_{1-42}$ could significantly increase the expression of inflammatory factors (IL-1β: $P<0.05$, IL-6: $P<0.01$, iNOS: $P<0.01$, COX-2: $P<0.01$, TNF-α: $P<0.01$, MCP-1: $P<0.01$ versus control group, Figure 1A–F). However, Ori could significantly decrease the levels of these pro-inflammatory cytokines induced by $A\beta_{1-42}$ (IL-1β: $P<0.05$, IL-6: $P<0.01$, iNOS: $P<0.01$, COX-2: $P<0.05$, TNF-α: $P<0.05$, MCP-1: $P<0.05$ versus Aβ group). Meanwhile, the mRNA level of IL-10 was decreased in AD group, and it was upregulated by Ori treatment (Figure 1G). In addition, Ori attenuated the protein levels of iNOS and COX-2 in the hippocampus of AD mice (Figure 2).

Ori Ameliorates Microglia and Astrocytes Activation in the Hippocampus of AD Mice

To verify whether Ori could inhibit $A\beta_{1-42}$ stimulated activation of microglia and astrocytes, Iba-1 and GFAP staining was performed. Iba-1 and GFAP were specific markers of activated microglia and astrocytes respectively. As shown in Figure 3, the expression of Iba-1 was significantly increased in the hippocampus of $A\beta_{1-42}$-induced AD mice ($P<0.01$), while treatment with Ori

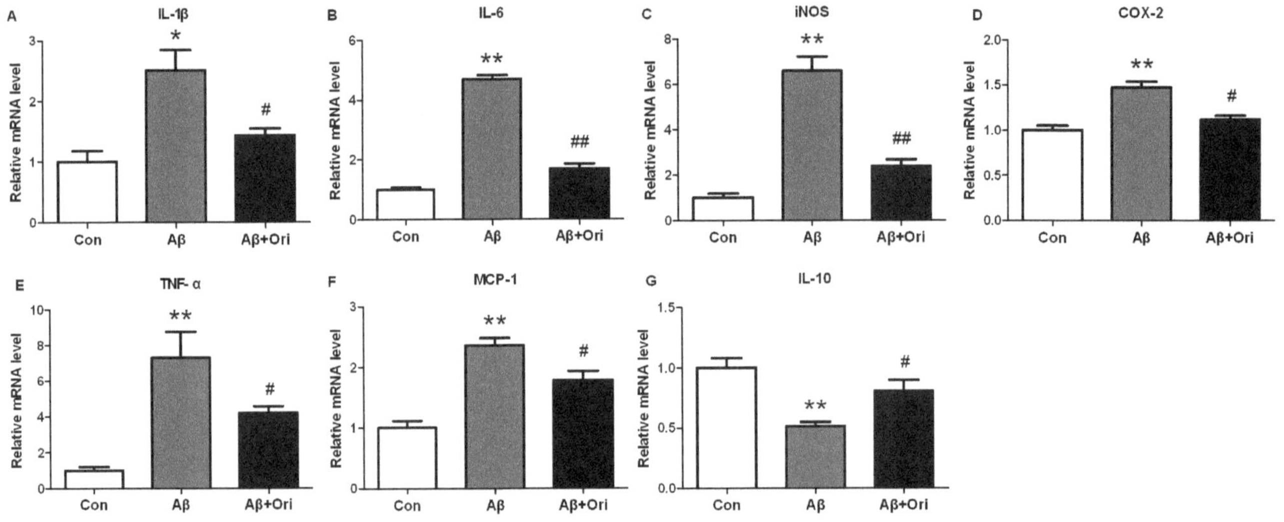

Figure 1. Ori reduces the inflammatory factors in $A\beta_{1-42}$ induced AD mice. The mRNA levels of IL-1β (A), IL-6 (B), iNOS (C), COX-2 (D), TNF-α (E), MCP-1 (F) and IL-10 (G) were measured in each group by Real-time PCR. GAPDH was used as an internal control. n = 6 mice per group. *$P<0.05$, **$P<0.01$ vs. control group; #$P<0.05$, ##$P<0.01$ vs. $A\beta_{1-42}$ induced AD mice.

significantly suppressed Iba-1 expression ($P<0.05$). Ori also reduced the GFAP expression in the hippocampus of AD mice ($P<0.05$).

Ori Inhibits $A\beta_{1-42}$-induced Activation of NF-κB p65 Signaling Pathway *in vivo*

NF-κBp65 signaling pathway is one of the most important pathways in modulating inflammation in AD. Therefore, we explored the role of Ori in $A\beta_{1-42}$-induced activation of NF-κB p65 signaling pathway *in vivo*. As shown in Figure 4, $A\beta_{1-42}$ treatment significantly increased the phosphorylation of IκBα ($P<0.01$). However, Ori treatment could decreased the phosphorylation of IκBα in the hippocampus of AD mice ($P<0.01$). In addition, Ori inhibited the $A\beta_{1-42}$-induced degradation of IκBα ($P<0.05$) and translocation of NF-κB p65 ($P<0.01$).

Ori Decreases Mitochondrial Injury in the Hippocampus of AD Mice

Since emerging evidence suggested that Aβ-induced inflammation may contribute to neuronal apoptosis in AD, we investigated the mitochondrial functions in the hippocampus of Ori-treated AD mice. As shown in Figure 5, Ori treatment inhibited the release of cytochrome c from the mitochondria to the cytoplasm ($P<0.01$). In addition, $A\beta_{1-42}$ increased the expression of Bax ($P<0.01$) and decreased the expression of Bcl-2 ($P<0.01$). However, Ori treatment could decrease the level of Bax ($P<0.05$) and increased the level of Bcl-2 ($P<0.01$), which indicated that Ori could attenuate the mitochondrial dysfunction induced by $A\beta_{1-42}$.

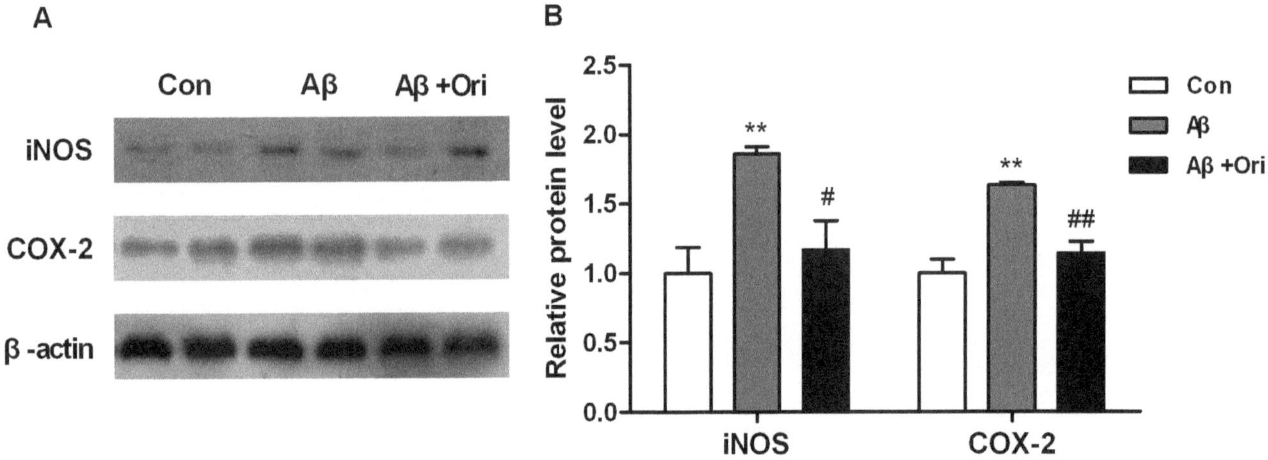

Figure 2. Effects of Ori on the protein levels of iNOS and COX-2 in $A\beta_{1-42}$ induced AD mice. (A) Representative images of western blotting showing Ori inhibited the expression of iNOS and COX-2 in $A\beta_{1-42}$ induced AD mice. (B) Quantitative analysis of iNOS and COX-2 expression. n = 3 mice per group. *$P<0.05$, **$P<0.01$ vs. control group; #$P<0.05$, ##$P<0.01$ vs. $A\beta_{1-42}$ induced AD mice.

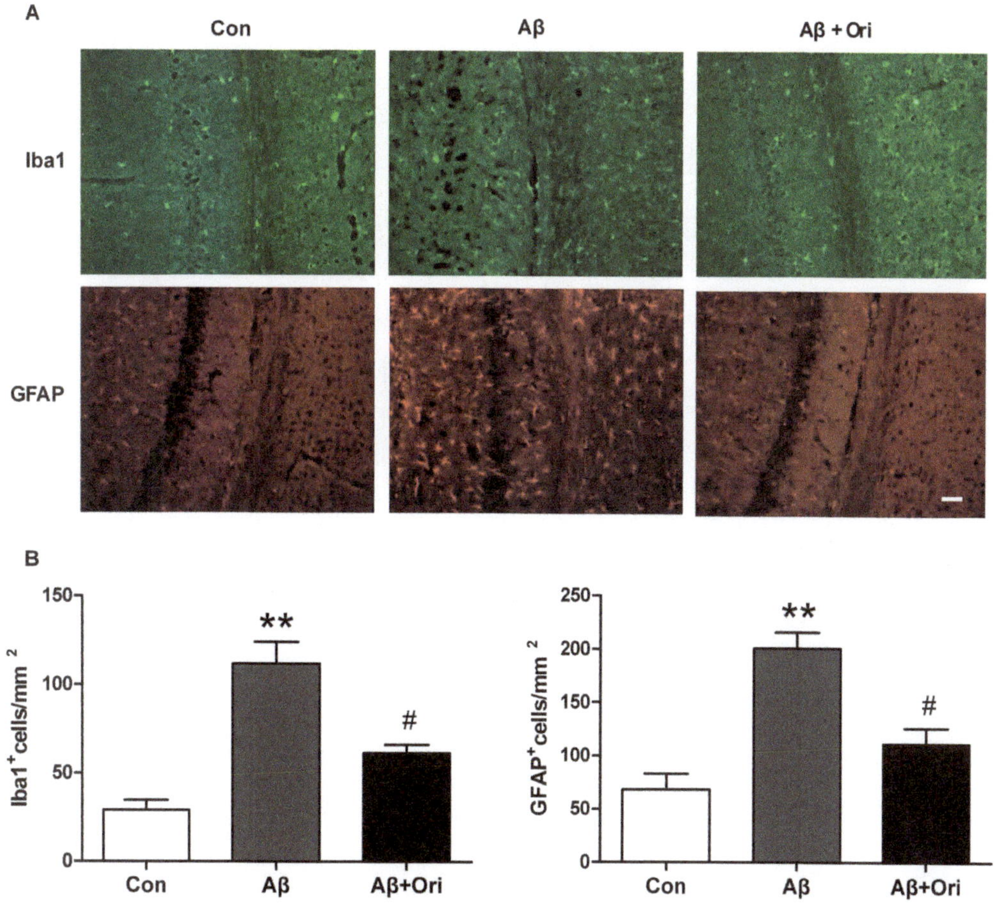

Figure 3. Ori suppresses glial activation in $A\beta_{1-42}$ induced AD mice. (A) Immunostaining for Iba1 and GFAP in the hippocampus of mice. (B) Quantitative analysis of Iba1 and GFAP staining. n = 6 mice per group. Scale bar = 50 μm. *P<0.05, **P<0.01 vs. control group; #P<0.05, ##P<0.01 vs. $A\beta_{1-42}$ induced AD mice.

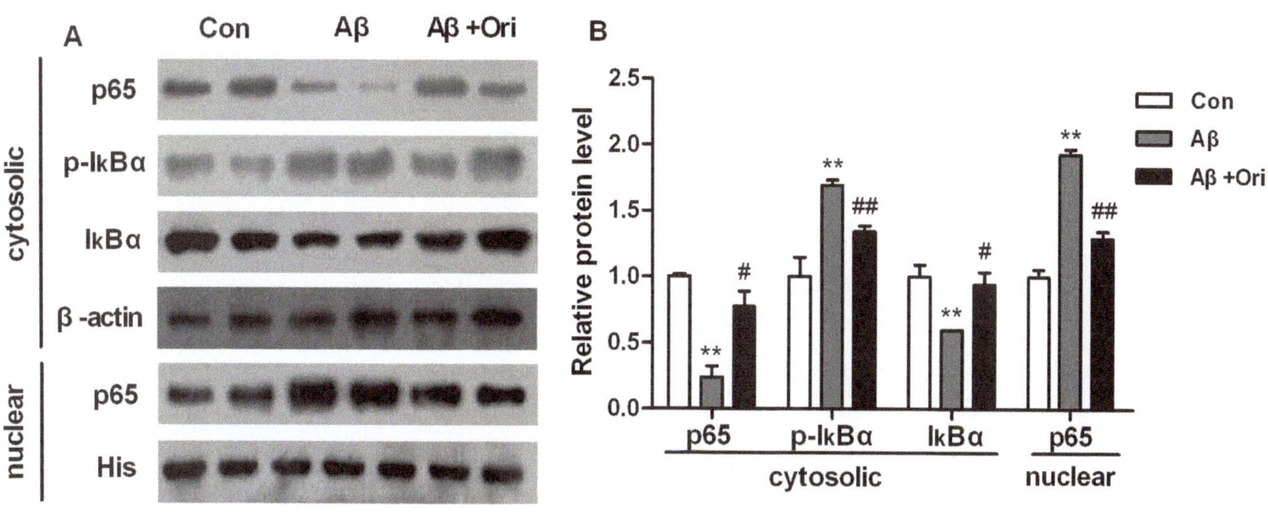

Figure 4. Ori inhibits $A\beta_{1-42}$ induced activation of NF-κB in $A\beta_{1-42}$ induced AD mice. (A) Representative image of western blotting of p65, p-IκBα, IκBα in the cytosolic and p65 in nuclear. (B) Quantitative analysis of Figure 4A. n = 6 mice per group. *P<0.05, **P<0.01 vs. control group; #P<0.05, ##P<0.01 vs. $A\beta_{1-42}$ induced AD mice.

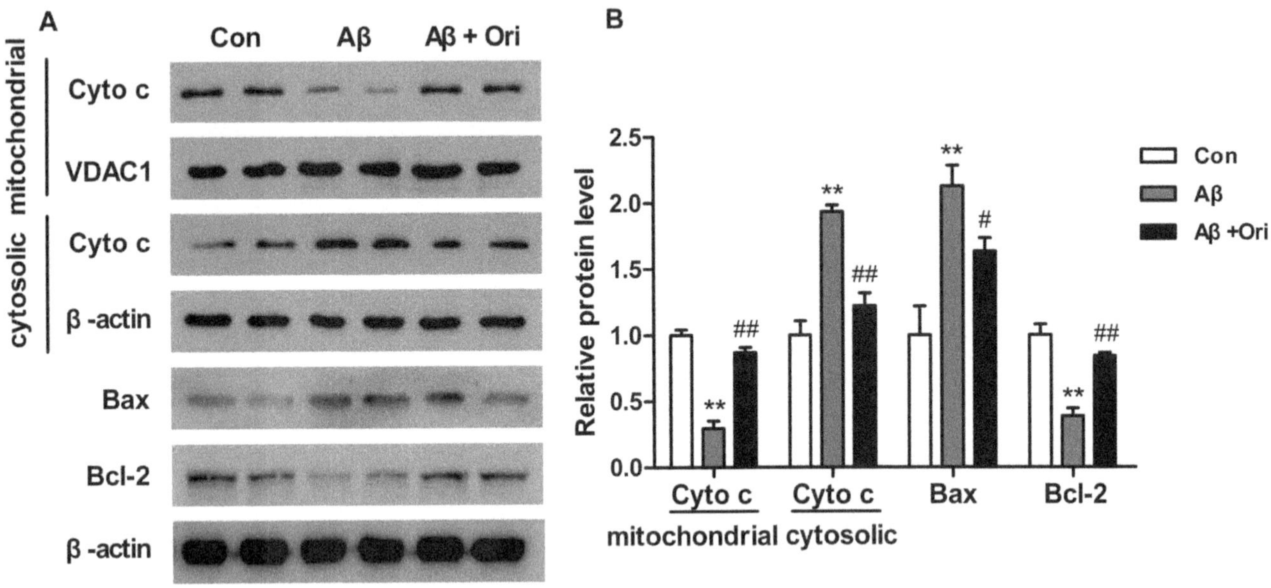

Figure 5. Ori decreases mitochondrial dysfunction in the hippocampus of $A\beta_{1-42}$ induced AD mice. (A) Representative images of western blotting of cytochrome c, Bax and Bcl-2. (B) Quantitative analysis of Figure 5A. n = 6 mice per group. *P<0.05, **P<0.01 vs. control group; #P<0.05, ##P<0.01 vs. $A\beta_{1-42}$ induced AD mice.

Ori Improves Cognitive Impairment in $A\beta_{1-42}$-induced AD Mice

To explore whether Ori could improve cognitive impairment in $A\beta_{1-42}$- induced AD mice, Morris water maze test was performed. As shown in Figure 6A, the mean escape latency of $A\beta_{1-42}$ induced AD mice was significantly increased compared with control group (P<0.01), while Ori-treated AD mice showed significant improvements compared with AD mice after the training periods (P<0.01). The searching distance by the Ori-treated AD mice was significantly decreased compared with that of AD mice (P<0.01, Figure 6B). Moreover, on the 6th day, the platform was removed and the probe trail was conducted. The number of platform crossings by the Ori-treated AD mice was significantly higher than that of AD mice (P<0.01, Figure 6C). In addition, there were no differences for swimming speed among these three groups (Figure 6D).

Discussion

AD is characterized by neurodegeneration and is the most common type of dementia. The Aβ deposition and formation of plaques in the brain have been thought as key events during the progression of AD [24]. In the present study, we demonstrated that Ori attenuated memory impairment in $A\beta_{1-42}$-induced AD mice. Furthermore, Ori could suppress the inflammatory response, and the underlying mechanism might be associated with the inhibition of NF-κB pathway.

Growing data from basic and clinical studies indicate that inflammation induced by Aβ is involved in neuronal degeneration in AD [25,26]. It has been reported that the levels of proinflammatory cytokines are significantly elevated in brains of AD patients, which suggests that inflammation might contribute to the pathogenesis of AD [27]. The deposition of Aβ can activate glial cells which will release a wide spectrum inflammatory cytokines, such as IL-6 and TNF-α [28]. Aβ-induced overproduction of cytokines could lead to neuronal dysfunction and eventually death in AD. Therefore, inhibiting the activation of glial cells and production of proinflammatory cytokines may contribute to neuroprotection. Previous study indicated that Iba-1 and GFAP was increased in the brain of AD patients [29,30]. In the present study, the levels of Iba-1 and GFAP were significantly decreased in the Ori-treated mice compared with AD mice, which suggested that Ori suppressed the activation of microglia and astrocytes. Consistently, the results indicated that Ori could inhibit the mRNA levels of IL-1β, IL-6, COX-2, iNOS, TNF-α, and MCP-1 induced by Aβ, and it also up-regulated the expression of IL-10. Collectively, the current findings suggested that Ori modulated inflammatory response by inhibiting the activation of glial cells, which ameliorated the cognitive impairment of $A\beta_{1-42}$-induced AD mice.

NF-κB has been regarded as the key regulator of inflammatory processes, and many studies have showed that suppression of NF-κB pathway ameliorates the neuroinflammation [31,32]. NF-κB is activated in brains of patients with AD and activated NF-κB is also detected in Aβ surrounding areas [33,34]. In the resting cells, NF-κB family composed of five members, p65 (RelA), RelB, c-Rel, p50/p105 and p52 which bound to the inhibitory proteins IκB, thereby maintaining NF-κB in an inactive form in the cytoplasm. Upon stimuli, IκB is phosphorylated by IKK (IκB kinase), which then is ubiquitinated and subsequent degraded, leading to translocation of NF-κB to the nucleus and binding to specific target genes, and increased the expression of proinflammatory factors [35]. Hydrogen sulfide inhibits neuroinflammation via suppressing NF-κB pathway and attenuates neuronal death in the hippocampus of Aβ-induced AD rats [36]. Moreover, experimental studies show that suppressing NF-κB could decrease production of Aβ [37,38]. This study demonstrated that Ori significantly inhibited NF-κB p65 nuclear translocation by attenuating $A\beta_{1-42}$-induced IκBα phosphorylation and degradation *in vivo*.

In summary, the present study shows that Ori, a typical compound of Rabdosia rubescens, attenuates cognitive impairment and inhibits inflammatory response in $A\beta_{1-42}$-induced AD mice. In addition, the anti-inflammatory effects of Ori might be

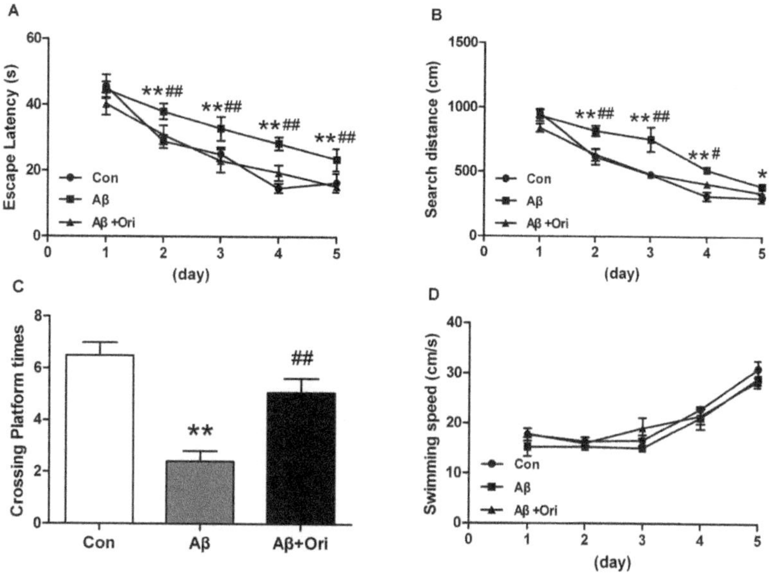

Figure 6. Ori attenuates learning and memory impairment in $A\beta_{1-42}$ induced AD mice in the Morris water maze test. (A) Escape latency for escape to a submerged platform in the training trails. **P<0.01 vs. control group; ##P<0.01 vs. Ori-treated AD mice. (B) Searching distance for escape to a submerged platform in the training trails. **P<0.01 vs. control group; #P<0.05, ##P<0.01 vs. Ori-treated AD mice. (C) Crossing platform times in the probe trail. **P<0.01 vs. control group; ##P<0.01 vs. $A\beta_{1-42}$ induced AD mice. (D) Swimming speed in the training trails. n = 6 mice per group.

due to inhibiting the NF-κB pathway. These findings suggest that Ori might be a potential agent for AD treatment.

Author Contributions

Conceived and designed the experiments: YX XLZ SLW. Performed the experiments: SLW HY LJY JLJ. Analyzed the data: SLW LQ HZ. Contributed reagents/materials/analysis tools: SLW HY LJY. Contributed to the writing of the manuscript: SLW HY LJY XLZ.

References

1. Batsch N, Mittelman M (2012) World Alzheimer Report 2012: Overcoming the stigma of dementia. London: Alzheimer's Disease International.
2. Kurt MA, Davies DC, Kidd M (1997) Paired helical filament morphology varies with intracellular location in Alzheimer's disease brain. Neurosci Lett 239: 41–44.
3. Price DL, Sisodia SS, Gandy SE (1995) Amyloid beta amyloidosis in Alzheimer's disease. Curr Opin Neurol 8: 268–274.
4. Zhang YY, Fan YC, Wang M, Wang D, Li XH (2013) Atorvastatin attenuates the production of IL-1beta, IL-6, and TNF-alpha in the hippocampus of an amyloid beta1–42-induced rat model of Alzheimer's disease. Clin Interv Aging 8: 103–110.
5. McGeer PL, McGeer EG (2013) The amyloid cascade-inflammatory hypothesis of Alzheimer disease: implications for therapy. Acta Neuropathol 126: 479–497.
6. Llano DA, Li J, Waring JF, Ellis T, Devanarayan V, et al. (2012) Cerebrospinal fluid cytokine dynamics differ between Alzheimer disease patients and elderly controls. Alzheimer Dis Assoc Disord 26: 322–328.
7. Jaturapatporn D, Isaac MG, McCleery J, Tabet N (2012) Aspirin, steroidal and non-steroidal anti-inflammatory drugs for the treatment of Alzheimer's disease. Cochrane Database Syst Rev 2: CD006378.
8. Couturier J, Paccalin M, Morel M, Terro F, Milin S, et al. (2011) Prevention of the beta-amyloid peptide-induced inflammatory process by inhibition of double-stranded RNA-dependent protein kinase in primary murine mixed co-cultures. J Neuroinflammation 8: 72.
9. Lyman M, Lloyd DG, Ji X, Vizcaychipi MP, Ma D (2014) Neuroinflammation: The role and consequences. Neurosci Res 79C: 1–12.
10. Wu J, Wang A, Min Z, Xiong Y, Yan Q, et al. (2011) Lipoxin A4 inhibits the production of proinflammatory cytokines induced by beta-amyloid in vitro and in vivo. Biochem Biophys Res Commun 408: 382–387.
11. Heneka MT, O'Banion MK, Terwel D, Kummer MP (2010) Neuroinflammatory processes in Alzheimer's disease. J Neural Transm 117: 919–947.
12. Lawrence T, Fong C (2010) The resolution of inflammation: anti-inflammatory roles for NF-κB. Int J Biochem Cell Biol 42: 519–523.
13. Boissiere F, Hunot S, Faucheux B, Duyckaerts C, Hauw JJ, et al. (1997) Nuclear translocation of NF-kappaB in cholinergic neurons of patients with Alzheimer's disease. Neuroreport 8: 2849–2852.
14. Kaltschmidt B, Uherek M, Volk B, Baeuerle PA, Kaltschmidt C (1997) Transcription factor NF-κB is activated in primary neurons by amyloid beta peptides and in neurons surrounding early plaques from patients with Alzheimer disease. Proc Natl Acad Sci U S A 94: 2642–2647.
15. Kim HG, Moon M, Choi JG, Park G, Kim AJ, et al. (2014) Donepezil inhibits the amyloid-beta oligomer-induced microglial activation in vitro and in vivo. Neurotoxicology 40: 23–32.
16. Ku CM, Lin JY (2013) Anti-inflammatory effects of 27 selected terpenoid compounds tested through modulating Th1/Th2 cytokine secretion profiles using murine primary splenocytes. Food Chem 141: 1104–1113.
17. Bu HQ, Liu DL, Wei WT, Chen L, Huang H, et al. (2014) Oridonin induces apoptosis in SW1990 pancreatic cancer cells via p53- and caspase-dependent induction of p38 MAPK. Oncol Rep 31: 975–982.
18. Bae S, Lee EJ, Lee JH, Park IC, Lee SJ, et al. (2014) Oridonin protects HaCaT keratinocytes against hydrogen peroxide-induced oxidative stress by altering microRNA expression. Int J Mol Med 33: 185–193.
19. Xu Y, Xue Y, Wang Y, Feng D, Lin S, et al. (2009) Multiple-modulation effects of Oridonin on the production of proinflammatory cytokines and neurotrophic factors in LPS-activated microglia. Int Immunopharmacol 9: 360–365.
20. Leung CH, Grill SP, Lam W, Han QB, Sun HD, et al. (2005) Novel mechanism of inhibition of nuclear factor-κB DNA-binding activity by diterpenoids isolated from Isodon rubescens. Mol Pharmacol 68: 286–297.
21. Zhao H, Wang SL, Qian L, Jin JL, Li H, et al. (2013) Diammonium glycyrrhizinate attenuates Abeta(1–42) -induced neuroinflammation and regulates MAPK and NF-κB pathways in vitro and in vivo. CNS Neurosci Ther 19: 117–124.
22. Han L, Yin K, Zhang S, Wu Z, Wang C, et al. (2013) Dalesconols B inhibits lipopolysaccharide induced inflammation and suppresses NF-κB and p38/JNK activation in microglial cells. Neurochem Int 62: 913–921.
23. Zhu X, Chen C, Ye D, Guan D, Ye L, et al. (2012) Diammonium glycyrrhizinate upregulates PGC-1alpha and protects against Abeta1-42-induced neurotoxicity. PLoS One 7: e35823.
24. Karran E1, Mercken M, De Strooper B. (2011) The amyloid cascade hypothesis for Alzheimer's disease: an appraisal for the development of therapeutics. Nat Rev Drug Discov 10: 698–712.
25. Rozemuller AJ, Jansen C, Carrano A, van Haastert ES, Hondius D, et al. (2012) Neuroinflammation and common mechanism in Alzheimer's disease and prion amyloidosis: amyloid-associated proteins, neuroinflammation and neurofibrillary degeneration. Neurodegener Dis 10: 301–304.

26. Meng QH, Lou FL, Hou WX, Liu M, Guo H, et al. (2013) Acetylpuerarin reduces inflammation and improves memory function in a rat model of Alzheimer's disease induced by Abeta1–42. Pharmazie 68: 904–908.
27. Gubandru M, Margina D, Tsitsimpikou C, Goutzourelas N, Tsarouhas K, et al. (2013) Alzheimer's disease treated patients showed different patterns for oxidative stress and inflammation markers. Food Chem Toxicol 61: 209–214.
28. Capiralla H, Vingtdeux V, Zhao H, Sankowski R, Al-Abed Y, et al. (2012) Resveratrol mitigates lipopolysaccharide- and Abeta-mediated microglial inflammation by inhibiting the TLR4/NF-κB/STAT signaling cascade. J Neurochem 120: 461–472.
29. Thangavel R, Stolmeier D, Yang X, Anantharam P, Zaheer A (2012) Expression of glia maturation factor in neuropathological lesions of Alzheimer's disease. Neuropathol Appl Neurobiol 38: 572–581.
30. Overmyer M, Helisalmi S, Soininen H, Laakso M, Riekkinen P Sr, et al. (1999) Astrogliosis and the ApoE genotype. an immunohistochemical study of postmortem human brain tissue. Dement Geriatr Cogn Disord 10: 252–257.
31. Wang C1, Li J, Liu Q, Yang R, Zhang JH, et al. (2011) Hydrogen-rich saline reduces oxidative stress and inflammation by inhibit of JNK and NF-κB activation in a rat model of amyloid-beta-induced Alzheimer's disease. Neurosci Lett 491: 127–132.
32. Zhang J, Zhen YF, Pu-Bu-Ci-Ren, Song LG, Kong WN, et al. (2013) Salidroside attenuates beta amyloid-induced cognitive deficits via modulating oxidative stress and inflammatory mediators in rat hippocampus. Behav Brain Res 244: 70–81.
33. Kaltschmidt B1, Uherek M, Volk B, Baeuerle PA, Kaltschmidt C (1997) Transcription factor NF-kappaB is activated in primary neurons by amyloid beta peptides and in neuronssurrounding early plaques from patients with Alzheimer disease. Proc Natl Acad Sci U S A 94: 2642–2647.
34. Huang Y1, Liu F, Grundke-Iqbal I, Iqbal K, Gong CX (2005) NF-kappaB precursor, p105, and NF-kappaB inhibitor, IkappaBgamma, are both elevated in Alzheimer disease brain. Neurosci Lett 373: 115–118.
35. Hayden MS, Ghosh S (2004) Signaling to NF-κB. Genes Dev 18: 2195–2224.
36. Fan H, Guo Y, Liang X, Yuan Y, Qi X, et al. (2013) Hydrogen sulfide protects against amyloid beta-peptide induced neuronal injury via attenuating inflammatory responses in a rat model. J Biomed Res 27: 296–304.
37. Paris D, Patel N, Quadros A, Linan M, Bakshi P, et al. (2007) Inhibition of Abeta production by NF-κB inhibitors. Neurosci Lett 415: 11–16.
38. Valerio A, Boroni F, Benarese M, Sarnico I, Ghisi V, et al. (2006) NF-κB pathway: a target for preventing beta-amyloid (Abeta)-induced neuronal damage and Abeta42 production. Eur J Neurosci 23: 1711–1720.

"I Try and Smile, I Try and Be Cheery, I Try Not to Be Pushy. I Try to Say 'I'm Here for Help' but I Leave Feeling… Worried": A Qualitative Study of Perceptions of Interactions with Health Professionals by Community-Based Older Adults with Chronic Pain

Amanda Clarke[1], Denis Martin[2]*, Derek Jones[1], Patricia Schofield[3], Geraldine Anthony[4], Paul McNamee[5], Denise Gray[5], Blair H. Smith[4]

1 School of Health, Community and Education Studies, Northumbria University, Newcastle, United Kingdom, **2** Health and Social Care Institute, Teesside University, Middlesbrough, United Kingdom, **3** School of Health and Social Care, University of Greenwich, London, United Kingdom, **4** Medical Research Institute, University of Dundee, Dundee, United Kingdom, **5** School of Medicine and Dentistry, University of Aberdeen, Aberdeen, United Kingdom

Abstract

Background: Over 50% of community-dwelling older adults experience chronic pain, which threatens their quality of life. Of importance to their pain management is older people's interaction with health professionals that, if unsatisfactory, may impair the outcome.

Aims: To add to the limited research specific to older people living with chronic pain in the community, we explored how they perceive their experiences of interacting with health professionals, seeking factors that might optimise these interactions.

Methods: Purposive sampling was used to recruit men and women >65 years with self-reported musculoskeletal chronic pain. Qualitative individual interviews and one group interview were undertaken with 23 participants. Data were transcribed verbatim and underwent Framework Analysis.

Results: Three themes were identified. *Seeking help* illustrates issues around why older people in the community may or may not seek help for chronic pain, and highlights the potential involvement of social comparison. *Importance of diagnosis* illustrates the desire for professional validation of their condition and an aversion to vague explanations based on the person's age. *Being listened to and being heard* illustrates the importance of empathic communication and understanding expectations, with due respect for the person's age.

Conclusions: In common with people of all ages, an effective partnership between an older person in pain and health professionals is essential if pain is to be reported, appropriately assessed and managed, because of the subjective nature of pain and its treatment responses. For older people with pain, perception about their age, by both parties in the partnership, is an additional factor that can unnecessarily interfere with the effectiveness of this partnership. Health professionals should engage with older adults to clarify their expectations about pain and its management, which may be influenced by perceptions about age; and to encourage expression of their concerns, which may also be affected by perceptions about age.

Editor: Diane Medved Harper, University of Missouri Kansas City School of Medicine, United States of America

Funding: This study was funded by the Medical Research Council as part of the Lifelong Health and Wellbeing programme. The funders had no role in the design, execution, analysis and interpretation of the data, or writing of the study.

Competing Interests: The authors have declared that no competing interests exist.

* Email: d.martin@tees.ac.uk

Introduction

Chronic non-malignant pain is associated with physical, emotional and social limitations [1] and is one of the most pervasive and costly health-care challenges globally [2]. Most of the burden of pain, however, rests on those personally affected. Older adults are particularly vulnerable: it affects more than 50% of those living in the community [3], prevalence increases with age, and its impact is compounded by age-related comorbidities [4,5].

Various observations have been made about older adults with chronic pain, including a determination to get on with life [6,7] believing that pain is an expected consequence of later life [8,9] and, consequently, assuming that seeking help is not an option [10]; and their lack of awareness of effective treatment options [11]. Particular observations have been made about encounters between older adults with chronic pain and health professionals (HPs). These include older adults assuming that professionals 'know best' [12,13]; negative interactions with HPs and a fear of medical treatment leading to older adults not seeking help at all [14]; a lack of knowledge on the part of HPs about pain in older age [15]; failure to assess pain and underestimation of pain in older age by both professionals and older individuals [15]; and HPs disbelieving older adults' accounts or believing that the accounts are exaggerated [16].

These observations clearly point towards problems in the interaction between older adults with chronic pain and HPs, problems that can affect their pain management and quality of life [17]. Such problems with interactions with health professionals are not in themselves necessarily unique to older people [18]. Also, any consideration of older people as a distinct group needs to acknowledge that age is a continuous variable with no obvious point at which populations become discretely separate. However, there are strong arguments that there are aspects of living with pain particularly shaped by living with advanced years [19].

Most of this knowledge is based on qualitative methods of enquiry, which is entirely appropriate given the match between such methods and the nature of the research questions, which focus on people's perceptions, experiences and opinions. Qualitative methods are, by nature, constrained in their ability to allow their findings to be transferred or extrapolated outwith the sample studied. Given the relatively limited amount of research in this area there is a need for more such studies to iteratively add to the knowledge being generated. Also, compared to studies on samples of older people in specialist care from pain clinics there has been little contribution to the knowledge base from studies in which samples are older people living in the community [20]. The aim of this paper, therefore, is to gain more insight into how older adults living with chronic pain in the community (and not attending pain clinics) perceive their encounters with healthcare professionals, with a view to informing and improving these interactions. To do this, we draw on data from a qualitative exploration of community-dwelling older adults' experiences of living with chronic pain.

Methods

Setting, recruitment and participants

Men and women were recruited from the community through media advertising and contacts with groups and organisations in North-East Scotland. Despite rigorous efforts to recruit individuals from Black and Minority Ethnic (BME) groups, the only BME individuals who opted into the study were seven people from a Chinese community group. Using purposive sampling we included all those who volunteered to participate if they were aged 65 or over, had self-reported musculoskeletal chronic pain for three months or longer, and could give informed consent.

Data collection

In a qualitative design we aimed to undertake two in-depth interviews with each participant (four to six weeks apart) using a topic guide (Table 1) based on the literature and discussions with our advisory group. The first interview focused on day-to-day living with pain. The second interview focused on the individual in order to follow-up and clarify emerging themes.

Out of the 23 participants recruited, 14 agreed to be interviewed twice. The nine who were interviewed only once comprised the seven Chinese participants, who declined to participate further, and two other men who were unable to participate further due to ill-health. Individual interviews were undertaken in participants' homes with all but the Chinese participants who preferred to participate together in a group interview at a community group. Although this diverted from our intention to conduct individual interviews, it was consistent with qualitative approaches, which aim to respond flexibly and sensitively to participants' needs in order to capture a range of experiences and views [21]. A worker at the Chinese community group acted as interpreter when needed. The group interview followed recommendations that respondents are questioned simultaneously for individual responses, rather than the dynamic, interactive responses of focus groups, with the emphasis on individual, rather than collective responses [21]. Each interview lasted approximately an hour, was digitally recorded with permission, and transcribed.

The interviews included general questions such as the opening question "Tell me about your pain", with subsequent probes such as "How do you feel other people respond about your pain?" A number of distinct overarching themes emerged including how people describe pain, their views on its assessment, and experiences of interactions with health professionals. The findings on describing pain and its assessment are reported elsewhere [22]. This paper focuses on the interactions with health professionals.

Analysis

To facilitate transparent data analysis amongst the research team, we were guided by the matrix-based principles of Framework Analysis, which involves a structured process of coding and sorting the transcribed data according to key issues and themes [23].Transcripts were read, re-read and coded using QSR NVivo version 9 to assist with sorting and retrieval of data. Codes were applied to the text independently by DG and AC.

The research team and advisory group (which included lay advisers) were consulted to enhance balanced interpretation and rigorous analysis of data. Divergent interpretations were discussed until a common thematic framework was agreed, which was then systematically applied to each transcript by DG (whilst being open to incorporating new themes). We moved back and forth between the full interview transcripts and the thematic framework to ensure that interpretations were valid and contextualised in participants' broader accounts. Table 2 shows the thematic chart with examples of its application to one transcript.

Ethical considerations

The study was approved by the North of Scotland Research Ethics Committee (09/SO802/93). Verbal and written informed consent was obtained before participants' first and second interviews and all data were anonymised.

Reflexivity

The team involved in the study comprises researchers from nursing, medicine, physiotherapy, occupational therapy medical and health economics backgrounds, and a practising General Practitioner (GP). The research was conducted as part of a large collaborative project on self-management for older people with pain: Engaging with Older People and their Carers to develop interventions for the self-management of Chronic Pain (EOPIC), the background to which is reported online (www.eopic@dundee.ac.uk).

Table 1. Interview Topic Guide.

Questions	Probing questions
Tell me about your pain?	What is the cause of your pain?
	How long have you had the pain?
	How would you describe your pain?
	Have you experienced pain before?
	Has the cause of your pain been diagnosed?
	Who provided the diagnosis?
	How do you feel about the diagnosis?
	Is your pain comparable to anything else?
	What is your first memory of pain?
Can you tell what it's like to live with pain?	What was your life like before the pain started?
	What effect has pain had on your life?
	How does pain make you feel?
	Do you think that getting older has affected your pain at all?
	Do you think your pain has affected the way you have aged?
What treatments have you been offered for pain?	Who offered the treatment?
	Is there anything else that you feel might help your pain?
What helps to relieve your pain?	What about prescribed medicine?
	What about complementary therapy?
	What about other?
What do you know about chronic pain?	Where did you find out this information?
	How helpful was information you received?
	If you wanted to find out more, how would you do that/who would you ask?
Any other comments?	

Table 2. Example of Thematic Chart.

Seeking help	*Only when pain persisted*: When the pain set in, I thought, 'I must see about this.' (Interview 1: 17–37).
	Reasons for not seeking help: Sometimes you'll say, 'why have I not investigated'… and I think 'stop complaining'. I think that's what you do when you're older. (Interview 1: 351–357). So I think you just don't speak about things because you don't want to be a moan, nobody's wanting to hear about somebody's aches and pains, so you just brush over them a bit. (Interview 1: 437–440). Their (hospital consultant) time is so precious. (Interview 2: 130).
The importance of diagnosis	*Increases worry*: There was an MRI scan, but again, very disappointing because I just thought 'oh know, they'll see really where this is', but they didn't' they didn't see anything. (Interview 1: 95–87 & 135; repeated Interview 2: 120–125.) I imagine all my body is getting to get like this. (Interview 1: 184; repeated Interview 2: 257).
	Invisibility of pain: I think it would give me peace of mind knowing, because all along, there's so many of my friends haven't a clue that I've got this. (Interview 1: 370–372).
	Feels like a fraud: Nobody realises I'm putting up with this, I feel like a fraud. (Interview 1: 831; Interview 2: 149–150).
	Lack of expectation: I don't expect (GP) can do anything about it now, no nothing. (Interview 2: 211–212).
Being listened to and being heard	*Effort involved in presenting to HPs*: I don't sort of go on about it, I just brief tell them and that's it. (Interview 2: 207–208).
	Being nice not enough: He was very sympathetic, but I don't want sympathy, I don't want people to feel sorry for me. (Interview 2: 159).
	(Different) Expectations: (Hospital consultant) They more or less said 'well there's no point in me having another appointment with you. You just felt 'that's so final.' (Interview 2: 123–124). (GP) said 'I think you should make up your mind that you're going to have to live with it.' (Interview 1: 64). (New Hospital Consultant) He said 'I can see that it would mean an awful lot to you if you knew exactly where that pain was coming from.' (Interview 1: 715–718).
	Knowing own body: I said (to GP), 'I'm wondering if it's related to anything with the problem I have in my leg?' and she just brushed passed it. (Interview 1: line 609–611; repeated Interview 2: 201–204 &210).
Notes	Sought help from GP only after experiencing back pain for a 'couple of years' – when pain extended down her leg. New hospital consultant recognised how important diagnosis was to her. She repeats issues around lack of diagnosis several times in both interviews. Appeared to be a conflict between not wanting to make a fuss but needing reassurance and someone to talk to about her concerns.

The example used here is Female 13, Aged 66, Caucasian, Undiagnosed back and leg pain ('nerve pain').

Results

Twenty-three participants (16 women, 7 men) were recruited aged from 66 to 89 years (median = 73 years). Of these four had university education, seven had college education, and the remaining 12 did not have any further educational qualifications. Eighteen lived in the city and the remaining participants lived in rural areas. Fourteen of these participants lived alone and the remaining nine lived with their spouse/partner.

Three themes emerged: *Seeking help*; *The importance of diagnosis*; and *Being listened to and being heard*. We present findings directly relating to participants' perceptions of interactions with GPs, nurses, physiotherapists, and hospital doctors. A range of quotes from different participants (here ascribed a code, F = female, M = male) was chosen that succinctly captured a theme across interviews.

It should be noted that no differences were found between Caucasian and Chinese participants' perceptions. However, Chinese participants chose to be interviewed as a group, once only and, at times, needed the help of an interpreter to clarify our questions and help them express their answers. Answers tended to be short, probing was difficult, and they might have been reluctant to discuss personal issues in the presence of their peers [24].

Theme: *Seeking help*

In the UK, GPs would be expected to be a particularly appropriate source of help for older adults who are frequent users of primary care [17]. Amongst participants, an insidious onset of pain seemed to contribute to delays in seeking help from GPs. Only when the pain became persistent, more noticeable and repetitive was help sought:

> When the pain set in, I said, "I must see about this" (F13).

A variety of reasons were offered for participants' reluctance to see their GP, although the concern not "to bother" physicians, or "waste" their time appeared paramount. One woman, who had experienced back pain for "many years" said she needed to be "really ill" before she went to a doctor (F17). Comparisons were made to other "elderly" people; participants felt that they were "lucky" not to be as bad as them. This appeared to add to their reticence to seek professional support since they were concerned not to be seen as "complainers" by visiting GPs "too often." For a few participants, decisions about seeking help seemed to be influenced by the belief that "nothing much" could be done about their pain since they associated it with getting older:

> It's something that, as you get older, you're going to have to live with (M19).

Managing the impact of pain concomitantly with engaging with HPs seemed to consume a great deal of emotional effort and self-protection and seemed also to account for delays in seeking help. Much effort was spent thinking about how they should present to HPs, reflecting their concern not to be seen as making a "fuss." Participants considered hard how they might present their accounts succinctly, without complaint or being over-assertive:

> I try and smile, I try and be cheery I try not to be pushy [laughs]. I try to say "I'm here for help" but I leave feeling… worried (F10).

Theme: *The importance of diagnosis*

Feelings of worry were exacerbated when no cause could be found for their pain:

> If it was a known pain, I could say "well that could be so and so…" When I get a pain that I can't put a name to … I worry… (F10).

Most participants discussed the importance of having a diagnosis and the frustration when none was apparent:

> "When I think about it, I think there must be some reason for this, why… you know?" (M3).

The invisibility of pain made the diagnosis particularly important. Commonly, participants worried about being seen as "a fraud" or "making it up." One woman described encounters with various HPs and her relief when her pain was "labelled":

> I felt people thought I was making it up, making a fuss about nothing. Eventually, something showed on the x-ray. They said "of course, you've got a painful hip" And I thought, "I've been telling you that for years". It was osteoarthritis. So I did get a label eventually (F14).

Another participant said that "the most disappointing thing" about her pain was not having a diagnosis. This led to a lack of expectation that things might improve in the future:

> As far as this leg is, I don't expect him [GP] to do anything about it now, no, nothing (F13).

In contrast, an 82 year-old woman expressed hope that her pain would be cured once diagnosed:

> I just keep thinking it's going to get better! I think maybe after I see this doctor, he'll find something that could be sorted (F11).

A few, however, felt it was insufficient to simply name their condition:

> The general [comment from doctors that] it must be a nerve problem that cannot be explained is frustrating (F13).

One woman was unimpressed by the consultant's diagnosis of sciatica since she felt she had not had the tests to support the claim:

> [He] breezed into the room like a gale of wind and said "what are you doing back here? There's nothing we can do for you!" … But I stuck to my guns and managed to extract an MRI scan for my knee (F15).

Another woman was so relieved at her diagnosis that she was unconcerned about the consultant's "blunt" approach:

> There was no sort of "I'm sorry to have to give you this diagnosis or"…. The nurse was a bit taken aback. She said

"are you okay? That was a bit harsh, wasn't it?" And I said "no, it's a relief to have a diagnosis" (F14).

An 81 year-old man was the exception in reflecting that the inability of doctors to give him a diagnosis for his pain was understandable given his age:

Maybe it's not their [doctors'] fault. As people get older, it's like an old car, it's breaking down a bit (M12).

Theme: *Being listened to and being heard*

Participants described becoming anxious and confused when they perceived that HPs had been disparaging and dismissive rather than supplying the information and support anticipated. This, it was felt, led to treatment that was based on assumptions, ("professionals tend to want to make up their own minds") rather than their own experiences and knowledge of their own bodies. Again, the importance of presentation – this time the participant's history – was emphasised:

You've to have your story very short and succinct, present it well. You've to get through to him [GP]. If he short circuits you, because he's a habit of putting his hand out to try and stop you speaking, you've got to shut up [laughs]! He does it all the time! You can never get your story out. ...I've had physio three times, but it doesn't help... nobody seems to listen to me (F15).

GPs who took time to listen were perceived as "traditional" or "family practitioners" who participants felt "fortunate" to have. One woman said, "I've a holistic GP practice,' elucidating "they really get to know the person". She also said she was "lucky" with her orthopaedic surgeons, "they were very approachable and listened." (F14). Another described experiencing "nothing but kindness from everyone, doctors, nurses, receptionists". She clarified that that this was because the nurses visited her at home and spent time listening to her (F8). Simply being "nice", however, was not welcomed if ineffective:

All the doctors are very nice, but they don't take any notice...They don't do anything (F10).

It was also apparent how participants' unmet expectations could affect the interaction:

Most [physiotherapists] are lovely girls. I went to lots of them and the doctors believe in it... I just can't. They give you a bit of elastic to pull on and chat away and say nice things, but I thought I'd get a manipulation or something (M12).

There was some ambiguity in participants' perceptions concerning whether their age affected HPs' approach to them. One woman felt aggrieved by hospital doctors talking to her daughter "over my head," which she attributed to her age (F8). The perceived reluctance of HPs to manage pain in all but a "conservative way" was felt also by some to be influenced by age:

Is it because I'm over 65, they're not doing anything about it? (M9)

It was reflected that the study had given some the first opportunity to talk at length about their pain. One man said:

Who's asked me? The GP, her attitude is "nothing very much you can do about it" (M9).

Others went further:

I think the attitude to people over 70 is wrong, just tablets, treat them conservatively...a lot of people have got a lot of life in them still ... (F15).

A few participants were unsure that HPs' approach was to do with their age, recognising that this was not always their peers' experience:

I get tablets, but [GP] wasn't willing to give me an operation. She didn't come out and say "your heart is maybe not very good" but I'd the feeling maybe that was my age [82], but a lot of people older than me get hips and knees and things. (F11).

One woman went further in suggesting that HPs sometimes made too many assumptions and should be more prepared to listen to older adults about their pain precisely because of their advanced age. She considered that older individuals are more conscious of their bodies and sensitive to when something is wrong such as pain:

Sometimes, doctors don't give people credit for knowing their bodies. We've lived in our bodies and as we get older, we've lived in them for a long time; we're aware of when things are not working as well as they should and it's sometimes difficult to convince them (F14).

Discussion

Our description of three main themes adds to the theoretical knowledge about the interaction between older people with chronic pain and their health professionals, providing insight into the perspectives of older people with chronic pain in the community. This perspective is relatively poorly represented compared to that of older people in specialist pain services. Clinically, these findings should help inform health professionals' approaches to older adults with chronic pain, specifically with respect to communication and managing expectations.

We reported how a reluctance to be judged by health professionals as wasting their time might delay seeking help for their pain. This observation is consistent with previous studies on pain in adults of different ages and a variety of clinical settings [11,12]. In our study, the advanced age of participants was a factor in this: rightly or wrongly there were presumptions that health professionals would be dismissive of their condition as simply a part of old age. We also observed self-judgement in this context of being reluctant to seek help, whereby people felt that they would be taking up health professionals' time that could be better used by people they viewed as more deserving of that opportunity. Their judgement appeared to involve, to some extent, suppositions that there were others worse-off than them. Again, the advanced age of participants was involved in this with opinions expressed that because of their age there was nothing that could be done to help compared to younger adults for whom a professional consultation would be more appropriate. This introduces the idea of social comparison influencing decisions to engage with health professionals.

Social comparison has been investigated to a limited extent in pain [25,26]. Its influence appears to be complex and dependent on the specific context. In our study, such comparisons appeared to add to people's reluctance to seek help or pursue treatment. Our interpretation is that the social comparisons we witnessed were harmful in the sense that they were involved in preventing people receiving something that may have helped. However, in research with older adults attending pain clinics comparisons with others were interpreted as distracting from the individual's pain and contributing to a feeling of wellbeing [6]. The scope of our study does not allow any concrete conclusions about this but it does introduce to the field the idea that social comparison may be an important phenomenon to explore further in research and to be aware of when interacting with older people with pain.

Once engaged with HPs, our participants put much effort into the presentation of self and their pain accounts. This adds to findings from previous studies on chronic illness in general amongst mixed aged groups rather than specifically relating to older adults with chronic pain [27]. The desire to present oneself in a positive manner may involve a mix of respect for the professionals' status and a strategy to avoid being judged as unnecessarily moaning. Inadvertently, however, this positive face could distract from the underlying reason for the consultation to seek help for a situation that they are having difficulty in coping with.

In our sample the desire for a diagnosis was evident. An ongoing search for diagnosis can be associated with a biomedical "cause and cure" understanding of chronic pain [28]. Findings elsewhere have suggested that many older adults attending pain clinics accept that their chronic pain is not curable [7,8]. This is indicative of a more biopsychosocial understanding of chronic pain compared to our sample. Education to facilitate a biopsychosocial understanding of pain is an expected feature of all but the most biomedically-focused pain clinics. Perhaps our sample, recruited from the community rather than pain clinics, had not had access to that education. Diagnosis has been identified as a frame of reference for individuals with chronic pain, clarifying and providing explanation for what they experience [29,30]. Without this scaffolding, anxiety and worry may creep in, as highlighted by our study and other research with working and mixed age groups [31]. The clinical and research communities may be moving towards viewing chronic pain as a long-term condition in its own right, defined in biopsychosocial terms. However, our data suggest that for many older adults affected there remains a high likelihood of a belief that pain is a symptom of an underlying condition, a belief that gives rise to a strong expectation of a medical diagnosis. The challenge to clinicians is to meet this expectation of diagnosis with a clear and plausible explanation consistent with a biopsychosocial model of pain, taking care to avoid their communication being interpreted as dismissive through vague language or language that implies age as an insurmountable barrier towards management of pain.

Good practices in communication were described, primarily where professionals demonstrated empathy with the person. Empathy has been described as underpinning satisfactory and successful consultations [32,33]. However, participants did not always feel that they were listened to or heard: physicians sometimes were perceived to have unhelpfully controlled pain communication by interrupting participants' reports of pain. This is in contrast to participants' desire for the opportunity to tell their story in sufficient detail and their antipathy towards being asked to give abbreviated descriptions of their pain and its effects [22]. Indeed, participating in our research presented some with the first opportunity to talk at length about their pain, as others have found [5,6,15]. It was also felt that credence was not given to older individuals' knowledge and experience of their own body. When partnership is encouraged in clinical decision-making this is, at least, a missed opportunity.

Our findings should be treated as illustrative rather than representative. The geographical location - NE Scotland - meant that possible influences and interplay of factors such as ethnicity, socio-economic circumstances or sites of pain could not be investigated in-depth. This phase of our study sought older adults' views only, so findings reflect their perspective, not the view of HPs who frequently report frustration in having inadequate time, training or resources to meet the support needs of chronic pain patients [34].

Older adults' confidence in reporting pain is likely to be increased if they are listened to and believed, if discussions about pain are actively facilitated, and their awareness of treatments and services is improved [15]. For an individualised approach to be realised, older adults' expectations about symptoms, treatment and management of their pain should be clarified, and they should be encouraged to express their concerns.

Acknowledgments

We are grateful to the lay members of our Advisory Group and to the individuals who took part in the interviews.

Author Contributions

Analyzed the data: DM DJ PS BS GA PM. Contributed reagents/materials/analysis tools: AC DG DM DJ BS PS PM GA. Wrote the paper: AC DM DJ PS GA PM DG BS. Used framework analysis for this research: AC DG. Conducted most of the data collection: AC DG. Wrote the first draft of this article: AC. Contributed to the data analysis and results: DM DJ BS PM PS. Conducted the interviews: AC DG.

References

1. Breivik H, Collett B, Ventafrida V, Cohen R, Gallagher D (2006) Survey of chronic pain in Europe: prevalence, impact on daily life, and treatment. Eur J Pain 10: 287–333.
2. IASP (2009) Global year against pain 2009–2010 musculoskeletal pain. Available http://www.iasp-pain.org/Advocacy/GYAP.aspx?ItemNumber=771 Accessed 2014 July 9.
3. Helme RD, Gibson SJ (2001) The epidemiology of pain in elderly people. Clin Geriatr Med 17: 417–431.
4. Jakobsson U, Klevsgard R, Westergren A, Rahm Hallberg I (2003) Old people in pain: a comparative study. J Pain Symptom Manage 26: 625–636.
5. Elliott AM, Smith BH, Penny KI, Smith WC, Chambers WA (1999) The epidemiology of chronic pain in the community. Lancet 354: 1248–1252.
6. Sofaer-Bennett B, Holloway I, Moore A, Lamberty J, Thorp T, et al (2007) Perseverance by older people in their management of chronic pain: a qualitative study. Pain Med 8: 271–280.
7. Sofaer B, Moore AP, Holloway I, Lamberty TJM, Thorpe TAS, et al (2005) Chronic pain as perceived by older people: a qualitative study. Age Ageing 34: 462–6109.
8. Sanders C, Donovan J, Dieppe P (2002) The significance and consequences of having painful and disabled joints in older age: co-existing accounts of normal and disrupted biographies. Sociol Health Ill 24: 227–253.
9. Grime J, Richardson JC, Ong B (2010) Perceptions of joint pain and feeling well in older people who reported being healthy: a qualitative study. Br J Gen Pract 60: 597–603.

10. Gignac MA, Davis AM, Hawker G, Wright JG, Mahomed N, et al (2006) "What do you expect? You're just getting older": a comparison of perceived osteoarthritis-related and aging-related health experiences in middle- and older-age adults. Arthritis Care Res 55: 905–912.
11. Hill J, Bird H (2007) Patient knowledge and misconceptions of osteoarthritis assessed by a validated self-completed knowledge questionnaire (PKQ OA). Rheumatology 46: 796–800.
12. Cooper K, Smith BH, Hancock E (2008) Patient-centeredness in physiotherapy from the perspective of the chronic low back pain patient. Physiotherapy 94: 244–252.
13. Zalon M (1997) Pain in frail, elderly women after surgery. Image J Nurs Sch 29: 21–26.
14. Roberto KA, Reynolds SG (2002) Older women's experiences with chronic pain: daily challenges and self-care practices. J Women Aging 14: 5–23.
15. Kumar A, Allcock N (2008) Pain in Older People: Reflections and Experiences From an Older Person's Perspective. London: Help the Aged.
16. Sofaer-Bennet B, Schofield PA, Cameron PA (2012) Chronic Pain in Older People. Geriatric Medicine. 42: 13–19.
17. Kristiansson MH, Brorsson A, Wachtler C, Troein M (2011) Pain, power and patience - a narrative study of general practitioners' relations with chronic pain patients. BMC Fam Pract 12: 31 doi:10.1186/1471-2296-12-31
18. Ong BN, Hooper H (2006) Comparing clinical and lay accounts of the diagnosis and treatment of back pain. Sociol Health Ill 28: 203–22.
19. Gagliese L (2009) Pain and aging: the emergence of a new subfield of pain research. J Pain 10: 343–353.
20. Schofield P, Clarke A, Jones D, Martin D, McNamee P, et al (2011) Chronic pain in later life: a review of current issues and challenges. Aging Health 7: 551–556.
21. Kvale S (1996) InterViews: An Introduction to Qualitative Research Interviewing. London: Sage Publications.
22. Clarke A, Anthony G, Gray D, Jones D, McNamee P, et al (2012) "I feel so stupid because I can't give a proper answer...." How older adults describe chronic pain: A qualitative study. BMC Geriatr 2012, 12: 78 doi:10:1186/1471-2318-12-78
23. Ritchie J, Spence L (1994) Qualitative data analysis for applied policy research. In: Bryman A, Burgess G, eds. Analysing Qualitative Data. London and New York: Routledge. pp. 172–194.
24. Leung K, Wu E, Lue B, Tang L (2004) The use of focus groups in evaluating quality of life components among elderly Chinese people. Qual Life Res 13: 179–190.
25. Jensen MP, Karoly P (1992) Comparative self-evaluation and depressive affect among chronic pain patients: an examination of selective evaluation theory. Cognit Ther Res 16: 297–308.
26. Jackson T, Phillips H (2011) Social comparison performance standards, threat, and tolerance for experimentally-induced pain. Eur J Pain 15: 1081–1086.
27. Ong BN, Jinks C, Morden A (2011) The hard work of self-management: Living with chronic knee pain. Int J Qual Stud Health Well-being 6: 7035 - DOI: 10.3402/qhw.v6i3.7035.
28. Toye F, Barker K (2011) Persistent non-specific low back pain and patients' experience of general practise: a qualitative study. Prim Health Care Res Dev 13: 72–84.
29. Corbett M, Foster NE, Ong BN (2007) Living with low back pain - stories of hope and despair. Soc Sci Med: 1584–1594.
30. Jutel A (2009) Sociology of diagnosis: a preliminary review. Sociol Health Ill 31: 278–299.
31. Walker J, Holloway I, Sofaer B (1999) In the system: the lived experience of chronic back pain from the perspectives of those seeking help from pain clinics. Pain 80: 621–628.
32. Mercer SW, Watt GCM, Reilly D (2001) Empathy is important for enablement. BMJ 322: 865.
33. Mercer SW, Reilly D (2004) A qualitative study of patients' views on the consultation at the Glasgow Homeopathic Hospital, an NHS integrative complementary and orthodox medical care unit. Patient Educ Couns 53: 13–18.
34. Stannard C, Johnson M (2003) Chronic pain management – can we do better? An interview-based survey in primary care. Curr Med Res and Opin. 19: 703–706.

Electroencephalographic Variation during End Maintenance and Emergence from Surgical Anesthesia

Divya Chander[1]*ⓢ, Paul S. García[2]ⓢ, Jono N. MacColl[3], Sam Illing[3], Jamie W. Sleigh[3]

1 Department of Anesthesiology, Perioperative and Pain Medicine, Stanford University School of Medicine, Stanford, California, United States of America, **2** Department of Anesthesiology, Atlanta VA Medical Center/Emory University, Atlanta, Georgia, United States of America, **3** Department of Anaesthesia, Waikato Clinical School, University of Auckland, Hamilton, New Zealand

Abstract

The re-establishment of conscious awareness after discontinuing general anesthesia has often been assumed to be the inverse of loss of consciousness. This is despite the obvious asymmetry in the initiation and termination of natural sleep. In order to characterize the restoration of consciousness after surgery, we recorded frontal electroencephalograph (EEG) from 100 patients in the operating room during maintenance and emergence from general anesthesia. We have defined, for the first time, 4 steady-state patterns of anesthetic maintenance based on the relative EEG power in the slow-wave (<14 Hz) frequency bands that dominate sleep and anesthesia. Unlike single-drug experiments performed in healthy volunteers, we found that surgical patients exhibited greater electroencephalographic heterogeneity while re-establishing conscious awareness after drug discontinuation. Moreover, these emergence patterns could be broadly grouped according to the duration and rapidity of transitions amongst these slow-wave dominated brain states that precede awakening. Most patients progressed gradually from a pattern characterized by strong peaks of delta (0.5–4 Hz) and alpha/spindle (8–14 Hz) power ('Slow-Wave Anesthesia') to a state marked by low delta-spindle power ('Non Slow-Wave Anesthesia') before awakening. However, 31% of patients transitioned abruptly from Slow-Wave Anesthesia to waking; they were also more likely to express pain in the post-operative period. Our results, based on sleep-staging classification, provide the first systematized nomenclature for tracking brain states under general anesthesia from maintenance to emergence, and suggest that these transitions may correlate with post-operative outcomes such as pain.

Editor: Uwe Rudolph, McLean Hospital/Harvard Medical School, United States of America

Funding: This work was supported by a collaborative grant from the James S. McDonnell Foundation, and departmental resources of the authors. The funders had no role in study design, data collection and analysis, decision to publish, or preparation of the manuscript.

Competing Interests: The authors have declared that no competing interests exist.

* Email: dchander@stanford.edu

ⓢ These authors contributed equally to this work.

Introduction

Both sleep and anesthesia have been tracked in the human electroencephalogram (EEG) since the 1950s [1–3], but a staging nomenclature based on specific EEG features has only been well-developed for natural sleep [4,5]. While there are also stereotyped EEG features, such as a shift in the spectrum toward lower frequencies (<14 Hz), that correlate with anesthesia-induced unresponsiveneses (the historical clinical marker of anesthetic adequacy) [6–11], a standardized nomenclature for anesthetic maintenance and emergence has never been universally accepted by clinicians. Recent focus has been placed on the spatial and temporal distribution of these frequency changes [12–15], and identifies an anteriorization of lower frequency power that correlates with the behavioral transition to loss of consciousness [8,9,16,17]. Studies in which volunteers have been exposed to slowly changing doses of propofol have described spectral power changes upon emergence that appear to be the inverse of induction, i.e. a decrease in power in these low frequency oscillations over the frontal EEG, followed by an increase in higher frequencies as the patient becomes behaviorally responsive to mild stimuli [8,9]. This is in contrast to the termination of natural sleep, which is typically preceded by cyclic transitions into progressively longer episodes of cortical activation [18]. Waking usually occurs from rapid eye movement (REM) sleep (reviewed in Steriade [19]).

Although sleep and anesthesia are not the same, significant overlap in neurotransmitters, circuitry and electrical patterns do exist [20,21], suggesting that anesthetics may achieve part of their hypnotic effect by acting on the normal sleep and arousal systems of the brain [22]. Pharmacologic enhancement of inhibitory signaling, mediated via the gamma aminobutyric acid type A ($GABA_A$) receptor, underlies the mechanisms of most commonly used anesthetic agents [23,24]. Similarly, a physiological GABAergic state also contributes to the thalamocortical oscillations characteristic of non-REM sleep [25], while pharmacologic inhibition of the $GABA_A$ receptor reverses sleepiness in hypersomnic patients [26]. It has been shown that sleep deprivation potentiates the efficacy of anesthetics [27], and these effects can be partially reversed by antagonists to adenosine, an endogenous ligand that accumulates during sleep pressure [28]. Furthermore, activation of subcortical endogenous arousal pathways (e.g. thalamus, basal forebrain, hypothalamus, brain stem) can reverse anesthesia in some animal models [29–36], significantly blurring the distinction between sleep and anesthesia. Perhaps most

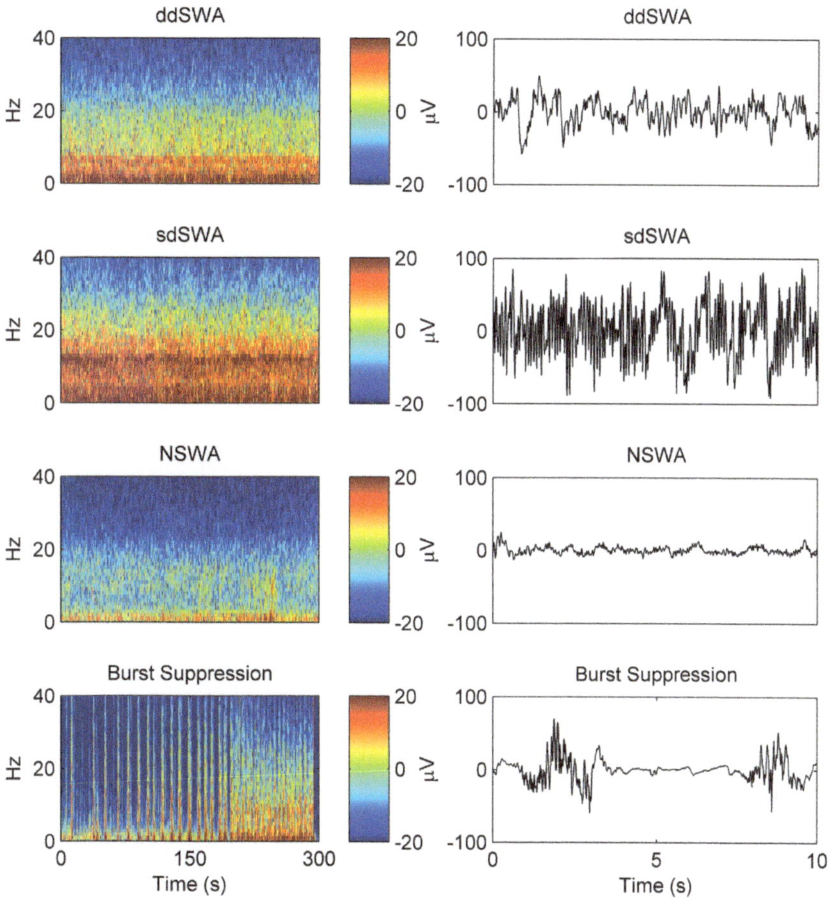

Figure 1. Spectral patterns at the end of maintenance under sevoflurane general anesthesia comprise 4 basic patterns. 'Slow-Wave Anesthesia' (SWA) is a spectral pattern in which there is both high delta and spindle power (>7 dB). Panel (A) shows the more common variant, or subclass, of the SWA spectrogram, calculated over 5 minutes prior to turning off the anesthetic, in which delta power is higher than spindle power (point #1 below the diagonal in Figure 2B) termed delta dominant SWA, or ddSWA. An example 10 second raw EEG tracing is take from this period and shown in the right column. Panel (B) is an SWA spectral variant/subclass in which spindle power is higher than delta power, termed spindle-dominant SWA, or sdSWA (point #2 above the diagonal in Figure 2B). Finally, a small subset of patients (5%) showed low amplitude power in both the spindle and delta frequency bands (C). We termed this pattern non Slow-Wave Anesthesia, or NSWA (point #3 in Figure 2B). For completeness, the spectrogram in panel (D) reflects a deeper anesthetic maintenance pattern, burst suppression, transitioning into a ddSWA pattern at approximately 1.5 minutes prior to End Maintenance. The representative 10 second EEG to its right is taken from the burst suppression period.

importantly, both non-REM (NREM) sleep and general anesthesia exhibit similar synchronization and slowing of the EEG [37,38]. Not surprisingly, the same range of lower frequency oscillations that indicate loss of consciousness are also used to separate natural sleep into specific stages [4,5,39,40]. Thalamocortical oscillations in the alpha band (8–14 Hz) are the electroencephalographic hallmark of the loss of perceptual awareness in synchronized sleep [41]. Generated by the reticular nucleus of the thalamus [42], these oscillations consist of waxing and waning of electrical potentials, and are often referred to as sleep spindles [43]. As sleep deepens, spindles are progressively reduced and replaced by slower oscillations (0.5–4 Hz) [44,45]. In contrast, REM sleep is characterized by profound inhibition of motor output, abolition of these low-frequency oscillations, and an EEG resembling the aroused brain [46]. Although the different sleep stages were arbitrarily and heuristically defined, based on EEG patterns described above [5,47], they have been successfully used by clinicians and researchers to relate sleep physiology to functional neuroanatomy [48], consolidation of memory [49–51], and sleep disorders [52,53].

We therefore designed a study with three objectives. The first was to catalogue and define a standardized nomenclature for the EEG during anesthetic maintenance, analogous to that used to describe natural sleep. The second was to characterize the evolution of the human EEG during emergence from general anesthesia during surgery, to determine if there was a single common path, or multiple pathways to re-establishing conscious awareness and interaction with the outside world. Our final goal was to determine if the path by which the patient emerged had any relationship to the quality of a patient's recovery.

We recorded the frontal EEG from 100 human subjects in the operating room, undergoing routine orthopedic surgery with general volatile anesthesia, prior to loss of consciousness, through the maintenance and recovery from anesthesia, until patients were able to be taken safely to the recovery room. Using spectral processing techniques, we propose a nomenclature of four basic EEG patterns, based on the relative dominance of low frequency oscillatory patterns seen during maintenance of general anesthesia (i.e. a degree of hypnosis considered to be commensurate with unconsciousness). We also identified four stereotypical trajectories

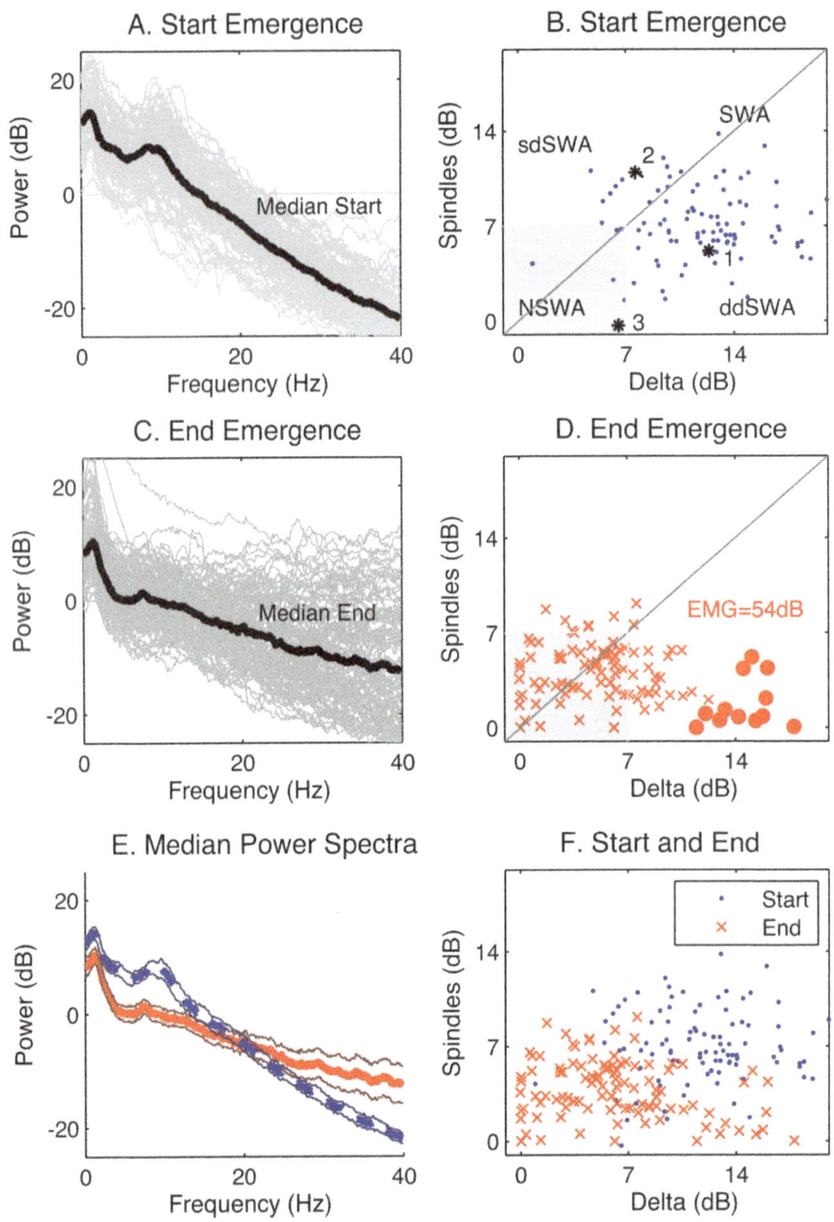

Figure 2. Emergence from general anesthesia is characterized by a loss in power in the slower spindle and delta frequency bands, and a recovery of power in the higher frequency bands. Power spectra and scatterplots of delta and spindle power (dB) for all patients, at the start (2A, 2B) and the end (2C, 2D) of emergence. The thick black lines are the median of the power spectra at each frequency for all patients. The median power spectra and 95% confidence intervals of the median, at the start and end, are shown in 2E. Patients were separated into two main spectral classes by thresholding spindle and delta power at 7 dB, whose boundary is marked by the gray box (see also Figure S1). Thus, the most common pattern, seen in 95% patients at Start Emergence, is characterized by high power (>7 dB) in both frequency bands, which we define as **'Slow-Wave Anesthesia (SWA)'**; the alternate pattern, defined as **'Non Slow-Wave Anesthesia (NSWA)'**, represents the 5% of patients that fall within the gray box. The fuzzy clusters in 2B are defined in the text: SWA = Slow-Wave Anesthesia, ddSWA = delta-dominant Slow-Wave Anesthesia, sdSWA = spindle-dominant Slow-Wave Anesthesia, NSWA = Non Slow-Wave Anesthesia (gray box). Red circles in 2D are those patients with a high delta power at End Emergence. All except one subject with high delta at End Emergence also had an EMG>40 dB. 2F is the same as 2B and 2D superimposed for ease of visual comparison.

that describe the progression toward conscious awareness during emergence. These emergence patterns do not consistently follow the averaged patterns of volunteers undergoing slow infusions of propofol described in prior studies [8,9], but in some instances do share similarities with sleep stages that precede awakening. Further, we noted that the trajectory taken to re-establish conscious awareness is not correlated to the brain state at the cessation of the anesthetic (End Maintenance), but the path taken to re-establishing awareness does appear to have some correlation with a subject's subsequent level of sedation and post-operative pain. Our work suggests that the central nervous system may not always re-establish connectivity in a canonical sequence after unconsciousness produced by general anesthesia during surgery. We hypothesize that these less typical emergence sequences under

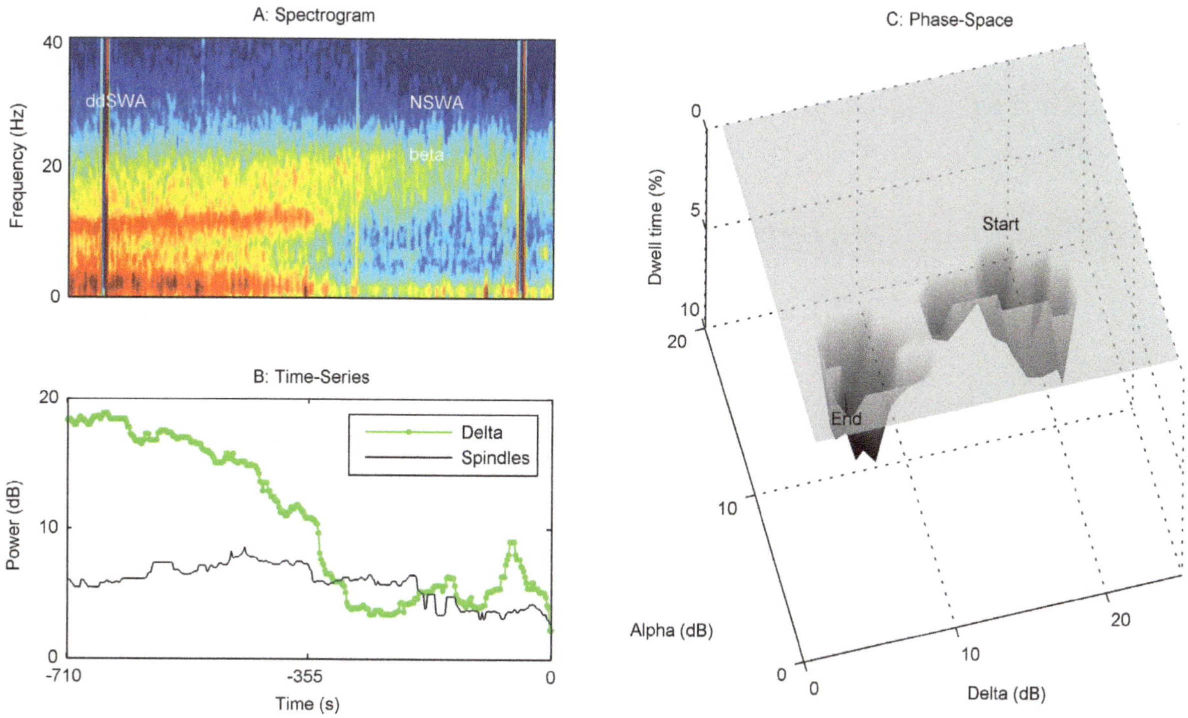

Figure 3. Emergence Trajectory 1, SWA → NSWA. The upper left panel (A) is the spectrogram from Start Emergence (measured in negative seconds) to End Emergence (time 0 seconds) for a representative patient (#81); this also corresponds to the time of anesthetic wash-out from the brain. Below it is a time series (B) that quantifies spindle and delta power (dB) over the same emergence period. To the right is a dwell time state-space plot (C). The evolution of spindle and delta power over the emergence trajectory from Start Emergence (upper right) to End Emergence (lower left) is shown where the depth of the contour (y-axis) reflects the time spent in each pixel of the state, as a percentage of the total emergence time. At the start of emergence, this patient remained for a signficant period in a slow-wave state (SWA) characterized by higher delta to spindle power ratio (ddSWA). There was a relatively abrupt transition period of approximately 60 seconds, to a second attractor characterized by lower delta and spindle power (NSWA) prior to waking-up. In our sample, 23% of patients had a similar trajectory.

anesthesia may predispose patients to undesirable wake-ups, in a similar way that parasomnias are exacerbated by disrupted sleep architecture [54].

Results

Patterns during maintenance in the human frontal electroencephalograph can be divided into four (4) basic spectral variants

In order to define a nomenclature for anesthetic maintenance, we analyzed the relative contribution amongst major oscillatory features found in the power spectra of the frontal electroencephalogram (EEG) of 100 patients undergoing routine orthopedic surgery under general anesthesia. The time at which the anesthetic was turned off was defined as the 'End Maintenance' or 'Start Emergence' point. A spectrogram of EEG data from a single frontal EEG electrode for 5 minutes prior to End Maintenance was computed for each individual patient. Visual inspection revealed clear peaks in the spectrogram within the delta and alpha bands of some patients, but these peaks showed considerable variation across the population (Figure 1A-D). The power spectra and a scatterplot of delta power against the oscillatory component of alpha power, computed over an 8 second EEG window (see Methods) for all 100 patients at Start Emergence, are shown in Figures 2A and 2B. The oscillatory component of alpha power was quantified by measuring the height of the alpha peak above the underlying broadband activity [55]. This has the advantage that it specifically targets the narrowband oscillatory component of this peak, and is less influenced by the underlying broadband ($1/f$) components of the EEG, making the alpha oscillatory power more orthogonal to the delta power. In this study we have chosen to borrow the term 'spindles' from the sleep literature to describe the specific oscillatory component in the alpha range from the overall composite alpha power [5]. Although the scatterplot in Figure 2B does not readily segregate into discrete clusters, we followed statistical convention and separated the patients into two main spectral classes by thresholding spindle and delta power at 7 dB. Because the bi-variate data appears to follow a unimodal distribution, the 7dB theshold reflects the boundary below which only 5% of the Start Emergence data lay, and the region within which most of the End Emergence data lay (Figure S1). Thus, the most common pattern, seen in 95% patients at Start Emergence, is characterized by high power (>7 dB) in both frequency bands, which we define as **'Slow-Wave Anesthesia (SWA)**;' this includes patients above the 7 dB boundary marked by the gray box. Some patients have a relatively equal distribution of spindle and delta power during SWA, lying on or near the unity diagonal (Figure 2B). However, it was more common in this patient sample for delta power to be greater than spindle power during SWA. This is represented by the preponderance of points lying below the diagonal in Figure 2B. We therefore propose the term **'delta-dominant Slow-Wave Anesthesia'** (**ddSWA**, Figure 1A) to describe this sub-classification. Conversely when spindle power is greater than delta power (i.e. points above the diagonal, Figure 2B), we propose the term **'spindle-dominant Slow-Wave Anesthesia'** (**sdSWA**, Figure 1B). In this sample, we

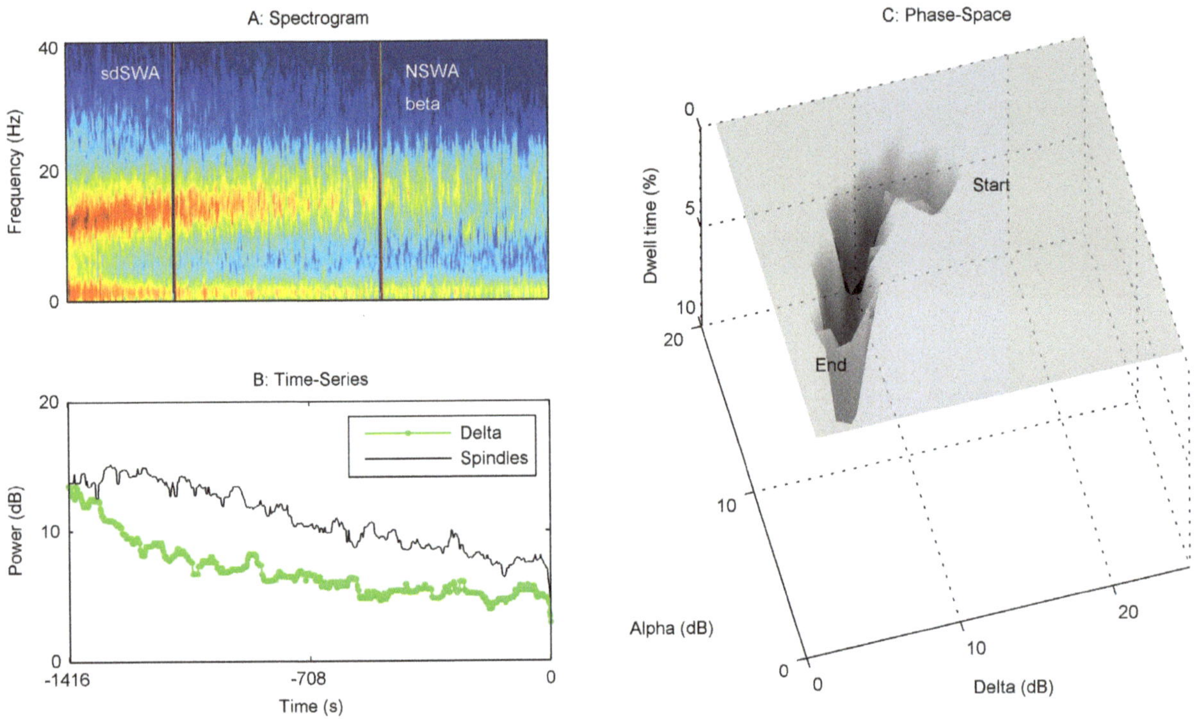

Figure 4. Emergence Trajectory 2, SWA→NSWA, continuous progression. The spectrogram (A) and time series (B) from Start Emergence to End Emergence for a representative patient (#36) are shown. To the right is dwell time state-space plot (C). This patient started in a slow-wave state (SWA). Over approximately 1.5 minutes, the patient transitioned into a state characterized by higher spindle power (sdSWA), and then showed a progressive decrease in delta and spindle power towards the NSWA region over about 20 minutes before waking. There was a converse increase in beta power as alpha/spindle power was diminished. No single deep attractor in state-space characterizes this patient's emergence path until reaching NSWA prior to wake-up. In our sample, 20% of patients had a similar trajectory.

noted a continuum of relative spindle and delta power between patients, and even within patients during the course of their anesthetic. Because of this we have purposely left the terms sdSWA and ddSWA somewhat loosely defined – they are convenient labels that indicate a patient (in SWA) has relatively stronger spindle or delta waves. These plots are generated over a short snap-shot in time; thus, a patient in a ddSWA pattern may gradually lose delta power and transition into an sdSWA pattern over the course of an anesthetic. Five percent (5%) of patients had Start Emergence EEGs with a very low spindle and delta power (<7 dB) – we termed these indeterminate patterns "**Non Slow-Wave Anesthesia**" (**NSWA**, Figure 1C). An example of another common maintenance pattern, that of burst suppression (transitioning into SWA) is shown in Figure 1D, for as complete a description as possible of spectral patterns encountered during surgical anesthesia. This pattern is more typically seen post-induction of general anesthesia (i.e. just after loss of consciousness is achieved with a bolus dose of propofol), but may be seen during the entire course of the maintenance phase of anesthesia.

Emergence from general anesthesia is characterized by a shift from a slow-wave pattern (SWA) to a more uniform distribution of power across all frequency bands

In order to characterize salient features of the EEG at the start (i.e. turning off anesthetic) and end of emergence (i.e. responsiveness to standard verbal stimulation), the power-spectral density (PSD) plots for individual patients were compared in each condition. The plots in the left column of Figure 2 show the power spectra for all patients (gray), derived from the 8 second EEG segments at the start (Figure 2A) and end of emergence (Figure 2C). There is considerable variation in individual patient spectral power, encompassing a 30 dB range (equivalent to an approximately five-fold variation in raw voltage) at both Start and End Emergence, with greater spread in the higher frequency bands (>14 Hz) during End Emergence. The thick black line in both Figures 2A and 2C are the median power spectra for each condition. Distinct peaks are present at Start Emergence/End Maintenance in the delta and spindle frequency bands. At End Emergence, the spindle peak is lost, and the delta peak diminishes in amplitude. The scatterplots in Figures 2B and 2D, in which delta and spindle power are plotted against one another for each patient, clearly show the downward shift in power in both these frequency bands (from 2B to 2D). There is a small subset of patients (12%) at End Emergence that maintains high delta power (red dots in Figure 2D); this subset is also the group that showed high EMG at End Emergence (>40 dB) suggesting that the high delta power is actually broad-band contamination of the EEG with frontalis muscle activity rather than true frontal cortical activity. For ease of comparison, the shifts in median power spectra at Start (blue) and End Emergence (red) are shown in Figure 2E, while the downward shift in spindle-delta power at Start (blue) and End Emergence (red) is summarized in Figure 2F. As a whole, the median power spectra at End Emergence demonstrates a more uniform distribution of power in the 20–40 Hz range, consistent with recent studies in human volunteers receiving propofol infusions [8,9], but with more variability as evidenced by broader confidence intervals.

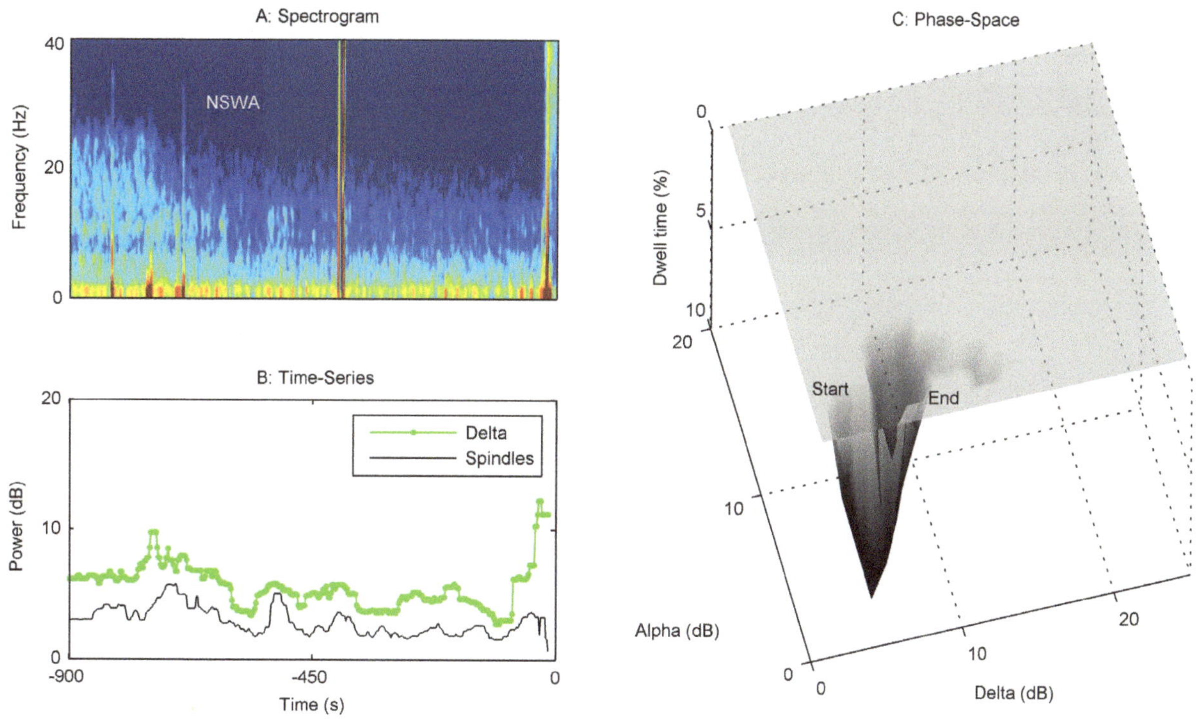

Figure 5. Emergence Trajectory 3, NSWA→Wakefulness. The spectrogram (A) and time series (B) from Start Emergence to End Emergence for a representative patient (#19) are shown. To the right is a dwell time state-space plot (C). This patient started and ended in a state characterized by a non slow-wave state (NSWA) attractor prior to waking up. The duration of emergence was long (15 minutes), and the attractor did not move significantly. In our sample, 16% of patients had a similar trajectory.

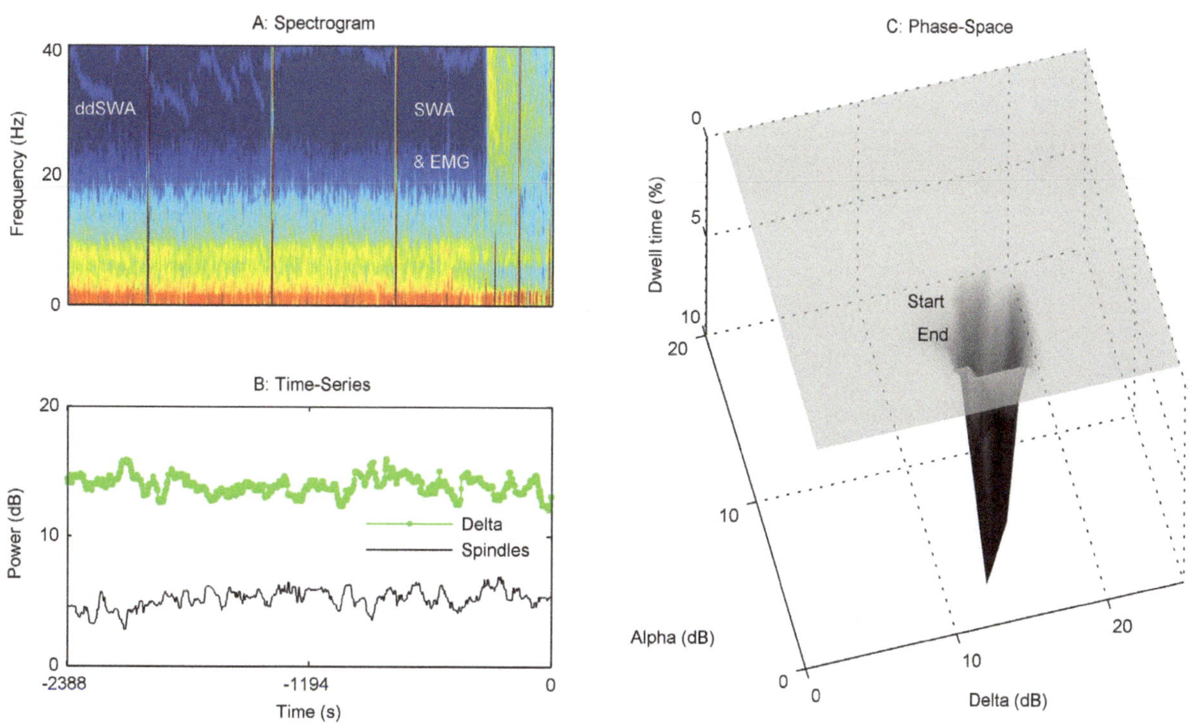

Figure 6. Emergence Trajectory 4, SWA→Wakefulness. The spectrogram (A) and time series (B) from Start Emergence to End Emergence for a representative patient (77) are shown. To the right is a dwell time state-space plot (C). This patient started and ended in a state characterized by a slow-wave state (SWA) attractor prior to waking up. Patients who woke up this abruptly from a slow-wave state of anesthesia were more likely to experience high pain in recovery. In our sample, 31% of patients had a similar trajectory.

Table 1. Level of Consciousness and Pain.

PACU-Cons Score	
0	Confused
1	Quickly alert (Ramsay score = 2 at 15 minutes)
2	Somnolent (Ramsay score = 3 or 4 at 15 minutes)
PACU-Pain Score	
0	Minimal (NRS = 0–3 and relaxed)
1	Moderate (NRS = 4–8 and relaxed or going back to sleep)
2	Severe (NRS = 8–10 or NRS>4 and signs of distress)

PACU = Post anesthesia care unit, Cons = consciousness, NRS = numerical rating scale

Evolution of trajectories from Start Emergence to End Emergence vary by patient

Figure 2 captures a static image of the state of the brain at the start and end of emergence. While a shift from one average state to another can be seen in Figure 2E, the variability of individual patient PSDs and spindle-delta power scatterplots suggests that the path from Start to End Emergence may not be identical or stereotyped. Clinically, this is often reflected in the length of time a patient takes to emerge from general anesthesia. We chose not to average patient trajectories, and instead looked for graphical methods to describe changes for individual patients. This involved construction of an 'emergence trajectory' for each patient. A spectrogram from Start to End Emergence was first calculated (Figure 3–6A), and a time series data of spindle and delta power extracted from the power spectrum (Figure 3–6B). Finally, we applied a dynamical systems approach to the data, creating a corresponding 3-D 'dwell time plot' for each patient's emergence trajectory (Figure 3–6C). These graphically depict how the relative spindle and delta power changes for each patient in response to the progressive decline in both anesthetic drug concentrations and the residuum of surgical nociception from the time the anesthetic is turned off until the patient responded to voice. In these 'phase-space' plots, spindle power is reflected on the y-axis, delta power on the x-axis, and the z-axis reflects the time spent in each 'pixel' of state-space as a percentage of the total emergence time ("dwell time"). From these surfaces, we can see that a continuous, progressive decrease in spindle and delta power was **not** the usual pattern of emergence. Instead the majority of patients tended to follow a more "punctated equilibrium" pattern, occupying restricted regions of the state-space for extended periods of time, before relatively rapidly moving to other areas of phase space, or to the waking state. At first approximation, these areas appear to functionally act as point attractors [56]. At Start Emergence, most (95%) of these point attractors can be classified as SWA, or a sub-classification (sdSWA or ddSWA), while at End Emergence, the majority (59%) are classified as NSWA. The path from Start Emergence to End Emergence took variable trajectories. These were roughly classified by the presence of one or two attractors, whether these attractors lay in the SWA or NSWA regions, and whether the transition to a new state was rapid or gradual through the phase-space. Figure 3 demonstrates a common emergence trajectory (23% of patients). It shows an initial attractor in the SWA region, which steps abruptly to a second attractor in NSWA space, followed by arousal. The second trajectory (20%) is similar to the first except it shows a more gradual transition between SWA and NSWA state space (Figure 4). Figure 5 describes a third trajectory (16%), a single attractor in NSWA, which reflects a patient who spends nearly the entire duration of emergence in NSWA before responding to voice. The fourth trajectory (31%) is characterized by a patient who woke up directly from SWA (Figure 6). About 10% of patients fell into indeterminate categories. We would note that during emergence many patients who start emergence in the ddSWA go on to lose their delta power and gained spindle power during their emergence; this resulted in nearly half (49%) of patients spending more than 25% of their time in the sdSWA region. This transition pattern is analogous to that seen in the progression from deep to lighter natural NREM stage 2 sleep. At the other extreme, 27% patients spend no time in the sdSWA region at all, as if NREM stage 2 sleep was skipped during the process of waking.

Evolution of trajectories from Start Emergence to End Emergence are correlated to nociceptive state and level of consciousness upon waking

We next examined whether there was an association with, the relative time spent in SWA vs. NSWA, and the *quality of emergence*. Two post-anesthesia scores were used to quantify level of consciousness and post-operative pain (Table 1). Because sedation can interfere with reported pain, we measured pain heuristically by combining self-reported pain score with non-reported signs of distress. We found an association between lower pain scores and the relative amount of time spent in NSWA during emergence (Figure 7). Those who spent a long time in a non slow-wave state prior to wake-up were more likely to waken with minimal pain (PACU-Pain = 0) than those who woke directly from a slow-wave state ($p = 0.037$, Chi-squared test; $p = 0.0017$ for delta power distribution, $p = 0.05$ for alpha power distribution; Kolmogorov-Smirnov test). This is reflected in the averaged dwell-time contour map for the low and high pain groups (Figure 8).

Associations amongst patient variables with delta and spindle power

The delta power at the start of emergence was negatively correlated with age ($r = -0.44$, $p<0.0001$), and positively correlated with the C_eMAC ($r = 0.24$, $p = 0.015$). Combined in a multiple regression model, these two variables explained 21% of the variability in delta power. Addition of anesthetic agent, regional block and gender insignificantly increased this to 24%. Delta power was not correlated with $C_eOpioid$. The spindle power was also negatively correlated with age ($r = -0.34$, $p = 0.0003$) and with duration of operation ($r = -0.29$, $p = 0.002$). When combined with the C_eMAC, the model explained 23% of the variation in spindle power. However older patients were also more likely to have longer operations ($r = 0.25$, $p = 0.01$), and receive less volatile anesthetic drug ($r = -0.19$, $p = 0.05$).

Associations amongst patient variables, emergence time, and post-operative pain

Emergence time was positively correlated with the duration of operation ($r = 0.24$, $p = 0.014$), and weakly influenced by the C_eMAC ($r = 0.18$, $p = 0.07$). Consistent with prior studies [57–60], male patients were slower to emerge ($p = 0.02$) than females. In this study, we found that different volatile drugs had no significant influence on emergence time, but the number of patients receiving desflurane or isoflurane was small. The multivariate model of emergence time is given below (the presence of a regional block is coded as 1, the absence as 0; the difference between the genders was included as a categorical variable [1/0]).

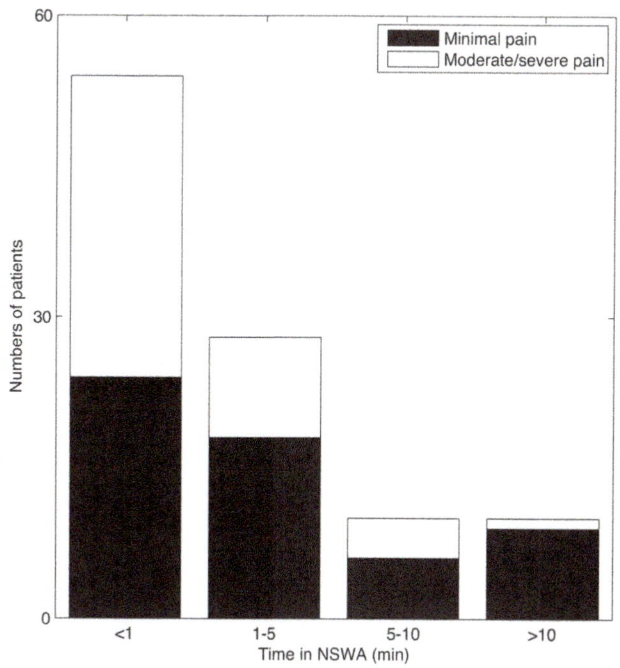

Figure 7. Increased time spent in a non slow-wave state (NSWA) during emergence is correlated with a lower nociceptive state. Patients had a variable duration of emergence from the time the anesthetic was turned off, ranging from 2 minutes to more than 10 minutes, as well as a variable dwell-time in the state of NSWA. When divided into 4 groups based on NSWA dwell-time, patients that spent more time in NSWA prior to emerging were more likely to have minimal pain (PACU-pain =0, Table 1). Of the group that spent>10 minutes in NSWA prior to wake-up, 90% had minimal pain. Of the group that spent less than a minute in NSWA prior to wake-up, 44% had minimal pain ($p = 0.037$, Chi-squared test).

$$Log[Emergence\ Time(min)] = 0.75 + 0.004 \times [Rregional\ Block] + 0.20 \times [C_e MAC] + 0.036 \times [Delta\ Power] + 0.05 \times [gender\ Male - Female] + 0.001 \times [Operation\ Duration(min)] \quad (1)$$

Although the model is statistically significant, these explanatory variables are not a very good explanation of the variation in emergence time, as the r^2 value was only 0.16.

When combined in the logistic regression model, the effect site concentration of opioid at the start of emergence, expressed in fentanyl equivalents (C_eOpioid), duration of NSWA, and male gender were the most significant associations with postoperative pain. A higher opioid concentration was associated with more pain. We attribute this unusual observation to the fact that patients who were expected to have more painful operations would have been given more (but presumably not enough) opioids intraoperatively. This model had a modest predictive capability (area under ROC $= 0.71$), but again the strength of association was quite weak ($r^2 = 0.11$).

$$Probability[Severe\ pain/Mild\ pain] = -0.23 + 1.08 \times [C_e Opioid] - 0.004 \times [NSWA] - 0.61 \times [gender\ Male - Female] \quad (2)$$

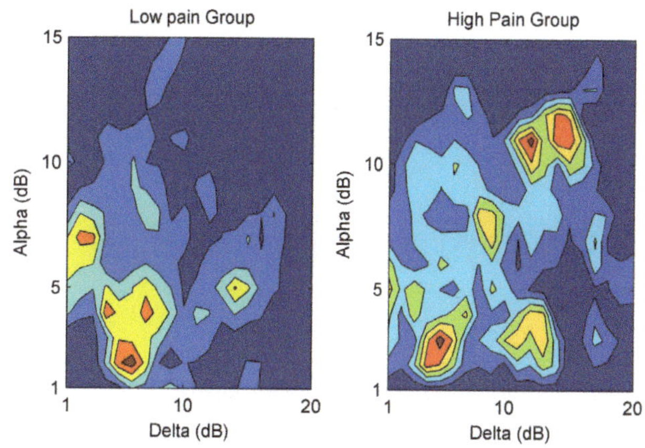

Figure 8. Patients with low pain scores (0) spend more time in a non slow-wave (NSWA) pattern during emergence while patients with higher pain scores (2) spend more time in a slow-wave pattern (SWA). This is reflected in the averaged trajectories through the spindle-delta state space for the low (left panel) and high pain (right panel) groups. The heat map from blue to red reflects least to most time.

Associations amongst patient variables and different EEG patterns of emergence

The heterogeneity in patterns of emergence seem to be largely determined by unknown intrinsic factors, and are not strongly related to the common clinical explanatory variables. We found no significant associations between the EEG emergence pattern group and simple clinical and demographic variables – namely postoperative pain, type of volatile anaesthetic drug, gender, the presence of a regional block, operation duration, or the C_eMAC. However those patients that started in SWA, but then spent a period of time in the NSWA attractor before transitioning to wakefulness tended to be younger (mean(SEM) 43(4) years vs. 58(3) years, $p = 0.015$) and have a higher C_eOpioid (0.80(0.09) vs. 0.44(0.08) ng/ml fentanyl equivalents, $p = 0.04$), than those who jumped directly from a SWA state to wakefulness. Thus the relationship between C_eOpioid, postoperative pain, and EEG emergence pattern, is complex and remains to be fully elucidated in larger studies.

EMG Activation During Emergence

The BIS EEG monitor attributes the power (dB) in the frequency range 70–110 Hz to the frontalis EMG signal, because it lies above the frequency band at which there is significant scalp EEG power. Typically the EMG power is low during general anaesthesia, and then rather abruptly increases in a stepwise fashion at various points during the emergence period. Often there are no overt clinical signs of an increase in muscle tone, or any gross motor movement. After examination of the EMG records, we chose the point at which the EMG power rose above 40 dB as a time point that reflected the activation of the EMG with reasonable face validity. The most striking feature was that the activation of the EMG often had quite a different time course to the EEG changes. The interval between EMG activation and End Emergence approximately followed an exponential probability distribution. For a quarter of the patients, their EMG became activated coincident with their waking (response to voice). Another one-half of patients woke within 74 seconds of EMG activation. However, a quarter of patients had a prolonged interval of at least 334 seconds between EMG activation and waking. The strongest

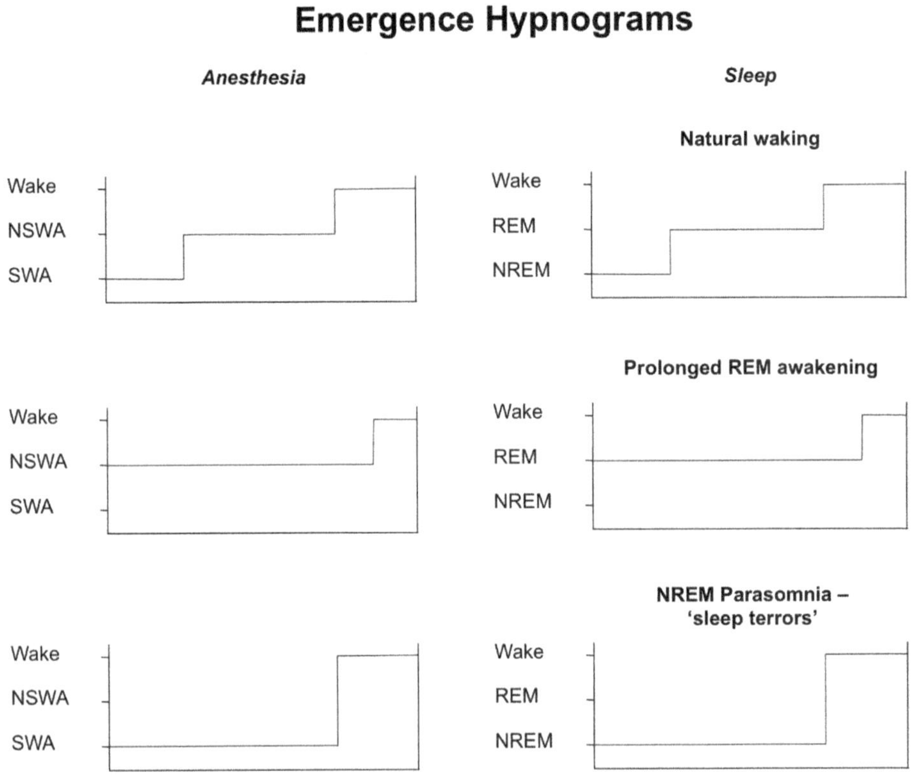

Figure 9. Hypnograms for emergence from general anesthesia and sleep. Temporal evolution of stages of arousal during emergence from general anesthesia (GA) are plotted in the left column, and from sleep in the right column. Each GA hypnogram on the left reflects an identified Emergence Trajectory as defined earlier in the text. These trajectories might be loosely correlated with arousal trajectories from various stages of sleep that are placed immediately to the right. SWA = Slow-Wave Anesthesia, NSWA = Non Slow-Wave Anesthesia; NREM = non-REM sleep, REM = REM sleep.

correlations were with duration of operation ($r = 0.23$, $p = 0.02$) and age ($r = 0.21$, $p = 0.03$).

Discussion

A Nomenclature for Distinguishing Between Anesthetic Maintenance States

In this study, we present a conceptual framework to discriminate four patterns of anesthetic maintenance comprised of two states, 'Slow-Wave Anesthesia' (SWA) and 'Non Slow-Wave Anesthesia' (NSWA), and two derivative sub-classes of the slow-wave state, 'delta-dominant' (ddSWA) and 'spindle-dominant' (sdSWA). These classes were defined by the relative contribution of delta (0.5–4 Hz) and spindle-alpha (8–14 Hz) power in their spectral signatures (Figure 2B). These sub-14 Hz oscillations that dominate the EEG during both NREM (slow-wave) sleep and general anesthesia have been shown to correspond to diminished responsiveness to mild stimuli in NREM sleep [41,61] and to more aversive stimuli during general anesthesia [9,62,63]. Because these oscillations can also be correlated with specific neural generators in a more generally hyperpolarized reticulothalamocortical circuit, they have been used for decades to classify stages of natural sleep. We were therefore able to capitalize on the methods by which sleep is staged and dynamically tracked over time (Figures 1, 9) to generate a new standardized taxonomy that could be used to describe the maintenace phase of general anesthesia. Although a pattern similar to the spindle-dominant slow-wave pattern (sdSWA) has been previously reported in studies in which volunteers are exposed to slowly changing levels of propofol anesthesia [8,64], the greater diversity of patterns we observed may be due to the lack of spectral averaging in our subjects, the greater diversity of the typical surgical population (e.g. baseline neurological status and co-morbidities, pre-operative medication status, baseline pain sensitivity), and the highly variable surgical environment (e.g. intraoperative medication administration, surgical stimulation, nociception).

A Description of Emergence Trajectories

We examined the transition from unconsciousness back to conscious awareness (i.e. responsiveness) after general anesthesia was terminated at the conclusion of surgery, from End Maintenance/Start Emergence to End Emergence. We found a general shift from the slow-wave pattern (SWA) to a more uniform distribution of power across frequency bands (NSWA). This trend was immediately visible and highly significant when the grand average of EEG spectra across the entire patient population was performed at the beginning and end of emergence (Figure 2E, $p < 0.05$). However, just as with the maintenance patterns, individual patient emergence trajectories from unconsciousness to waking were more variable than averaged trajectories [8,9] (Figure 2F, Figures 3–6). We speculate that inactivation of endogenous sleep networks, activation of redundant arousal networks, and the nociceptive residuum experienced by the patient, contribute to this variability. In order to minimize non-surgical noxious stimuli, an LMA was used as the airway device, and auditory and tactile stimulation during emergence was limited (see Methods); we

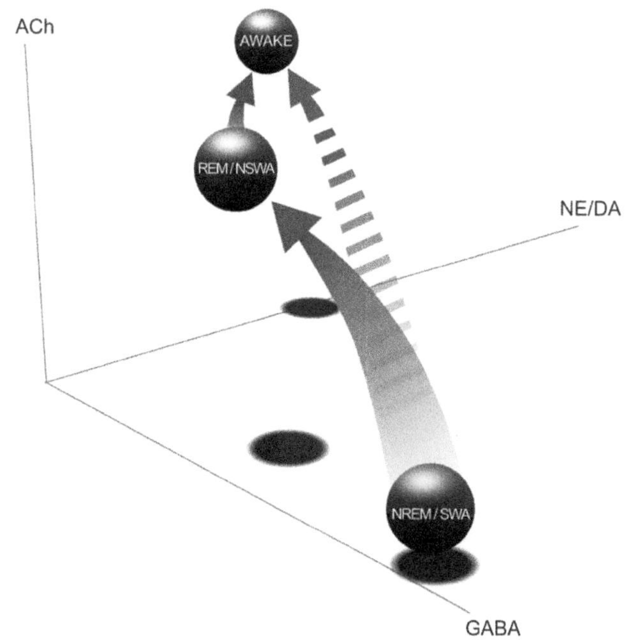

Figure 10. A putative (shared) 3-D neurotransmitter state space for emergence from sleep and general anesthesia. Based on spectral power and underlying neural generators, stages of anesthesia and stages of sleep may be analagous, especially on the path from thalamocortical hyperpolarization to waking. During natural NREM sleep, levels of GABA are high, while REM is characterized by high levels of both GABA and acetylcholine (ACh). As the brain passes from REM to waking, levels of GABA diminish, and monoamines such as norepinephrine and dopamine start to increase. The progression on the more typical anesthetic-emergence trajectory from SWA -> NSWA -> waking may reflect a similar shift in neurotransmitter balance as shown in this diagram (solid arrow). The "non-preferred" pathway of emergence that transitions directly from SWA -> waking (somewhat analagous to NREM -> waking) is represented by the broken arrow. NREM = non-REM sleep, REM = rapid eye movement sleep, SWA = Slow-Wave Anesthesia, NSWA = Non Slow-Wave Anesthesia, GABA = GABA-aminobutyric acid, ACh = acetylcholine, NE = norepinephrine, DA = dopamine.

therefore do not attribute this variability to tracheal or general environmental stimulation. More importantly, these diverse emergence patterns suggest that recovery from general anesthesia does not necessarily mirror the induction process, and may reflect a behavioral state barrier, which depends in part on the balance of activation in endogenous sleep and arousal pathways [31,65–67].

Using a dynamical systems approach, we grouped 100 observed emergence trajectories in state-space into categories based on the apparent number of attractors during emergence, the time each subject occupied that stable attractor state, and the time required to transition between attractor states (Figures 3–6). As with any empirical study, the exact dynamical system classification of the attractor topology is provisional. Although the attractors resembled simple point attractors, more detailed studies of the EEG dynamics might reveal some high dimensional chaotic or limit cycle structure within these attractors. With those provisos, almost half (43%) of patients exhibited a canonical sequence: loss of delta, followed by loss of spindles, and then a period of NSWA (characterized by the absence of low frequency oscillatory peaks in the EEG and behavioral unresponsiveness), before waking. In contrast, approximately one-third (31%) of subjects skip the NSWA stage and transition directly from SWA to wakefulness (Trajectory 4), and 16% do not achieve SWA at any stage during end maintenance or emergence (Trajectory 3). We also observed a sharp increase in electromyographic power (EMG) that often precedes the return of consciousness, but is not a necessary prerequisite.

Connections between Emergence Trajectories and Post-operative Recovery

The time spent in NSWA prior to wake-up (defined on the dwell-time plots from Figures 3–6) was modestly predictive of subsequent pain (Figures 7–8). Patients who spent little of their emergence time in NSWA, were more likely to have high pain, and express a degree of agitation in recovery. (A similarly sudden transition from slow wave sleep directly to wakefulness is associated with some sleep pathologies such as night terrors [53,68], see also FIgure 9). These patients often had more frontal EMG activation during emergence, which in itself was weakly associated with a higher pain score in the PACU. Frontalis muscle activation (EMG) in patients can in itself confound the results. The EMG signature is broad-band and can potentially contaminate, distort or obscure the underlying EEG signal. Conversely EMG activation is a valuable indication of motor system activation as part of the emergence sequence from anesthesia, and we found it to be largely independent of the return of consciousness, as defined by recovery of responsiveness to voice. This observation is in accord with other work suggesting that components of motor systems are relatively resistant to the effects of anesthesia, and that recovery of motor tone is not captured by changing information in the EEG which tends to reflect the hypnotic axis [69]. Different central nervous subsystems may not always reconnect in a well-defined sequence after general anesthesia is discontinued; in some instances, alternate paths or sequences for bringing various brain arousal nuclei or networks on-line preceding the return of consciousness may predispose patients to undesirable wake-ups, in the same way that parasomnias are exacerbated by disrupted sleep architecture [54]. Our measurements also do not assess recovery along the axis of memory, another subsystem affected by anesthetics and sleep.

The evolution of trajectories from Start to End Emergence can be captured in an emergence hypnogram for general anesthesia

Figure 9 graphically depicts the evolution of each of the emergence trajectory patterns (Figures 3–6) and compares these patterns to arousal from specific stages of sleep. Carrying the analogy between waking from natural sleep and emergence from general anesthesia further, we propose using a hypnogram to capture the emergence trajectories from general anesthesia (left column) seen in Figures 3–6, where the length of the horizontal line at each stages reflects the relative dwell-time in the state-space plot (panel C of Figures 3–6). These can be compared to the sequences of emergence from natural sleep, seen in the right column, in the more classic version of the emergence hypnogram. A transition from SWA to NSWA before waking may correspond most closely to the waking from natural sleep. Waking from very prolonged NSWA may not have a correlate in normal sleep (prolonged REM awakening), but may instead reflect certain hypersomnia subtypes [70]. The emergence trajectory of an abrupt transition from SWA to wakefulness can be compared to arousal during NREM sleep, often associated with parasomnias or sleep disturbances resulting from fragmented sleep [53,54].

Table 2. Demographic Data.

Age (yrs)	48(19)
Gender (F/M)	48/52
Duration of surgery (min)	99(68)
Duration of emergence (min)	12.4 [8.4 to 18.9]
Sevo/Des/Isoflurane	81/8/11
C_eMAC_s	10.79 [0.66 to 0.98]
C_eMAC_e	0.06 [0.001 to 0.08]
$C_e$fentanyl$_e$ (ng/ml)	0.54 [0.31 to 0.78]
PACU-Cons (0/1/2)	17/42/41
PACU-Pain (0/1/2)	56/15/29

C_e denotes effect site concentration of the drug, and the subscripts 's' and 'e' denote the start and end of emergence. MAC indicates units of age adjusted Minimum Alveolar Concentration, PACU-Cons and PACU-Pain are defined in the text and in Table 1.

The Neurochemical Relationship Between Sleep Circuitry And General Anesthesia

The degree of thalamocortical hyperpolarization depends on the balance of activity in neurotransmitters systems [71,72]. While there are many regional and nuclear brain differences, NREM sleep tends to be dominated by high GABAergic and low cholinergic and monoaminergic tone, while REM sleep is dominated by both GABAergic and cholinergic tone, and low levels of monoamines [73,74]. We postulate that the presence of spindles and delta oscillations within the stage we define as SWA also reflects overwhelming GABAergic tone and low cholinergic tone, consistent with the mechanism of action of many of our volatile and intravenous anesthetics. The exact sequence of neuromodulator activation during emergence from anaesthesia is unknown, and is probably the main cause for the heterogeneity that we observed in the emergence trajectories. As anesthetic washes out of the brain, the residual GABAergic effects of the drug may be antagonized by depolarizing cholinergic (or aminergic) systems, pushing the brain into the NSWA state. The reason for transition from this point to waking is unclear, but probably involves a switch from high GABAergic tone to high monoaminergic and orexinergic tone, allowing the patient to fully emerge and reconnect with the external world. These pathways may be visualized in a 3-D neurotransmitter diagram for NREM/SWA, REM/NSWA, and waking states (Figure 10). The solid arrow signals a "preferred" wake-up sequence in which a patient moves from SWA to NSWA prior to waking, and experiences a higher degree of conscious awareness and a lower degree of pain and agitation in recovery (i.e. the classic cycle of NREM to REM to waking). The "non-preferred" sequence – in which the brain transitions directly from SWA to waking state – is reflected by the broken arrow, which if compared to sleep, would characterize a parasomnic or less desirable trajectory to re-establishing conscious awareness.

Underlying Neurobiology of EEG Signatures of Emergence and their Relationship to Sleep

Both sleep and general anesthesia share many similarities, including specific nuclei, circuitry, and neurotransmitter systems. Physiological recordings [75–76] and modeling [64,77] suggest that the oscillatory components of the alpha band (spindles between 8–14 Hz) in the frontal EEG during sleep and anesthesia are generated by hyperpolarizing neurons of the reticular nucleus of the thalamus, in the permissive environment of depressed ascending cholinergic and monoaminergic brainstem activity [75], which switches them to a burst firing mode [78–80]. Spindles predominate in NREM stage 2 sleep, and are more commonly observed during general anesthesia when analgesics are administered to diminish noxious stimulation [63]. NREM stage 3 sleep reflects an even greater degree of thalamocortical hyperpolarization as spindle activity diminishes and slower delta oscillations (0.5–1 Hz) begin to dominate [40]. Because our data demonstrate a positive correlation between anesthetic dose and relative delta power [81] we suggest that NREM stage 3 sleep may be similar to a ddSWA pattern under anesthesia, and NREM stage 2 sleep to an sdSWA pattern. This notion is further supported by the observation that at the midpoint of emergence (with decreasing anesthetic dose) there is an increase in the number of subjects categorized as sdSWA.

A progressive depolarization within the corticothalamic system accompanies the ordered transition to waking from natural sleep. This state is termed REM and is typically the stage of sleep from which most individuals awaken. Similarly, most subjects emerging from general anesthesia appear to move progressively from SWA to NSWA. Can NSWA be likened to REM sleep? Approximately 25% of patients report dream mentation if queried immediately upon waking, and it was more common for the group who reported dreaming to be in NSWA (i.e. have low power in the $<$ 14 Hz range) prior to waking [55]. Thus, SWA and NSWA may directly correspond to different levels of activation in the two distinct networks of conscious awareness (i.e. awareness of environment and awareness of self) described by others [82]. NSWA may reflect an unresponsive state in which some form of internally-directed consciousness has been established (e.g. fronto-parietal connectivity), but there is still insufficient brain function to connect externally. This is consistent with the concept of an unconnected (i.e. with the external world) or covert consciousness, which has been seen using carefully controlled propofol infusions in human volunteers with combined fMRI/EEG [9]. The thalamocortical network is rendered insensate to external inputs, yet activation to stimuli is still observed in cortical areas such as the precuneus. The role of the thalamus is less clear. It plays an important role in sleep, but its contribution to anesthesia has been questioned [83], and thalamic deactivation may not be the cause of unconsciousness but rather a consequence, via a functional thalamic de-afferentation from diminished cortical connectedness [84,85].

One significant limitation to this study is that we only used a frontal EEG electrode strip for our recordings. Our data is therefore constrained to data gathered from accessible frontal leads (corresponding approximatley to FPz, FP1/2 from a traditional 10–20 montage) without simultaneous recording from parietal, temporal or occipital regions. We therefore could not consider other markers of loss and return of consciousness such as global coherence [8,16] or the degree of connectedness and communication between different cortical regions [11,13–15,86]. However, EEG power is largely anteriorized upon loss of consciousness under general anesthesia [11,16,17,87], making the frontal leads reasonable markers for spectral changes that can be observed at the single electrode level. Use of commercially available EEG electrodes that can be easily placed on a patient's forehead intraoperatively as part of the placement of routine monitors also increases the likelihood that our methods for tracking and staging depth of consciousness could be used more routinely by clinicians making real-time decisions in the operating room. Our data indicate that a long period of NSWA before waking is associated with less pain than a direct transition from SWA to waking. Without further prospective randomized clinical studies, it is unclear whether it would actually be clinically useful to specifically titrate anesthetic (or analgesic) drugs to target any particular intraoperative spectral pattern. Apart from the effect of age on spectral power, we found relatively weak correlations between clinical variables and spectral pattern. This would suggest that the spectral pattern for each patient is largely determined by other unknown (possibly inherited) factors. Nevertheless we would hope that this study provides a methodological framework in which these questions could be answered.

Conclusions

The unconsciousness that accompanies general anesthesia during surgery is marked by several, distinct, oscillatory patterns in the EEG. Because these share features with those observed in natural sleep, it is possible that the underlying neural generators are conserved. Building upon a classification system used to stage sleep, we provide, for the first time, a standardized EEG-based nomenclature by which anesthetic maintenance can be staged and followed intraoperatively. We also applied a dynamical systems approach to characterize the return to consciousness after discontinuation of the anesthetic. We found that recovery of consciousness varies amongst individuals, and that deviations from a canonical sequence of SWA to NSWA occur. Further, the functional path by which the brain re-establishes conscious awareness is correlated with preferred wake-ups (e.g. diminished pain). We have created a descriptive means by which endogenous sleep rhythms and general anesthesia can be compared. Subsequent usage of this nomenclature should further our understanding of the overlapping neural mechanisms of sleep and anesthesia. As the homeostatic, learning and memory benefits of sleep are beginning to be characterized [88], future work may identify targets to improve post-operative cognitive health. The latter is of increasing concern as patients, researchers, and physicians become more apprehensive about the potential for anesthesia to cause or exacerbate adverse neurocognitive sequelae.

Methods

Ethics Statement

Studies were approved by the Northern Y Regional Ethics Committee of New Zealand (NTY/11/EXP/077), and written informed consent obtained from each patient. Free and public access to the de-identified data is available from the website: www.accesshq.org.

Patient Selection

We studied 100 adult patients presenting for routine orthopedic surgery under general anesthesia at Waikato Hospital, New Zealand, from November 2011 to January 2013. Data collection was restricted to patients eligible for laryngeal mask airway (LMA) management, considered less stimulating than an endotracheal tube [89], in order to minimize confounding effects of airway irritation, a strong non-surgical arousal stimulus, on the EEG. We specifically included patients who would be expected to have a wide range of post-surgical pain levels (some augmented with regional nerve blocks). We excluded patients with pre-existing psychiatric illness, chronic substance abuse, chronic pain, or obesity (BMI>35). Patient demographics are represented in Table 2.

Surgical Procedure and Data Collection

In order to determine the spread of emergence patterns at the conclusion of routine clinical anesthesia, we did not restrict the course of administration of the general anesthetic with the exception of limiting the airway device to an LMA, allowing it proceed according to the clinician's judgment. Patients were induced with a bolus dose of intravenous fentanyl (50–200 µg) followed by propofol (80–200 mg). Patients were maintained on a volatile general anesthetic (VA) of the clinician's choice - sevoflurane, desflurane, or isoflurane - delivered in a mixture of air and oxygen. No neuromuscular blocking drugs were used. Intraoperative analgesia was provided by intravenous morphine (0–25 mg); analgesic adjuncts of paracetamol (1 gm, n = 34), parecoxib (40 mg, n = 39), tramadol (100–200 mg, n = 22) or clonidine (60–120 µg, n = 18) were given as needed. 21 patients received a peripheral nerve block for post-operative analgesia; 14 of these were femoral blocks, done for reduction of postoperative muscle spasm for lower limb joint replacements. Because of the mutineuronal innervation of the knee and hip, most of these nerve blocks achieved incomplete analgesia. Of the others (mainly ankle blocks and brachial plexus blocks), 5 patients had pain scores of 0 on awakening – indicative of a completely successful block.

We used standard American Society of Anesthesiology [90] monitors (pulse oximeter, non-invasive blood pressure cuff, electrocardiogram, capnograph) to measure intraoperative oxygen saturation, hemodynamics, and end-tidal gas concentrations (O_2, CO_2, VA). In addition to these routine parameters, the times of surgery, tourniquet inflation and release, and drug administration were recorded.

A 2-lead EEG prefrontal electrode strip was placed on the patient's forehead, as per the manufacturer's recommendations (BIS, Covidien Vista). Frontal EEG data (sampling rate 128 Hz) was collected for the duration of the anesthetic, prior to induction through the end of emergence. The frontal EEG waveforms on the BIS sensor strip correlate approximately to the FPz and FP1/2 leads of standard 20 electrode EEG montage. Both electrodes are referenced by an additional electrode over the eyebrow. A separate lead over the temporalis muscle is used as an EMG electrode. Suitable electrode impedance (<5 kOhm) was confirmed using the manufacturer's automatic checking routine. To provide a mechanism to correlate external events with the patient's EEG, the times of surgical incision, cessation of the volatile anesthetic agent, and the exact moment of awakening were marked on the EEG record by tapping the electrodes 4 times in ~1.5 seconds to create a clear stimulus artifact. The patients were allowed to waken without excessive stimulation beyond the usual noise and activity of the operating room and post anesthesia care unit (PACU) environment (e.g. removal and replacement of monitors, background talking). Sustained awakening was confirmed by a positive response to verbal command ("Mrs. X, your operation is over, open your eyes."). 'Emergence' from general anesthesia was specifically defined as the time between the cessation of administration of the maintenance hypnotic drug (VA) and the point at which the patient became responsive to verbal command. Raw EEG and EMG data for each patient were downloaded post-operatively for further analysis.

Drug Effects

The decreasing effect-site concentrations (C_e) of the different volatile anesthetic drugs were estimated as a fraction of age adjusted MAC [91] at Start and End Emergence, and the estimated effect-site concentrations of the intraoperative opioids (fentanyl and morphine) were calculated using standard compartmental pharmacokinetic modeling [92,93]. In order to compare opioid effects across patients, and to take into account the fact that many patients had received both morphine and fentanyl intraoperatively, we expressed the morphine concentrations as fentanyl concentration equivalents (C_e *fentanyl*), assuming a conversion factor of 50. This data is also summarized in Table 2.

Evaluation of post-emergence level of consciousness and pain

It is common for patients to experience fluctuations in both level of consciousness and pain in the early postoperative period. These changes are hard to capture and analyze [94]. Accordingly we used simple, heuristically derived, descriptions of level of consciousness (PACU-Cons) and pain (PACU-Pain) as described in Table 1. We believe that these classifications have the advantage of capturing the clinically relevant, qualitative aspects of the recovery period. The PACU-Cons score is based on the change in the Ramsay Score over the first 15 minutes in the PACU [95]. The severity of the pain was quantified using a composite of the standard integer numerical verbal rating scale (NRS) – where 0 is no pain and 10 the worst imaginable pain. Because of the questionable validity of the fine gradations in these semi-quantitative scores, the PACU-Pain score bins the numerical rating scale into 'minimal', 'moderate' and 'severe' pain groups [96], which appear to have reasonable clinical validity. However, we also scored the degree of objective distress that the patient manifested, and used this added information to modify these scores as described in Table 1. The first pain score was obtained when the patient had achieved a level of consciousness at which they could maintain a brief conversation. These pain queries were then repeated every 15 minutes. If they were in pain, patients were treated with increments of 1–2 mg IV morphine, 25–50 μg of fentanyl, or 50–100 mg IV tramadol in the PACU, and then discharged to the ward according to institutional criteria based on the Aldrete score [97].

Spectral Processing, Statistical and Analytical Methods

All data was analyzed using custom scripts written in MATLAB (Mathworks, Natick, Massachusetts). The amplitude and frequency structure of the EEG signal was initially described by the mean power in the traditional frequency bands: delta (0.5–4 Hz), theta (5–7 Hz), alpha (8–14 Hz), and beta (15–25 Hz). The power in each band was then logarithmically transformed so that all spectral power was expressed in units of dB (10× logarithm base 10, referenced to 1 $\mu V^2/Hz$). These band-powers were then smoothed using a 30 second median smoothing filter. In addition we recorded the EMG output (dB) from the Vista monitor. We then extracted EEG features (the delta and alpha bands) that reflected the largest changes in spectral power seen in the prefrontal channels during emergence. Spindle power was specifically derived by measuring the height of the alpha peak above the underlying broadband activity to target the narrowband oscillatory component of this peak [55].

To follow these changes dynamically, we displayed the EEG using typical spectrograms and time series plots of salient features (spindle, delta and EMG power). Spectrograms of the EEG data were made using the 'mtspecgramc.m' function and PSDs using the 'mtspectrumsegc.m' function of the Chronux toolbox (http://chronux.org) [98] on 8 second segments, with 6 second (75%) overlap and tapers of 13 and 8. This segment length was chosen to balance the time required to reliably estimate power in the delta band, while still being short enough to allow for changes in the detection of waveforms within a clinically relevant time frame. 95% confidence intervals for the median PSD for each condition (Start and End Emergence) were calculated using a jackknife estimation method. To create 3-D individualized dwell-time plots for each patient's emergence trajectory (Figures 3–6, panel C), spindle and delta power were plotted against one another in x-y plane, while depth on the z-axis reflected the total amount of time a patient remained in each x-y pixel of the spindle-delta state space as a fraction of total emergence time. This allowed us to capture the changing relationship between oscillations over time, and permitted comparisons across different patients with differing lengths of emergence.

Correlations between pairs of variables were quantified using Pearson's correlation co-efficient (r) if they followed a normal distribution (Kolmogorov-Smirnoff test), otherwise Spearman's rank correlation was used. The multivariate analysis of the interrelationships between all the variables in an observational study is subject to unknown confounding factors. Following conservative statistical practice, we limited the total number of explanatory variables for each model to 5, in order to have 20 data points to estimate the parameter for each variable with reasonable precision. We used multiple linear regression models, with stepwise forward selection, to discover which group of variables were most significantly associated with the continuous outcome variables: namely delta and alpha power at Start Emergence, and emergence time (which was logarithmically transformed to achieve a normal probability distribution). We used similar techniques, but using logistic regression, for binary outcome variables (pain group).

A patient's post-operative nociceptive status was loosely correlated with the emergence trajectory. In order to display those average trajectories, we combined the phase-space data (spindle vs. delta power) for all patients in the low (PACU-Pain = 0) and high (PACU- Pain = 2) groups (Figure 8). More stereotypical patterns were reflected in data points remaining tightly constrained in the 2-D phase space. More variable EEG emergence trajectories were reflected in points spread out over a large area of the 2-D phase space. Cumulative time spent in each area of the phase space was reflected in a color heat map from blue (little time) to red (large amount of time).

Supporting Information

Figure S1 This 3-D histogram of spindle and delta power at Start Emergence, calculated on a single 8 second epoch for each patient (z-axis), reveals this data follows a unimodal distribution. Following statistical convention, patients were separated into two main spectral classes by thresholding spindle and delta power at 7 dB. This theshold reflects the boundary below which only 5% of the Start Emergence data lay, and the region within which most of the End Emergence data lay. Patients who began emergence (i.e. at the termination of general anesthetic delivery) above the 7 dB threshold (above the gray box) were termed to be in Slow-Wave Anesthesia (SWA). Those within the gray box, or below 7 dB, were termed to be in Non Slow-Wave Anesthesia (NSWA).
(TIF)

Author Contributions

Conceived and designed the experiments: DC PSG JWS. Performed the experiments: JWS JNM SI. Analyzed the data: JWS DC PSG. Contributed reagents/materials/analysis tools: JWS DC. Wrote the paper: DC PSG JWS.

References

1. Courtin RF, Bickford RG, Faulconer A Jr. (1950) The classification and significance of electro-encephalographic patterns produced by nitrous oxide-ether anesthesia during surgical operations. Proc Staff Meet Mayo Clin 25: 197–206.
2. Kiersey DK, Bickford RG, Faulconer A Jr. (1951) Electro-encephalographic patterns produced by thiopental sodium during surgical operations; description and classification. Br J Anaesth 23: 141–152.
3. Clark DL, Rosner BS (1973) Neurophysiologic effects of general anesthetics. I. The electroencephalogram and sensory evoked responses in man. Anesthesiology 38: 564–582.
4. Dement W, Kleitman N (1957) Cyclic variations in EEG during sleep and their relation to eye movements, body motility, and dreaming. Electroencephalogr Clin Neurophysiol 9: 673–690.
5. Rechtschaffen A, Kales A (1968) A manual of standardized terminology, techniques, and scoring system for sleep stages of human subjects. University of California, Los Angeles: Brain Information Service/Brain Research Institute.
6. Hudson RJ, Stanski DR, Saidman LJ, Meathe E (1983) A model for studying depth of anesthesia and acute tolerance to thiopental. Anesthesiology 59: 301–308.
7. Long CW, Shah NK, Loughlin C, Spydell J, Bedford RF (1989) A comparison of EEG determinants of near-awakening from isoflurane and fentanyl anesthesia. Spectral edge, median power frequency, and delta ratio. Anesth Analg 69: 169–173.
8. Purdon PL, Pierce ET, Mukamel EA, Prerau MJ, Walsh JL, et al. (2013) Electroencephalogram signatures of loss and recovery of consciousness from propofol. Proc Natl Acad Sci U S A 110: E1142–1151.
9. Ni Mhuircheartaigh R, Warnaby C, Rogers R, Jbabdi S, Tracey I (2013) Slow-wave activity saturation and thalamocortical isolation during propofol anesthesia in humans. Sci Transl Med 5: 208ra148.
10. Gugino LD, Chabot RJ, Prichep LS, John ER, Formanek V, et al. (2001) Quantitative EEG changes associated with loss and return of consciousness in healthy adult volunteers anaesthetized with propofol or sevoflurane. Br J Anaesth 87: 421–428.
11. John ER, Prichep LS, Kox W, Valdes-Sosa P, Bosch-Bayard J, et al. (2001) Invariant reversible QEEG effects of anesthetics. Conscious Cogn 10: 165–183.
12. Breshears JD, Roland JL, Sharma M, Gaona CM, Freudenburg ZV, et al. (2010) Stable and dynamic cortical electrophysiology of induction and emergence with propofol anesthesia. Proc Natl Acad Sci U S A 107: 21170–21175.
13. Lee U, Ku S, Noh G, Baek S, Choi B, et al. (2013) Disruption of frontal-parietal communication by ketamine, propofol, and sevoflurane. Anesthesiology 118: 1264–1275.
14. Ku SW, Lee U, Noh GJ, Jun IG, Mashour GA (2011) Preferential inhibition of frontal-to-parietal feedback connectivity is a neurophysiologic correlate of general anesthesia in surgical patients. PLoS One 6: e25155.
15. Boly M, Moran R, Murphy M, Boveroux P, Bruno MA, et al. (2012) Connectivity changes underlying spectral EEG changes during propofol-induced loss of consciousness. J Neurosci 32: 7082–7090.
16. Cimenser A, Purdon PL, Pierce ET, Walsh JL, Salazar-Gomez AF, et al. (2011) Tracking brain states under general anesthesia by using global coherence analysis. Proc Natl Acad Sci U S A 108: 8832–8837.
17. Vijayan S, Ching S, Purdon PL, Brown EN, Kopell NJ (2013) Thalamocortical mechanisms for the anteriorization of alpha rhythms during propofol-induced unconsciousness. J Neurosci 33: 11070–11075.
18. Steriade M, Timofeev I (2003) Neuronal plasticity in thalamocortical networks during sleep and waking oscillations. Neuron 37: 563–576.
19. Steriade M (2004) Acetylcholine systems and rhythmic activities during the waking—sleep cycle. Prog Brain Res 145: 179–196.
20. Zecharia AY, Nelson LE, Gent TC, Schumacher M, Jurd R, et al. (2009) The involvement of hypothalamic sleep pathways in general anesthesia: testing the hypothesis using the GABAA receptor beta3N265M knock-in mouse. J Neurosci 29: 2177–2187.
21. Nelson LE, Guo TZ, Lu J, Saper CB, Franks NP, et al. (2002) The sedative component of anesthesia is mediated by GABA(A) receptors in an endogenous sleep pathway. Nat Neurosci 5: 979–984.
22. Franks NP (2008) General anaesthesia: from molecular targets to neuronal pathways of sleep and arousal. Nat Rev Neurosci 9: 370–386.
23. Bonin RP, Orser BA (2008) GABA(A) receptor subtypes underlying general anesthesia. Pharmacol Biochem Behav 90: 105–112.
24. Garcia PS, Kolesky SE, Jenkins A (2010) General anesthetic actions on GABA(A) receptors. Curr Neuropharmacol 8: 2–9.
25. Huntsman MM, Porcello DM, Homanics GE, DeLorey TM, Huguenard JR (1999) Reciprocal inhibitory connections and network synchrony in the mammalian thalamus. Science 283: 541–543.
26. Rye DB, Bliwise DL, Parker K, Trotti LM, Saini P, et al. (2012) Modulation of Vigilance in the Primary Hypersomnias by Endogenous Enhancement of GABAA Receptors. Sci Transl Med 4: 161ra151.
27. Tung A, Szafran MJ, Bluhm B, Mendelson WB (2002) Sleep deprivation potentiates the onset and duration of loss of righting reflex induced by propofol and isoflurane. Anesthesiology 97: 906–911.
28. Tung A, Herrera S, Szafran MJ, Kasza K, Mendelson WB (2005) Effect of sleep deprivation on righting reflex in the rat is partially reversed by administration of adenosine A1 and A2 receptor antagonists. Anesthesiology 102: 1158–1164.
29. Berridge CW, Bolen SJ, Manley MS, Foote SL (1996) Modulation of forebrain electroencephalographic activity in halothane-anesthetized rat via actions of noradrenergic beta-receptors within the medial septal region. J Neurosci 16: 7010–7020.
30. Alkire MT, McReynolds JR, Hahn EL, Trivedi AN (2007) Thalamic microinjection of nicotine reverses sevoflurane-induced loss of righting reflex in the rat. Anesthesiology 107: 264–272.
31. Kelz MB, Sun Y, Chen J, Cheng Meng Q, Moore JT, et al. (2008) An essential role for orexins in emergence from general anesthesia. Proc Natl Acad Sci U S A 105: 1309–1314.
32. Solt K, Cotten JF, Cimenser A, Wong KF, Chemali JJ, et al. (2011) Methylphenidate actively induces emergence from general anesthesia. Anesthesiology 115: 791–803.
33. Chemali JJ, Van Dort CJ, Brown EN, Solt K (2012) Active emergence from propofol general anesthesia is induced by methylphenidate. Anesthesiology 116: 998–1005.
34. Taylor NE, Chemali JJ, Brown EN, Solt K (2013) Activation of D1 dopamine receptors induces emergence from isoflurane general anesthesia. Anesthesiology 118: 30–39.
35. Vazey EM, Aston-Jones G (2014) Designer receptor manipulations reveal a role of the locus coeruleus noradrenergic system in isoflurane general anesthesia. Proc Natl Acad Sci U S A 111: 3859–3864.
36. Solt K, Van Dort CJ, Chemali JJ, Taylor NE, Kenny JD, et al. (2014) Electrical Stimulation of the Ventral Tegmental Area Induces Reanimation from General Anesthesia. Anesthesiology.
37. Sleigh JW, Andrzejowski J, Steyn-Ross A, Steyn-Ross M (1999) The bispectral index: a measure of depth of sleep? Anesth Analg 88: 659–661.
38. Tung A, Lynch JP, Roizen MF (2002) Use of the BIS monitor to detect onset of naturally occurring sleep. J Clin Monit Comput 17: 37–42.
39. Walters AS, Lavigne G, Hening W, Picchietti DL, Allen RP, et al. (2007) The scoring of movements in sleep. J Clin Sleep Med 3: 155–167.
40. Silber MH, Ancoli-Israel S, Bonnet MH, Chokroverty S, Grigg-Damberger MM, et al. (2007) The visual scoring of sleep in adults. J Clin Sleep Med 3: 121–131.
41. Dang-Vu TT, Bonjean M, Schabus M, Boly M, Darsaud A, et al. (2011) Interplay between spontaneous and induced brain activity during human non-rapid eye movement sleep. Proc Natl Acad Sci U S A 108: 15438–15443.
42. Steriade M, Deschenes M, Domich L, Mulle C (1985) Abolition of spindle oscillations in thalamic neurons disconnected from nucleus reticularis thalami. J Neurophysiol 54: 1473–1497.
43. Steriade M, McCormick DA, Sejnowski TJ (1993) Thalamocortical oscillations in the sleeping and aroused brain. Science 262: 679–685.
44. McCormick DA, Pape HC (1990) Properties of a hyperpolarization-activated cation current and its role in rhythmic oscillation in thalamic relay neurones. J Physiol 431: 291–318.
45. Dossi RC, Nunez A, Steriade M (1992) Electrophysiology of a slow (0.5–4 Hz) intrinsic oscillation of cat thalamocortical neurones in vivo. J Physiol 447: 215–234.
46. Jones BE (1991) Paradoxical sleep and its chemical/structural substrates in the brain. Neuroscience 40: 637–656.
47. Moser D, Anderer P, Gruber G, Parapatics S, Loretz E, et al. (2009) Sleep classification according to AASM and Rechtschaffen & Kales: effects on sleep scoring parameters. Sleep 32: 139–149.
48. Dang-Vu TT, Schabus M, Desseilles M, Sterpenich V, Bonjean M, et al. (2010) Functional neuroimaging insights into the physiology of human sleep. Sleep 33: 1589–1603.
49. Gais S, Molle M, Helms K, Born J (2002) Learning-dependent increases in sleep spindle density. J Neurosci 22: 6830–6834.
50. Rasch B, Buchel C, Gais S, Born J (2007) Odor cues during slow-wave sleep prompt declarative memory consolidation. Science 315: 1426–1429.
51. Molle M, Eschenko O, Gais S, Sara SJ, Born J (2009) The influence of learning on sleep slow oscillations and associated spindles and ripples in humans and rats. Eur J Neurosci 29: 1071–1081.
52. Morgenthaler TI, Kapur VK, Brown T, Swick TJ, Alessi C, et al. (2007) Practice parameters for the treatment of narcolepsy and other hypersomnias of central origin. Sleep 30: 1705–1711.
53. Howell MJ (2012) Parasomnias: an updated review. Neurotherapeutics 9: 753–775.
54. Espa F, Ondze B, Deglise P, Billiard M, Besset A (2000) Sleep architecture, slow wave activity, and sleep spindles in adult patients with sleepwalking and sleep terrors. Clin Neurophysiol 111: 929–939.
55. Leslie K, Sleigh J, Paech MJ, Voss L, Lim CW, et al. (2009) Dreaming and electroencephalographic changes during anesthesia maintained with propofol or desflurane. Anesthesiology 111: 547–555.
56. Hilborn RC (2000) Chaos and nonlinear dynamics: an introduction for scientists and engineers. Oxford; New York: Oxford University Press.

57. Gan TJ, Glass PS, Sigl J, Sebel P, Payne F, et al. (1999) Women emerge from general anesthesia with propofol/alfentanil/nitrous oxide faster than men. Anesthesiology 90: 1283–1287.
58. Myles PS, McLeod AD, Hunt JO, Fletcher H (2001) Sex differences in speed of emergence and quality of recovery after anaesthesia: cohort study. BMJ 322: 710–711.
59. Hoymork SC, Raeder J (2005) Why do women wake up faster than men from propofol anaesthesia? Br J Anaesth 95: 627–633.
60. Bajaj P, Raiger LK, Jain SD, Kumar S (2007) Women emerge from general anesthesia faster than men. Middle East J Anesthesiol 19: 173–183.
61. Steriade M, Contreras D, Curro Dossi R, Nunez A (1993) The slow (<1 Hz) oscillation in reticular thalamic and thalamocortical neurons: scenario of sleep rhythm generation in interacting thalamic and neocortical networks. J Neurosci 13: 3284–3299.
62. Rampil IJ, Matteo RS (1987) Changes in EEG spectral edge frequency correlate with the hemodynamic response to laryngoscopy and intubation. Anesthesiology 67: 139–142.
63. MacKay EC, Sleigh JW, Voss LJ, Barnard JP (2010) Episodic waveforms in the electroencephalogram during general anaesthesia: a study of patterns of response to noxious stimuli. Anaesth Intensive Care 38: 102–112.
64. Ching S, Cimenser A, Purdon PL, Brown EN, Kopell NJ (2010) Thalamocortical model for a propofol-induced alpha-rhythm associated with loss of consciousness. Proc Natl Acad Sci U S A 107: 22665–22670.
65. Steyn-Ross ML, Steyn-Ross DA, Sleigh JW (2004) Modelling general anaesthesia as a first-order phase transition in the cortex. Prog Biophys Mol Biol 85: 369–385.
66. Friedman EB, Sun Y, Moore JT, Hung HT, Meng QC, et al. (2010) A conserved behavioral state barrier impedes transitions between anesthetic-induced unconsciousness and wakefulness: evidence for neural inertia. PLoS One 5: e11903.
67. Joiner WJ, Friedman EB, Hung HT, Koh K, Sowcik M, et al. (2013) Genetic and anatomical basis of the barrier separating wakefulness and anesthetic-induced unresponsiveness. PLoS Genet 9: e1003605.
68. Besset A, Espa F (2001) [Disorders of arousal]. Rev Neurol (Paris) 157: S107–111.
69. Illman H, Antila H, Olkkola KT (2010) Reversal of neuromuscular blockade by sugammadex does not affect EEG derived indices of depth of anesthesia. J Clin Monit Comput 24: 371–376.
70. (2005) International Classification of Sleep Disorders: Diagnostic and Coding Manual (ICSD-2). 2 ed. Westchester NY: American Academy of Sleep Medicine.
71. Basheer R, Sherin JE, Saper CB, Morgan JI, McCarley RW, et al. (1997) Effects of sleep on wake-induced c-fos expression. J Neurosci 17: 9746–9750.
72. Saper CB, Scammell TE, Lu J (2005) Hypothalamic regulation of sleep and circadian rhythms. Nature 437: 1257–1263.
73. Lydic R, Baghdoyan HA (2005) Sleep, anesthesiology, and the neurobiology of arousal state control. Anesthesiology 103: 1268–1295.
74. Van Dort CJ, Baghdoyan HA, Lydic R (2008) Neurochemical modulators of sleep and anesthetic states. Int Anesthesiol Clin 46: 75–104.
75. Keifer JC, Baghdoyan HA, Lydic R (1996) Pontine cholinergic mechanisms modulate the cortical electroencephalographic spindles of halothane anesthesia. Anesthesiology 84: 945–954.
76. Fuentealba P, Timofeev I, Steriade M (2004) Prolonged hyperpolarizing potentials precede spindle oscillations in the thalamic reticular nucleus. Proc Natl Acad Sci U S A 101: 9816–9821.
77. Gottschalk A, Haney P (2003) Computational aspects of anesthetic action in simple neural models. Anesthesiology 98: 548–564.
78. Contreras D, Curro Dossi R, Steriade M (1993) Electrophysiological properties of cat reticular thalamic neurones in vivo. J Physiol 470: 273–294.
79. Ferenets R, Lipping T, Suominen P, Turunen J, Puumala P, et al. (2006) Comparison of the properties of EEG spindles in sleep and propofol anesthesia. Conf Proc IEEE Eng Med Biol Soc 1: 6356–6359.
80. Kroeger D, Amzica F (2007) Hypersensitivity of the anesthesia-induced comatose brain. J Neurosci 27: 10597–10607.
81. Mulholland CV, Somogyi AA, Barratt DT, Coller JK, Hutchinson MK, et al. Association of innate immune single nucleotide polymorphisms with the electroencephalogram during desflurane general anaesthesia. Journal of Molecular Neuroscience: In press.
82. Vanhaudenhuyse A, Demertzi A, Schabus M, Noirhomme Q, Bredart S, et al. (2011) Two distinct neuronal networks mediate the awareness of environment and of self. J Cogn Neurosci 23: 570–578.
83. Alkire MT, Hudetz AG, Tononi G (2008) Consciousness and anesthesia. Science 322: 876–880.
84. Ferrarelli F, Massimini M, Sarasso S, Casali A, Riedner BA, et al. (2010) Breakdown in cortical effective connectivity during midazolam-induced loss of consciousness. Proc Natl Acad Sci U S A 107: 2681–2686.
85. Massimini M, Ferrarelli F, Sarasso S, Tononi G (2012) Cortical mechanisms of loss of consciousness: insight from TMS/EEG studies. Arch Ital Biol 150: 44–55.
86. Imas OA, Ropella KM, Ward BD, Wood JD, Hudetz AG (2005) Volatile anesthetics disrupt frontal-posterior recurrent information transfer at gamma frequencies in rat. Neurosci Lett 387: 145–150.
87. Tinker JH, Sharbrough FW, Michenfelder JD (1977) Anterior shift of the dominant EEG rhytham during anesthesia in the Java monkey: correlation with anesthetic potency. Anesthesiology 46: 252–259.
88. Tononi G, Cirelli C (2014) Sleep and the price of plasticity: from synaptic and cellular homeostasis to memory consolidation and integration. Neuron 81: 12–34.
89. Brimacombe J (1995) The advantages of the LMA over the tracheal tube or facemask: a meta-analysis. Can J Anaesth 42: 1017–1023.
90. (2010) American Society of Anesthesiologists Standards for Basic Anesthetic Monitoring. ASA House of Delegates (Standards and Practice Parameters Committee).
91. Whitlock EL, Villafranca AJ, Lin N, Palanca BJ, Jacobsohn E, et al. (2011) Relationship between bispectral index values and volatile anesthetic concentrations during the maintenance phase of anesthesia in the B-Unaware trial. Anesthesiology 115: 1209–1218.
92. Shafer SL, Varvel JR, Aziz N, Scott JC (1990) Pharmacokinetics of fentanyl administered by computer-controlled infusion pump. Anesthesiology 73: 1091–1102.
93. Villesen HH, Banning AM, Petersen RH, Weinelt S, Poulsen JB, et al. (2007) Pharmacokinetics of morphine and oxycodone following intravenous administration in elderly patients. Ther Clin Risk Manag 3: 961–967.
94. De Jonghe B, Cook D, Appere-De-Vecchi C, Guyatt G, Meade M, et al. (2000) Using and understanding sedation scoring systems: a systematic review. Intensive Care Med 26: 275–285.
95. Haenggi M, Ypparila H, Takala J, Korhonen I, Luginbuhl M, et al. (2004) Measuring depth of sedation with auditory evoked potentials during controlled infusion of propofol and remifentanil in healthy volunteers. Anesth Analg 99: 1728–1736.
96. Mei W, Seeling M, Franck M, Radtke F, Brantner B, et al. (2010) Independent risk factors for postoperative pain in need of intervention early after awakening from general anaesthesia. Eur J Pain 14: 149 e141–147.
97. Aldrete JA (1998) Modifications to the postanesthesia score for use in ambulatory surgery. J Perianesth Nurs 13: 148–155.
98. Mitra P, Bokil B (2008) Observed Brain Dynamics. New York: Oxford University Press.

Negative Body Image Associated with Changes in the Visual Body Appearance Increases Pain Perception

Michihiro Osumi[1,2*], Ryota Imai[1], Kozo Ueta[1], Satoshi Nobusako[1], Shu Morioka[1]

1 Department of Neurorehabilitation, Graduate School of Health Science, Kio University, Nara, Japan, **2** Neurocognitive Rehabilitation Center, Setsunan General Hospital, Osaka, Japan

Abstract

Changing the visual body appearance by use of as virtual reality system, funny mirror, or binocular glasses has been reported to be helpful in rehabilitation of pain. However, there are interindividual differences in the analgesic effect of changing the visual body image. We hypothesized that a negative body image associated with changing the visual body appearance causes interindividual differences in the analgesic effect although the relationship between the visual body appearance and analgesic effect has not been clarified. We investigated whether a negative body image associated with changes in the visual body appearance increased pain. Twenty-five healthy individuals participated in this study. To evoke a negative body image, we applied the method of rubber hand illusion. We created an "injured rubber hand" to evoke unpleasantness associated with pain, a "hairy rubber hand" to evoke unpleasantness associated with embarrassment, and a "twisted rubber hand" to evoke unpleasantness associated with deviation from the concept of normality. We also created a "normal rubber hand" as a control. The pain threshold was measured while the participant observed the rubber hand using a device that measured pain caused by thermal stimuli. Body ownership experiences were elicited by observation of the injured rubber hand and hairy rubber hand as well as the normal rubber hand. Participants felt more unpleasantness by observing the injured rubber hand and hairy rubber hand than the normal rubber hand and twisted rubber hand ($p<0.001$). The pain threshold was lower under the injured rubber hand condition than with the other conditions ($p<0.001$). We conclude that a negative body appearance associated with pain can increase pain sensitivity.

Editor: Matthew Longo, Birkbeck, University of London, United Kingdom

Funding: This work was supported by the Sasakawa Scientific Research Grant from The Japan Science Society. http://www.jss.or.jp/ikusei/sasakawa/. MO received the funding. Grant Agreement Number 25-613. The funders had no role in study design, data collection, and analysis, decision to publish, or preparation of the manuscript.

Competing Interests: The authors have declared that no competing interests exist.

* Email: p0511109@univ.kio.ac.jp

Introduction

"Pain" is a subjective experience. It not only occurs when a peripheral organ is damaged but also is easily influenced by the central nervous system [1]. Therefore, pain is modulated by attention [2], expectation [3], emotion [4], social factors [5], and emotional facial expressions [6], Recently, the perceived pain level was modulated by introducing a pain stimulus and showing visual information, such as various facial expressions or pictures of a romantic partner at the same time [7]. Also, according to a report by Longo et al. [8], individuals felt less pain when they looked at their own bodies than when they looked at an object. This analgesic effect had been identified by nociceptive laser-evoked potentials recorded by an electroencephalogram [8]. Also, it was reported that brain activity-related pain was lower when looking at a body than an object [9]. More recently, it has been said that body ownership can increase the analgesic effect of looking at the body. For example, Romano et al. reported that during states of illusory self-identification with the avatar, looking at the body was effective in modulating physiological responses to painful stimuli [10]. Also, Martini et al. reported that the pain threshold was increased when looking at a virtual body, which participants felt was their own body, than looking at an oblique cylinder [11]. Similarly, there have been reports of the modulation of pain perception by looking at a rubber hand that was felt to be one's own hand. Mohan et al. reported that the same activity did not induce analgesia [12]. However, Hegedus et al. found that looking at a rubber hand that was felt to be one's own hand induced analgesia, which identified and remedied the problem of how to give pain stimulation experienced in Mohan's experiment [13]. In this way, it was clarified that body ownership can increase the analgesic effect of looking at the body. On the other hand, some studies reported that looking at a distorted body image (in size and color) had an even greater pain modulating effect than a regular body image [14,15]. Mancini et al. reported that individuals felt less pain when their own bodies appeared large in a concave mirror, but felt increased pain when their bodies appeared shrunken in a convex mirror [14]. Romano et al. reported that looking at an enlarged version of their own body decreased physiological responses to painful stimuli [16]. Martini et al. used a virtual reality system that colored the visual body appearance red or blue. The participants felt stronger pain when their body appeared red while they felt less pain when the body appeared blue [15]. Such visual body image-based interventions have been applied to patients with chronic pain who have complex regional pain syndrome, phantom limb pain, chronic back pain, and osteoarthritis [17–20]. For example, phantom limb pain was decreased by individuals observing their shrunken body in a funny mirror. Of note, however, is that manipulation of visual body images has not produced reliable intervention effects. For example, Preston et al. reported that the appearance of extended fingers had an analgesic effect in some osteoarthritis patients while the appearance of shortened fingers had the same effect for others [20]. Although the pain and edema in complex regional pain syndrome were increased by looking at one's own body magnified [17], in other cases the same visual distortion led to pain reduction [14]. Results varied when summarizing reports of the analgesic effect of looking at a distorted body appearance. However, the reasons have not been shown. Mirror visual feedback by looking at one's own body is one of the rehabilitation tools. Although mirror therapy is effective for pain [21–23], there have been reports of adverse effects, for example, increased pain [24,25], Hagenberg et al. reported that "emotional reaction" is the most common adverse effect of mirror visual feedback [26]. Osumi et al. also reported that individuals who had a negative emotion toward to a distorted body appearance felt increased pain while looking at a distorted body appearance [27]. In this way, negative emotion toward one's body image (negative body image) is one factor in preventing an analgesic effect by looking at a distorted body appearance. However, there are different forms of a negative body image. A negative body image is now believed to include anxiety arising from looking at one's own body, embarrassment from being seen by others, and recognition of one's own body not conforming to an established idea of a desirable appearance [28]. Regarding anxiety arising from looking at one's own body, looking at one's injured body increased brain activity-related pain [29,30]. As to embarrassment from being seen by others, in experiments involving individuals with bulimia nervosa there was increased brain activity-related pain, for example, that of the anterior cingulate cortex or medial prefrontal cortex when they viewed their own fat bodies [31]. Concerning one's body not conforming to the established idea of what a body should look like, discomfort with simulating sensorimotor incongruence evoked brain activity-related pain [32,33]. Based on these studies, we hypothesized that the three species of negative body image would increase physical pain because they could increase brain activity-related pain. But it is considered that those who have a negative body image are sensitive to pain. The objective of this study therefore was to identify specific types of negative body image that would worsen a perceived pain level.

Materials and Methods

Ethics Statement

The experimental protocol was approved by the Kio University Ethics Committee (approval number: H24-19) and the study protocol conformed to the Declaration of Helsinki. Participants gave written consent to participate after receiving an explanation of the procedures involved.

Participants

A total of 25 healthy right-handed students (9 males, 16 females; mean age, 21.61 years; SD, 0.56) participated in this study. Prior to the experiment, the experimental procedure was explained to them. The purpose of the experiment, however, was not explained to prevent the participants from having any bias.

Rubber Hand Illusion

A rubber hand illusion was used to evoke a negative body image associated with one's own body. The rubber hand illusion is a body ownership illusion in which individuals start to feel that the fake hand is their own hand when a hidden real hand and a rubber hand placed in front of them are touched simultaneously [34]. In recent years, it has been used to let individuals experience a wide variety of perceptions. For example, a rubber hand with no fourth finger allows individuals to experience a phantom fourth finger [35]. Also, a black rubber hand allows non-black individuals to experience what it is like to have dark skin [36]. For this study, special rubber hands designed to evoke a negative body image were created. Study participants were then led to develop a sense of ownership over these hands so that they would experience a negative body image about their own bodies. In this study, "rubber hand" refers to both the forearm and hand. Examples of a negative body image include anxiety that arises when individuals see what has happened to their bodies; inferiority that arises when they compare themselves with others; embarrassment that arises when they are seen by others; and an emotion that arises when their appearance does not conform to an established idea of a desirable physical appearance [26]. For the purpose of this study, the following types of rubber hands were created (Fig. 1): (a) a normal rubber hand that would not make the participants feel uncomfortable (normal rubber hand: Normal); (b) an injured rubber hand to make the participants feel uncomfortable by the sight of an injury (injured rubber hand: Injured); (c) a hairy rubber hand to make the participants feel uncomfortable about being seen by others (hairy rubber hand: Hairy); and (d) a distorted rubber hand to make the participants feel uncomfortable because their body does not conform to the established idea of what a body should look like (distorted rubber hand: Distorted). In addition, for each type of rubber hand, we provided both illusion and no illusion conditions.

Participants sat on a chair and placed the left index finger on a spot marked on the table. On the table, a board was installed parallel to the sagittal plane to keep participants from seeing their own hand. In the illusion condition, a rubber hand was then placed on the table with its left index finger 15 cm away to the right of the real left index finger and also vertically aligned with the left armpit when seen from the front (Fig. 2). In the no illusion condition, the posture of the rubber hand was slightly incongruent

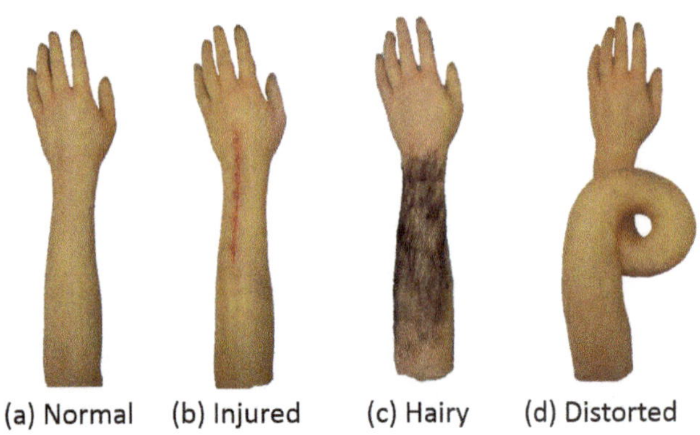

Figure 1. Rubber hands used in the experiments. We used 4 rubber hands that represented the following conditions: (a) did not evoke a negative body image, (b) evoked a pain-related negative body image, (c) evoked a negative body image due to non-conformance of a socially accepted appearance, and (d) evoked a negative body image due to non-conformance of the concept of a normal body.

with the real hand, though anatomically possible (rotated by 20–30°) in order to maximize the reduction of the illusion. The method of Hegedüs et al. was used as a reference to setting this no illusion condition [24]. In both the illusion and no illusion conditions, a bath towel was put over the proximal end of the rubber hand as well as the left arm and shoulder of participants so they could not see how the real and fake hands were arranged in this area. Participants were instructed not to move the left hand and to keep looking at the rubber hand during the experiment.

Pain Stimulation Device and Pain Threshold Measurement

Pain thresholds were measured by applying stimuli to the back of the left forearm (10 cm from the left wrist) by a thermal stimulator (UDH-105, UNIQUE MEDICAL, Tokyo, Japan). The thermal probe was 20 mm in size and was directly placed on the measurement point. Measurement was conducted in accordance with the study by Yarnitsky et al. [37]. The thermal stimulus started at 32°C with a 1°C increment per second. The temperature at which the participant felt the stimulus as painful was recorded as the pain threshold. Participants were instructed to press the switch on the remote control in the right hand the moment they felt pain so that the temperature would not be increased further (Fig. 2). Note that thermal stimuli were introduced a few times to an area (center of the back of a hand) not subject to the threshold measurement so that participants could become sufficiently accustomed to the pain caused by thermal stimuli prior to the experiment.

Procedure

This procedure involved 8 different conditions: Normal rubber hand (illusion/no illusion), Injured rubber hand (illusion/no illusion), Hairy rubber hand (illusion/no illusion), and Distorted rubber hand (illusion/no illusion). These conditions were randomized across subjects. The experiment consisted of 4 sequences of experimental steps for the 8 conditions presented by the rubber hands. Each sequence was designed to include an index finger location task, pain threshold measurement, and a rubber hand illusion questionnaire. Fig. 3 shows a diagram of the sequence of the experiments.

All sequences were performed identically and included the index finger location task to examine the effectiveness of the illusion of body ownership over the rubber hand and the rubber hand illusion questionnaire (RHI Questionnaire).

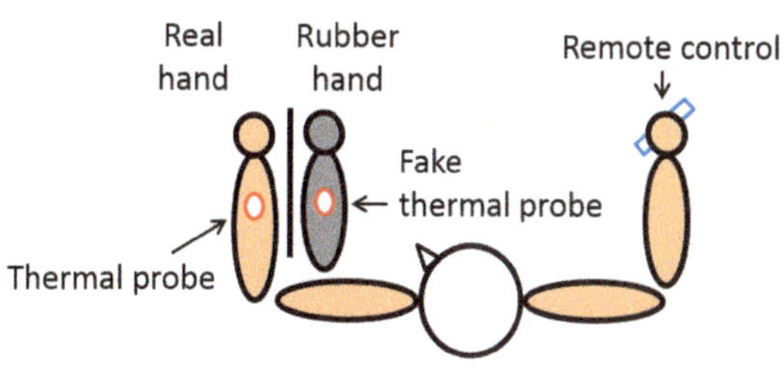

Figure 2. Experimental setting for pain threshold measurement. A thermal probe was placed on the participant's forearm and a fake thermal probe was placed on the forearm of the rubber hand. The participant was instructed to stare at the rubber hand during the pain threshold measurement. The experimenter increased the temperature of the stimulus by 1°C per second. The participant used a remote control in his/her right hand to stop the temperature from increasing any further the moment pain was felt. The temperature was recorded as the pain threshold.

The first step of a sequence was the index finger location task. An acrylic board and cloth were used to prevent participants from seeing the real hand and rubber hand. Then, the experimenter who was seated in front of the participant slowly moved experimenter's index finger from the left side of the participant (20 cm to the left of the real index finger) toward the midline. Participants were instructed to verbally inform the experimenter when they thought that the experimenter's index finger was above their left index finger. The experimenter recorded the reported position.

The second step was a rubber hand illusion. In the illusion condition, the illusion was created using 2 paintbrushes, stimulating both the rubber hand and the real hand for 5 minutes on the same locations and at the same time. In the no illusion condition, both the rubber hand and the real hand were stimulated for 5 minutes on different locations and at different times. The participant was instructed not to move his/her left hand and to keep looking at the rubber hand.

After the rubber hand illusion or no illusion task, the third step was another index finger location task, which was performed in the same way as the first index finger location task. The distance between the participant's reported location of the index finger before and after the rubber hand illusion was recorded as the proprioceptive drift and used in the analysis as the perceived effectiveness of the body ownership illusion. A larger value meant that the location of the real index finger reported by the participant was closer to that of the rubber hand. In other words, a larger value meant that the rubber hand illusion was more effective [38].

The fourth step was the pain threshold measurement on the back of the participant's hidden left forearm. A mock probe was placed on the rubber hand in order to make the participant feel that the pain came from the rubber hand (Fig. 2). In the experiment, the pain threshold was measured 4 times with a 1-minute interval between measurements. The number of measurements of pain threshold and the time of the interval were determined by reference to an experiment devised by Mancini [14] who used a pain stimulation device similar to our device. The average of the 4 measurements was used as the pain threshold value in the analysis.

After the pain threshold measurement, the final step was administration of the RHI Questionnaire and ratings of unpleasantness. The RHI questionnaire items were created based on the questionnaire developed by Longo et al. [39]. The participant used a 7-point Likert scale from −3 (strongly disagree) to +3 (strongly agree) to rate the following 4 statements: "When a rubber hand was stroked by a paintbrush, it felt as if the paintbrush stroked the same place on my hand," "When a rubber hand was stroked by a paintbrush, it felt as if the paintbrush touched my hand," "It felt as if the rubber hand was my own hand," and "It felt like my left hand moved to the right (towards the rubber hand)." The RHI Questionnaire was administered under both the illusion and no illusion conditions. The ratings given to the 4 questions were averaged for each condition. The obtained values were then compared. Also, the participants rated 3 kinds of unpleasantness using a numerical rating scale from 0 (no unpleasantness) to 10 (worst possible unpleasantness). The numerical rating was done only for the illusion condition. The participants rated "unpleasantness associated with injury," "unpleasantness associated with embarrassment" and "unpleasantness associated with nonconformance to the ideal body shape" for the 4 kinds of rubber hand.

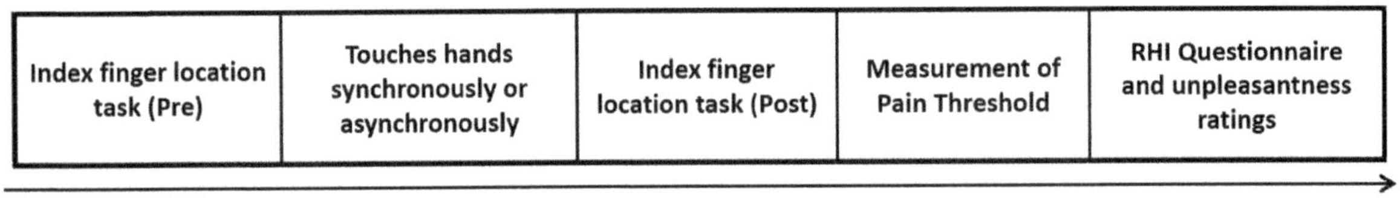

Figure 3. Experimental procedure. The experiment consisted of 4 sequences of experimental steps for each of the 8 conditions presented by the rubber hands. Each sequence was designed to include an index finger location task, pain threshold measurement, a rubber hand illusion questionnaire, and unpleasantness rating.

Statistical Analysis

Because the values for the perceived effectiveness of the illusion, proprioceptive drift, and pain threshold did not have normal distribution in Shapiro-Wilk tests, two-factorial ANOVA was not used. So, the perceived effectiveness of the illusion, proprioceptive drift, and pain threshold were analyzed using the Friedman test across rubber hand conditions under both illusion and no illusion conditions. In both of these cases, Wilcoxon signed-rank tests were used for post hoc analyses and the Bonferroni correction was used to adjust the p-values obtained in the post hoc analyses. In the present study, results using the illusion condition were compared among 4 rubber hand conditions; in addition, results from each rubber hand condition were compared between illusion and no illusion conditions. A total of 10 comparisons were made, and the significance level was set at $P<0.005$. Unpleasant feelings evoked by the illusion were compared across rubber hand conditions for each item separately using the Friedman test, with Wilcoxon signed-rank tests used for post hoc analyses. Bonferroni correction was used for the 4 items and the significance level was set at $P<0.0083$. SPSS ver. 17.0 (SPSS, Chicago, IL, USA) was used for statistical processing.

Results

Table 1 shows the proprioceptive drift, perceived effectiveness of the illusion and pain threshold for each condition.

Proprioceptive Drift

In comparisons of proprioceptive drift for the 4 rubber hand conditions under illusion conditions, the Friedman test showed a significant main effect ($\chi^2=15.22$, $P=0.002$). Under the no illusion condition, the Friedman test showed no significant main effect ($\chi^2=2.08$, $P=0.557$). The post-hoc test showed that the proprioceptive drift for the distorted condition under the illusion condition was significantly lower than for normal, injured, and hairy conditions under the illusion condition ($p<0.001$) (Fig. 4a and Table 1). For all 4 rubber hand conditions, there were significant differences between the illusion and no illusion conditions ($p<0.001$) (Fig. 4a and Table 1). These results mean that under the distorted conditions the distance between the actual and perceived locations of the index finger during the rubber hand illusion was shorter than for the other conditions.

Perceived Effectiveness of the Illusion

In the comparison of perceived effectiveness of the illusion for the 4 rubber hand conditions under illusion conditions, the Friedman test showed a significant main effect ($\chi^2=28.76$, $P<0.001$). In the comparison under no illusion conditions, the Friedman test showed no significant main effect ($\chi^2=4.35$, $P=0.226$). The post-hoc test showed that the perceived effectiveness of the illusion was significantly lower for the distorted condition under the illusion condition than for the normal, injured, and hairy conditions ($p<0.001$) (Fig. 4b and Table 1). Under the all rubber hand conditions, there were significant differences between the illusion and the no illusion conditions ($p<0.001$) (Fig. 4b and Table 1). These results mean that compared to other conditions, the rubber hand illusion under the distorted condition was perceived to be less effective.

Unpleasant Feeling Evoked by the Illusion

In the item "unpleasantness associated with embarrassment", the Friedman test and post-hoc test showed that the unpleasantness associated with embarrassment under the hairy condition was significantly stronger than for normal, injured and distorted conditions ($X^2=48.13$, $p<0.001$; Hairy rubber hand: $M=3.24$, $SE=0.59$; Normal rubber hand: $M=0.00$, $SE=0.00$; Injured rubber hand: $M=0.08$, $SE=0.08$; Distorted rubber hand: $M=0.24$, $SE=0.20$) (Fig. 5). In the item of "unpleasantness associated with injury", the Friedman test and the post-hoc test showed that unpleasantness associated with the injured condition was significantly stronger than for normal, hairy and distorted conditions ($X^2=49.29$, $p<0.001$; Injured rubber hand: $M=3.44$, $SE=0.56$; Normal rubber hand: $M=0.00$, $SE=0.00$; Hairy rubber hand: $M=0.28$, $SE=0.20$; Distorted rubber hand: $M=0.00$, $SE=0.00$) (Fig.5). In the item "unpleasantness associated with nonconformance", the Friedman test and post-hoc test showed that the unpleasantness associated nonconformance under the hairy condition was significantly stronger than for normal, injured and distorted conditions ($X^2=14.21$, $p<0.0083$; Hairy rubber hand: $M=3.28$, $SE=0.59$; Normal rubber hand: $M=1.00$, $SE=0.46$; Injured rubber hand: $M=1.16$, $SE=0.39$; Distorted rubber hand: $M=1.32$, $SE=0.41$) (Fig. 5).

Pain Threshold

In the comparison of the pain threshold for the 4 rubber hand conditions under illusion conditions, the Friedman test showed a significant main effect ($X^2=9.34$, $P=0.025$). Such a comparison under no illusion conditions showed that the Friedman test indicated no significant main effect ($X^2=1.72$, $P=0.63$) (Fig. 6 and Table 1). The post-hoc test showed that the pain threshold for the injured condition in the illusion condition was significantly lower than for normal, hairy and distorted conditions ($p<0.005$) (Fig. 6 and Table 1). Under the injured rubber hand condition, the Wilcoxon signed-rank test showed that the pain threshold with the illusion condition was lower than with the no illusion condition ($P<0.005$) (Fig. 6 and Table 1), but there were no significant differences under normal, hairy and distorted conditions ($p>0.005$).

Discussion

In examining the influence of a negative body image on pain threshold through the rubber hand illusion, the injured and hairy

Table 1. Value of drift (SE), subjective degree of illusion (SE), and pain threshold (SE) under each condition.

	Normal		Injured		Hairy		Distorted	
	illusion	no illusion	illusion	no illusion	illusion	no illusion	Illusion	no illusion
Value of drift (cm)	2.25 (0.22)	0.19 (0.07)	2.58 (0.31)	0.10 (0.70)	2.41 (0.32)	0.14 (0.06)	1.16 (0.32)	0.19 (0.05)
Subjective degree of illusion	2.27 (0.13)	-2.54 (0.12)	2.02 (0.16)	-2.48 (0.16)	1.92 (0.16)	-2.64 (0.11)	0.8 (0.21)	-2.68 (0.11)
Pain threshold (°C)	43.11 (0.32)	43.37 (0.29)	42.01 (0.40)	43.43 (0.32)	43.08 (0.28)	43.35 (0.29)	42.92 (0.33)	43.41 (0.29)

rubber hands created the same level of body ownership illusion as the normal rubber hand. They also evoked a more negative body image than the normal rubber hand. As the result of unpleasant feelings evoked by the illusion (Fig. 5), participants felt specifically "unpleasantness associated with injury" in the injured rubber hand condition and participants felt specifically "unpleasantness associated with embarrassment" and "unpleasantness associated with nonconformance to the ideal body shape" with the hairy rubber hand condition. The experiment further showed that the pain threshold was lower when the participants were under the illusion of body ownership over the injured rubber hand compared to the illusion of body ownership over the other types of rubber hand.

Effectiveness of the Illusion and Negative Body Image under Various Experimental Conditions

In the current experiments, the injured and hairy rubber hands created the same level of body ownership illusion as the normal rubber hand and also evoked a more negative body image than the normal rubber hand. The distorted rubber hand produced a less effective body ownership illusion than the other types of rubber hands and also failed to evoke any negative body image.

Many experiments have explored the necessary elements for creating a rubber hand illusion. According to these studies, a rubber hand must not only be stimulated at the same time and at the same location as the real hand but must also have corporeality [40], be anatomically identical to the real hand [41], and be arranged at the same angle as the real hand [42] to create an illusion. The distorted rubber hand was not anatomically identical to a real hand and also lacked corporeality, which would seem to have made it less likely for the distorted rubber hand to create an illusion. A recent study reported that a rubber hand could create a body ownership illusion without being influenced by its skin color as long as it was anatomically identical to a real hand [36]. The injured and hairy rubber hands had different skin appearances but were anatomically identical to a real hand. This seems to be the reason why these rubber hands created the same level of body ownership illusion as the normal rubber hand.

The illusion of body ownership over the injured and hairy rubber hands evoked a stronger unpleasant feeling than the normal rubber hand. A wide variety of psychological changes have been reported to occur during the process in which an illusion of body ownership over a rubber hand is created. For example, a 'bizarre and strange' feeling arose when an illusion of body ownership was created for a normal rubber hand [43]. Also, an illusion of body ownership over a rubber hand with a missing fourth finger evoked an unpleasant feeling such as pain [35]. Furthermore, there was a report of even a psychosocial change in which implicit racial biases held against people with dark skin turned into a positive feeling after individuals experienced an illusion of body ownership over a black rubber hand [44]. In the injured rubber hand condition, participants felt specifically "unpleasantness associated with injury". With the hairy rubber hand condition, participants felt specifically "unpleasantness associated with embarrassment" and "unpleasantness associated with nonconformance to the ideal body shape". The initial hypothesis for the study was that participants would feel only "unpleasantness associated with embarrassment" under the hairy rubber hand condition, but they also felt"unpleasantness associated with nonconformance to the ideal body shape". We inferred that the reason for this result was that participants in this study were not actually hairy because participants included young adults and women. However, we could cause participants to feel"unpleasantness associated with the injury" and"unpleasantness

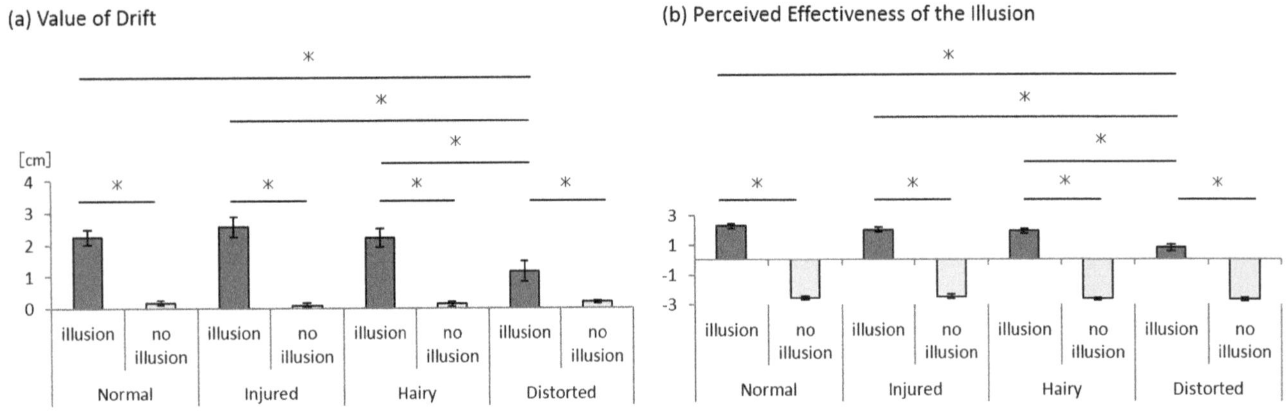

Figure 4. Value of drift (a) and subjective degree of illusion (b) under each condition. The post-hoc test showed that the value of drift and perceived effectiveness of the illusion under the distorted condition were significantly lower than under the normal, injured, and hairy conditions. Error bars indicate ± SE. * p<0.005.

associated with embarrassment" by feeling body ownership of the injured or hairy rubber hand.

The distorted rubber hand therefore failed to meet the prerequisite for being compared with other types of rubber hand because it was unlikely to create a body ownership illusion and did not evoke any unpleasant feeling. The injured and hairy rubber hands, on the other hand, were able to lead the participants to a psychological state of "negative body image about one's own body" by creating the same level of body ownership illusion as the normal rubber hand and also by evoking a stronger unpleasant feeling than the normal rubber hand.

Pain Felt Under Each Experimental Condition

Under the normal rubber hand condition, there were no significant differences in pain threshold between the illusion and no illusion conditions. In a previous study, the effect of seeing a new dummy that embodied one's own body was unclear [11–13,45]. In a previous study, it was unclear whether the effect of seeing embodied new dummy or virtual bodies [11–13,45]. This difference in results is thought to be due to a difference in the experimental method. Among the various differences in experimental methods, the most important difference is whether there is"visual capture of pain". When visual input predicts pain, there is anticipatory recruitment of the related brain region and enhanced pain perception [46]. Mohan et al. reported that the pain threshold did not change even with the rubber hand illusion [12]. They suggested that the heat probe on the rubber hand might have facilitated the "visual capture of pain". This "visual capture of pain" evoked prediction of pain and enhanced sensitivity to pain [46]. In the present study, the dummy heat probe was placed on the rubber hand, and, as a result, seeing the dummy heat probe evoked prediction of pain. We thought that seeing the dummy heat probe was the reason the pain threshold did not differ significantly between illusion and no illusion conditions. However, it was very important that participants felt the illusion of body ownership and felt unpleasantness regarding a particular kind of rubber hand in order to achieve this present experimental objective. It was reported that synchronizing pain and visual stimuli evoked the rubber hand illusion as well as synchronizing tactile and visual stimuli [47]. From this study it can be considered that if there were no dummy heat probe on the rubber hand incongruity would occur between pain and visual stimuli and

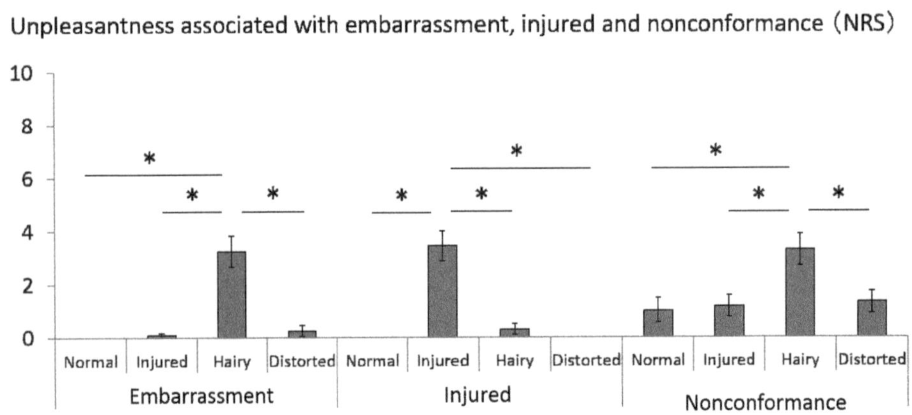

Figure 5. Unpleasantness associated with embarrassment, injury and nonconformance (NRS) under each condition. The post-hoc test showed that the hairy condition had a significantly greater impact than the normal, injured and distorted conditions for the item of unpleasantness associated with embarrassment. The post-hoc test showed that the injured condition had a significantly greater impact than normal, hairy and distorted conditions for the item of unpleasantness associated with injury while the hairy condition had a significantly greater impact than normal, injured and distorted conditions for unpleasantness associated with embarrassment. Error bars indicate ± SE. * p<0.0083.

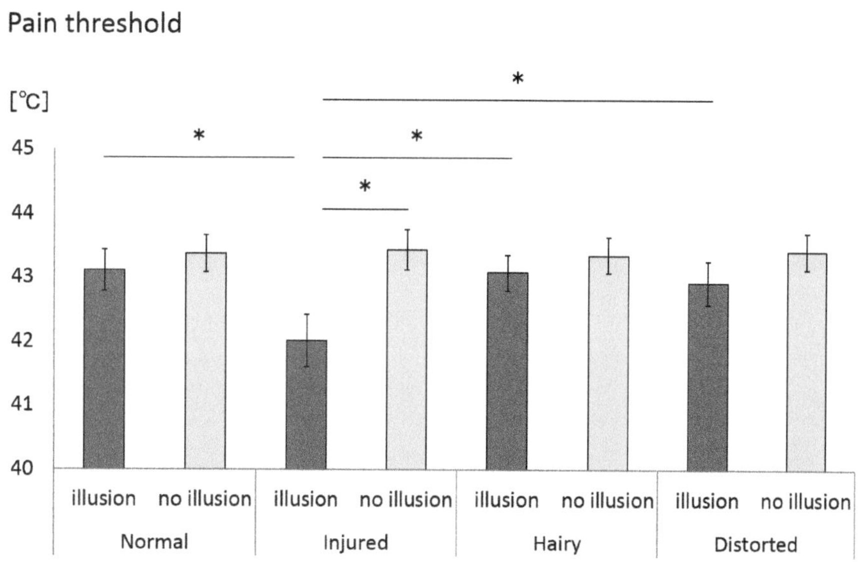

Figure 6. Pain threshold under each condition. The arm pain threshold was significantly lower under the injured condition than for the normal, hairy, and distorted conditions. Error bars indicate ± SE. * $p<0.005$.

participants would not feel the illusion of body ownership of the rubber hand. Therefore, we used a dummy heat probe on the rubber hand when pain thresholds were measured.

The study found that the pain threshold was lower when the participant was under the illusion of body ownership over the injured rubber hand than when under the illusion of body ownership over other types of rubber hand. The initial hypothesis for the study was that the pain threshold would decrease when an unpleasant body image was evoked. What the study indicated, however, was that the pain threshold decreased only for the injured rubber hand even though both the hairy and injured rubber hand equally evoked an unpleasant feeling. Looking at one's own body is considered to produce an analgesic effect through the psychological effect of eliminating uncertainty about danger as well as any anxiety associated with it, thereby preventing pain sensitivity from becoming stronger [48]. Moseley et al., for example, instructed the participating patients with complex regional pain syndrome suffering from significant swelling to see their affected hands through binoculars and reported that the patients experienced increased pain under the illusion that the swelling had worsened [17]. Martini et al. used a virtual reality system to color the hands of the study participants red and instructed them to look at their colored hands. The participants felt that the pain worsened because that coloration reminded them of inflammation [15]. These examples suggest that the absence of negative perceptual experiences associated with pain is essential for the analgesic effect of looking at one's own body. In this study, both the injured and hairy rubber hands evoked an unpleasant feeling, but only the injured rubber hand resulted in worsening of pain. This result implies that, instead of a negative body image changing the pain threshold, pain worsens only when a pain-related negative body image is associated with a particular body part. In recent years, medical intervention for chronic pain patients through manipulation of a visual body appearance has been reported to be effective [17,18,20]. According to our experimental result, however, pain could worsen if a patient has pain-related unpleasant feelings toward the visual body image. Therefore, in clinical settings, it is desirable to provide a visual body appearance that reminds patients of reduced pain. For example, visual feedback that reminds a person of "cold" would be desirable for causalgia. Similarly, visual feedback that reminds a person of "stretching" would be desirable for pain accompanying stiffened limbs. Examination of these assumptions is our future clinical research theme.

This study has some limitations. First, emotional changes in the participants were measured only by a numerical rating scale, and it was not clear whether or not autonomic nervous responses actually occurred. It is necessary in the future to measure them, including skin conductance and heart rate. Second, only the sensory aspect of pain, or the pain threshold, was measured. Since pain also has cognitive and emotional aspects, the influence of pain on these aspects is a future research task. Third, the study did not clarify what kind of change in the central nervous system caused changes in pain. This is because brain activities were not measured by a brain function imaging device. This question should be clarified in the future through functional magnetic resonance imaging and/or electroencephalography. Lastly, all of the study participants were Japanese, so we did not consider the cultural background.

Supporting Information

Table S1 Outcomes of the study.
(XLSX)

Author Contributions

Conceived and designed the experiments: MO RI KU. Performed the experiments: MO RI. Analyzed the data: MO. Contributed reagents/materials/analysis tools: MO RI KU. Contributed to the writing of the manuscript: MO SN SM.

References

1. Bingel U, Schoell E, Büchel C (2007) Imaging pain modulation in health and disease. Curr Opin Neurol 20: 424–431.
2. Kong J, Gollub RL, Rosman IS, Webb JM, Vangel MG, et al. (2006) Brain activity associated with expectancy-enhanced placebo analgesia as measured by functional magnetic resonance imaging. J Neurosci 26: 381–388.
3. Valet M, Sprenger T, Boecker H, Willoch F, Rummeny E, et al. (2004) Distraction modulates connectivity of the cingulo-frontal cortex and the midbrain during pain–an fMRI analysis. Pain 109: 399–408.
4. Schweinhardt P, Kalk N, Wartolowska K, Chessell I, Wordsworth P, et al. (2008) Investigation into the neural correlates of emotional augmentation of clinical pain. Neuroimage 40: 759–766.
5. Eisenberger NI, Jarcho JM, Lieberman MD, Naliboff BD (2006) An experimental study of shared sensitivity to physical pain and social rejection. Pain 126: 132–138.
6. Senkowski D, Kautz J, Hauck M, Zimmermann R, Engel AK (2011) Emotional facial expressions modulate pain-induced beta and gamma oscillations in sensorimotor cortex. J Neurosci. 2011 31: 14542–14550.
7. Yoshino A, Okamoto Y, Onoda K, Shishida K, Yoshimura S, et al. (2012) Sadness enhances the experience of pain and affects pain-evoked cortical activities: an MEG study. J Pain 13: 628–635.
8. Longo MR, Betti V, Aglioti SM, Haggard P (2009) Visually induced analgesia: seeing the body reduces pain. J Neurosci 29: 12125–12130.
9. Longo MR, Iannetti GD, Mancini F, Driver J, Haggard P (2012) Linking pain and the body: neural correlates of visually induced analgesia. J Neurosci 32: 2601–2607.
10. Romano D, Pfeiffer C, Maravita A, Blanke O (2014) Illusory self-identification with an avatar reduces arousal responses to painful stimuli. Behav Brain Res 261: 275–281.
11. Martini M, Perez-Marcos D, Sanchez-Vives MV (2014) Modulation of pain threshold by virtual body ownership. Eur J Pain [Epub ahead of print].
12. Mohan R, Jensen KB, Petkova VI, Dey A, Barnsley N, et al. (2012) No pain relief with the rubber hand illusion. PLOS One 7: e52400.
13. Hegedüs G, Darnai G, Szolcsányi T, Feldmann A, Janszky J, et al. (2014) The rubber hand illusion increases heat pain threshold. Eur J Pain [Epub ahead of print].
14. Mancini F, Longo MR, Kammers MP, Haggard P (2011) Visual distortion of body size modulates pain perception. Psychol Sci 22: 325–330.
15. Martini M, Perez-Marcos D, Sanchez-Vives MV (2013) What color is my arm? Changes in skin color of an embodied virtual arm modulates pain threshold. Front Hum Neurosci 7: 438.
16. Romano D, Maravita A (2014) The visual size of one's own hand modulates pain anticipation and perception. Neuropsychologia 57: 93–100.
17. Moseley GL, Parsons TJ, Spence C (2008) Visual distortion of a limb modulates the pain and swelling evoked by movement. Curr Biol 18: R1047–1048.
18. Ramachandran VS, Brang D, McGeoch PD (2009) Size reduction using Mirror Visual Feedback (MVF) reduces phantom pain Neurocase 15: 357–360.
19. Diers M, Zieglgänsberger W, Trojan J, Drevensek AM, Erhardt-Raum G, et al. (2013) Site-specific visual feedback reduces pain perception. Pain 154: 890–896.
20. Preston C, Newport R (2011) Analgesic effects of multisensory illusions in osteoarthritis. Rheumatology (Oxford) 50: 2314–2315.
21. Sumitani M, Miyauchi S, McCabe CS, Shibata M, Maeda L, et al. (2008) Mirror visual feedback alleviates deafferentation pain, depending on qualitative aspects of the pain: a preliminary report. Rheumatology (Oxford) 47: 1038–1043.
22. Cacchio A, De Blasis E, De Blasis V, Santilli V, Spacca G (2009) Mirror therapy in complex regional pain syndrome type 1 of the upper limb in stroke patients. Neurorehabil Neural Repair 23: 792–799.
23. McCabe CS, Haigh RC, Ring EF, Halligan PW, Wall PD, et al. (2003) A controlled pilot study of the utility of mirror visual feedback in the treatment of complex regional pain syndrome (type 1). Rheumatology 42: 97–101.
24. Darnall BD, Li H (2012) Home-based self-delivered mirror therapy for phantom pain: a pilot study. J Rehabil Med 44: 254–260.
25. Chan BL, Witt R, Charrow AP, Magee A, Howard R, et al. (2007) Mirror therapy for phantom limb pain. N Engl J Med 357: 2206–2207.
26. Hagenberg A, Carpenter C (2014) Mirror Visual Feedback for Phantom Pain: International Experience on Modalities and Adverse Effects Discussed by an Expert Panel: A Delphi Study. PM R S1934-1482(14)00018-5.
27. Osumi M, Imai R, Ueta K, Nakano H, Nobusako S, et al. (2014) Factors associated with the modulation of pain perception by visual distortion of body size. Front Hum Neurosci 8: 137.
28. Gallagher S (2005) How the body shapes the mind. Oxford University Press. 17–39 p.
29. Ehrsson HH, Wiech K, Weiskopf N, Dolan RJ, Passingham RE (2007) Threatening a rubber hand that you feel is yours elicits a cortical anxiety response. Proc Natl Acad Sci U S A 104: 9828–9833.
30. González-Franco M, Peck TC, Rodríguez-Fornells A, Slater M (2014) A threat to a virtual hand elicits motor cortex activation. Exp Brain Res 232: 875–887.
31. Spangler DL, Allen MD (2012) An fMRI investigation of emotional processing of body shape in bulimia nervosa. Int J Eat Disord 45: 17–25.
32. McCabe CS, Haigh RC, Halligan PW, Blake DR (2005) Simulating sensory-motor incongruence in healthy volunteers: implications for a cortical model of pain. Rheumatology (Oxford) 44: 509–516.
33. Nishigami T, Nakano H, Osumi M, Tsujishita M, Mibu A, et al. (2014) Central neural mechanisms of interindividual difference in discomfort during sensori-motor incongruence in healthy volunteers: an experimental study. Rheumatology (Oxford) [Epub ahead of print].
34. Botvinick M, Cohen J (1998) Rubber hands 'feel' touch that eyes see. Nature 391: 756.
35. Lewis E, Lloyd DM, Farrell MJ (2013) The role of the environment in eliciting phantom-like sensations in non-amputees. Front Psychol 3: 600.
36. Farmer H, Tajadura-Jiménez A, Tsakiris M (2012) Beyond the colour of my skin: how skin colour affects the sense of body-ownership. Conscious Cogn 21: 1242–1256.
37. Yarnitsky D, Sprecher E, Zaslansky R, Hemli JA (1995) Heat pain thresholds: normative data and repeatability. Pain 60: 329–332.
38. Kammers MP, de Vignemont F, Verhagen L, Dijkerman HC (2009) The rubber hand illusion in action. Neuropsychologia 47: 204–211.
39. Longo MR, Schüür F, Kammers MP, Tsakiris M, Haggard P (2008) What is embodiment? A psychometric approach. Cognition 107: 978–998.
40. Tsakiris M, Carpenter L, James D, Fotopoulou A (2010) Hands only illusion: multisensory integration elicits sense of ownership for body parts but not for non-corporeal objects. Exp Brain Res 204: 343–352.
41. Tsakiris M, Haggard P (2005) The rubber hand illusion revisited: visuotactile integration and self-attribution. J Exp Psychol Hum Percept Perform 31: 80–91.
42. Costantini M, Haggard P (2007) The rubber hand illusion: sensitivity and reference frame for body ownership. Conscious Cogn 16: 229–240.
43. Valenzuela Moguillansky C, O'Regan JK, Petitmengin C (2013) Exploring the subjective experience of the "rubber hand" illusion. Front Hum Neurosci 7: 659.
44. Maister L, Sebanz N, Knoblich G, Tsakiris M (2013) Experiencing ownership over a dark-skinned body reduces implicit racial bias. Cognition 128: 170–178.
45. Hänsel A, Lenggenhager B, von Känel R, Curatolo M, Blanke O (2011) Seeing and identifying with a virtual body decreases pain perception. Eur J Pain 15: 874–879.
46. Senkowski D, Höfle M, Engel AK (2014) Crossmodal shaping of pain: a multisensory approach to nociception. Trends Cogn Sci 18: 319–327.
47. Capelari ED, Uribe C, Brasil-Neto JP (2009) Feeling pain in the rubber hand: integration of visual, proprioceptive, and painful stimuli. Perception 38: 92–99.
48. Mancini F (2013) Focus on pain in the blind. Pain 154: 1906–1907.

20

Meloxicam and Buprenorphine Treatment after Ovarian Transplantation Does Not Affect Estrous Cyclicity and Follicular Integrity in Aged CBA/J Mice

Anna H. Le, Luis A. Bonachea, Shelley L. Cargill*

Department of Biological Sciences, San José State University, San José, California, United States of America

Abstract

Angiogenesis, the formation of new blood vessels, is important for the survival of ovarian transplants and the restoration of ovarian functions. Without angiogenesis, transplanted ovarian tissue becomes more susceptible to tissue damage and necrosis. Administration of analgesics for pain management has been shown to decrease angiogenesis, which can influence transplant success especially in aged animals. Aging and the effects of hypoxia after transplantation decrease reproductive viability of the ovarian transplant; therefore, it is important to understand the additional effects of analgesics on aged animal models. The present study investigated the effects of two analgesics, buprenorphine, an opiate, and meloxicam, a non-steroidal anti-inflammatory drug (NSAID), on the reproductive indicators related to estrous cyclicity and follicular integrity after ovarian transplantation of young ovaries into aged CBA/J mice. These aged females did not show any different reproductive responses when treated with either buprenorphine or meloxicam. No significant differences were observed in estrous cycle length, the onset of estrous cycling, the regularity of estrous cycles, and the proportion of viable follicles and total number of follicles per ovarian sample across treatment groups.

Editor: Shree Ram Singh, National Cancer Institute, United States of America

Funding: This work was supported by: California State University Research Funds to SC; Junior Faculty Career Development Grant to SC; John and Betty Davison Fellowship to AL. The funders had no role in study design, data collection and analysis, decision to publish, or preparation of the manuscript.

Competing Interests: The authors have declared that no competing interests exist.

* Email: shelley.cargill@sjsu.edu

Introduction

Angiogenesis, the development of new blood vessels, is important during normal tissue development and healing. Angiogenesis, therefore, is an important determinant in the outcomes of organ transplantation as tissues require a continuous supply of nutrients, oxygen, and hormones as well as a route for removal of wastes in order to maintain viability. Angiogenic processes in normal tissue, as opposed to tumors, decrease into adulthood but occur regularly in the adult female reproductive system [1], [2]. In female rodents, angiogenesis is particularly important for the estrous cycle, which regulates varying levels of estrogen and progesterone for ovarian functions [3], [4], [5].

While the use of analgesics is advised in survival surgeries to minimize pain and discomfort in research animals, analgesics can reduce angiogenesis [6], [7], [8], [9], [10]. Although not all of the interactions of analgesics and angiogenesis have been elucidated, the putative anti-angiogenic effects of the two classes of analgesics, opiates and NSAIDs, have been investigated in some *in vivo* and *in vitro* studies [6], [7], [8], [9], [10].

In a previous aging study, the transplantation of ovaries from young CBA mice into aged, late-reproductive female mice significantly increased the remaining life expectancy of the recipients [11]. In that experiment, nearly all transplantations performed were successful, as was indicated by the restoration of estrous cyclicity. Further experiments were performed, with all procedural details kept consistent except for the additional use of post-surgery buprenorphine [12]. However, unpublished data from the same experiment suggested several unsuccessful transplants, as indicated by the lack of estrous cyclicity after surgery. It is possible that the post-surgical administration of analgesics negatively influenced transplantation success by decreasing angiogenesis and thereby decreasing the blood supply to the transplant [6], [7], [8], [9], [10].

Aging has long been acknowledged in its role in decreased female fertility [13], [14]. Angiogenesis becomes deficient with age [15] and may negatively influence reproductive function. Aged 40–48 week old female ICR mice showed a higher frequency of oocytes with DNA fragmentation, implying increased apoptotic cells compared with young 7–8 week old mice and 20–24 week old mice [13]. Estrous cycles become extended in aged mice, often leading to the cessation of cycling [14]. In addition to the effects of aging, ischemic injury due to transplantation may cause decreased viability of ovarian transplants [16], [17]. It has been demonstrated that ovarian size and the number of follicles were dramatically decreased after orthotopic grafting in mice [16]. Although mice have also demonstrated the restoration of reproductive cycling after transplantation, distinguishable estrous cycles were not always clear [17]. The use of aged models that are subject to treatment with analgesics for ovarian transplantation may have compounding effects on reproductive function. This highlights the importance of evaluating analgesic effects in aged transplant recipients to understand its impact in future transplantation studies in aged animals.

The effects of two analgesics, buprenorphine and meloxicam, on ovarian transplant success in aged females were evaluated and compared using follicular analysis, ovarian size, and estrous cyclicity post-surgery as indicators of transplant viability. A decrease in the viability of the transplant would indicate decreased angiogenesis [4], [5]. As the two different classes of analgesics have different mechanisms of action, the two analgesics may have different effects on angiogenesis and transplant viability [18], [19], [20].

Materials and Methods

Ethics Statement

This study was carried out in strict accordance with the recommendations in the Guide for the Care and Use of Laboratory Animals of the National Institutes of Health. All experimental procedures were approved by the Institutional Animal Care and Use Committee at San Jose State University (Protocol #959). Surgery was performed under sodium pentobarbital anesthesia, and all efforts were made to minimize suffering.

Mice

Adult CBA/J strain female mice (Jackson Laboratory, Sacramento, CA) were housed under controlled conditions of temperature (21±2°C), humidity (minimum 50%) and lighting (12L:12D, lights on at 0700 hours) in accordance to the University Animal Care guidelines with approval by the San José State University Institutional Animal Care and Use Committee. Animals received feed (Purina Mouse Chow 5008: 23.5% protein, 6.5% fat; Purina Mills. St Louis, MO) and water (deionized) *ad libitum*. Through power analysis, we determined that a sample size of nine focal animals per treatment group would be needed to detect a one-tailed mean difference between groups in the range of 1.5–2 standard deviations from the control animals for a single response. A sample size of 10 animals per group was chosen to account for the roughly 5% transplant failure rate and 5% seizure loss rate observed in previous studies (pers. obs.). For every experimental animal, a donor female was used to supply transplant ovaries, giving a total of 60 female mice anticipated for use in this study. As a note for other researchers, while CBA/J mice are known to be prone to seizures [21], we did not anticipate the high percentage of animals that died of seizures before the end of the study (n = 4, roughly 13%). Prior to surgery, three females died due to seizures and were excluded from the study. As a result, 27 recipient and 27 donor females were used in the transplantation procedures. Recipient and donor females were group housed with 5 animals per 26×17×13-cm cage until surgery. After surgery, each recipient female was housed individually in a 26×17×13-cm cage for the duration of the experiment. Male mice were housed in cages adjacent to female mice to promote estrous cycling in females [22].

Surgical Procedures and Vaginal Cytology

Bilateral ovariectomies of and ovarian transplantations to recipients at 11 months of age were carried out as previously described [23] with the following exception: the ovarian bursa was closed with one suture of 7-0 Ethilon nylon filament (Ethicon, San Angelo, TX) instead of the 6-0 suture [23]. The transplanted ovaries were from 2-month old females of the same strain [23]. Reproductive data in the form of vaginal cytology were collected via vaginal lavage daily at 0730 hours for one month when the recipient females were 5 months old (pre-surgery), for 14 days immediately prior to ovarian transplantation surgery, and daily starting three days after ovarian transplantation surgery for approximately 75 days (73–76 days) until the end of the experiment. All vaginal cytology data were assessed as wet mounts without staining. Donor mice were housed in close proximity to males for 1–3 weeks prior to use and were at an age considered to be reproductively competent [11] [12]. Donor mice estrous cyclicity was confirmed after surgery, as all ovarian transplant recipients cycled within 10 days after receiving the transplant. At recipient female ovariectomy, complete removal of all recipient ovarian tissue was visually confirmed under stereomicroscopy. At sacrifice, the presence of only transplanted ovarian tissue was visually confirmed under stereomicroscopy, and upon removal for analysis, no residual ovarian fragments from the ovariectomized recipient ovary were observed.

Analgesic Administration

For administration of drug treatments after surgeries, meloxicam, buprenorphine, and 0.9% saline (no analgesics) were randomly assigned to nine females each. Two saline-treated females died during the course of the experiment. One female died during the transplantation process due to anesthesia complications. CBA/J mice are susceptible to seizures, which may have been the cause of an approximately 1 month post-surgery premature death for the second female [21]. Both of these females from the saline control group were excluded from the study, for a new *n* of seven. After the unplanned losses in the saline group, the final sample size of n = 7 for the saline group would have allowed us to detect a difference as small as 1.9 SD from the mean of the saline group. The meloxicam treatment group received IP meloxicam (Boehringer Ingelheim, St. Joseph, MO) doses of 5 mg/kg of body weight, the buprenorphine treatment group received IP buprenorphine (Reckitt Benckiser Healthcare, Hull, England) doses of 0.05 mg/kg of body weight, and the saline-control group received IP 0.9% saline (Vedco, Inc., St. Joseph, MO) with the same volumes given with analgesic treatments. The analgesic doses administered were in accordance of veterinary recommendations and previous studies [12], [24], [25], [26]. These treatments were administered every 12 hours for 48 hours post-surgery, with the first dose of treatment administered at the end of surgery prior to recovery from anesthesia.

Fixation and Preservation of Ovaries

All female mice were randomly reassigned a new identification number for subsequent follicular analysis and sacrificed by cervical dislocation. Immediately after sacrifice, one ovary from each female was placed into optimal cutting temperature (OCT) medium (Sakura Finetek, Torrance, CA) and frozen over isopentane (Fisher Scientific, Fair Lawn, NJ) and dry ice (Praxair Distribution Inc., San Jose, CA). The fixed and frozen ovaries were transported overnight by FedEx to IHC World (Ellicott City, MD) to be sectioned using a cryostat. Serial consecutive sections of 6 μm thickness were placed onto glass microscope slides (TruBond, Woodstock, MD) and shipped to San Jose, CA. Upon receipt of the shipment, slides were immediately stored in −80°C until staining with hematoxylin and eosin. Nine consecutive sections per ovary were used for follicular analysis. Analyses made from these nine tissue sections are referred to as a single ovarian sample.

Histological Staining and Assessment

After removal of slides from −80°C storage, slides were warmed to room temperature, fixed in ice cold acetone (Fisher Scientific,

Santa Clara, CA) and rinsed twice in phosphate buffered saline (PBS). The primary stain, Mayer's hematoxylin (Thermo Fisher Lab Vision, Fremont, CA), was applied for five seconds, then rinsed under running tap water for 30 seconds. Slides were counterstained with 0.5% eosin Y in 95% ethanol (Allied Chemical & Dye Corp, New York, NY) for two minutes and rinsed with distilled water by dipping the slide ten times. Slides were dehydrated using 95% ethanol followed by 100% ethanol (Fisher Scientific, Pittsburgh, PA), cleared using xylene (Fisher Scientific, Fair Lawn, NJ) and a coverslip was applied using SecureMount^{TM} mounting medium (Fisher Scientific, Kalamazoo, MI).

Hematoxylin and eosin stained slides were utilized for determination of follicle numbers and the mean cross sectional area from each ovarian sample. Follicular data were collected from images captured on a Leica ICC550HD camera (JH Technologies, Fremont, CA) that had been fitted on a Leica DM500 microscope (JH Technologies, Fremont, CA) at a total magnification of 100X. Cross sectional area per ovarian sample was measured in ImageJ software (National Institutes of Health, Bethesda, MD).

Both viable and atretic follicles were counted from serial sections of each ovarian sample and viable follicles were analyzed as a proportion of the total number of follicles counted. To avoid duplication of follicle numbers, only the follicles with nuclei present in the section were counted. If a follicle did not have a nucleus present on any of the sections, the relative position of the follicle was noted to ensure the follicle was counted only once. Follicular classifications were determined based on previously described classifications [1], [27]. Representative follicle types in this study are depicted in Figure 1.

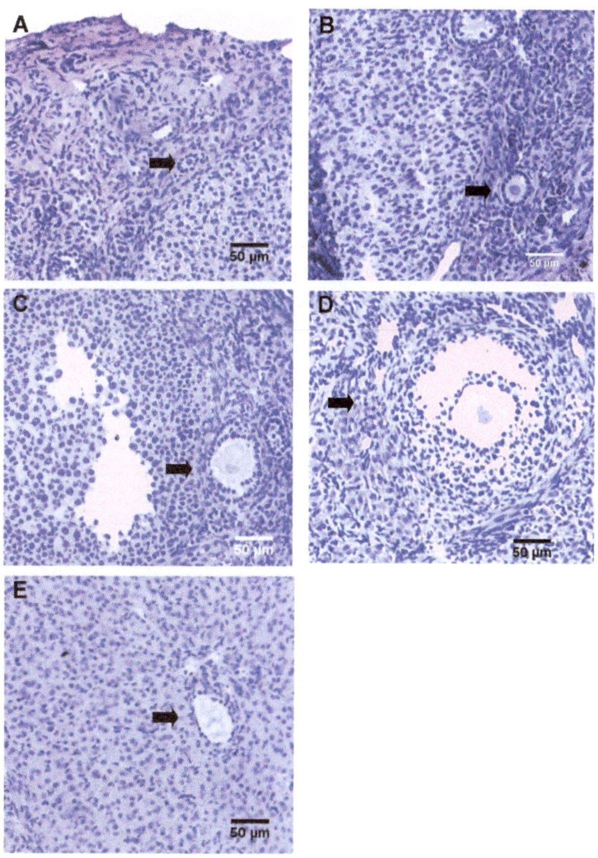

Figure 1. Representative follicle types, H&E stain, 100X total magnification. (A) primordial follicle, (B) primary follicle, (C) secondary follicle, (D) antral follicle, (F) atretic follicle. Corresponding follicles are marked by arrows.

Statistical Analyses

All vaginal smear data and follicular analyses were recorded and analyzed blind with respect to treatment. Prior to vaginal cytology analyses and follicular analyses, all animals were randomly reassigned a new identification number, which was not disclosed to the person observing the slides or performing estrous stage classification.

Estrous cycle length was determined by counting the number of days from proestrus to the next proestrus [15], [28], [29]. The 75 days of post ovarian transplantation vaginal smears were divided into three blocks of 25 days: Block 1 (days 1–25 after surgeries), Block 2 (days 26–50 after surgeries), and Block 3 (days 51–75 after surgeries). The mean estrous cycle length across treatment groups was analyzed for all 75 days and for each block. In addition, the onset of estrous cycle was determined by the number of days after surgery to the first proestrus. Finally, the estrous cycles from each animal were classified into three categories: regular (4–5 days in length with either 1–2 days of estrus or 2–3 days of diestrus), extended (3–4 consecutive days of estrus or 4–5 consecutive days of diestrus), and abnormal (more than 4 consecutive days of estrus or more than 6 consecutive days of diestrus) [28].

Estrous cycle lengths (days) for all 75-days post-surgery and the onset of estrous cycle (days) across treatment groups were compared using Kruskal-Wallis ANOVA as the data failed the Shapiro-Wilk Test for normality. The estrous cycle lengths (days) for the three blocks were rank transformed and analyzed using MANOVA as the data were not normally distributed as determined by the Shapiro-Wilk Test. Whether or not individuals from each treatment group cycled until the end of the study was compared using a Chi-square Test of Independence. The differences in the number of regular, extended, and abnormal cycles between treatments were rank transformed and compared using MANOVA as the data failed the Shapiro-Wilk Test for normality. Classifications of estrous cycles were also compared using the Chi-square Test of Independence for differences in the percentage of females between treatments that exhibited abnormal cycles *versus* those that did not. A separate Chi-square Test of Independence was used to test the differences in the percentage of females between treatments that did and did not exhibit extended cycles. Percentage of viable follicles and the total number of follicles counted per ovarian sample were compared using MANOVA. The cross sectional area per ovarian sample of each treatment group was compared using Kruskal-Wallis ANOVA as the data failed the Levene's Test for Homogeneity of Variances.

Results

Estrous Cyclicity

Estrous cycle length was not significantly different across groups (Kruskal-Wallis ANOVA: $\chi^2 = 0.92$, df = 2, $p = 0.63$; Figure 2A). The median estrous cycle length for the saline-control was 7.7 days ($n = 6$, $Q_1 = 7.3$, $Q_3 = 8.1$), for the buprenorphine-treated was 6.9 days ($n = 8$, $Q_1 = 6.2$, $Q_3 = 9.1$), and for the meloxicam-treated was 7.2 days ($n = 8$, $Q_1 = 6.1$, $Q_3 = 8.3$). One female from each treatment group was excluded from analysis due to abnormal cycle lengths (>3 standard deviations from the sample mean).

The cycle lengths during Block 1 (days 1–25 after surgeries), Block 2 (days 26–50), and Block 3 (days 51–75) were not

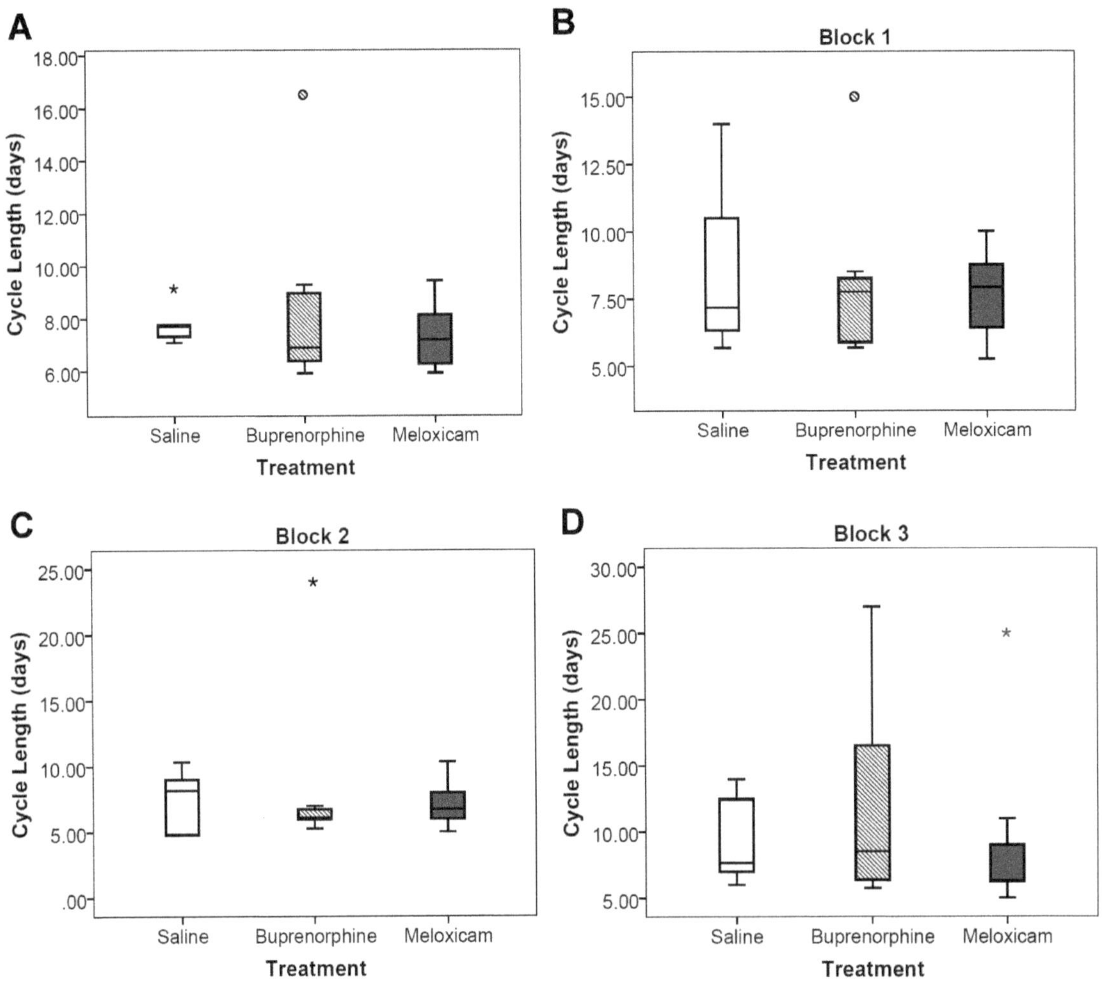

Figure 2. Boxplots of the estrous cycle length in days taken from daily vaginal cytology for each time block after surgery. (A) all 75 days (Kruskal-Wallis ANOVA: $\chi^2 = 0.92$, df = 2, $p = 0.63$). (B) block 1, days 1–25 after surgery. (C) block 2 days 26–50 after surgery. (D) block 3, days 51–75 after surgery. $N = 22$, saline ($n = 6$), buprenorphine ($n = 8$), meloxicam ($n = 8$). (Rank transformed, MANOVA: F(6,34) = 0.27, $p = 0.95$). The horizontal line in each box interior represents the median, the upper and lower whiskers show the maximum and minimum values, the upper hinge represents the 75th percentile, the lower hinge represents the 25th percentile, "o" represents an outside value, and asterisk (*) represents a far outside value.

significantly different across treatment groups in any of the three time blocks (Rank transformed, MANOVA: F(6,34) = 0.27, $p = 0.95$; Figure 2B, 2C, 2D). The median cycle length during Block 1 was 7.2 days for the saline-control ($n = 6$, $Q_1 = 6.2$, $Q_3 = 11.4$), 7.8 days for the buprenorphine-treated ($n = 8$, $Q_1 = 5.8$, $Q_3 = 8.4$), and 7.9 days for the meloxicam-treated ($n = 8$, $Q_1 = 6.4$. $Q_3 = 8.9$). During Block 2, the median cycle length was 8.2 days for saline ($Q_1 = 4.8$, $Q_3 = 9.3$), 6.1 days for buprenorphine ($Q_1 = 6.0$, $Q_3 = 6.9$), and 6.8 days for meloxicam ($Q_1 = 5.9$, $Q_3 = 8.0$). During Block 3, the median cycle length was 7.7 days for saline ($Q_1 = 6.8$, $Q_3 = 12.9$), 8.5 days for buprenorphine ($Q_1 = 6.2$, $Q_3 = 18.8$), and 6.3 days for meloxicam ($Q_1 = 6.3$, $Q_3 = 10.0$). One female from each treatment group was excluded from analysis due to no cycling in at least one of the blocks.

There was no significant difference in the time until the onset of estrous cycling between groups (Kruskal-Wallis ANOVA: $\chi^2 = 3.64$, df = 2, $p = 0.16$). Median number of days to the onset of cycling was 9.0 days for the saline-control ($n = 7$, $Q_1 = 7.00$, $Q_3 = 12.00$), 6.0 days for the buprenorphine-treated ($n = 9$, $Q_1 = 5.00$, $Q_3 = 9.00$), and 7.0 days for the meloxicam-treated ($n = 9$, $Q_1 = 5.50$, $Q_3 = 7.50$). The onset of cycling was seen as early as 5 days post-surgery and the mean onset of estrous cycling across all treatment groups was 10 days ($SD = 10.52$) post-surgery. All females across all treatment groups exhibited estrous cyclicity after ovarian transplantation indicating successful transplantation for all recipient females.

Estrous cycle analysis showed no significant relationship between treatment and duration of cycling (whether or not a female cycled until the end of the study, Day 75) (Chi-square Test of Independence: $\chi^2 = 3.87$, df = 2, $p = 0.15$). Two females from the buprenorphine-treated group exhibited early cessation of cycling (approximately 20 days before sacrifice), while the other seven buprenorphine-treated females (77.8%) cycled until the end of the study. All females (100%) from the saline-control and meloxicam-treated groups cycled until the end of the study.

There was no significant difference across treatments in the number of regular, extended, or abnormal cycles exhibited in the 75 days post-surgery (Rank transformed, MANOVA: F(6,40) = 0.60, $p = 0.73$; Figure 3). The saline group ($n = 7$) exhibited a median of 4 regular cycles ($Q_1 = 3.0$, $Q_3 = 6.0$), 1 extended cycle ($Q_1 = 0.0$, $Q_3 = 3.0$), and 2 abnormal cycles ($Q_1 = 1.0$, $Q_3 = 3.0$). The buprenorphine group ($n = 9$) exhibited

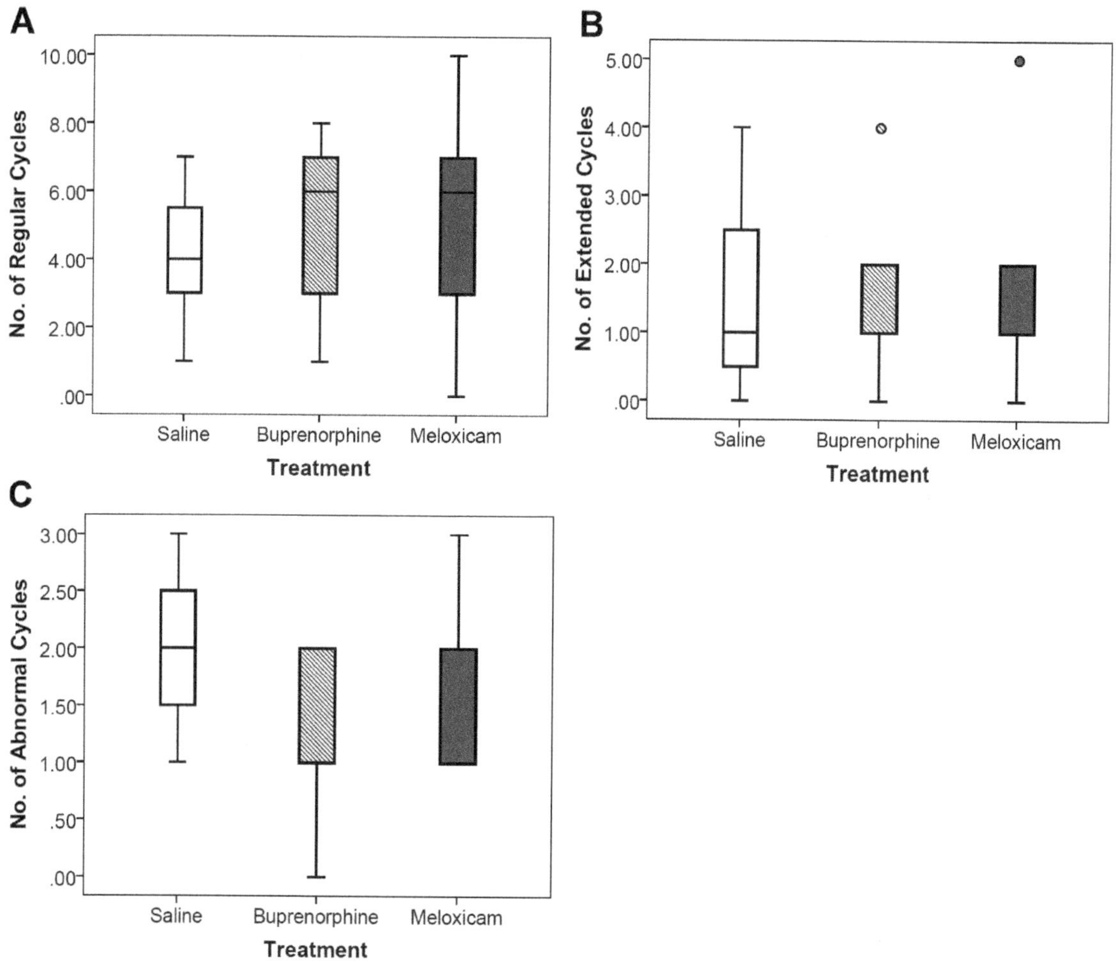

Figure 3. Boxplots of the estrous cycle classifications for each treatment. (A) regular, defined by 4–5 days in length. (B) extended, defined by 3–4 consecutive days of estrus or 4–5 consecutive days of diestrus. (C) abnormal, defined by having >4 days consecutive days of estrus or >6 consecutive days of diestrus. $N = 25$, saline ($n = 7$), buprenorphine ($n = 9$), meloxicam ($n = 9$). (Rank transformed, MANOVA: $F(6,40) = 0.60$, $p = 0.73$). The horizontal line in each box interior represents the median, the upper and lower whiskers show the maximum and minimum values, the upper hinge represents the 75th percentile, the lower hinge represents the 25th percentile, "o" represents an outside value, and asterisk (*) represents a far outside value.

a median of 6 regular cycles ($Q_1 = 3.0$, $Q_3 = 7.0$), 1 extended cycle ($Q_1 = 1.0$, $Q_3 = 2.0$), and 2 abnormal cycles ($Q_1 = 0.5$, $Q_3 = 2.0$). The meloxicam group ($n = 9$) exhibited a median of 6 regular cycles ($Q_1 = 3.0$, $Q3 = 6.0$), 1 extended cycle ($Q_1 = 0.5$, $Q_3 = 2.0$), and 2 abnormal cycles ($Q_1 = 1.0$, $Q_3 = 2.5$).

All females in the saline-control ($n = 7$) group and the meloxicam-treated group ($n = 9$) exhibited abnormal estrous cycles (more than 4 consecutive days of estrus or more than 6 consecutive days of diestrus) compared with seven females (77.8%) in the buprenorphine-treated ($n = 9$) group. The percentages of each treatment exhibiting abnormal estrous cycles as opposed to not

Table 1. Percentage of females from each treatment exhibiting the three categories of estrous cycles: regular, extended, and abnormal.

Treatment	n	Females with Regular Cycles (%)	Females with Extended Cycles (%)	Females with Abnormal Cycles (%)
Saline	7	100	71.4	100
Buprenorphine	9	100	77.8	77.8
Meloxicam	9	88.9	77.8	100

Regular cycles defined by cycle lengths of 4–5 days, extended cycles defined by 3–4 days of consecutive estrus or 4–5 days of diestrus, and abnormal cycles defined by >4 days or consecutive estrus or >5 days of diestrus, (Chi-square Test of Independence, Regular $\chi^2 = 1.85$ and $p = 0.40$, Extended $\chi^2 = 0.11$ and $p = 0.95$, Abnormal $\chi^2 = 3.87$ and $p = 0.15$).

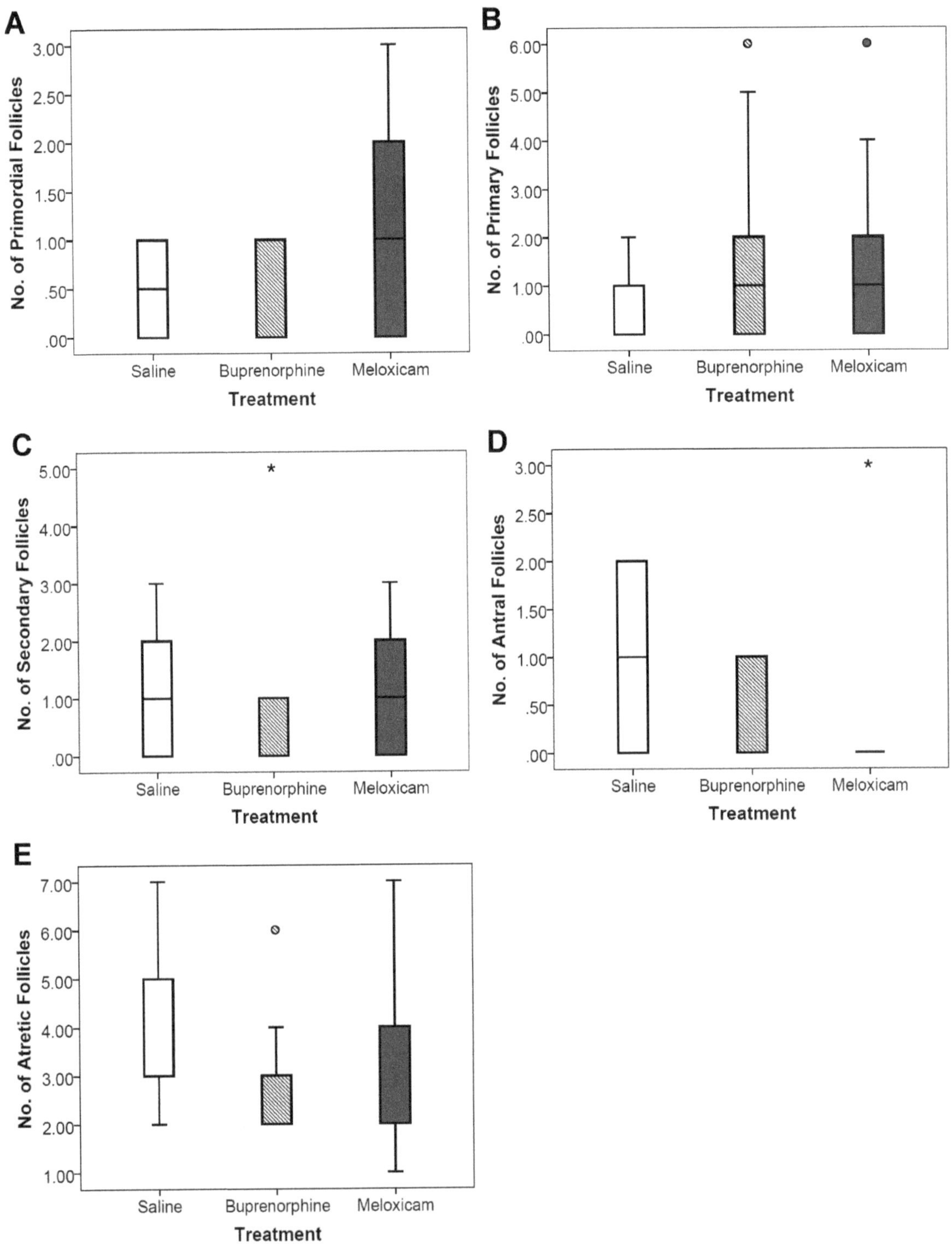

Figure 4. Boxplots of the number of each follicle type per ovarian sample (each ovarian sample consists of nine tissue sections). $N = 24$, saline ($n = 6$), buprenorphine ($n = 9$), meloxicam ($n = 9$). (Rank transformed, MANOVA: $F(10,34) = 0.45$, $p = 0.91$). (A) primordial follicles. (B) primary follicles. (C) secondary follicles. (D) early antral follicles. (E) antral follicles. (F) atretic follicles. The horizontal line in each box interior represents the median, the upper and lower whiskers show the maximum and minimum values, the upper hinge represents the 75th percentile, the lower hinge represents the 25th percentile, "o" represents an outside value, and asterisk (*) represents a far outside value.

exhibiting abnormal cycles were not significantly different (Chi-square Test of Independence: $\chi^2 = 3.87$, df = 2, $p = 0.15$, Table 1). Five saline-control, seven buprenorphine-treated, and seven meloxicam-treated females exhibited extended estrous cycles (3–4 consecutive days of estrus or 4–5 consecutive days of diestrus). The proportions of each treatment group exhibiting extended estrous cycles was also not significant (Chi-square Test of Independence: $\chi^2 = 0.11$, df = 2, $p = 0.95$, Table 1). All saline-

Table 2. The proportion of viable follicles and the total number of follicles per ovarian sample for each treatment.

Treatment	n	Proportion of Viable Follicles per ovarian sample	Total No. of Follicles per ovarian sample
Saline	6	0.48±0.18	7.3±2.07
Buprenorphine	9	0.44±0.26	6.9±5.09
Meloxicam	9	0.51±0.24	7.6±4.33

Data are shown as mean ± SD. Each ovarian sample consists of nine tissue sections. The total number of follicles per ovarian sample includes counts from viable and atretic follicles. (MANOVA, F(4,40) = 0.10, $p = 0.98$).

control and buprenorphine-treated females and eight meloxicam-treated females exhibited at least one regular estrous cycle (Chi-square Test of Independence: $\chi^2 = 1.85$, df = 2, $p = 0.40$, Table 1).

Histological Analysis

One female from the saline-control group was excluded from all histological analyses, as tissue sections from this female were lacking ovarian tissue. The number of each follicle type across treatment groups was not significantly different (Rank transformed, MANOVA: F(10,34) = 0.45, $p = 0.91$; Figure 4). Treatment did not have any significant effect on the proportion of viable follicles and the number of total follicles observed per ovarian sample (MANOVA: F(4,40) = 0.10, $p = 0.98$; Table 2). The mean proportion of viable follicles was approximately 47.8% for the saline-control group, 43.7% for the buprenorphine-treated group, and 50.9% for the meloxicam-treated group. The mean total number of follicles (including viable and atretic follicles) counted from each ovarian sample was 7.3 for the saline-control, 6.9 for the buprenorphine-treated, and 7.6 for the meloxicam-treated groups.

No significant differences were observed in the cross-sectional area of the ovary across treatments (Kruskal-Wallis ANOVA: $\chi^2 = 0.76$, df = 2, $p = 0.69$). The median cross sectional area of the saline-control group was 1.33 mm^2 ($n = 6$, $Q_1 = 0.91$, $Q_3 = 1.62$), of the buprenorphine-treated group was 1.64 mm^2 ($n = 9$, $Q_1 = 0.91$, $Q_3 = 2.00$), and of the meloxicam-treated group was 1.40 mm^2 ($n = 9$, $Q_1 = 1.30$, $Q_3 = 1.69$).

Discussion

Indicators of ovarian transplant success, estrous cyclicity, and viability of follicles revealed no significant differences between treatment groups. Previous studies have found that both opiates and NSAIDs negatively affect angiogenesis with some conflicting results regarding increased or decreased angiogenesis with opiate treatments [6], [8], [9], [30], [31]. Most of these studies have employed high doses of analgesics for prolonged periods, which do not represent the veterinary recommended doses utilized in the current study [6], [8], [9], [27], [28]. The results from this study indicate that recommended doses for a moderate time period do not negatively affect the transplanted ovary in aged females beyond what is expected by the surgical process itself.

Neovascularization of an ovarian heterotopic autotransplant could be observed as soon as three days after transplantation in mice and two days in rats [32], [33], [34]. Restoration of ovarian cycling has been reported to occur as soon as 10–14 days after transplantation of whole ovary transplants and ovarian grafts [16], [17], [35]. However, after transplantation of whole ovaries in this study, as opposed to transplantation of ovarian grafts in previous studies, the onset of estrous cycle occurred as early as five days post-surgery with a mean of 10 days for all females.

Animal models of ovarian transplantations are especially sensitive to the effects of aging. In the present study, ovaries from 2-month old females were transplanted into 11-month old females. The CBA/J mice used in the current study have a lifespan of 647 days [36] with a decline in fecundity at approximately 11 months of age [37]. Total follicle numbers in young 6–8 week old C3H/HeNCrlBR and B6129SF1/J ovaries that had been grafted into 6–8 week old B6C3F1/J and B6129SF1/J recipients was lower than intact ovary total follicle numbers and have been estimated to be about 100 follicles per ovary [16] due to the hypoxia experienced with ovarian transplantation [5]. Also of importance is that gonadotropin levels decrease with age, reducing gonadotropic input to the ovaries [38], [39]. In middle-aged rodents, a significant decrease was seen in the levels of LH during an LH surge as well as a delayed occurrence of the LH surge compared with young rodents [39]. GnRH levels may not change with age, but the LH response to GnRH decreases with age [38]. These age-associated factors could lead to decreased follicular development and thus to decreased follicular counts in the aged recipients of this study. These factors may have contributed to the early cessation of cycling seen in two of the buprenorphine-treated animals. It is also possible that those two animals experienced decreased vascularization of the transplanted ovary but it is unclear whether this can be attributed to the analgesic buprenorphine.

The effects of analgesics on ovarian transplant success in aged females require further investigation. This study suggests that at the recommended veterinary doses [12], [24], [25], [26], the two analgesics studied do not decrease angiogenesis to the extent that there are alterations in estrous cycle length or the proportion of viable follicles and the total number of follicles per ovary. This would imply that the veterinary recommended doses of analgesic do not induce additional damage after ovarian transplantation nor significantly affect the function of the transplanted ovary. Thus, the recommended dosages for buprenorphine and meloxicam may be beneficial to decrease surgical pain in mice without negatively affecting ovarian transplant survival as assessed by estrous cycle length and follicle count.

Acknowledgments

We thank Michael Sneary and Rachael French for sharing their scientific expertise and Gary B. Anderson for his insightful review of the manuscript.

Author Contributions

Conceived and designed the experiments: SC AL. Performed the experiments: AL SC. Analyzed the data: AL LB. Contributed reagents/materials/analysis tools: AL SC LB. Contributed to the writing of the manuscript: AL SC LB.

References

1. Bassett DL (1943) The changes in the vascular pattern of the ovary of the albino rat during the estrous cycle. Am J Anat 73(2): 251–291.
2. Shweiki D, Itin A, Neufeld G, Gitay-Goren H, Keshet E (1993) Patterns of expression of vascular endothelial growth factor (VEGF) and VEGF receptors in mice suggest a role in hormonally regulated angiogenesis. J Clin Invest 91(5): 2235–2243.
3. Fevold HL, Hisaw FL, Leonard SL (1931) The gonad stimulating and the luteinizing hormones of the anterior lobe of the hypophesis. Am J Physiol 97(2): 291–301.
4. Israely T, Dafni H, Granot D, Nevo N, Tsafriri A, et al. (2003) Vascular remodeling and angiogenesis in ectopic ovarian transplants: a crucial role of pericytes and vascular smooth muscle cells in maintenance of ovarian grafts. Biol Reprod 68(6): 2055–2064.
5. Kim SS, Yang HW, Kang HG, Lee HH, Lee HC, et al. (2004) Quantitative assessment of ischemic tissue damage in ovarian cortical tissue with or without antioxidant (ascorbic acid) treatment. Fertil Steril 82(3): 679–685.
6. Hsiao PN, Chang MC, Cheng WF, Chen CA, Lin HW, et al. (2009) Morphine induces apoptosis of human endothelial cells through nitric oxide and reactive oxygen species pathways. Toxicol 256(1): 83–91.
7. Jones MK, Wang H, Peskar BM, Levin E, Itani RM, et al. (1999) Inhibition of angiogenesis by nonsteroidal anti-inflammatory drugs: insight into mechanisms and implications for cancer growth and ulcer healing. Nat Med 5(12): 1418–1423.
8. Lam CF, Chang PJ, Huang YS, Sung YH, Huang CC, et al. (2008) Prolonged use of high-dose morphine impairs angiogenesis and mobilization of endothelial progenitor cells in mice. Anesth Analg 107(2): 686–692.
9. Liu HC, Anday JK, House SD, Chang SL (2004) Dual effects of morphine on permeability and apoptosis of vascular endothelial cells: morphine potentiates lipopolysaccharide-induced permeability and apoptosis of vascular endothelial cells. J Neuroimmunol 146(1): 13–21.
10. Zúñiga J, Fuenzalida M, Guerrero G, Illanes J, Dabancens A, et al. (2003) Effects of steroidal and non steroidal drugs on the neovascularization response induced by tumoral TA3 supernatant on CAM from chick embryo. Biol Res 36(2): 233–240.
11. Cargill SL, Carey JR, Müller HG, Anderson G (2003) Age of ovary determines remaining life expectancy in old ovariectomized mice. Aging Cell 2(3): 185–190.
12. Mason JB, Cargill SL, Anderson GB, Carey JR (2009) Transplantation of young ovaries to old mice increased life span in transplant recipients J Gerontol A Biol Sci Med Sci 64(12): 1207–1211.
13. Fujing Y, Ozaki K, Yamamasu S, Ito F, Matsuoka I, et al. (1996) DNA fragmentation of oocytes in aged mice. Mol Hum Reprod 11(7): 1480–1483.
14. Nelson JF, Felicio LS, Randall PK, Sims C, Finch CE (1982) A longitudinal study of estrous cyclicity in aging C57BL/6J mice: I. Cycle frequency, length and vaginal cytology. Biol Reprod 27(2): 327–339.
15. Rivard A, Fabre JE, Silver M, Chen D, Murohara T, et al. (1999) Age-dependent impairment of angiogenesis. Circulation 99(1): 111–120.
16. Liu L, Wood GA, Morikawa L, Ayearst R, Fleming C, et al. (2008) Restoration of fertility by orthotopic transplantation of frozen adult mouse ovaries. Hum Reprod 23(1): 122–128.
17. Gunasena KT, Villines PM, Critser ES, Critser JK (1997) Live births after autologous transplant of cryopreserved mouse ovaries. Hum Reprod 12(1): 101–106.
18. Kamei J, Saitoh A, Suzuki T, Misawa M, Nagase H, et al. (1995) Buprenorphine exerts its antinociceptive activity via μ1-opioid receptors. Life Sci 56(15): PL285–PL290.
19. Tarnawski AS, Jones MK (2003) Inhibition of angiogenesis by NSAIDs: molecular mechanisms and clinical implications. J Mol Med 81: 627–636.
20. Vane JR, Botting RM (1996) Mechanism of action of anti-inflammatory drugs. Scand J Rheumatol 25: 9–21.
21. Fuller JL, Sjursen Jr FH (1967) Audiogenic seizures in eleven mouse strains. J Hered 58(3): 135–140.
22. Whitten WK (1956) Modification of the oestrous cycle of the mouse by external stimuli associated with the male. J Endocrinol 13(4): 399–404.
23. Cargill SL, Medrano JF, Anderson GB (1999) Infertility in a line of mice with the high growth mutation is due to luteal insufficiency resulting from disruption at the hypothalamic-pituitary axis. Biol Reprod 61: 283–287.
24. Flecknell P (2009) Laboratory Animal Anesthesia. Burlington: Academic Press. 300 p.
25. Plumb DC (2002) Veterinary Drug Handbook. White Bear Lake: Iowa State Press. 1208 p.
26. Wright-Williams SL, Courade JP, Richardson CA, Roughan JA, Flecknell PA (2007) Effects of vasectomy surgery and meloxicam treatment of faecal corticosterone levels and behaviour in two strains of laboratory mouse. Pain 130: 108–118.
27. Myers M, Britt KL, Wreford NGM, Ebling FJP, Kerr JB (2004) Methods for quantifying follicular numbers within the mouse ovary. Reprod 127(5): 569–580.
28. Goldman JM, Murr AS, Cooper RL (2007) The rodent estrous cycle: characterization of vaginal cytology and its utility in toxicological studies. Birth Defects Res B Dev Reprod Toxicol 80(2): 84–97.
29. Lohff JC, Christian PJ, Marion SL, Arrandale A, Hoyer PB (2005) Characterization of cyclicity and hormonal profile with impending ovarian failure in a novel chemical-induced mouse model of perimenopause. Comp Med 55(6): 523–527.
30. Dai X, Song H, Cui S, Wang T, Liu Q, et al. (2010) The stimulative effects of endogenous opioids on endothelial cell proliferation, migration, and angiogenesis in vitro. Eur J Pharmacol 628: 42–50.
31. Gupta K, Kshirsagar S, Chang L, Schwartz RS, Law PY, et al. (2002) Morphine stimulates angiogenesis by activating proangiogenic and survival-promoting signaling and promotes breast tumor growth. Cancer Res 62: 4491–4498.
32. Dissen GA, Lara HE, Fahrenbach WH, Costa ME, Ojeda SR (1994) Immature rat ovaries become revascularized rapidly after autotransplantation and show a gonadotropin-dependent increase in angiogenic factor gene expression. Endocrinol 134(3): 1146–1154.
33. Nugent D, Newton H, Gallivan L, Gosden RG (1998) Protective effect of vitamin E on ischaemia-reperfusion injury in ovarian grafts. J Reprod Fertil 114(2): 341–346.
34. Wang Y, Chang Q, Sun J, Dang L, Ma W, et al. (2012) Effects of HMG on revascularization and follicular survival in heterotopic autotransplants of mouse ovarian tissue. Reprod Biomed Online 24(6): 646–653.
35. Harris M, Eakin RM (1949) Survival of transplanted ovaries in rats. J Exp Zool 112(1): 131–163.
36. Yuan R, Tsaih SW, Petkova SB, Evsikova CM, Xing S, et al. (2009) Aging in inbred strains of mice: study design and interim report on median lifespans and circulating IGF1 levels. Aging Cell 8: 277–287.
37. Gosden RG. (1975) Ovarian support of pregnancy in ageing inbred mice. J Reprod Fert 42: 423–430.
38. Arias P, Carbone S, Szwarcfarb B, Feleder C, Rodríguez M, et al. (1996) Effects of aging on N-methyl-D-aspartate (NMDA)-induced GnRH and LH release in female rats. Brain Res 740(1): 234–238.
39. Cooper RL, Conn PM, Walker RF (1980) Characterization of the LH surge in middle-aged female rats. Biol Reprod 23(3): 611–615.

21

Persistent At-Level Thermal Hyperalgesia and Tactile Allodynia Accompany Chronic Neuronal and Astrocyte Activation in Superficial Dorsal Horn following Mouse Cervical Contusion Spinal Cord Injury

Jaime L. Watson, Tamara J. Hala, Rajarshi Putatunda, Daniel Sannie, Angelo C. Lepore*

Department of Neuroscience, Farber Institute for Neurosciences, Sidney Kimmel Medical College at Thomas Jefferson University, Philadelphia, Pennsylvania, United States of America

Abstract

In humans, sensory abnormalities, including neuropathic pain, often result from traumatic spinal cord injury (SCI). SCI can induce cellular changes in the CNS, termed central sensitization, that alter excitability of spinal cord neurons, including those in the dorsal horn involved in pain transmission. Persistently elevated levels of neuronal activity, glial activation, and glutamatergic transmission are thought to contribute to the hyperexcitability of these dorsal horn neurons, which can lead to maladaptive circuitry, aberrant pain processing and, ultimately, chronic neuropathic pain. Here we present a mouse model of SCI-induced neuropathic pain that exhibits a persistent pain phenotype accompanied by chronic neuronal hyperexcitability and glial activation in the spinal cord dorsal horn. We generated a unilateral cervical contusion injury at the C5 or C6 level of the adult mouse spinal cord. Following injury, an increase in the number of neurons expressing ΔFosB (a marker of chronic neuronal activation), persistent astrocyte activation and proliferation (as measured by GFAP and Ki67 expression), and a decrease in the expression of the astrocyte glutamate transporter GLT1 are observed in the ipsilateral superficial dorsal horn of cervical spinal cord. These changes have previously been associated with neuronal hyperexcitability and may contribute to altered pain transmission and chronic neuropathic pain. In our model, they are accompanied by robust at-level hyperaglesia in the ipsilateral forepaw and allodynia in both forepaws that are evident within two weeks following injury and persist for at least six weeks. Furthermore, the pain phenotype occurs in the absence of alterations in forelimb grip strength, suggesting that it represents sensory and not motor abnormalities. Given the importance of transgenic mouse technology, this clinically-relevant model provides a resource that can be used to study the molecular mechanisms contributing to neuropathic pain following SCI and to identify potential therapeutic targets for the treatment of chronic pathological pain.

Editor: Guglielmo Foffani, Hospital Nacional de Parapléjicos, Spain

Funding: This work was funded by the NIH (1R01NS079702 to A.C.L.) and the Craig H. Neilsen Foundation (#190140 to A.C.L.). The funders had no role in study design, data collection and analysis, decision to publish, or preparation of the manuscript.

Competing Interests: The authors have declared that no competing interests exist.

* Email: Angelo.Lepore@jefferson.edu

Introduction

Spinal cord injury (SCI) is a debilitating condition with widespread symptoms that affect patient quality of life. As many as 327,000 SCI patients are currently living in the United States, and approximately 12,000 new cases are reported each year [1]. Clinical studies propose that 64–82% of SCI patients experience some form of pathological pain following injury, and this pain has been associated with mood changes as well as difficulty with work and social activities [2]. Neuropathic pain constitutes a significant percentage of pain resulting from SCI; 41% of patients encounter at-level and 34% experience below-level neuropathic pain [3] following injury. Although SCI most often involves an acute injury to the spinal cord, the resulting pathological pain is often chronic and can increase in severity over time [4]. Thus, SCI-related neuropathic pain and its treatment is an important focus of spinal cord research.

In this study, we wanted to identify the molecular changes accompanying the alterations of at-level pain sensitivity in a mouse model of cervical contusion SCI. We induced SCI in the mouse and measured changes in pain behavior, specifically thermal hyperalgesia and tactile allodynia. Additionally, we studied the expression of various proteins in the dorsal horn of the spinal cord that may contribute to neuropathic pain and the cell types expressing these proteins. Importantly, we chose to utilize a mouse model of SCI that is clinically relevant but has not previously been used to study neuropathic pain.

Currently, mouse models of SCI-induced neuropathic pain are available, but do not address cervical contusion injury. According to the National Spinal Cord Injury Statistical Center, the majority of SCI patients in the United States experience injury to the cervical regions of the spinal cord [1], but most rodent SCI models involve injury to thoracic regions. Therefore, we chose to target our SCI to the cervical region of the spinal cord.

Additionally, contusion-type injury is most common in human patients [5] and is a popular model of SCI in rodents [6]. The respiratory and other dysfunctions that commonly accompany cervical contusion injuries make this model difficult to study [7]. To date, our group [8], [9], [10] and others [11] have used models of cervical contusion SCI in the mouse and rat to study motor deficits following injury. In the study of neuropathic pain, however, contusive injury to the cervical regions of the spinal cord has not been utilized in mice. Instead, transection, compression, contusion and other procedures are used primarily at thoracic levels to induce SCI in mice for studying neuropathic pain [6]. Here, we designed a model of moderate hemicontusive injury to the cervical spinal cord in the mouse that does not develop significant respiratory or other life-threatening complications for the study of neuropathic pain.

The development of neuropathic pain following SCI involves the disruption of neurons involved in nociception in the dorsal horn of the spinal cord. Under normal circumstances, neurons in the superficial laminae of the dorsal horn are responsible for pain transmission from peripheral nociceptors to the thalamus and, ultimately, the sensory cortex. Upon injury to the spinal cord, however, local changes can occur that alter how nociceptive neurons respond to peripheral stimuli [12]. These changes, termed central sensitization, can underlie pathological pain behaviors such as allodynia and hyperalgesia [12], [13].

One mechanism involved in central sensitization is the hyperexcitability of pain transmission neurons. Neuronal hyperexcitability results in an increase in the response of neurons to electrical input or even the firing of neurons in the absence of input. Hyperexcitability is characterized by spontaneous neuronal activity, aberrant responses to subthreshold stimuli, and increased transmission of suprathreshold input [12], [13]. In SCI, pain projection neurons in the dorsal horn can become more easily excited by noxious as well as non-noxious stimuli, resulting in pathological pain transmission. Changes to the neuron itself, as well as to its extracellular environment, can alter the neuron's electrophysiological profile, increasing its resting membrane potential and/or decreasing its action potential threshold. As one example of a mechanism underlying central sensitization, increased activity of transcription factors can trigger changes in gene expression that lead to long-term alterations in neuronal function and excitability. For instance, ΔfosB, a commonly used marker of persistent neuronal activation, has been associated with plasticity of pain transmission circuits in inflammatory pain, possibly through downstream targets such as CDK5 [14], [15].

Underlying hyperexcitability and central sensitization in SCI are changes in glial activation and glutamate transporter function. Astrocytes play an essential role in the central nervous system, providing support to neurons, regulating the uptake of glutamate and other factors from the extracellular space, and modulating synapse formation and function [13], [16]. Soon after insult, astrocytes can become activated (marked by glial fibrillary acidic protein (GFAP)) and possibly even proliferative and act to minimize the effects of the injury by reestablishing the blood brain barrier, releasing antioxidants, and protecting the lesion site from detrimental molecules. Activation of astrocytes, however, can also be harmful to neighboring neurons; when persistently active, astrocytes can contribute to neuronal hyperexcitability through the release of factors such as proinflammatory molecules, nitric oxide, and ATP [13], [17], [18].

The loss of glutamate transporters by activated astrocytes and the resulting imbalance in glutamate homeostasis may also contribute to the development of post-SCI neuropathic pain. Under normal conditions, glutamate is cleared from the synapse via glutamate transporters, such as GLT1 and GLAST, located in the plasma membrane of neurons and, more often, astrocytes. However, elevated release of glutamate from presynaptic neurons and/or injured neurons and glia or from damage to the glutamate transporter system can cause an excess of glutamate to linger in synaptic and extra-synaptic locations [13]. This disruption in glutamate homeostasis leads to overactivation of glutamate receptors, which can in some instances result in increased Ca^{2+} concentrations in the postsynaptic neuron. These changes can have negative impacts on cell health and function and alter the activation state of the neuron [19], [20], [21]. In SCI, glutamate excitotoxic damage to inhibitory interneurons can also indirectly boost the excitability of nociceptive neurons in the dorsal horn [18]. In this way, the loss of GLT1 in astrocytes observed following injury by our group [22], [23], [24] and others [25], [26] may contribute to central sensitization and neuropathic pain.

Recently published data from our group showed changes in neuronal and astrocyte activation as well as GLT1 expression in the superficial dorsal horn following cervical contusion SCI-induced hyperalgesia in the rat [24]. The study characterized a moderate hemicontusion injury to cervical regions of the rat spinal cord, which resulted in ipsilateral hyperalgesic behavior. Accompanying hyperalgesia were chronic increases in ΔfosB expression in neurons, astrocyte activation and proliferation in addition to a loss of GLT1 both at the site of the injury and in intact spinal cord caudal to the contusion site [24].

In the current study we characterize increases in pain sensitivity in a mouse model of cervical contusion SCI and the accompanying molecular alterations in the dorsal horn of the spinal cord. Our model exhibits at-level thermal hyperalgesia and tactile allodynia in addition to increases in neuronal and astrocyte activation and a decrease in astrocyte glutamate transporter expression in the superficial dorsal horn. Alterations in pain behavior, as well as neuronal and glial activation and glutamate transport expression in the dorsal horn, have not previously been characterized in mice receiving cervical contusion SCI. Thus, this study provides an observation of the molecular and behavioral changes that occur following cervical SCI in the mouse that can be used to further study the mechanisms underlying neuropathic pain in SCI.

Methods

Animal Studies

Ethics Statement. All animal care and treatment were conducted in strict accordance with the *European Communities Council Directive* (2010/63/EU, 86/609/EEC and 87-848/EEC) and the *NIH Guide for the Care and Use of Laboratory Animals*. Experimental protocols were approved by the Thomas Jefferson University Institutional Animal Care and Use Committee.

Animals. Fifty-six male C57BL/6 mice (25–30 g; The Jackson Laboratory, USA) and 26 transgenic BAC-GLT1-eGFP reporter mice [27] were used. The BAC-GLT1-eGFP reporter mice were created by Regan et al. [27]. The transgene in these mice involves cDNA for eGFP inserted into the start codon of a mouse BAC encompassing the entire GLT-1 gene. Thus, in these mice, eGFP expression is driven by the GLT1 promoter. Mice were housed 5 per cage in a controlled light-dark environment in the Thomas Jefferson University Animal Facility and were given food and water *ad libitum*. To prevent suffering, a combination of ketamine/xylazine and isofluorane was used to anesthetize animals during surgical procedures.

SCI Models. We chose to utilize two models in the C57BL/6 mice in this study; one with injury at the C5 level and another with injury at the C6 level. We did this to show that contusion injury to various levels of the cervical spinal cord has the potential to produce at-level neuropathic pain. Mice were anesthetized initially with ketamine (100 mg/kg) and xylazine (5 mg/kg) injected intraperitoneally, and the anesthetic plane was maintained with 1% isofluorane for the duration of the surgery. The body was immobilized by taping the forelegs to a fixation plate, and the head was immobilized by the isofluorane nose cone. The skin and muscle overlying the spinal column were retracted from levels C3 to T1, and spinal cord was exposed by unilateral laminectomy from the midline blood vessel to the lateral edge of the vertebral lamina at the level of C5 or C6. The spinal column was stabilized at the C3 and T1 spinous processes by microforceps attached to the fixation plate and the far right and left corners. C57BL/6 mice received unilateral contusion injuries at the exposed portion of the spinal cord using the Infinite Horizon Impactor (Precision Systems and Instrumentation; Lexington, KY) with an impactor tip of 0.7 mm in diameter, a force of 40 kilodynes, two seconds of dwell time, and an approximately perpendicular impact angle, parameters similar to our previously published cervical contusion SCI paradigms [8], [9], [10]. Injury parameters for BAC-GLT1-eGFP mice included a 1.0 mm diameter tip, 50 kilodyne force, and no dwell time at the C5 level. Control animals received unilateral laminectomy but not contusion injury to the spinal cord. Following injury, the forceps were removed and the muscle layers were secured with a sterile 4-0 silk suture. Sterile wound clips were used to close the skin, and 1 ml of lactated Ringers solution and 0.1 mg/kg of buprenorphine-HCl were administered subcutaneously.

Unilateral Hargreaves Thermal Test. A modified version of the Hargreaves test for thermal hyperaglesia, based on previously established methods [28], was conducted for the forepaws of each animal. This test detects sensitivity to thermal nociceptive stimuli by determining the latency to withdrawal of the paw from an infrared stimulus of a particular intensity. Prior to surgery, baseline measures were collected once weekly for two weeks. Following contusion SCI or laminectomy, each animal was tested weekly for six weeks. Before the first baseline test, the animals were acclimated to the testing room for an hour each day for five days. Prior to each session, mice were also acclimated to the testing room for an hour. Individually, the mice were restrained manually by the scruff only and placed on a thin glass pane, with one of the forepaws directly above the source of the infrared stimulus (UgoBasile; Comerio, VA). The animals continued to be restrained, but movement of the forepaw was unimpeded. The stimulus was initiated, and a fiber optic sensor on the movable infrared heat source measured the time to forepaw withdrawal. Forepaw withdrawal was defined as a quick movement of the paw away from the infrared stimulus often accompanied by licking of the forepaw. Spontaneous movements of the forepaw were not considered forepaw withdrawal and resulted in discarding the data and repeating the trial. Three trials were conducted for each forepaw of each animal, alternating the left and right forepaws, with an inter-trial interval of 120 seconds.

von Frey Filament Test. Semmes-Weinstein monofilaments (Stoetling Company; Dale, IL) ranging from 1.65 grams to 4.56 grams of force were utilized to measure tactile allodynia using the up-down method. Testing occurred twice prior to surgery to obtain baseline data and once weekly for six weeks after injury. Acclimation procedures were the same as those used for the Hargreaves test. Each mouse experienced ten trials per testing day with an inter-trial interval of 120 seconds. The first trial of each testing day utilized a filament of 3.84 grams. A single trial involved directing a monofilament at the center of the plantar surface of the forepaw of interest and application until the filament buckled. Mice were not restrained for this testing. The response of the mouse was then recorded as a positive or negative withdrawal response. The filament application was considered to produce a positive response if the mouse rapidly withdrew its forepaw, which was mostly accompanied by vocalization and/or licking of the forepaw. If the response was positive, the filament used in the next trial would be the next smaller filament. If instead the response was negative, the next larger filament would be used in the next trial. Withdraw threshold was determined as the lowest filament/force that evoked a positive withdrawal response in greater than 50% of the trials with that particular filament.

Grip Strength Testing. Grip strength was measured by the DFIS-2 Series Digital Force Gauge (Columbus Instruments, OH) [26], used previously by our group [8]. Attached to the force gauge is a triangular metal pull bar that allows for the transduction of force from the mouse to the gauge. The Digital Force Gauge measures the strength with which the mouse is able to grasp and hold onto a thin metal bar. Three baseline measures spread across two weeks were obtained prior to surgery, and mice were tested once weekly for six weeks following injury. In each trial, the mouse was allowed to grab the bar with one forepaw and was then quickly pulled away from the gauge so its grip was released, providing a measurement of the force with which the mouse gripped the bar. During each testing session, three trials for each forepaw were performed with an inter-trial interval of at least 60 seconds.

Histological Analyses

Tissue Processing. Mice were sacrificed at two days or two or six weeks following injury or laminectomy by anesthetic overdose and transcardial perfusion with 0.9% saline followed by 4% paraformaldehyde. The spinal cord was harvested following perfusion, fixed in 4% paraformaldehyde at room temperature for 24 hours, washed in 0.1M phosphate buffer at 4°C for 24 hours and then cryoprotected in 30% sucrose in 0.1M phosphate buffer at 4°C for three days. The cervical/rostral thoracic spinal cord was dissected from the rest of the cord, embedded in freezing medium, and flash-frozen with dry ice. Embedded tissue was cut transversely by cryostat at a thickness of 30 μm and mounted directly onto slides. Slides were stored at −20°C.

Motor Neuron Counts. A representative sample (i.e. every fifth section) of spinal cord tissue was used to locate the injury epicenter. Slides were thawed at room temperature for an hour and stained with 0.5% Cresyl violet acetate/Eriochrome cyanine. For each section, large motor neurons ventral to the central canal in the grey matter were counted for the ipsilateral and contralateral sides [9]. The motor neuron cell bodies were identified by their size and characteristic morphology. The injury epicenter was defined as the section with the fewest large motor neurons in the ipsilateral ventral grey matter.

Immunohistochemistry. Immunohistochemical analysis was performed both ipsilaterally and contralaterally to the unilateral injury at the injury epicenter as well as 1.05 mm caudal to the epicenter (Figure 1A–B). Sectioned tissue was thawed and dried at room temperature for an hour and then washed in TBS. Sections were blocked in 10% normal goat serum/0.2% Triton/TBS at room temperature for one hour followed by primary antibody incubation in 2% goat serum/0.5% Triton/TBS at 4°C overnight. Secondary antibody was incubated in 2% goat serum/0.5% Triton/TBS at room temperature for two hours. Primary and secondary antibodies used were rabbit polyclonal ΔfosB (IHC 1:100; Santa Cruz, USA) [30], rabbit polyclonal Ki67 (IHC 1:200; Abcam, USA) [31], mouse monoclonal GFAP (IHC 1:400, Sigma Aldrich, USA) [32], rabbit polyclonal GLT1 (IHC 1:800, kindly

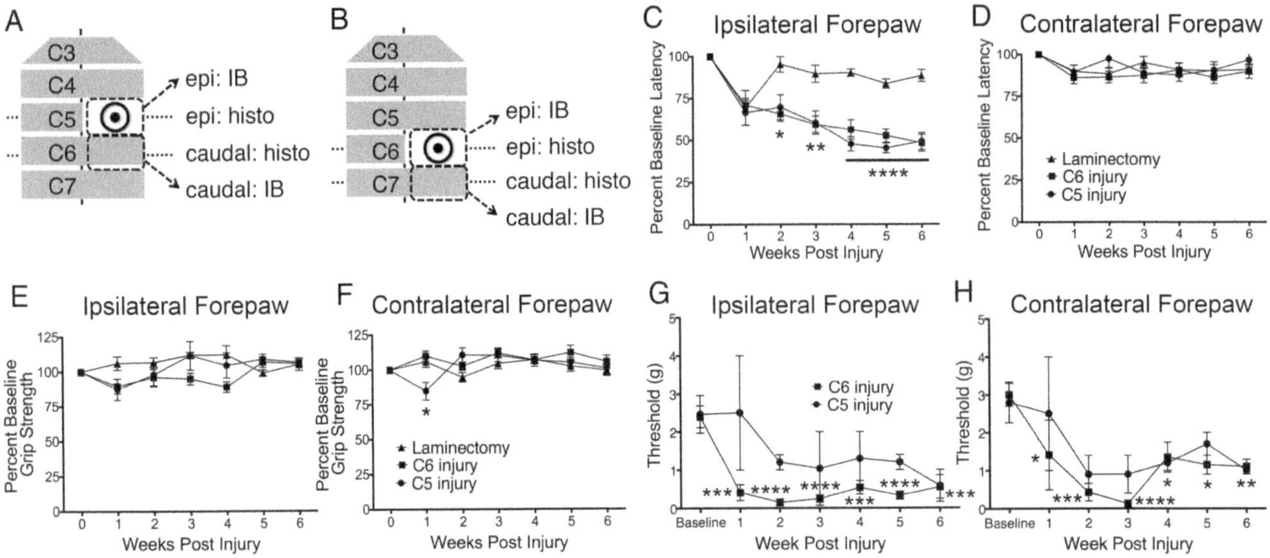

Figure 1. Animals receiving unilateral cervical contusion SCI exhibited persistent thermal hyperalgesia and tactile allodynia in the forepaw. Cervical contusion SCI was administered at the C5 or C6 level of the spinal cord while uninjured control animals received only laminectomy at the C6 level. Tissue from the level of laminectomy or epicenter of the injury and from the region immediately caudal was harvested for either immunoblotting or histology (A–B). Thermal hyperalgesia was measured using a modified version of the Hargreaves test. Animals receiving contusion injury showed a decrease in latency to withdrawal in the ipsilateral forepaw, measured as a percentage of baseline latency, compared to control animals (C). This difference was first observed at two weeks after injury and persisted until the animals were sacrificed at six weeks after injury. No change in withdrawal latency was seen in injured vs. uninjured animals in the contralateral forepaw (D). Animals receiving SCI were also tested for tactile allodynia using von Frey filament testing. In animals receiving C6 injury, but not C5 injury, a significant decrease compared to pre-injury baseline in the force threshold required to elicit a withdrawal response was evident both ipsilaterally (E) and contralaterally (F) for each of the six weeks following injury. The decrease in ipsilateral forepaw withdrawal latency and bilateral force threshold in injured animals occurred in the absence of changes in grip strength in either forepaw (G–H). Epi = epicenter; IB = immunoblotting; histo = histology; * = $p<0.05$; ** = $p<0.01$; **** = $p<0.0001$.

provided by Jeffrey Rothstein's lab at Johns Hopkins University) [29],, mouse monoclonal CD11b (IHC 1:4,000, AbD Serotec, USA), rhodamine-conjugated goat-anti-rabbit IgG (1:100; Jackson Immuno, USA) and FITC-conjugated goat-anti-mouse IgG (1:100; Jackson Immuno, USA).

Fluorescence Imaging and Quantification. Imaging and quantification of fluorescence immunostaining and BAC-GLT1-eGFP tissue were performed using a Zeiss Imager M2 upright fluorescence microscope [23]. Images were taken and analyses performed on saved PNG images for analyses. All immunostaining was quantified in the most superficial laminae (I–II) or lamina III of the spinal cord dorsal horn (Figure 2F–G). Laminae I–III were delineated by beginning at the most lateral portion of the dorsal horn, drawing a horizontal line across the gray matter, and following the outline of the gray matter back to the lateral extension of the dorsal horn. The border between laminae I–II and lamina III was identified by the change in tissue morphology represented by darker tissue in laminae I–II and lighter tissue in lamina III. Quantification analyses were performed using Metamorph software (Molecule Devices; Sunnyvale, CA). ΔfosB- and Ki67-positive cells were quantified by counting the stained nuclei in the superficial laminae. GFAP and GLT1 staining was more diffusely distributed and was therefore quantified in laminae I–II as an integrated intensity, or the sum of the intensity of pixels over a region, at constant exposure, brightness, and contrast. In BAC-GLT1-eGFP tissue, quantification was performed for laminae I–II and lamina III. eGFP-positive cells were counted separately for these regions [23].

Biochemical Analyses

Tissue Harvesting. Sacrifice occurred at two or six weeks after injury or laminectomy. Following anesthetic overdose, animals were perfused with 0.9% saline and the cervical spinal cord removed, dissected, and flash-frozen in dimethylbutane. The spinal cord was sub-dissected to collect the ipsilateral cord at the level of the injury and the segment directly caudal to the injury (Fig. 1A–B). To identify the regions of interest, the muscles were first removed to expose the spinal column. The laminectomy area was located, and the contralateral vertebral lamina was removed. Microdissection scissors were used to cut the spinal cord along the midline, and a 1.0 mm piece of tissue between the remaining laminae was collected. Flash-frozen tissue was stored at −80°C.

Western Blotting. Tissue samples were homogenized on ice in 50 μl of RIPA buffer containing 50 mM TRIS-HCl pH 7.6, 150 mM NaCl, 2 mM EDTA, 0.1% SDS, 0.01% NP-40, and Protease Inhibitor Cocktail (Roche Diagnostics, Indianapolis, IN). Protein concentration was determined by the Bradford assay, and equal amounts of protein were run on 4–12% Bis-Tris gels and transferred to nitrocellulose membranes. Odyssey blocking buffer (Li-Cor; Lincoln, NE) was used to block the membranes at room temperature for one hour. Primary antibodies for GLT1 (1:2,000) and actin (1:2,000; Abcam) were diluted in Odyssey blocking buffer and membranes were incubated at 4°C overnight. The membranes were then probed with IRDye-conjugated goat anti-rabbit or goat anti-mouse IgG (1:20,000; Li-Cor) at room temperature for one hour. Imaging was performed by the Li-Cor Odyssey infrared imaging system, and GLT1 band intensity was measured and normalized to actin band intensity using ImageJ software [22].

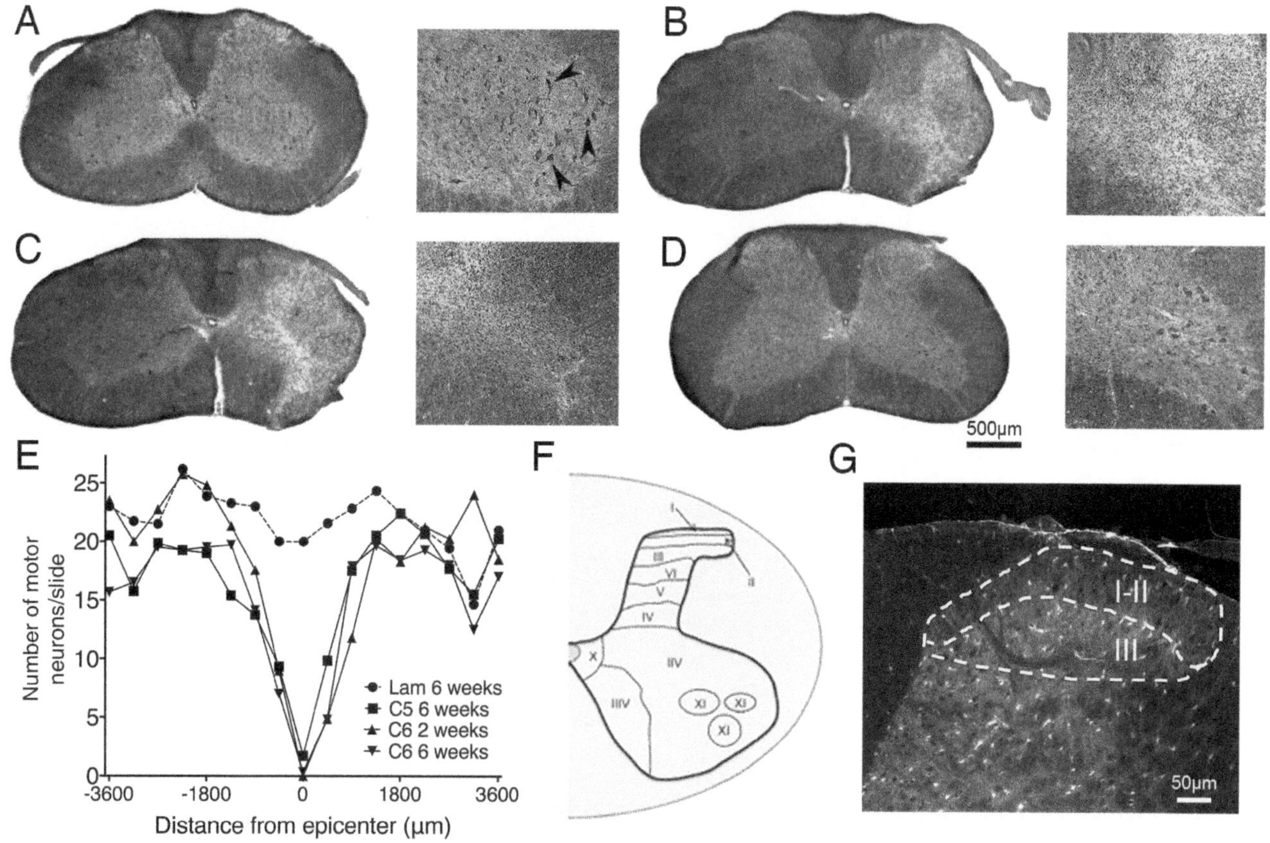

Figure 2. Unilateral contusion SCI induced a loss of ventral horn motor neurons at the injury epicenter. Harvested tissue was stained with Cresyl violet and Eriochrome cyanine. At the level of the laminectomy, uninjured control animals (A) exhibited large motor neurons in the ventral horn (arrowheads). At six weeks post-injury, animals receiving unilateral C5 (B) or C6 (C) contusion SCI showed a loss of these motor neurons at the injury epicenter but not 1.0 mm caudal to the injury (D). The spread of ventral horn motor neuron loss was approximately 1.0 mm rostrally and 1.0 mm caudally (2.0 mm total) from the epicenter (E). Immunohistochemical analyses of the injury models were performed in laminae I–II and lamina III of the cervical spinal cord dorsal horn (F–G). Lam = laminectomy.

Statistical Analyses

All data are presented as mean ± SEM. Statistical analyses were performed using GraphPad Prism (GraphPad Software, Inc.; La Jolla, CA). Bar graphs are presented as averages with error bars representing standard error. The Hargreaves test and von Frey threshold data were analyzed using a two-way ANOVA with repeated measured to compare the means within each group (laminectomy, C5 injury, or C6 injury) at each time point. The immunohistochemical and biochemical data were assessed with one-way ANOVA, comparing each group (laminectomy, C6 2 weeks, or C6 6 weeks) to one another. Statistical significance is defined as $p<0.05$ for all analyses.

Results

Robust and persistent forepaw thermal hyperalgesia and tactile allodynia were observed following unilateral cervical contusion SCI

Here we present a model of unilateral cervical contusion SCI in the mouse that exhibits persistent changes in pain behavior in the absence of motor deficits. Following baseline behavior testing, animals received unilateral laminectomy and contusion injury of 40 kilodyne of force with two seconds of dwell time at either the C5 (Fig. 1A) or C6 (Fig. 1B) level of the spinal cord. Control animals underwent laminectomy without injury. In both injury models, no grossly observable deficits in respiratory or other vital functions were present.

Beginning one week after injury, thermal hyperalgesia, tactile allodynia and grip strength were measured in laminectomy ($n = 8$) and injured animals (C5: $n = 8$; C6: $n = 10$) for six weeks. A modified version of the Hargreaves test was utilized to measure sensitivity to noxious thermal stimuli in the ipsilateral and contralateral forepaws. In both injured and uninjured animals, forepaw withdrawal upon noxious thermal stimulation was deliberate and was often accompanied by licking or scratching of the paw. Two-way ANOVA was used to compare withdrawal latency between animals with C5 injury, C6 injury, and laminectomy only at each time point. Post-injury measurements of latency to forepaw withdrawal are reported as a percentage of the baseline average for each animal. In laminectomy-only animals, withdrawal latency non-significantly decreased in the ipsilateral forepaw at one week post-injury but returned to and persisted at baseline levels until six weeks after injury (Fig. 1C). Beginning two weeks after injury and persisting for the length of testing, ipsilateral forepaw withdrawal latencies for animals receiving unilateral contusion SCI at the C5 or C6 level were significantly reduced compared to uninjured laminectomy animals (Fig. 1C). In the contralateral forepaw, no significant changes amongst the three experimental groups were seen (Fig. 1D).

In addition, tactile allodynia was assessed in C5 injured and C6 injured animals. The threshold force required to elicit a withdrawal response in each of the forepaws was measured by the von Frey test. In the C6 injury group, but not as robustly in the C5 injury group, tactile allodynia was evident (Fig. 1E–F). Animals were tested prior to injury to obtain baseline data and were then assessed for six weeks following injury. When values for each testing week were compared to pre-injury baseline data, animals receiving C6 injury exhibited a significant decrease in threshold force both ipsilaterally (Fig. 1E) and contralaterally (Fig. 1F). Although the data were not significant for animals receiving C5 injury, there was a similar trend in decreased response threshold.

While thermal and mechanical sensitivity increased in injured animals, this was not associated with changes in grip strength. Grip strength results were analyzed by two-way ANOVA to identify significance between each group at each time point. For the ipsilateral forepaw, no changes were observed between injured and uninjured animals for the six weeks following surgery (Fig. 1G). A significant decrease in contralateral grip strength for animals receiving injury at the C5 level was seen one week after injury compared to laminectomy or C6 injury (Fig. 1H). However, because the change occurred so soon after surgery and grip strength recovered to baseline levels by the next testing session, a spinal shock mechanism may be responsible for this unexpected change.

Together, the Hargreaves, von Frey, and grip strength data suggest hypersensitivity to noxious thermal and tactile stimuli in the absence of altered grip strength, indicating that the observed changes in forepaw withdrawal resulted from aberrant pain processing rather than motor deficits.

Unilateral cervical contusion SCI produced an injury characterized by a focal loss of ventral horn motor neurons

The animals that received unilateral contusion SCI exhibited loss of large motor neurons in the ventral grey matter as well as a disruption of lateral grey matter, dorsolateral funiculus, and ventrolateral funiculus of the ipsilateral hemicord (Fig. 2B–C). In laminectomy-only animals (n = 8), large motor neurons of distinct morphology were present throughout the ipsilateral ventral horn (Fig. 2A). These motor neurons were absent or their numbers were greatly reduced, however, at the injury site in animals receiving C5 (Fig. 2B; n = 8) or C6 (Fig. 2C; 2 weeks: n = 8; 6 weeks: n = 10) injury. This effect was limited to the injury site, as motor neuron populations and white matter were intact in regions rostral and caudal to the injury (Fig. 2D). Additionally, no loss of motor neurons was observed on the contralateral side of the spinal cord at any point along the rostral-caudal axis (data not shown). Thus, the anatomical disruption sustained by injured animals was restricted to the injury site ipsilaterally.

In order to quantify the contusion injury sustained by the animals and identify the injury epicenter along the rostral-caudal axis, sections were stained with Cresyl violet acetate/Eriochrome cyanine and motor neurons in the ventral horn were counted. The epicenter of the injury was determined by the extent of motor neuron loss, and the motor neuron counts were plotted by distance from this site (Fig. 2E). Significance was determined using one-way ANOVA to compare motor neuron counts between each group. Compared to laminectomy animals, a significant decrease in ventral horn motor neurons was observed for animals receiving injury at either cervical level and at both time points. The spread of both C5 and C6 injuries was approximately 2.0 mm (1.0 mm rostrally and 1.0 mm caudally from the epicenter) with a gradual decrease in motor neurons immediately rostral and caudal to the epicenter. The epicenter identified by this method was used for further immunohistochemical analyses of the neuronal and glial populations of the spinal cord dorsal horn, which were performed in laminae I–II and laminae III (Fig. 2F–G).

Chronic neuronal activation in the superficial laminae of the dorsal horn resulted from contusion SCI

Because injury at either the C5 or C6 level produced thermal hyperalgesia and tissue damage to a similar extent, we chose to move forward with a single model, the C6 injury, for further analyses. ΔfosB, a truncated splice version of the immediate early gene c-fos, is a transcription factor and marker of persistent neuronal activation. Chronic upregulation of this gene has been implicated in plasticity and inflammatory pain [14], [15] and has the potential to contribute to neuropathic pain. To study the extent of ΔfosB expression in our SCI model, we sacrificed animals at two weeks and six weeks after injury (n = 7–10) or six weeks after laminectomy (n = 8). Immunohistochemistry for ΔfosB was performed at the injury epicenter and 1.0 mm caudal to the injury in laminae I–II.

We found that ΔfosB-positive cells exhibited a defined pattern of nuclear staining in the superficial laminae. In our SCI model, we observed a persistent increase in the number of Δfos-expressing cells, suggesting chronic neuronal activation following cervical contusion injury. One-way ANOVA was used to compare the number of ΔfosB-positive cells between each group. Following laminectomy, limited-to-no ΔfosB expression was seen in the dorsal horn (Fig. 3A). Two weeks after injury (Fig. 3B), there was an increase in ΔfosB-positive cells on the ipsilateral side at and caudal to the injury epicenter. At six weeks (Fig. 3C), ΔfosB was upregulated bilaterally in the superficial laminae at the injury epicenter and 1.0 mm caudal. These changes are quantified in Figure 3D. The greatest increase in ΔfosB expression was observed at six weeks, suggesting that its expression was persistent and cumulative over time. Additionally, the expression of ΔfosB in the injured animals was specific to the dorsal horn of the spinal cord. There were few to no ΔfosB-positive cells in other regions of the spinal cord, including the ventral horn. This suggests that the effects of our injury paradigm on chronic neuronal activation were focal to the dorsal horn, an important region of the spinal cord for pain transmission and modulation.

Astrocytes were activated and proliferated in the dorsal horn of the spinal cord following cervical contusion SCI

Astrocytes play important protective and homeostatic roles in both the immediate and delayed response to CNS injury. Chronic activation in the spinal cord, however, can contribute to neuronal hyperexcitability of pain transmission neurons that underlies neuropathic pain [12], [13]. When astrocytes become activated, they express distinct proteins and in some cases proliferate [21]. In order to measure the spatial and temporal change in astrocyte activation in our model of SCI, we used immunohistochemistry to stain for GFAP, expressed by activated astrocytes, and Ki67, a marker of cellular proliferation. As in the previous immunohistochemical analyses, animals were studied two or six weeks after injury (n = 7–10) or six weeks after laminectomy (n = 8). For each analysis, one-way ANOVA was utilized to identify significance between the three groups.

Figure 4B shows the distinct morphology of activated astrocytes observed following injury compared to uninjured control (Fig. 4A). We found that injury induced diffuse GFAP expression throughout the gray matter of the spinal cord; therefore, we quantified astrocyte expression in laminae I–II by measuring GFAP intensity.

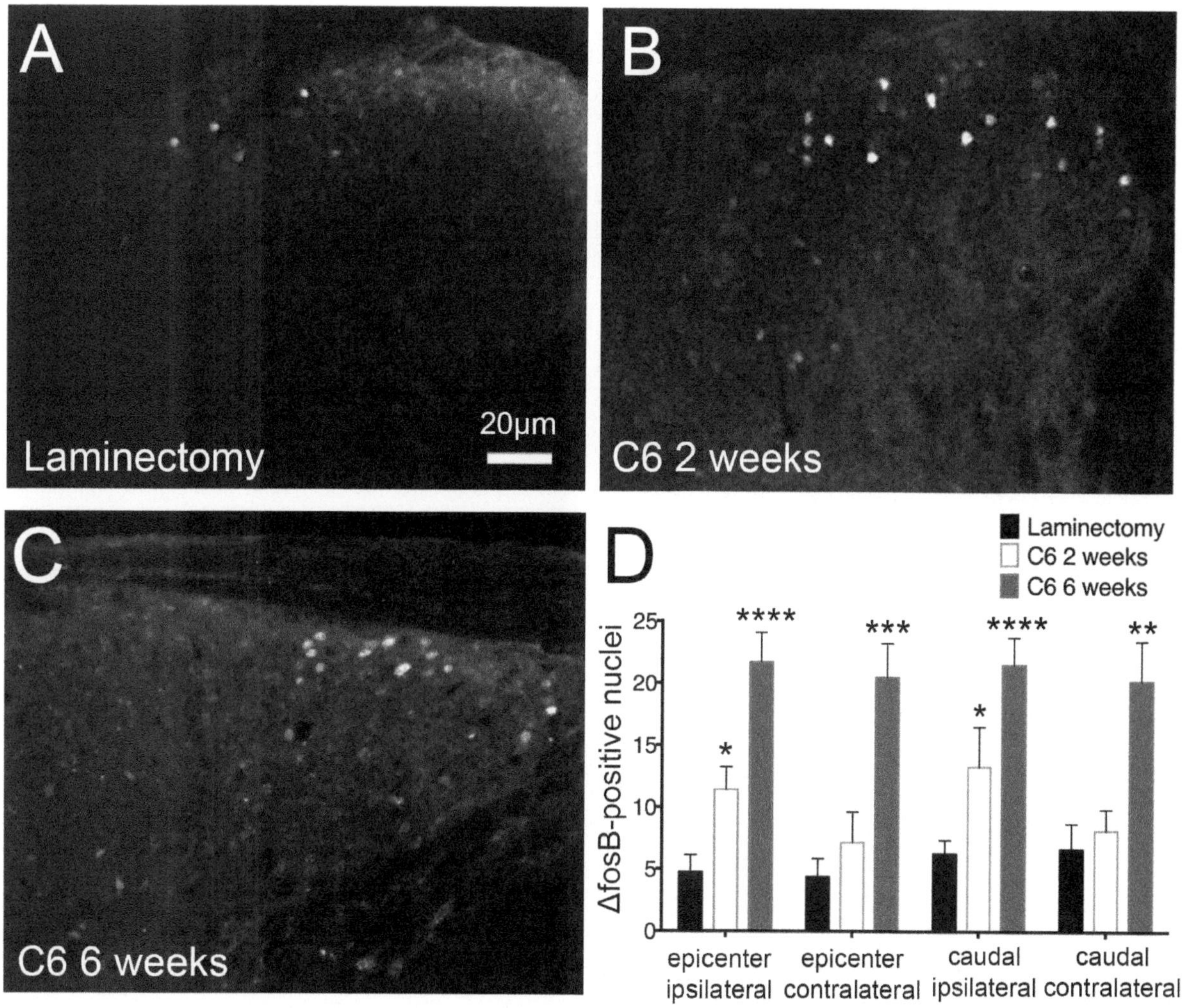

Figure 3. Chronic neuronal activation in the dorsal horn resulted from cervical contusion SCI. ΔfosB staining was used to measure the extent of persistent neuronal activation in the spinal cord. Following injury, ΔfosB-positive nuclei (arrowheads) were evident in laminae I–II (A–C). At all regions, laminectomy control animals (A) showed little-to-no ΔfosB expression (D). Two weeks after C6 injury (B), a significant increase in numbers of ΔfosB expressing cells in the superficial laminae of the ipsilateral dorsal horn was observed at the injury epicenter and caudal to the injury (D). ΔfosB levels were further increased at all regions in animals sacrificed six weeks post-injury (C, D). * = $p<0.05$; ** = $p<0.01$; *** = p 0.001; **** = $p<0.0001$.

Compared to laminectomy (Fig. 4C), GFAP intensity was significantly greater at both time points in animals receiving contusion SCI (Fig. 4D–E). These changes were observed ipsilaterally at the injury epicenter, with no alterations in GFAP expression at the other regions analyzed (Fig. 4F). GFAP expression was highest two weeks after injury, which suggests that, while post-injury astrocyte activation is chronic, it may lessen over time.

We next sought to study the extent of astrocyte proliferation in the dorsal horn to further support our assertion that astrocytes respond to the spinal cord insult we induced. We confirmed using confocal microscopy that, after injury, the majority of Ki67-expresing cells in the superficial were GFAP-positive astrocytes (Fig. 5A). Basally, proliferating cell numbers, and thus Ki67 expression, in the spinal cord were low (Fig. 5B). Two weeks following injury (Fig. 5C), the superficial laminae expressed a robust increase in bilateral Ki67 that was also seen in the ipsilateral dorsal horn caudal to the injury (Fig. 5E). At six weeks (Fig. 5D), an increase in Ki67 was also observed but did not reach the levels seen at two weeks.

We identified the phenotypes of these Ki67-positive proliferative cells. First, we quantified microglial activation in the superficial dorsal horn by immunostaining for CD11b (Fig. 5G–I). Like astrocytes, microglia play a role in both immediate and delayed responses to injury to the spinal cord and may contribute to the development of pathological pain (13). Compared to laminectomy (Fig. 5G), the intensity of CD11b expression was greater in animals with C6 SCI at both two (Fig. 5H–I) and six (Fig. 5I) weeks after injury. This increase was significant at the injury site both ipsilaterally and contralaterally, as well as caudal to the injury on the ipsilateral side (Fig. 5I).

We also quantified the percentage of Ki67-positive cells that were either GFAP-positive or CD11b-positive. This allowed us to determine if the proliferative cells are, in fact, astrocytes (GFAP-positive) or microglia (CD11b-positive). One-way ANOVA was used to identify significance in Ki67 and GFAP or CD11b colocalization. In laminectomy animals, the percentage of cells

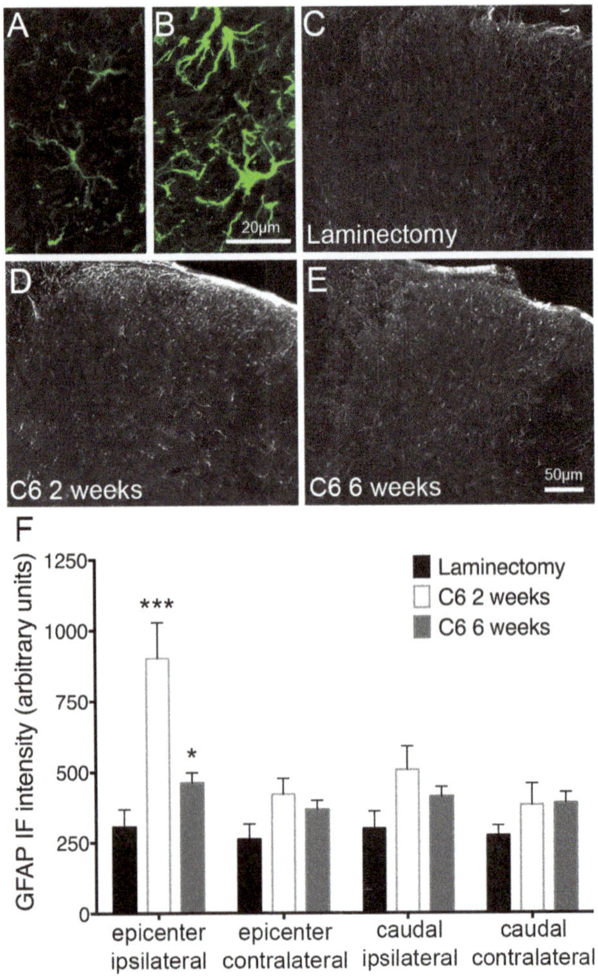

Figure 4. Astrocytes were activated and proliferated in the dorsal horn following cervical contusion SCI. Astrocyte activation in the superficial dorsal horn was characterized by quantification of GFAP expression in laminae I–II. (A) and (B) show representative images of dorsal horn GFAP expression at high magnification in laminectomy and injured animals, respectively. At the injury epicenter, compared to uninjured control animals (C), an increase in GFAP expression in the ipsilateral dorsal horn was evident at two (D) and six weeks (E) following injury. No significant changes in GFAP expression were observed at the other regions studied (F). IF = immunofluorescence; * = $p<0.05$; *** = $p<0.001$.

that are positive for both Ki67 and GFAP or CD11b is zero because there are no Ki67-positive cells present (Fig. 5F). At both two weeks and six weeks after C6 injury, there is a significant increase in the percentage of Ki67-positive cells that are also GFAP-positive or CD11b-positive (Fig. 5F). No significant difference exists between the percentage of Ki67-positive cells that are GFAP-positive or those that are CD11b-positive (Fig. 5F). Thus, both astrocytes and microglia are proliferative following cervical contusion SCI. These data further support the notion that activated astrocytes are present in the spinal cord following injury but retreat over time and/or that proliferation is mostly an early process of astrocyte activation post-SCI. The effects of astrocyte activation can be lasting, however, through the release of factors, for example, that can contribute to hyperexcitability.

Cervical contusion SCI led to reduced expression of GLT1 in the superficial dorsal horn of the spinal cord

The most abundant glutamate transporter in the CNS is GLT1, and its greatest expression is in astrocytes [33]. Through GLT1 and other glutamate transporters, astrocytes clear excitatory amino acids from the synapse after they are released, regulating glutamate's duration of action, controlling normal synaptic communication, and protecting cells from excitotoxic effects [33]. After SCI, we and others [23], [24], [25], [26] have reported a loss in astrocyte GLT1 expression. In this study, we utilized two animal models to study localized decreases in GLT1 in the context of neuropathic pain in the superficial dorsal horn.

In BAC-GLT1-eGFP reporter mice, the GLT1 promoter drives expression of eGFP [27]. Following injury, we sacrificed animals at two days (n = 7), two weeks (n = 9), and six weeks (n = 8) and quantified eGFP-positive cells separately in laminae I–II and lamina III. We used one-way ANOVA to compare the number of eGFP-positive cells at each time point. In uninjured animals (Fig. 6D; n = 6), eGFP expression was robust and widespread throughout the grey and white matter. Furthermore, almost all of the GFAP-expressing astrocytes in these regions co-localized with eGFP-positive cells (Fig. 6A–B). eGFP-positive cells were decreased, however, at two days, two weeks, and six weeks (Fig. 6E) at various regions in the spinal cord. Despite the increase in GFAP expression after injury, there were few cells co-expressing eGFP and GFAP, suggesting a loss of GLT1 expression in activated astrocytes (Fig. 6C). At the injury epicenter, eGFP expression was downregulated at two days ipsilaterally (Fig. 6F) and at all time points contralaterally in laminae I–II (Fig. 6G). In lamina III, a decrease in eGFP-positive cells was observed bilaterally at the injury epicenter (Fig. 6F–G). Caudal to the injury, we report a decrease in eGFP at all time points in laminae I–II and at two days and six weeks in lamina III (Fig. 6H). No changes in the contralateral dorsal horn caudal to the injury were observed (Fig. 6I).

In wild-type C57BL/6 animals, we employed immunohistochemical staining for GLT1 after C6 injury (n = 7–10) or laminectomy (n = 8). One-way ANOVA was used to identify significant differences in GLT1 staining between laminectomy, injured animals at 2 weeks, and injured animals at six weeks. Compared to laminectomy-only animals (Fig. 7A), animals receiving injury two weeks (Fig. 7B) or six weeks (Fig. 7C) prior to analysis showed a decrease in diffuse GLT1 protein expression in laminae I–II. These changes were seen at all regions analyzed (Fig. 7D). We further quantified the extent of GLT1 protein expression in injured (n = 7–8) and uninjured animals (n = 7) using immunoblotting techniques. At the injury epicenter, we observed a decrease in GLT1 protein in the ipsilateral hemicord at both time points after injury (Fig. 7E). Caudal to the injury, however, this glutamate transporter loss was not observed (Fig. 7F).

These data seem to contradict the immunohistochemical results we reported above. Thus, we performed immunohistochemical quantifications in regions outside of the superficial dorsal horn to try to identify the source of these contradictory results. At six weeks after injury, there is a significant loss of GLT1 expression in the ventral horn ipsilaterally at the epicenter compared to laminectomy animals (Fig. 7G). No significant change is seen in the ventral horn or white matter ipsilaterally caudal to the injury (Fig. 7G). These data suggest that, focally at the injury site, GLT1 loss occurs in multiple anatomical regions. However, caudal to the injury, the decrease in GLT1 expression may be more specific to the superficial dorsal horn (Fig. 7G). The changes in GLT1 from the immunoblotting data may not be evident due to the lack of anatomical specificity.

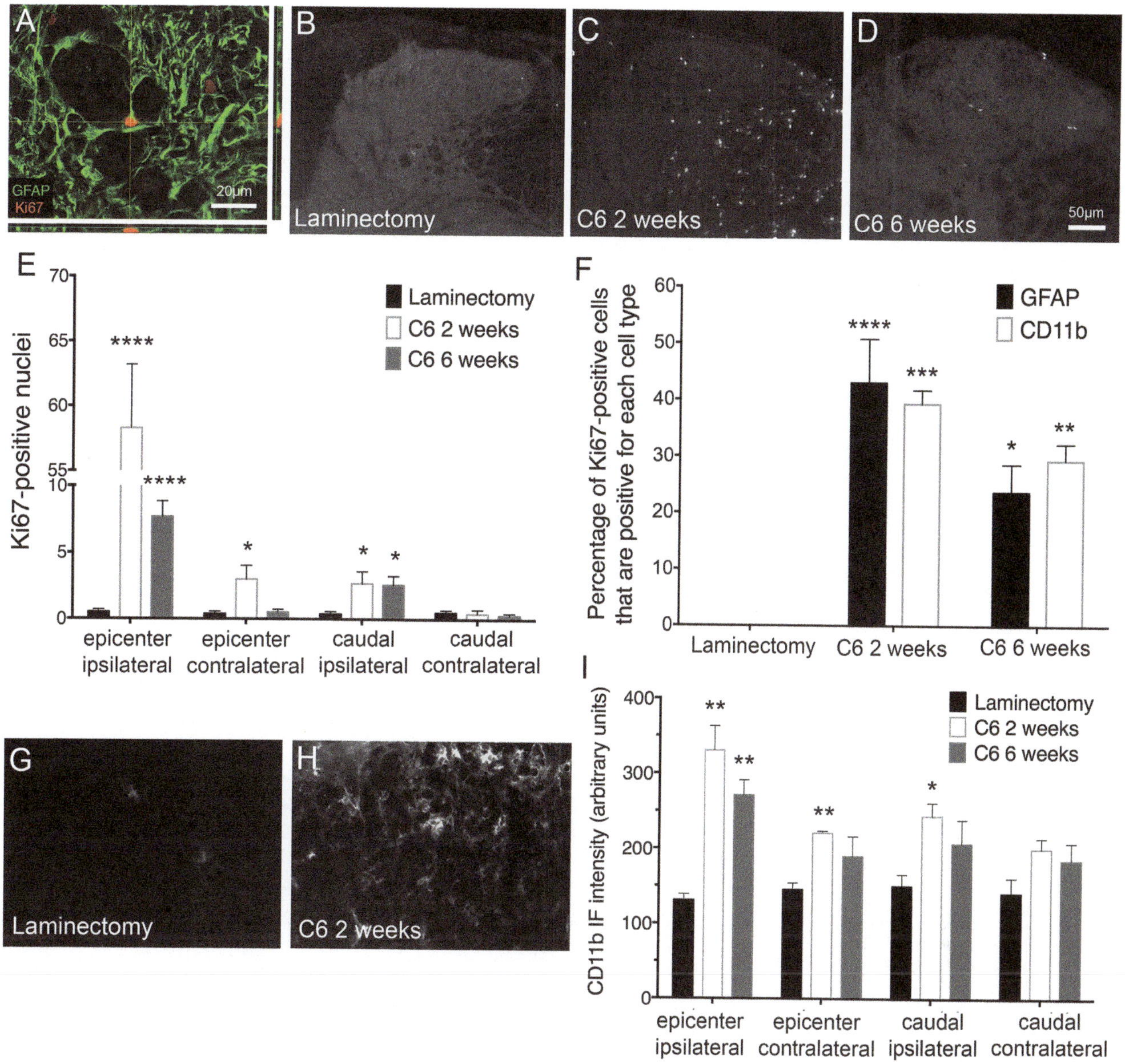

Figure 5. Enhanced cell proliferation, including proliferation of astrocytes, was evident after cervical contusion SCI. In the superficial laminae of the injured ipsilateral dorsal horn, we observed cells co-expressing GFAP and Ki67 (A), representing activated and proliferating astrocytes. In laminectomy control animals, little to no cell proliferation was evident (B). However, the number of Ki67-positive cells was significantly increased at two weeks (C) and six weeks (D) after injury on the ipsilateral side both at the level of and caudal to the injury (E). Additionally, at two weeks, there was a significant increase in proliferating cells contralaterally at the injury site (E). At both two and six weeks, a significant percentage of Ki67-positive cells were also either GFAP-positive or CD11b-positive (F). Compared to laminectomy (G), the intensity of CD11b expression in the superficial dorsal horn was greater in animals with C6 SCI at both two (H–I) and six (I) weeks after injury. This increase was significant at the injury site both ipsilaterally and contralaterally, as well as caudal to the injury on the contralateral side (I). * = $p<0.05$; ** = $p<0.01$; **** = $p<0.0001$.

Discussion

Here we describe changes in neuronal, astrocyte and microglial activation and GLT1 expression accompanying at-level thermal hyperalgesia in a cervical contusion SCI mouse model. In our model, robust and persistent thermal hyperalgesia and tactile allodynia are evident beginning one-two weeks after injury. Additionally, cervical contusion SCI induces an upregulation of ΔfosB, a marker of neuronal activity, in the superficial laminae of the dorsal horn. Astrocyte and microglial activation and proliferation, as measured by increases in GFAP, CD11b and Ki67 immunostaining, are also increased in these regions. We also observe a decrease in GLT1 expression and the number of GLT1-expressing cells in this model. These molecular changes that accompany hyperalgesia and allodynia in this study may contribute to the development of this aberrant pain response and represent important targets for better understanding the development of and treating neuropathic pain in SCI.

Hyperalgesia, defined as an increase in sensitivity to noxious stimuli, whether due to a decrease in pain threshold or an increase in response to stimuli above the pain threshold [36], is common in humans and is associated with sensory changes resulting from

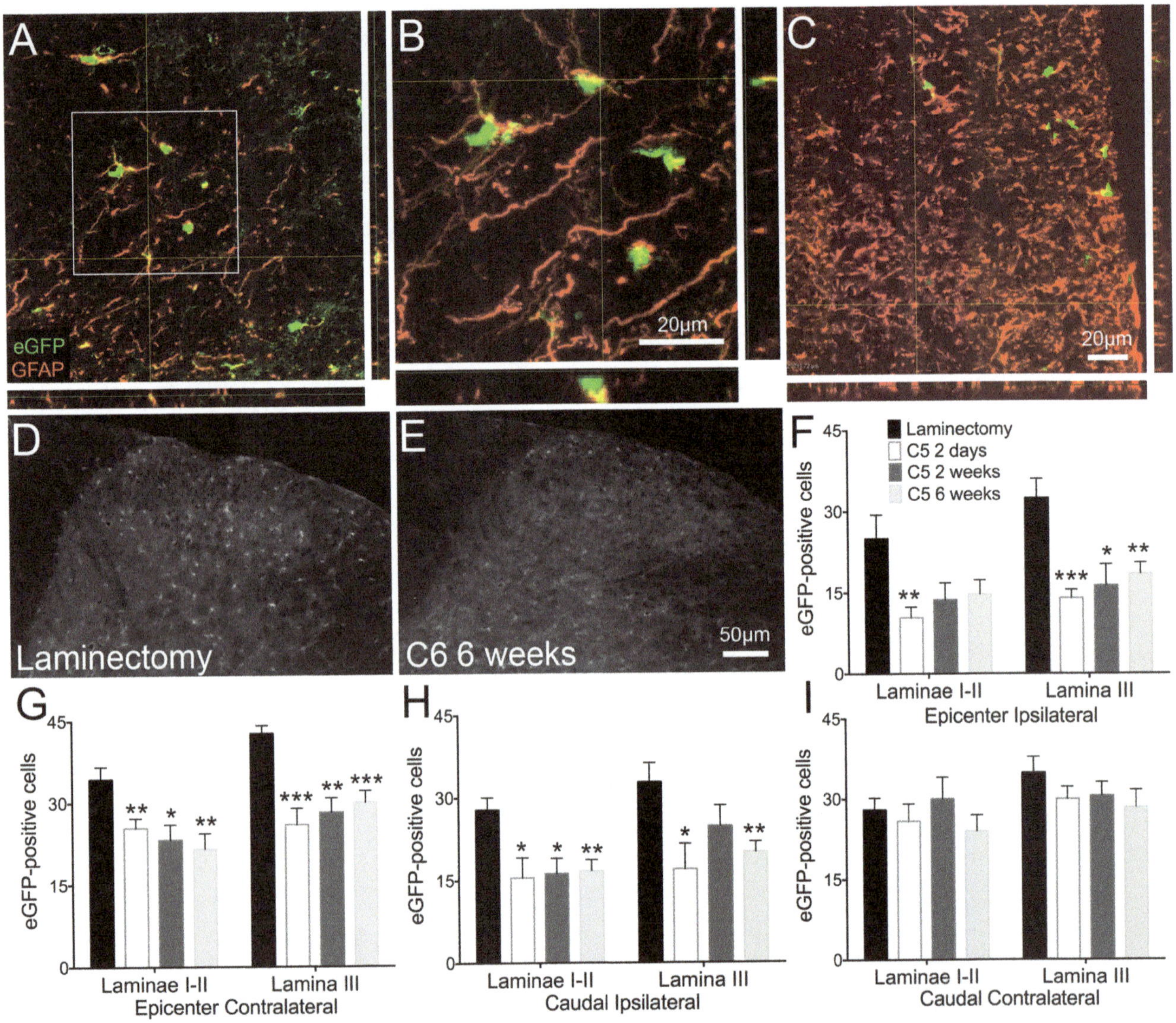

Figure 6. Astrocyte GLT1 promoter activity was reduced in injured BAC-GLT1-eGFP transgenic reporter mice. Following cervical contusion SCI, GLT1 expression/promoter activity, represented by eGFP-positive cells, was decreased in the superficial dorsal horn. In laminectomy animals, there were low levels of GFAP, although many of the cells that were GFAP-positive also expressed GLT1 (A–B). Following injury, however, an increase in GFAP was observed, but fewer of these activated astrocytes co-expressed GLT1 (C). Laminectomy control animals (D) had greater numbers of eGFP-positive cells compared to animals that received contusion injury two days, two weeks, or six weeks (E) prior to analysis. This decrease in GLT1 expression was observed at the injury epicenter in both the ipsilateral (F) and contralateral (G) superficial laminae as well as caudal to the injury on the ipsilateral side (H). No change in the number of eGFP-positive cells was found caudal to the injury on the contralateral side (I). * = $p<0.05$; ** = $p<0.01$; *** = p 0.001.

neuronal hyperexcitability [34], [35]. In mice, hyperalgesia in response to thermal stimuli can be measured using the Hargreaves test, in which a noxious infrared heat stimulus is placed under the paw and the paw withdrawal is recorded. In the models presented here, we observe thermal hyperalgesia in the ipsilateral forepaw beginning two weeks following cervical contusion SCI and persisting for the duration of the experiment. This is consistent with data from other groups, which report the development of hyperalgesia between two and three weeks after contusion SCI at various spinal levels in the mouse [37], [38] [39]. In the rat, our group and others observed thermal hyperalgesia as early as one week after cervical contusion injury [24], [40].

Like injured animals, laminectomy control animals show a decrease in withdrawal latency one week after surgery in the ipsilateral forepaw. This finding was unexpected, but not previously unreported. The development of post-laminectomy pain has been studied in the context of the extent of laminectomy, spinal deformation, and the loss of spinal stability following surgery [41], [42]. Researchers also showed that minimal laminectomy can induce transient hyperalgesic behavior at about one week after surgery [41]. While the cause of this pain behavior is unknown, it could reflect peripheral changes or spinal deformity rather than central sensitization or only transient central sensitization.

The ipsilateral development of thermal hyperalgesia in the mouse after SCI is consistent with the injury we see histologically. At the site of the injury, we observe a loss of ventral horn motor neurons and a disruption of normal tissue anatomy on the ipsilateral but not contralateral side. This suggests a disruption of

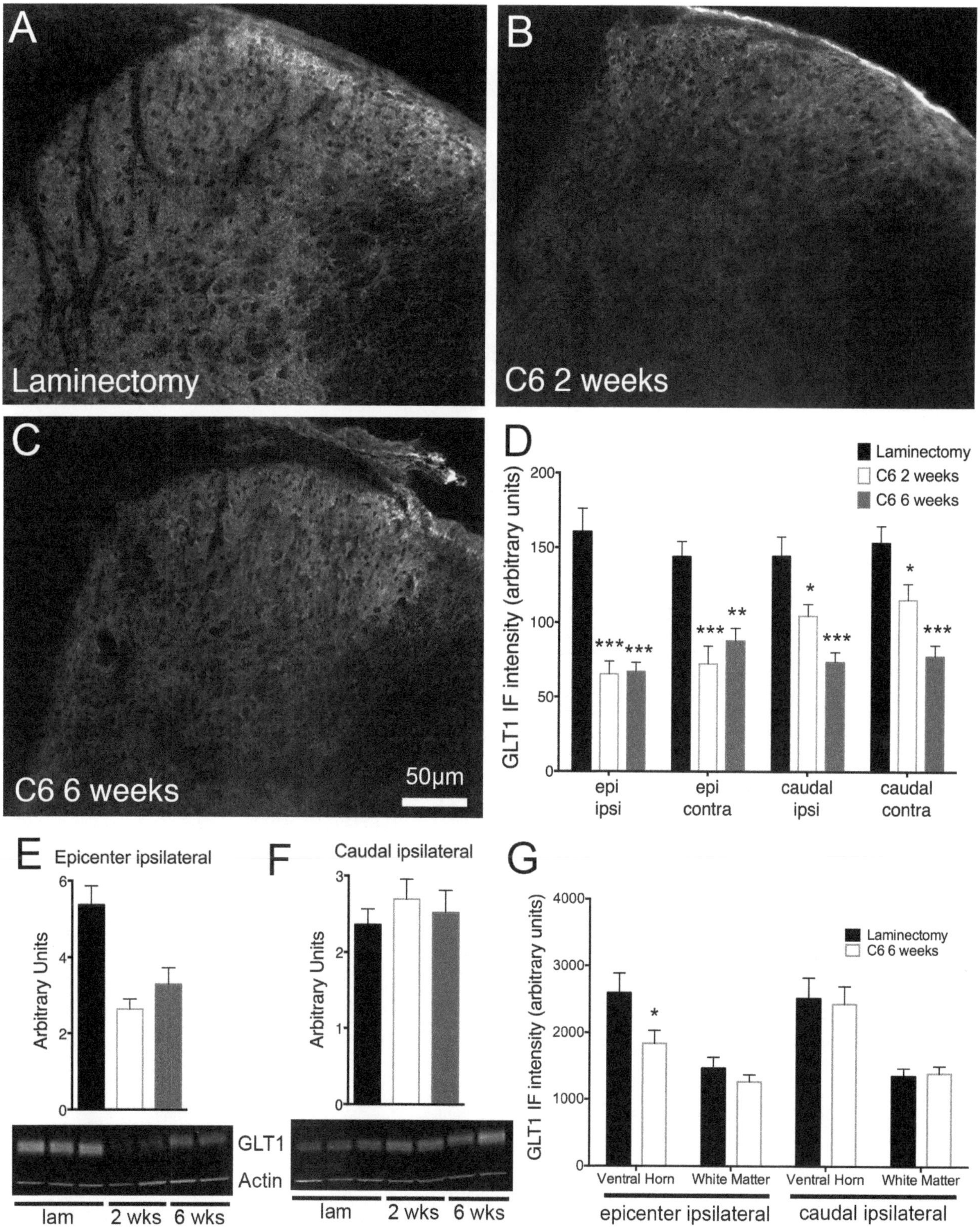

Figure 7. Cervical contusion SCI resulted in decreased astrocyte GLT1 expression in the dorsal horn. Immunohistochemical analysis revealed a decrease in GLT1 protein expression two (B) and six weeks (C) after cervical contusion SCI compared to laminectomy (A). This downregulation of the glutamate transporter was seen in the superficial dorsal horn on both sides of the spinal cord both at the injury site and caudal to the injury (D). Immunoblots of spinal cord tissue also showed a significant loss of GLT1 expression on the ipsilateral side at both time points following injury. However, this difference was seen only at the epicenter (E) and not caudal to the injury (F). Representative immunoblots are shown for each region (E–F). Analysis of GLT1 levels in regions of the spinal cord other than the superficial laminae at six weeks after injury reveal a loss of GLT1 expression in the ventral horn at the epicenter with no changes caudal to the injury (G). IF = immunofluorescence; epi = epicenter; ipsi = ipsilateral; contra = contralateral; lam = laminectomy; * = $p<0.05$; ** = $p<0.01$; *** = p 0.001.

pain transmission circuitry on the side of the injury, which may contribute to the hyperalgesia in the ipsilateral forepaw displayed by injured animals. The unilateral extent of the injury is also consistent with previous findings from our group; we previously reported damage to the ipsilateral dorsolateral and ventrolateral funiculi that did not extend bilaterally following moderate unilateral cervical SCI [10].

Unlike other studies [40], [44], we observe thermal hyperalgesia ipsilaterally but not contralaterally to the site of the injury. This discrepancy may reflect the modified version of the Hargreaves test that we utilized compared to these other groups. The Hargreaves test is most often used to measure thermal hyperalgesia in the hindpaw rather than the forepaw. Despite attempts to perform the Hargreaves test without restraint, including changes to the environment and longer acclimation times, we were unable to obtain reliable results. To overcome these difficulties, we restrained the mice in a way that did not impede forepaw movement but ensured that the mice remained still long enough to respond to the thermal stimulus. This method was introduced previously by Menendez, Lastra, Hidalgo, and Baamonde [28] for the study of hyperalgesia in the mouse forepaw. While the restraint improved the reliability of our thermal hyperalgesia measures, however, it may have affected the sensitivity of the mice to pain, which could have influenced the results we observed contralaterally.

Interestingly, while the hyperalgesia behavior changes we see are limited to the injured side of the spinal cord, we observe some molecular changes both ipsilaterally and contralaterally. ΔfosB and Ki67 expression is increased and GLT1 levels are decreased contralaterally after injury. The one alteration that is present ipsilaterally but not contralaterally is the activation of astrocytes. One possible explanation for the lack of hyperalgesic behavior in the contralateral forepaw is that the molecular changes we see are all required to elicit changes in pain behavior. There may be some interaction between activated neurons and glia that can disrupt pain transmission in the superficial laminae of the spinal cord following injury. Without activation of glia, pain transmission may continue normally.

Using von Frey filament testing, we assessed tactile allodynia following SCI. Allodynia, defined as a pain response to a previously non-noxious stimulus, is a common form of neuropathic pain [34]. In our model, we were able to identify allodynia following injury compared to baseline in the C6 injury group, but a similar significant effect was not observed in animals receiving C5 injury. We observed persistent tactile allodynia in both forepaws, which unlike the thermal testing results coincides with the anatomy of the histological findings.

Both hyperalgesia and allodynia are evoked pain behaviors in that they require a stimulus, whether noxious or non-noxious. We did not, however, study spontaneous pain, meaning pain that occurs in the absence of an external stimulus [43]. Spontaneous pain could potentially result, for example, from spontaneous activity in dorsal horn nociceptive neurons. Furthermore, while we measured at-level pain in the forepaw, we did not investigate below-level pain, which describes pain in dermatomes caudal to the level of injury and has been observed in the hindpaws of rats receiving cervical contusion SCI [40].

In this study, changes in pain behavior are exhibited in the absence of changes in motor behavior, as measured by grip strength. Because measures of evoked pain, such as the Hargreaves test and von Frey test, rely on motor activity (i.e. forepaw withdrawal) as a response, any dysfunction in motor behavior could affect test outcomes. The decrease in grip strength seen in the contralateral forepaw of C5 injury animals at one-week post injury was unexpected and could reflect transient local changes to the cervical spinal cord rather than a global alteration of pain transmission circuitry. Importantly, grip strength returns to baseline levels after this first week, at which point hyperalgesia and allodynia have developed.

Despite the maintenance of forepaw grip strength, we observed a significant loss of ventral horn motor neurons at the injury epicenter on the ipsilateral side following injury. One likely explanation for this disconnect is that our current injury model is milder and results in less motor neuron loss compared to our previous unilateral cervical contusion model in the mouse [9], which did produce persistent forelimb motor dysfunction. There is presumably some level of motor neuron loss necessary to result in quantifiable motor deficits.

At the molecular level, changes in ΔfosB and GLT1 were observed in the superficial dorsal horn of the injured spinal cord of our SCI model. Alterations in the expression of these proteins may contribute to central sensitization of pain transmission neurons in the cervical spinal cord. Central sensitization, including post-translational and transcriptional changes to dorsal horn neurons, affects the output of nociceptive neurons and the way in which peripheral stimuli are perceived. Thus, the observed changes may contribute to the hyperalgesic and allodynic phenotypes seen in our cervical contusion SCI.

C-fos is a member of the Fos family of transcription factors, which are induced quickly and transiently by a variety of stimuli. Because its expression is stimulated by an influx of calcium into neurons, c-fos acts as a marker of neuronal activity [45]. Previously, researchers have shown an induction of c-fos expression in the dorsal horn of the spinal cord following exposure to noxious stimuli in various forms [46],[47], [48], [49], [50]. ΔfosB is a truncated splice variant of the Fos family member, FosB. Unlike c-fos, which is expressed quickly but returns to basal levels within hours after stimulation, ΔfosB is induced gradually and is stable, so it accumulates over time and persists on the order of weeks or months [50]. ΔfosB has been implicated in a number of processes in the nervous system, including addiction, plasticity, and stress [45], [50] but may also play a role in neuronal changes associated with pain [14], [15].

In our SCI model, we see long-term elevation in the levels of ΔfosB in the superficial dorsal horn of the spinal cord, suggesting persistently increased activation of these neurons. These results are in accordance with another study that reported an increase in ΔfosB expression following pain induction, specifically carrageenan-induced inflammation [14]. Additionally, we previously reported an increase in ΔfosB expression in the rat following cervical contusion SCI [24]. While ΔfosB expression is significantly increased ipsilaterally at two weeks after injury, there is an even greater increase that spreads bilaterally at the six-week time point. This is consistent with the protein's stability and tendency to accumulate over time [46]. Furthermore, this persistent expression of the protein in the dorsal horn suggests an increase in the activity of these nociceptive neurons, possibly due to an increase in spontaneous firing and/or synaptic input, which may contribute to central sensitization. Thus the expression of ΔfosB that we see in our injury model is likely in accordance with its role in pain and plasticity.

In the nucleus accumbens and cortex, identified targets of ΔfosB include GluA2 and GluN1. In these regions, ΔfosB has been shown to upregulate these two proteins [50]. These targets are subunits of the glutamate receptors AMPAR and NMDAR, and their upregulation may contribute to increased glutamatergic transmission. Excessive stimulation of glutamate receptors can lead to hyperexcitability directly by increased activation of dorsal horn neurons and indirectly via glutamate excitotoxic loss of inhibitory interneurons [18]. It is unknown whether ΔfosB also targets these AMPAR and NMDAR subunits in the spinal cord following SCI. However, researchers have reported changes in GluA1 trafficking and expression in spinal neurons following central and peripheral injury and pain [51], [52], [53] as well as an upregulation of GluN1 and GluN2A in the ventral horn as a result of contusion SCI [54]. Despite this potential connection between ΔfosB and glutamate receptor subunits, ΔfosB does not definitively measure hyperexcitability. Instead, a continuation of this experiment to provide more conclusive evidence of the hyperexcitability could include electrophysiological measures of dorsal horn neurons.

Also following injury, we observe an increase in GFAP, a protein upregulated in activated astrocytes, in the dorsal horn of the spinal cord. We see this change at both time points, but it is more pronounced two weeks after injury. These data are in accordance with our group and others who have shown localized increases in markers of astrocyte activation following SCI [23], [24], [55], [56]. The observed increase in GFAP is seen only at the injury epicenter on the ipsilateral side, suggesting that this change is region-specific and may not play a role in potential above- or below-level changes, at least in our model.

The increase in activated astrocytes in our model of SCI could potentially have negative effects on the injured spinal cord and pain transmission circuitry. Often, activated astrocytes in the context of SCI and other injuries are considered detrimental because of their role in the formation of the glial scar, which can inhibit axon regeneration and plasticity, and the release of pro-inflammatory and other harmful molecules that can alter the excitability of neurons. Astrocytes, however, play many beneficial roles in the CNS, such as maintaining extracellular ion and neurotransmitter homeostasis, providing neurotrophic factor support, aiding in metabolic functions, and regulating the formation and maintenance of synapses [57].

Interestingly, while at-level thermal hyperalgesia is maintained through six weeks after injury, GFAP levels decrease slightly by this time point. Activated astrocytes play a significant role in the structural and molecular maintenance of the injury site [13], [17], [18], [57], [58]. The repair process following spinal cord injury, however, occurs in various phases, including acute, sub-acute, and chronic. While the effects of the glial scar and other repair processes can last months or years, not all of the molecules contributing to post-injury repair may be present at all stages. Thus, some astrocytes may return to the basal state in the days or weeks following injury, explaining the decrease in GFAP we see at six weeks compared to two weeks. Another explanation for the persistence of thermal hyperalgesia and tactile allodynia despite GFAP levels decreasing is that the loss of GLT1 also persists and contributes more strongly to the development of neuropathic pain after SCI. Alternatively, there may be irreversible damage to the spinal cord at this point that the inactivation of astrocytes may have no effect on.

Considering the various roles that astrocytes play following injury, it is important not only to study the reactive state of astrocytes in our model but also the effects of our injury on important homeostatic and protective functions of astrocytes. In light of this, we decided to investigate how our injury paradigm alters a centrally important function of astrocytes in the CNS, the uptake of glutamate through GLT1. Several groups have reported decreases in GLT1 levels following SCI [22], [23], [24], [25], [26], but the role of such changes has not been studied extensively in the context of neuropathic pain. To study GLT1 expression, we utilized both C57BL/6 wild-type and BAC-GLT1-eGFP reporter mice as well as both immunohistochemistry and western blotting. In our mouse cervical contusion SCI model, GLT1 levels are diminished in the dorsal horn at both time points at the epicenter and caudally on the ipsilateral side, suggesting a significant compromise in glutamate clearance in the injured spinal cord. Unlike with wild-type mice, in BAC-GLT1-eGFP mice, we see no change in the caudal contralateral region of the dorsal horn. This is likely due to a slightly different injury used in these two mouse paradigms.

Western blotting reveals that GLT1 protein levels are decreased ipsilaterally at the epicenter. However, no change in GLT1 levels is observed at the caudal ipsilateral region, which is contrary to the results we report using immunohistochemistry. This discrepancy likely reflects the difference in spatial resolution between these two techniques. Using immunohistochemistry, analyses of very specific regions, such as the superficial dorsal horn, are possible. For western blotting, however, we use a piece of tissue that encompasses an entire spinal cord level, including both the dorsal and ventral horn and surrounding white matter tracts. For our immunohistochemical analyses of the injured spinal cord, we examined the most superficial laminae of the dorsal horn, laminae I–II, as well as laminae III.

Importantly, co-localization analyses of GFAP and GLT1-eGFP at high-magnification reveal that, in control animals, most of the GLT1-positive cells are also GFAP-positive astrocytes. However, after injury, while the number of GFAP-positive cells is increased, the number and percentage of these astrocytes also expressing GLT1 is greatly reduced. This suggests that the loss of GLT1 that is observed in our animals occurs mostly in astrocytes, supporting our proposal that astrocytes activated after injury are deficient in glutamate clearance.

Like astrocytes, microglia play a major role in both immediate and delayed responses to injury to the spinal cord and may contribute to the development of pathological pain [13]. We also noted significant microglial activation in the superficial dorsal horn following cervical contusion SCI. Unlike astrocyte reactivity, we observed microglial activation not just at the ipsilateral epicenter region, but also at contralateral epicenter and caudal ipsilateral locations. Though we focused mostly on astrocyte changes, including down-regulation of GLT1 expression, it is likely that microglial activation also played a significant role in the persistent neuropathic pain phenotype observed in this study.

Here we present a model of unilateral cervical contusion SCI in the mouse that is representative of typical injury seen clinically in humans [1], [5]. The model exhibits at-level neuropathic pain accompanied by relevant molecular changes in the superficial dorsal horn. The protein expression changes suggest the presence of activated and proliferating astrocytes and a loss of GLT1 function, which may contribute to central sensitization, and underlie the development of neuropathic pain. We have identified a number of proteins that are altered by SCI and accompany thermal hyperalgesia and tactile allodynia, but their roles in the development of neuropathic pain have yet to be fully elucidated. Further research with the model may include identifying the factors and processes underlying the formation and maintenance of neuropathic pain in the spinal cord as well as recognizing targets for the treatment of chronic pathological pain resulting from SCI and similar injuries. Importantly, the availability of this model in the mouse allow for the use of valuable transgenic tools.

Acknowledgments

We would like to thank Drs. Luis Menéndez and Ana Baamonde for their assistance in the thermal testing procedures. We would also like to thank Dr. Jeannie Chin, Dr. Anupam Hazra and Brain Corbett for their advice and technical help with ΔFosB immunohistochemistry. Additionally, J.W.

would like to thank the members of her thesis committee, Dr. Piera Pasinelli and Dr. Lorraine Iacovitti, for their guidance and support.

Author Contributions

Conceived and designed the experiments: JLW ACL. Performed the experiments: JLW TJH RP DS ACL. Analyzed the data: JLW TJH RP DS ACL. Wrote the paper: JLW ACL.

References

1. National Spinal Cord Injury Statistical Center, University of Birmingham, Alabama (2013) Spinal cord injury facts and figures at a glance. Available: https://www.nscisc.uab.edu/PublicDocuments/fact_figures_docs/Facts%202013.pdf.
2. de Miguel M, Kraychete DC (2009) Pain in patients with spinal cord injury: A review. Rev Bras Anestheiol 59: 350–357.
3. Siddall PJ, McClelland JM, Rutkowski SB, Cousins MJ (2003) A longitudinal study of the prevalence and characteristics of pain in the first 5 years following spinal cord injury. Pain 103: 249–257.
4. Ravenscroft A, Ahmed YS, Burnside IG (2000) Chronic pain after SCI: A patient survey. Spinal Cord 38: 611–614.
5. McDonald JW, Becker D (2003) Spinal cord injury: Promising interventions and realistic goals. Am J Phys Med Rehabil 82: S38–S49.
6. Nakae A, Nakai K, Yano K, Hosokawa K, Shibata M, et al. (2011) The animal model of spinal cord injury as an experimental pain model. J Biomed Biotechnol 2011: 939023.
7. Kundi S, Bicknell R, Ahmed Z (2013) Spinal cord injury: Current mammalian models. Am J Neurosci 4: 1–12.
8. Nicaise C, Hala TJ, Frank DM, Parker JL, Authelet M, et al. (2012) Phrenic motor neuron degeneration compromises phrenic axonal circuitry and diaphragm activity in a unilateral cervical contusion model of spinal cord injury. Exp Neurol 235: 539–552.
9. Nicaise C, Putatunda R, Hala TJ, Regan KA, Frank DM, et al. (2012) Degeneration of phrenic motor neurons induces long-term diaphragm deficits following mid-cervical spinal contusion in mice. J Neurotrauma 29: 2748–2760.
10. Nicaise C, Frank DM, Hala TJ, Authelet M, Pochet R, et al. (2013) Early phrenic motor neuron loss and transient respiratory abnormalities after unilateral cervical spinal cord contusion. J Neurotrauma 30: 1092–1099.
11. Streijger F, Beernink TM, Lee JH, Bhatnagar T, Park S, et al. (2013) Characterization of a cervical spinal cord hemicontusion injury in mice using the infinite horizon impactor. J Neurotrauma 30: 869–883.
12. Latremoliere A, Woolf CJ (2009) Central sensitization: A generator of pain hypersensitivity by central neural plasticity. J Pain 10: 895–926.
13. Hulsebosch CE, Hains BC, Crown ED, Carlton SM (2009) Mechanisms of chronic central neuropathic pain after spinal cord injury. Brain Res Rev 60: 202–213.
14. Luis-Delgado OE, Barrot M, Rodeau JL, Ulery PG, Freund-Mercier MJ, et al. (2006) The transcription factor deltafosB is recruited by inflammatory pain. J Neurochem 98: 1423–1431.
15. Pareek TK, Kulkarni AB (2006) Cdk5: A new player in pain signaling. Cell Cycle 5: 585–588.
16. Clarke LE, Barres BA (2013) Emerging roles of astrocytes in neural circuit development. Nat Rev Neurosci 14: 311–321.
17. Karimi-Abdolrezaee S, Billakanti R (2012) Reactive astrogliosis after spinal cord injury: Beneficial and detrimental effects. Mol Neurobiol 46: 251–264.
18. Nakagawa T, Kaneko S (2010) Spinal astrocytes as therapeutic targets for pathological pain. J Pharmacol Sci
19. Chen CJ, Liao SL, Kuo JS (2000) Gliotoxic action of glutamate on cultured astrocytes. J Neurochem 74: 1557–1565.
20. Mark LP, Prost RW, Ulmer JL, Smith MM, Daniels DL, et al. (2001) Pictorial review of glutamate excitotoxicity: Fundamental concepts for neuroimaging. AJNR Am J Neuroradiol 22: 1813–1824.
21. Doble A (1999) The role of excitotoxicity in neurodegenerative disease: Implications for therapy. Pharmacol Ther 81: 163–221.
22. Lepore AC, O'Donnell J, Kim AS, Yang EJ, Tuteja A, et al. (2011) Reduction in expression of the astrocyte glutamate transporter, GLT1, worsens functional and histological outcomes following traumatic spinal cord injury. Glia 59: 1996–2005.
23. Lepore AC, O'Donnell J, Bonner JF, Paul C, Miller ME, et al. (2011) Spatial and temporal changes in promoter activity of the astrocyte glutamate transporter GLT1 following traumatic spinal cord injury. J Neurosci Res 89: 1001–1017.
24. Putatunda R, Hala TJ, Chin J, Lepore AC (2014) Chronic at-level thermal hyperalgesia following rat cervical contusion spinal cord injury is accompanied by neuronal and astrocyte activation and loss of the astrocyte glutamate transporter, GLT1, in superficial dorsal horn. Brain Res: in press.
25. Vera-Portocarrero LP, Mills CD, Ye Z, Fullwood SD, McAdoo DJ, et al. (2002) Rapid changes in expression of glutamate transporters after spinal cord injury. Brain Res 927: 104–110.
26. Olsen ML, Campbell SC, McFerrin MB, Floyd CL, Sontheimer H (2010) Spinal cord injury causes a wide-spread, persistent loss of Kir4.1 and glutamate transporter 1: Benefit of 17 beta-oestradiol treatment. Brain 133: 1013–1025.
27. Regan MR, Huang YH, Kim YS, Dykes-Hoberg ML, Jin L, et al. (2007) Variations in promoter activity reveal a differential expression and physiology of glutamate transporters by glia in the developing and mature CNS. J Neurosci 27: 6607–6619.
28. Menendez L, Lastra A, Hidalgo A, Baamonde (2002) Unilateral hot plate test: a simple and sensitive method for detecting central and peripheral hyperalgesia in mice. J Neurosci Methods 113: 91–97.
29. Lepore AC, Rauck B, Dejea C, Pardo AC, Rao MS, et al. (2008) Focal transplantation-based astrocyte replacement is neuroprotective in a model of motor neuron disease. Nat Neurosci 11: 1294–1301.
30. Perrotti LI, Weaver RR, Robison B, Renthal W, Maze I, et al. (2008) Distinct patterns of DeltaFosB induction in brain by drugs of abuse. Synapse 62: 358–369.
31. Lepore AC, Dejea C, Carmen J, Rauck B, Kerr DA, et al. (2008). Selective ablation of proliferating astrocytes does not affect disease outcome in either acute or chronic models of motor neuron degeneration. Exp Neurol 211: 423–432.
32. Lepore AC, Fischer I. (2005) Lineage-restricted neural precursors survive, migrate, and differentiate following transplantation into the injured adult spinal cord. Exp Neurol 194: 230–242.
33. Maragakis NJ, Rothstein JD (2001) Glutamate transporters in neurologic disease. Arch Neurol 58: 365–370.
34. Jorum E, Warncke T, Stubhaug A (2003) Cold allodynia and hyperalgesia in neuropathic pain: The effect of N-methyl-D-aspartate (NMDA) receptor antagonist ketamine–double-blind, cross-over comparison with alfentanil and placebo. Pain 101: 229–235.
35. Gwak YS, Hulsebosch CE (2011) Neuronal hyperexcitability: A substrate for central neuropathic pain after spinal cord injury. Curr Pain Headache Rep 15: 215–222.
36. Sandkuhler J (2009) Models and mechanisms of hyperalgesia and allodynia. Physiol Rev 89: 707–758.
37. Hoschouer EL, Basso DM, Jakeman LB (2010) Aberrant sensory responses are dependent on lesion severity after spinal cord contusion injury in mice. Pain 148: 328–342.
38. Mesiner JG, Marsh AD, Marsh DR (2010) Loss of GABAergic interneurons in laminae I–III of the spinal cord dorsal horn contributes to reduced GABAergic tone and neuropathic pain after spinal cord injury. J Neurotrauma 27: 729–737.
39. Hoschouer EL, Yin FQ, Jakeman LB (2009) L1 cell adhesion molecule is essential for the maintenance of hyperalgesia after spinal cord injury. Exp Neurol 216: 22–34.
40. Detloff MR, Wade ER Jr, Houle JD (2013) Chronic at- and below-level pain after moderate unilateral cervical spinal cord contusion in rats. J Neurotrauma 30: 884–890.
41. Kosta V, Kojundzic SL, Sapunar LC, Sapunar D (2012) The extent of laminectomy affects pain-related behavior in a rat model of neuropathic pain. Eur J Pain 13: 243–248.
42. Busic Z, Kostic S, Kosta V, Carija R, Puljak L, et al. (2012) Postlaminectomy stabilization of the spine in a rat model of neuropathic pain reduces pain-related behavior. Spine 15: 1874–1882.
43. Djouhri L, Koutsikou S, Fang X, McMullan S, Lawson SN (2006) Spontaneous pain, both neuropathic and inflammatory, is related to frequency of spontaneous firing in intact C-fiber nociceptors. J Neurosci 26:1281–1292.
44. Christensen MD, Everhart AQ, Pickelman JT, Hulsebosch CE (1996) Mechanical and thermal allodynia in chronic central pain following spinal cord injury. Pain 68: 97–107.
45. Bullitt E (1990) Expression of c-fos-like protein as a marker for neuronal activity following noxious stimulation in the rat. J Comp Neurol 296: 517–530.
46. Abbadie C, Honore P, Besson JM (1994) Intense cold noxious stimulation of the rat hindpaw induces c-fos expression in lumbar spinal cord neurons. Neuroscience 59: 457–468.
47. Jinks SL, Simons CT, Dessirier JM, Carstens MI, Antognini JF, et al. (2002) C-fos induction in rat superficial dorsal horn following cutaneous application of noxious chemical or mechanical stimuli. Exp Brain Res 145: 261–269.
48. Yi DK, Barr GA (1995) The induction of Fos-like immunoreactivity by noxious thermal, mechanical and chemical stimuli in the lumbar spinal cord of infant rats. Pain 60: 257–265.
49. Bester H, Beggs S, Woolf CJ (2000) Changes in tactile stimuli-induced behavior and c-Fos expression in the superficial dorsal horn and in parabrachial nuclei after sciatic nerve crush. J Comp Neurol 428: 45–61.
50. McClung CA, Ulery PG, Perrotti L, Zachariou V, Berton O, et al. (2004) DeltaFosB: A molecular switch for long-term adaptation in the brain. Brain Res Mol Brain Res 132: 146–154.
51. Galan A, Laird JM, Cervero F (2004) In vivo recruitment by painful stimuli of AMPA receptor subunits to the plasma membrane of spinal cord neurons. Pain 112: 315–323.
52. Katano T, Furue H, Okuda-Ashitaka E, Tagaya M, Watanabe M, et al. (2008) N-ethylmaleimide-sensitive fusion protein (NSF) is involved in central sensitization in the spinal cord through GluR2 subunit composition switch after inflammation. Eur J Neurosci 27: 3161–3170.

53. Larsson M, Broman J (2008) Translocation of GluR1-containing AMPA receptors to a spinal nociceptive synapse during acute noxious stimulation. J Neurosci 28: 7084–7090.
54. Grossman SD, Wolfe BB, Yasuda RP, Wrathall JR (2000) Changes in NMDA receptor subunit expression in response to contusive spinal cord injury. J Neurochem 75: 174–184.
55. Iwasaki R, Matsuura Y, Ohtori S, Suzuki T, Kuniyoshi K, et al. (2013) Activation of astrocytes and microglia in the C3-T4 dorsal horn by lower trunk avulsion in a rat model of neuropathic pain. J Hand Surg Am 38: 841–846.
56. Cho DC, Cheong JH, Yang MS, Hwang SJ, Kim JM, et al. (2011) The effect of minocycline on motor neuron recovery and neuropathic pain in a rat model of spinal cord injury. J Korean Neurosurg Soc 49: 83–91.
57. Pekny M, Nilsson M (2005) Astrocyte activation and reactive gliosis. Glia 50: 427–434.
58. Rolls A, Schechter R, Schwartz M (2009) The bright side of the glial scar in CNS repair. Nat Rev Neurosci 10: 235–241.

The Effect of Treatment History on Therapeutic Outcome: Psychological and Neurobiological Underpinnings

Simon Kessner[1], Katarina Forkmann[2], Christoph Ritter[1,2], Katja Wiech[3,4], Markus Ploner[5], Ulrike Bingel[1,2]*

1 Department of Neurology, University Medical Center Hamburg-Eppendorf, Hamburg, Germany, **2** Department of Neurology, University Hospital Essen, University Duisburg-Essen, Essen, Germany, **3** Nuffield Department of Clinical Neurosciences, John Radcliffe Hospital, University of Oxford, Oxford, United Kingdom, **4** Oxford Centre for Functional Magnetic Resonance Imaging of the Brain, Nuffield Department of Clinical Neurosciences, John Radcliffe Hospital, University of Oxford, Oxford, United Kingdom, **5** Department of Neurology, Technische Universität München, Munich, Germany

Abstract

It is increasingly recognized that the efficacy of medical treatments is determined in critical part by the therapeutic context in which it is delivered. An important characteristic of that context is treatment history. We recently reported first evidence for a carry-over of treatment experience to subsequent treatment response across different treatment approaches. Here we expand on these findings by exploring the psychological and neurobiological underpinnings of the effect of treatment experience on future treatment response in an experimental model of placebo analgesia with a conditioning procedure. In a combined behavioral and neuroimaging study we experimentally induced positive or negative experiences with an analgesic treatment in two groups of healthy human subjects. Subsequently we compared responses to a second, different analgesic treatment between both groups. We found that participants with an experimentally induced negative experience with the first treatment showed a substantially reduced response to a second analgesic treatment. Intriguingly, several psychological trait variables including anxiety, depression and locus of control modulate the susceptibility for the effects of prior treatment experiences on future treatment outcome. These behavioral effects were supported by neuroimaging data which showed significant differences in brain regions encoding pain and analgesia between groups. These differences in activation patterns were present not only during the pain phase, but also already prior to painful stimulation and scaled with the individual treatment response. Our data provide behavioral and neurobiological evidence showing that the influence of treatment history transfers over time and over therapeutic approaches. Our experimental findings emphasize the careful consideration of treatment history and a strictly systematic treatment approach to avoid negative carry-over effects.

Editor: André Mouraux, Université catholique de Louvain, Belgium

Funding: This work was supported by grants from the German Research Foundation (BI 789/2-1, www.dfg.de) and the Federal Ministry of Education and Research (01GQ0808, www.bmbf.de). The funders had no role in study design, data collection and analysis, decision to publish, or preparation of the manuscript.

Competing Interests: The authors have declared that no competing interests exist.

* Email: ulrike.bingel@uk-essen.de

Introduction

Experimental and clinical observations suggest that treatment outcome is not solely determined by the genuine characteristics of a treatment (e.g., pharmacological properties), but also depends in critical part on the therapeutic context in which it is delivered [1]. A key element of treatment context is the prior experience with a treatment that is known to modulate treatment efficacy [2,3]. The pivotal role of this factor for the therapeutic outcome is most apparent in experimental placebo analgesia studies involving a conditioning component [4–7]. In these studies the administration of a placebo treatment is combined with a conditioning procedure (e.g., reduction of pain stimulus intensity) in which participants experience analgesia and thereby learn the efficacy of the treatment. Subsequent responses to the same placebo treatment are substantially enhanced after this positive learning experience. Importantly, the impact of prior experience on treatment outcome is not limited to placebo (i.e., inert) treatments. Prior experience also modulates the efficacy of a subsequently applied active treatment, presumably by inducing treatment-specific expectations, via (pharmacological) conditioning or a combination of both mechanisms; for review see [3]. To date, this influence of prior treatment experience has only been studied *within the same treatment* approach. However, in clinical practice treatments are commonly replaced by another approach (e.g., a drug with a different pharmacological profile), particularly if symptoms show no or insufficient improvement. Whether the experience with one treatment approach can 'carry over' to a subsequent, different treatment, is currently unknown.

To allow for the assessment of treatment history effects irrespective of pharmacological peculiarities, analgesia was modeled experimentally by using an analgesic placebo paradigm. Positive or negative experience with an analgesic patch treatment was experimentally induced using a conditioning procedure [8]. On day 3, the analgesic effect of a second placebo treatment

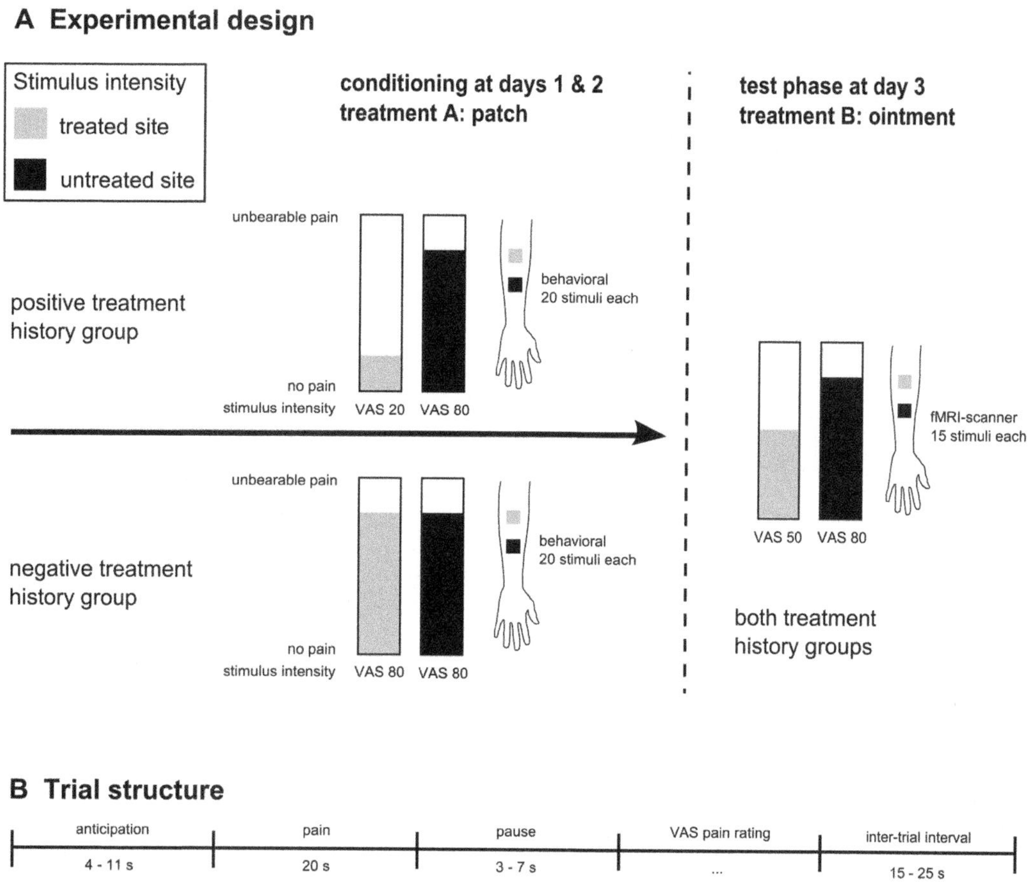

Figure 1. The experimental design comprised a group-specific conditioning phase with treatment A and a test phase using treatment B (A). The experiment took place on three consecutive days. On days one and two either a positive or negative treatment experience was induced by combining an inert patch treatment with a conditioning procedure. On day three the analgesic response to a second analgesic treatment applied as an ointment was assessed. Bars indicate the stimulation intensities of applied heat pain stimuli for the conditioning and the test session. In the conditioning session on days one and two (left-hand side) an inert patch (treatment A) was attached to the left forearm and after a waiting period of 20 minutes a series of 20 heat pain stimuli was applied to the untreated (black) and the treated site (gray) in randomized order. In the positive treatment history group, a low stimulus intensity (VAS 20) was applied to the patch treated site to mimic analgesia while an intensity of VAS 80 was applied to the untreated site. In the negative treatment history group the same stimulation intensity of VAS 80 was applied to the untreated and the treated site. The test phase performed with fMRI on day three was identical for both groups. Participants were instructed that another analgesic with a different pharmacological profile would be administered and an inert white ointment was applied to the participants' left forearm (treatment B). After a waiting period of 20 min two series of 15 painful heat stimuli were applied to the treated site and the untreated site in a randomized order. In both groups, a stimulus intensity of VAS 80 was applied to the untreated site and a stimulus intensity of VAS 50 was applied to treated site to mimic the analgesic effect of treatment B. **Trial structure of each pain stimulus (B).** Each trial consisted of three phases: anticipation, pain, and rating. The anticipation phase began when the white crosshair that was displayed on the computer screen turned into a red crosshair, indicating that a painful stimulation would follow shortly. Subjects had to press a button as quickly as possible when the crosshair changed color. After a variable delay a 20 s painful thermal stimulus was administered. Three to seven seconds after the thermal stimulation, subjects had to rate the pain intensity using a VAS. The trial was completed by a 15–25 seconds baseline during which a white crosshair was displayed.

introduced as an ointment with an unrelated pharmacological profile was compared between the positive and the negative treatment history group. Functional magnetic resonance imaging (fMRI) was performed as a physiological measure of analgesia and to characterize the brain mechanisms underlying the influence of treatment history on treatment outcome. We hypothesized that the individuals' experience with the first treatment carries over to the next treatment approach and thereby modulates subjective as well as objective indicators of subsequent treatment efficacy.

As previously reported in a short research letter [9], we found that the therapeutic effect of the second treatment approach (indexed by pain intensity ratings) was significantly higher in the positive compared to the negative treatment history group. This behavioral finding was corroborated by fMRI data indicating smaller treatment induced changes in posterior insula activity in the negative compared to the positive group. Additionally, the positive group showed stronger activity in the right dorsolateral prefrontal cortex during painful stimulation.

Here we expand on these findings by further exploring the psychological and neurobiological underpinnings of the effect of treatment experience on future treatment response. We hypothesized that individual psychological variables such as anxiety and depressiveness may influence the effects of the treatment itself and/or treatment history. Further we aimed at exploring the relationship between pain regulatory responses during pain anticipation and the effects of treatment history on pain related activity during thermal stimulation [10]. Finally, we provide a detailed discussion of all data, their potential implications for clinical practice and scientific questions to be addressed in future studies.

Methods

Participants

Forty healthy volunteers (all right handed, mean age: 26 years; range: 22 to 36 years, 20 male) participated in the study and were randomly assigned to either the positive or negative treatment experience group. The groups did not differ significantly with respect to age and gender. All participants had normal heat pain thresholds on their left forearm where painful stimuli were applied [11]. None of them was taking any medication except oral contraceptives. Participants had no known history of neurological or psychiatric diseases, including recurrent or chronic pain. The study was conducted in accordance with the Declaration of Helsinki and had been approved by the local ethics committee (Ärztekammer Hamburg, Ethik-Kommission, Hamburg, Germany). All participants gave written informed consent to participate and were free to withdraw from the study at any time. After the end of the study, participants were debriefed about the actual aim of the study and that only placebo treatments had been used. Due to technical failure of the thermode, data of one participant had to be discarded. The final data analysis is therefore based on 39 subjects (19 in the positive group).

Experimental procedures

The experiment took place on three consecutive days. On days 1 and 2, either a positive or a negative treatment experience was induced by combining an inert patch treatment with a *conditioning procedure* [8]. During the *test phase* performed on day 3 the analgesic response to a second analgesic treatment applied as an ointment was assessed behaviorally and using fMRI, see Fig. 1 A.

Conditioning phase (days 1 and 2)

Participants were recruited with the understanding that the purpose of the study was to investigate brain mechanisms responsible for inter-individual differences in the efficacy of analgesics. Upon arrival for the first session, subjects were informed about the experimental procedures and written informed consent was obtained. All instructions were read to the participants to ensure a standardized procedure. To assess participants' anxiety, depression and locus of control, participants filled in the State Trait Anxiety Inventory [12,13], the Center for Epidemiologic Studies Depression Scale [14]; German version: ADS-K [15], and the IPC questionnaire about locus of control [16,17]; German version: [18].

For the noxious stimulation, a contact heat stimulus delivery thermode (30×30 mm^2, ATS-Thermode, Pathway System, Medoc) was attached to the middle inner aspect of the left forearm. First, the individual heat pain threshold at the site of stimulus application was determined using the Method of Limits [19]. Subsequently, participants were familiarized with the equipment and pain rating procedure by presenting several stimuli of different temperature levels to the left forearm. The participants were asked to rate each pain stimulus on a Visual Analog Scale (VAS, [100 parts; endpoints labeled as "no pain" and "unbearable pain"]). The VAS was displayed on a computer screen using the experimental control program Presentation (www.neurobs.com). In the MR scanner the VAS was displayed via a video projector and a mirror on the head coil. Outside the scanner, subjects used computer mouse buttons to rate each pain stimulus. During the fMRI scan, a button box was used instead of a computer mouse. Second, a temperature calibration was performed to determine the individual temperatures to evoke pain levels of 20, 50 and 80 on the VAS. To this end, a pseudo-randomized sequence of 16 thermal stimuli (duration: 20 seconds) of different temperature levels was applied. Participants were instructed to rate the intensity of each stimulus on the VAS. Based on these ratings, stimulation intensities corresponding to subjective pain intensity ratings of VAS 20, 50 and 80 were determined by means of regression analysis to ensure a perception-locked stimulation across subjects.

Next, negative or positive treatment experience was induced by a conditioning procedure. To this end, an inert skin patch (treatment A) was attached to the left forearm. The 7×5 cm^2 patch consisted of a white cotton tissue with an inert sticky layer that was attached to the skin. Participants were informed that after a short period during which the drug would be absorbed the analgesic effect of the drug was expected to last for at least one hour. After 20 minutes the patch was removed. A rectangle was drawn around the treated site after the patch had been removed. This ensured that the subjects knew whether the treated or the untreated site would be stimulated next. Furthermore, participants were verbally instructed which site would be stimulated in the next block. During the actual conditioning session, a series of each 20 heat pain stimuli (duration 20s, ITI 40s) was applied to the treated or an untreated site in randomized order. The intensity of the stimuli on the treated site differed between subjects depending on the assignment to the 'negative' or the 'positive' treatment history group. In the positive treatment history group, a low stimulus intensity (VAS 20) was applied to the patch treated site to mimic analgesia while an intensity of VAS 80 was applied to the untreated site. This manipulation was unbeknownst to the participants. In contrast, the negative treatment history group received the same stimulation intensity of VAS 80 on the untreated and the treated site. In order to reinforce the positive or negative drug experience with the patch this conditioning procedure was performed twice and thus repeated on two consecutive days in both groups.

Each trial consisted of three phases: anticipation, pain, and rating. The anticipation phase began when the white crosshair that was displayed on the computer screen turned into a red crosshair, indicating that a painful stimulation would follow shortly. Subjects had to press a button as quickly as possible when the crosshair changed color. After a variable delay (7.5s$\pm$3.5), a 20s painful thermal stimulus was administered (1.5s ramp up, 17s plateau, 1.5s ramp down). A variable delay (5s$\pm$2) followed the thermal stimulation before subjects had to rate the level of pain during the trial using a VAS. A variable inter-trial interval (ITI; 20s$\pm$5) followed during which a white crosshair was displayed (see Fig. 1 B).

Test phase (day 3)

The test phase was identical for both groups. On day 3, both groups were instructed that another analgesic with a different pharmacological profile would be administered. Subsequently, an inert white ointment was applied to the participants' left forearm (treatment B). Subjects were told that the cream contained a different analgesic agent than the one that had been applied on days 1 and 2. In order to emphasize the difference between the two 'drugs', an ointment was chosen rather than a patch. The ointment was removed 20 min after administration. Thereafter, subjects were positioned in the MRI scanner and two series of 15 painful heat stimuli each were applied to the treated site and the untreated site. The order was randomized across subjects, i.e., in half of the participants the untreated site was stimulated first, while in the other half the treatment site was stimulated first. As in the conditioning session, a stimulus intensity of VAS 80 was applied to the untreated site. In both groups, a stimulus intensity of VAS 50 was applied at the ointment treated site. This procedure was chosen to mimic the effects of a novel analgesic treatment. The analgesic effect of this second treatment (as indexed by pain ratings) was compared between the positive and the negative treatment history group. In addition, functional magnetic resonance imaging (fMRI) was performed to assess pain-related brain activity as a physiological measure of analgesia. Importantly, both groups underwent exactly the same procedure of treatment with the ointment (treatment B). The only difference between the groups was their different prior experience with treatment A.

FMRI data acquisition

MR scanning during the test phase was performed on a 3 Tesla system (TimTrio, Siemens) equipped with a 32-channel head coil. A total of 42 axial slices per volume were acquired in top-down order using a gradient-echo echo-planar-imaging (EPI) T2*-sensitive sequence with the following parameters: TR = 2580 ms; TE = 26 ms; voxel size = $2\times2\times2$ mm^3; gap between slices = 1 mm; flip angle = 90°; field of view = 220×220 mm^2; time of acquisition = 30 minutes. After the functional measurement, an individual high-resolution anatomical image was obtained for each participant using a T1-weighted magnetization-prepared rapid acquisition gradient-echo (MPRAGE) sequence (TR = 2300 ms; TE = 2.98 ms; voxel size = $1\times1\times1$ mm^3; flip angle = 9°; field of view = 256×256 mm^2; time of acquisition = 7.23 minutes).

Analysis of behavioral data

Behavioral data (e.g. pain ratings, reaction times etc.) were automatically recorded and logged by the experimental control program Presentation. All behavioral data analyses were conducted using SPSS 18.0.

Behaviorally, the individual analgesic effect of the second analgesic treatment was defined as the difference between the pain ratings for the untreated site and the treated site. The mean analgesic effect was compared between treatment history groups using two-sample T-Tests. Pearson correlation coefficients were calculated to examine the relationship between the different experimental effects and questionnaire data.

Results with p-values<0.05 are considered statistically significant. All statistical analyses were performed using two-tailed testing. Results are presented as mean ± standard error unless indicated otherwise.

Image processing and statistical analysis

Image processing and statistical analysis of fMRI data was performed using SPM8 (http://www.fil.ion.ucl.ac.uk/spm/) [20,21]. After removing the first 6 volumes to compensate for T1 saturation effects, preprocessing included slice timing, realignment to the first volume, unwarping (correction for interaction of movements and field inhomogeneities), normalization to standard MNI space and finally smoothing with an 8 mm Gaussian kernel with full-width at half-maximum (FWHM). Data were also subjected to high-pass filtering (cut-off period: 128 s) and correction for temporal autocorrelations (based on a first-order autoregressive model).

Data analysis was performed using a general linear model approach. For each subject the first level design matrix included 2 experimental runs (i.e., stimulation of the treated and the untreated site) each of which had 4 regressors that modelled the predicted blood oxygen level dependent (BOLD) responses to the different events that comprised one pain trial. The painful stimulation was divided into an early and a late phase based on previous results regarding neural placebo effects [6,10]. First level models therefore comprised the following regressors: (i) the pain anticipation phase, (ii) the early phase of painful thermal stimulation, (iii) the late phase of painful stimulation and (iv) the pain rating procedure. All regressors were obtained by convolving the duration of the event with the canonical hemodynamic response function implemented in SPM.

After model estimation, the ensuing first-level contrast images from each subject were used for second-level analyses applying SPM's flexible factorial model that comprised the factors group (negative vs. positive), condition (untreated vs. treated site) and the individual subject factor. Inferences were made by entering the appropriate contrast into an ANOVA using a flexible factorial design and correcting for possible non-sphericity of the error term.

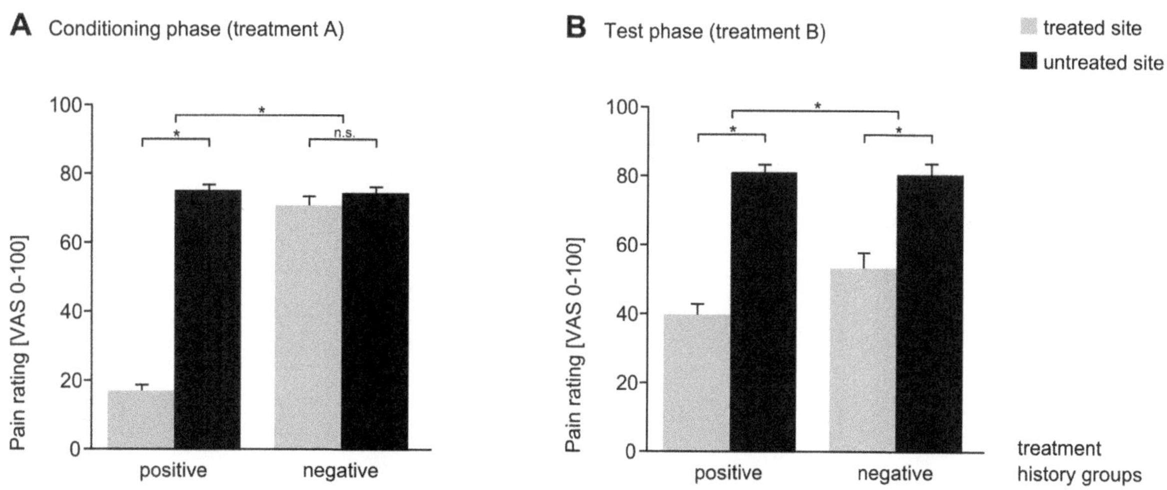

Figure 2. Behavioral effects during conditioning and test phase. Treatment experience during the conditioning session (**A**). Pain ratings (mean VAS score ± SEM) indicate a successful manipulation of the treatment experience for both groups with the placebo patch (treatment A). The effect of treatment history on treatment outcome - response to second treatment (**B**). Pain ratings indicate that the therapeutic effect (mean pain VAS score ± SEM) of the ointment treatment (treatment B) was significantly lower in the negative than in the positive treatment history group. See the difference between groups in gray bars. Error bars indicate standard error of the mean. * = p<0.01.

Table 1. FMRI results.

Region	**MNI-coordinates in mm**						**Voxel level (T)**
	right			**left**			**right/left**
	X	**Y**	**Z**	**X**	**Y**	**Z**	
(A) Main effect of painful stimulation (pooled across all four experimental conditions)							
Posterior insula	50	−8	10	−52	−8	8	21.6**/12.1**
S II	36	−18	20	−36	−20	14	21.2**/15.9**
DLPFC	46	48	12	−46	32	22	21.1**/8.2**
Middle insula	56	0	4	−54	−4	4	18.7**/11.2**
Anterior insula	44	16	6	−36	22	6	16.2**/12.6**
SMA	6	18	52				15.6**
Cerebellum	30	−64	−44	−34	−60	−44	7.7**/12.8**
MCC	8	−8	42	−10	24	38	10.0**/9.8**
Head of caudate	10	12	10	−10	12	8	9.6**/8.4**
Occipital lobe	10	−92	2	−8	−92	−6	8.3**/9.3**
Thalamus	16	−10	6	−10	−6	0	8.2**/5.6**
PAG	10	−30	−8				8.1**
S I	30	−36	64				7.8**
Amygdala	32	−2	−16	−34	−2	−22	7.7**/5.5**
(B) Main effect of condition [untreated site>treated site]							
Amygdala				−16	−2	−8	3.4*
Insula	40	8	2	−44	6	2	3.0†/3.4*
MCC	2	8	42				3.1†
(C) Main effect of group [Negative>Positive group]							
Medial frontal gyrus	50	44	20				5.9**
Occipital pole	2	−94	16	−16	−88	−4	5.3†5.1†
Superior parietal lobe	16	−66	64				4.4†
Amygdala	8	−4	−20	−8	−4	−20	4.1*/3.9*
S II	50	−16	16				3.5*
(D 1) Interaction in complete pain phase [Positive group $_{[untreated>treated\ site]}$>Negative group $_{[untreated>treated\ site]}$]							
Insular cortex	48	−8	10	−40	−8	−4	4.0*/3.6*
(D 2) Interaction in late pain phase [Positive group $_{[untreated>treated\ site]}$>Negative group $_{[untreated>treated\ site]}$]							
Insular cortex	48	−6	8	−46	−10	0	3.6*/3.1†
(E 1) Interaction in complete pain phase [Positive group $_{[treated>untreated\ site]}$>Negative group $_{[treated>untreated\ site]}$]							
Amygdala				−22	−2	−26	3.7*
Head of caudate				−18	10	−16	3.6*
Subgenual ACC				−10	8	−12	3.4*
Orbitofrontal cortex	22	14	−22	38	44	−20	3.2†/2.9†
(E 2) Interaction in late pain phase [Positive group $_{[treated>untreated\ site]}$>Negative group $_{[treated>untreated\ site]}$]							
Striatum/subgenual ACC				−12	6	−14	3.5*
DLPFC	42	38	40				3.2*
Amygdala	32	4	−30				3.2†
Orbitofrontal cortex	20	16	−20				2.8†
(F 1) Negative group during anticipation phase [T-test: negative correlation with treatment effect during pain]							
Insular cortex	44	−6	−4	−44	−2	−4	4.3*/5.5*
Thalamus	20	−6	2	−20	0	4	4.9*/4.2†
Cerebellum	6	−42	−14	−4	−42	−12	3.7†/4.5†
(F 2) Positive group during anticipation phase [T-test: positive correlation with treatment effect during pain]							
PAG	2	−20	−16	−2	−20	−16	5.4*/4.0*
Medial frontal gyrus				−8	34	48	5.2†
Cerebellum	32	−82	−26				5.1†

Table 1. Cont.

Region	MNI-coordinates in mm						Voxel level (T)
	right			left			right/left
	X	Y	Z	X	Y	Z	
DLPFC	36	34	42	−32	26	44	4.1*/4.2*
dACC	6	36	8	−8	42	18	3.7†/4.0*
Midbrain	16	−10	−10	16	−10	−10	3.7†

Areas of brain activation (BOLD responses from fMRI) during test phase (treatment B).
S I = primary somatosensory cortex, S II = secondary somatosensory cortex, DLPFC = dorsolateral prefrontal cortex, SMA = supplementary motor area, MCC = middle cingulate cortex, PAG = periaqueductal gray, dACC = dorsal anterior cingulate cortex;
(**) p<0.05 whole brain corrected,
(*) p<0.05 small volume corrected using respective a-priori region of interest,
(†) p<0.001 uncorrected.

Our analysis comprised five steps. First, we tested whether the noxious stimulation had activated brain regions implicated in pain processing and perception (main effect of pain). For this analysis, pain-related responses were pooled across all four conditions of the 2×2 factorial design.

Next, we tested for differences in pain-related responses depending on the stimulation site (main effect of treatment). Given that the analgesic treatment effect was mimicked by applying a reduced stimulus intensity corresponding to VAS 50 on the treated site compared to the untreated site (VAS 80), we expected activity changes in brain areas known to code pain intensity in this contrast.

Third, we tested for the main effect of treatment history by comparing pain related responses between the negative and the positive group.

Forth, we tested whether the difference in pain-related responses between the treated and the untreated site differed depending on treatment history group (interaction).

Finally, we tested for group-specific activity patterns and the relationship between pain regulatory responses during pain anticipation and the reduction of pain related activity during thermal stimulation. To this end, the difference in parameter estimates for the untreated and treated condition during painful stimulation was extracted from a 4 mm radius sphere centered on the insular peak voxel (as a neurobiological marker for the individual treatment effect) and used as a covariate for brain responses during the anticipation phase.

We report p-values at a level of $p \leq 0.05$ which have been corrected for multiple comparisons, as obtained both from whole brain correction (marked with two asterisks [**]) and from small volume correction (one asterisk [*]) from a-priori regions of interest. Correction was based on spheres centred around the peak coordinates (ignoring laterality) obtained from previous studies [10,22–25] or using an anatomical mask [26,27] in case of the dorsolateral prefrontal cortex. These regions include brain areas known to be involved in pain processing (brainstem (3/−35/−17), thalamus (12/−12/4), basal ganglia (8/14/−10), posterior (48/−4/16) and anteromedial (34/0/−6) insula and secondary somatosensory cortex (49/−19/18) [28]) and its modulation (subgenual (10/10/−10) and dorsal (8/34/18) anterior cingulate cortex, dorsolateral prefrontal cortex (Brodmann area 9 [29]), amygdala (16/−6/−15; 24/−2/−18) and hippocampus (21/−21/−9) [30,31]). Activation in cortical areas was corrected using 15 mm radius spheres, subcortical areas were corrected using 10 mm radius spheres. For exploratory purposes we also report uncorrected results on a more lenient threshold of $p \leq 0.001$ [†].

Results

Note that part of the behavioral data have been published elsewhere [9].

Behavioral data

All participants had normal thresholds to heat pain at the site of stimulus application (volar forearm, 45.8°C±2.7). The mean temperatures for the test stimuli that corresponded to a pain sensation of 20, 50 and 80 on the VAS as determined in the calibration session were 44.1°C±1.3, 45.9°C±1.1 and 46.9°C±0.9, respectively.

Mean pain ratings during the *conditioning phase* differed between groups. Pain ratings on the VAS were 17.3±1.9 on the treated site and 75.5±1.8 on the untreated site in the positive group and 71.1±2.8 on the treated site and 74.8±1.9 on the untreated site in the negative group. Pain relief from the placebo patch (treatment A) was significantly greater in the positive group (Δ VAS = 58.2) compared to the negative group (Δ VAS = 3.7, $t_{37} = -13.9$, $p<0.001$), indicating a successful manipulation of treatment experience (Fig. 2 A).

In the *test phase*, the analgesic effect of the second, different treatment was compared between the positive and the negative treatment history group. This analysis revealed that the therapeutic effect of the ointment (treatment B) was significantly greater in the positive treatment history group than in the negative group (positive group: Δ VAS = 41.3, negative group: Δ VAS = 27.1, $t_{37} = -2.9$, $p = 0.007$, (Fig. 2 B). Positive group: VAS 40.0±3.3 on the treated site and VAS 81.3±2.4 on the untreated site, negative group: VAS 53.6±4.6 on the treated site and VAS 80.7±3.4 on the untreated site [9]). Note, that physically identical stimulation temperatures were used in both groups (mean applied temperature: 45.9°C±0.2 at the treated and 46.9°C±0.1 at the untreated site).

Across all participants, the analgesic benefit from the second analgesic treatment was negatively correlated with individual trait anxiety ($r = -0.4$, $p<0.05$).

Within the positive group, a negative correlation between depression score (ADS-K) and treatment response was observed ($r = -0.53$, $p<0.05$). Furthermore, in the negative group, a correlation analysis of the psychological characteristic 'locus of control' and the individual treatment response showed that

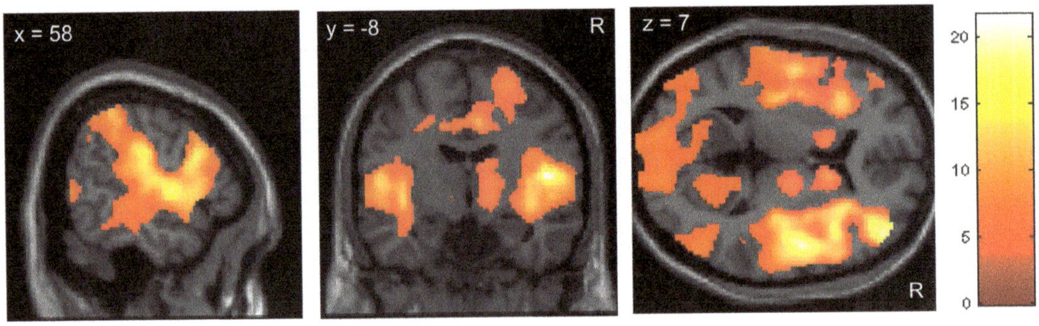

Figure 3. Pain-related BOLD response (main effect of pain). The 20 s thermal stimulus induced significant activation (t-score) of pain-processing regions including the thalamus, striatum, insula, S I, S II, MCC and prefrontal cortices. The image is thresholded at $p<0.05$ FWE whole brain correction. For a complete list of activated brain areas see Table 1 A.

subjects with a more external locus of control benefited even less from the analgesic treatment ($r = -0.68$, $p<0.05$).

FMRI

We first identified brain areas which responded to the painful thermal stimulation, pooled across all four experimental conditions. The results show that the painful stimuli significantly activated the well-known cerebral pain network [28], including the primary and secondary somatosensory cortices (S I, S II), the insula and the midcingulate cortex (MCC). Subcortical responses were recorded in the thalamus, basal ganglia, brainstem and cerebellum (Table 1 A and Fig. 3).

Comparing pain-related responses to stimulation on the untreated and the treated site (main effect of treatment) across both treatment history groups revealed stronger activity in the bilateral insular cortex, MCC and amygdala for the untreated compared to the treated site, reflecting the higher stimulation intensity on this site during the test phase (Table 1 B).

The main effect of group revealed stronger pain-related activity in the amygdala, S II and frontal cortex in the negative compared to the positive group. Furthermore, this group showed stronger activity in the occipital and superior parietal lobes (Table 1 C).

We then tested whether BOLD responses to pain reflect the behavioral differences in analgesia to the second treatment. We expected less reduction of pain-related activity on the treated compared to the untreated site in the negative treatment history group compared to the positive group. Indeed, the interaction contrast [Positive group $_{[\text{untreated}>\text{treated site}]}$>Negative group $_{[\text{untreated}>\text{treated site}]}$] revealed bilateral activity in the posterior insular cortex, which was stronger at the right side, corresponding to painful stimulation performed on the left forearm (Table 1 D1 and Fig. 4), as shown in [9]. This response pattern was evident during both pain phases (early and late).

Furthermore, we aimed to identify brain regions that mediated the increased analgesic response to the second treatment in the positive compared to the negative treatment history group. We therefore investigated the opposite 'group-by-condition-interaction' contrast [Positive group $_{[\text{treated}>\text{untreated site}]}$>Negative group $_{[\text{treated}>\text{untreated site}]}$] and expected that brain areas involved in the descending modulation of pain mediated the analgesic benefit from treatment B in the positive treatment history group. Indeed, we found that the stronger analgesic effect in the positive compared to the negative treatment history group was associated with activity within the striatum and anterior cingulate cortex (ACC) during both pain phases and in the right dorsolateral prefrontal cortex (DLPFC) during the late pain phase [9]. These areas are key regions of descending pain modulation (Table 1 E1, E2 and Fig. 5 B).

Intriguingly, a positive correlation between the activity in pain-inhibitory areas such as periaqueductal gray (PAG), ACC and DLPFC during the anticipation phase (treated – untreated) and the pain reduction in the posterior insula during the pain phase was observed within the positive treatment history group. This indicates that activity in the descending pain modulatory system during anticipation is associated with more analgesic benefit during pain (Table 1 F2 and Fig. 6).

In the negative group we found a negative correlation between activity in pain processing regions such as the insula and the thalamus during the anticipation phase (treated – untreated) and the pain reduction in the posterior insula during pain. This suggests that less analgesic benefit during pain is associated with increased anticipatory responses in pain related areas in this group (Table 1 F1 and Fig. 7).

Discussion

This study explored how prior experience with one treatment can influence the response to a second subsequently applied different treatment. This was studied in an experimental model of analgesia using an analgesic patch as the first treatment (treatment A) and an analgesic ointment treatment as the second analgesic treatment (treatment B). We found that, in comparison to those subjects with a positive treatment history, participants who experienced no analgesia from the first treatment continued to show a substantially reduced response to a second, different analgesic treatment. These findings therefore indicate that prior treatment experience critically influences the efficacy of a treatment and most importantly, that this influence transfers over time and over therapeutic approach.

Behavioral effects were substantiated by neuroimaging data showing significant activation differences in brain regions coding pain and analgesia between groups. Specifically, the adverse effect of a negative treatment history on analgesia was paralleled by stronger activation in bilateral posterior insular cortices. Activity in this brain region has consistently been shown to correlate with afferent nociceptive input and perceived pain intensity [32] and can therefore be taken as a physiological marker of analgesia. These data provide strong evidence that the differences in analgesia depending on prior treatment history are not the result of report bias, but reflect altered processing of ascending nociceptive input.

Furthermore, we found that the stronger analgesic effect of the second treatment (treatment B) in the positive treatment history

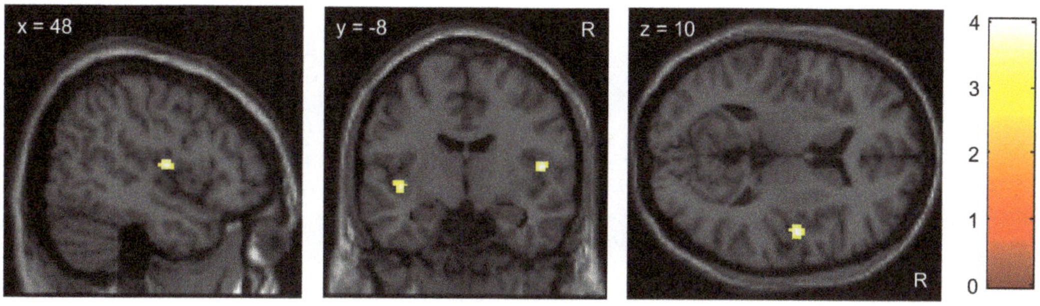

Figure 4. The effect of treatment history on analgesic outcome is reflected in pain-related responses in the posterior insula. FMRI revealed less reduction of pain-related BOLD activity (t-scores) on the treated compared to the untreated site following a negative treatment history compared to a positive treatment history. Activation related to the 'group-by-condition-interaction' contrast *[Positive group [untreated>treated site]> Negative group [untreated>treated site]],* for details see Table 1 D1. For visualization purposes the images are thresholded at $p<0.005$.

group was associated with increased engagement of the right dorsolateral prefrontal cortex (DLPFC) and the anterior cingulate cortex (ACC). This activity not only occurred during painful stimulation but also during the anticipation phase where it scaled with the subsequent reduction of insular activity. The DLPFC and ACC are key structures for top-down modulation of pain through different cognitive factors [33], including placebo and nocebo related modulations of pharmacological effects [34]. Although the multiple ROIs used for small volume correction potentially increased the rate of type 1 error, our data suggest that the descending pain modulatory mechanisms that complement the specific analgesic effect (modelled here by a simple temperature reduction) mediates the effect of treatment history and thereby determines the overall analgesic treatment outcome. This notion is further supported by the observation that activity in the descending pain modulatory system during pain anticipation is positively correlated with the reduction of pain related activity in the posterior insula in the positive treatment history group.

Our neuroimaging data further substantiate findings from previous studies suggesting that specific treatment effects and factors related to the treatment context (i.e. treatment expectancy or treatment experience) ultimately converge at the neurobiological level and can critically modulate the overall treatment outcome [34,35].

These results significantly extend previous findings by showing that the influence of treatment history transfers over time and over therapeutic approach. The experience with the patch treatment substantially modulated the response to the subsequent ointment treatment, with impaired analgesic efficacy following negative treatment experience and enhanced efficacy after the positive treatment experience.

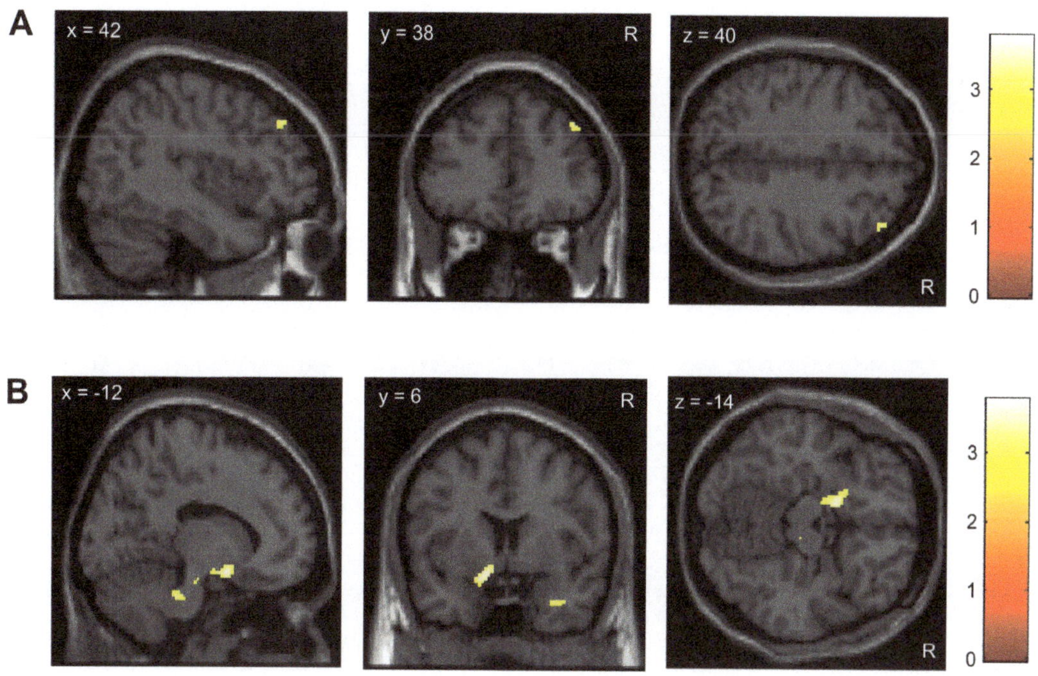

Figure 5. Increased analgesic response to new treatment following a positive treatment history is associated with higher pain related activity in the right dorsolateral prefrontal cortex (DLPFC, A) and the striatum (B). Images show BOLD responses (t-scores) to painful heat stimulation related to the 'group-by-condition-interaction' contrast *[Positive group [treated>untreated site]>Negative group [treated> untreated site]],* for details see Table 1 E2. For visualization purposes the images are thresholded at $p<0.005$.

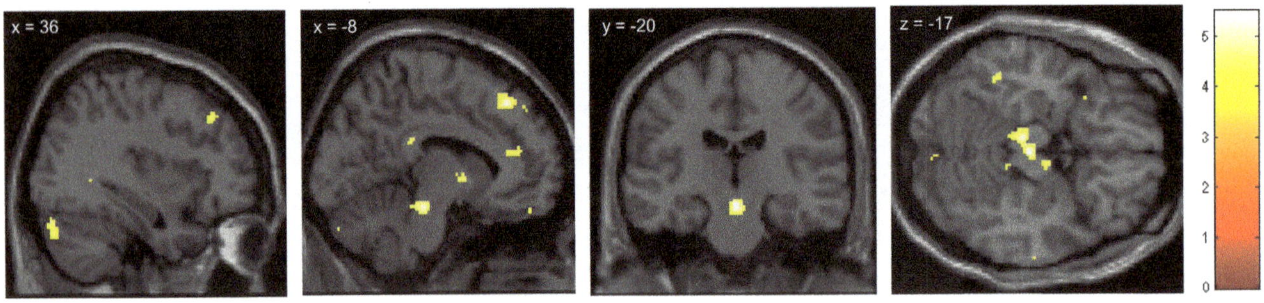

Figure 6. Increased treatment response in the positive group is associated with increased activity of pain regulatory networks during the anticipation of pain. Images show BOLD activity (t-scores) during the anticipation phase (t-test: positive correlation of anticipatory activity *[treated>untreated site]* with the treatment response in the posterior insula for the positive group). Stronger reductions of pain-related activity in the posterior insula during pain stimulation is preceded by stronger activity in pain inhibitory regions such as the PAG, DLPFC and rACC during pain anticipation before the actual pain stimulation is applied. For visualization purposes the images are thresholded at $p<0.005$. For details see Table 1 F2.

The results of our study are relevant for several reasons. We provide evidence for the transfer of conditioning effects over different treatment approaches using an experimental longitudinal approach. Because these conditioned effects affect not only responses within the same treatment but also affect subsequent different treatments we refer to these effects as "carry-over effects".

Data from pharmacological cross-over studies (i.e., drug trials in which subjects receive an active drug and a placebo in a randomized order) have previously suggested the carry-over of treatment effects from placebo to active treatments and vice versa. In a double-blind cross-over study on the effect of an antihypertensive drug, the placebo did not affect the patients' hypertension when administered first [36]. Yet, when placebos were administered after a week-long use of atenolol, they produced a significantly greater antihypertensive response than a 'no treatment' condition. Sequence effects of drug efficacy have also been proposed for analgesic treatments of musculoskeletal pain by [37] indicating that not only the placebo medication was more effective following active and effective treatment, but also that the active drug was less effective when it followed an ineffective placebo treatment. Similar sequence effects have recently been reported for the analgesic effect of active compared to sham rTMS for chronic pain [38]. It can, however, not be ruled out that these findings were confounded by residual drug (treatment) effects, the natural course of the underlying disease and expectancy-related effects due to unblinding. Because our study was undertaken in a controlled experimental setting and comprised behavioral and neuroimaging outcome measures it provides strong objective evidence for a carry-over effect in treatment outcome. Importantly, as analgesia was modelled experimentally by using a placebo paradigm, our findings are not related to any drug-specific pharmacological effects and may therefore apply to any treatment.

Our findings on this carry-over effect may have wide implications for medical practice and clinical trial designs. Treatment experiences are ubiquitous in clinical care, particularly in patients suffering from chronic diseases. Carry-over effects might therefore be particularly relevant in chronic conditions where treatments often fail repetitively and negative treatment experiences accumulate along the course of the disease. Our results advocate the careful assessment of treatment history and a strictly systematic treatment approach to avoid negative carry-over effects, as any treatment failure may hamper or even abolish future treatment response. In a similar vein, our results may even challenge common step care approaches in which treatment failure has to precede the prescription of next-in-line interventions [39].

Given that inter-individual differences are a major challenge for medical treatments, we also assessed whether clinically relevant personality traits affect treatment response in general, or specifically with respect to prior treatment experience. We found that higher anxiety levels were associated with lower treatment

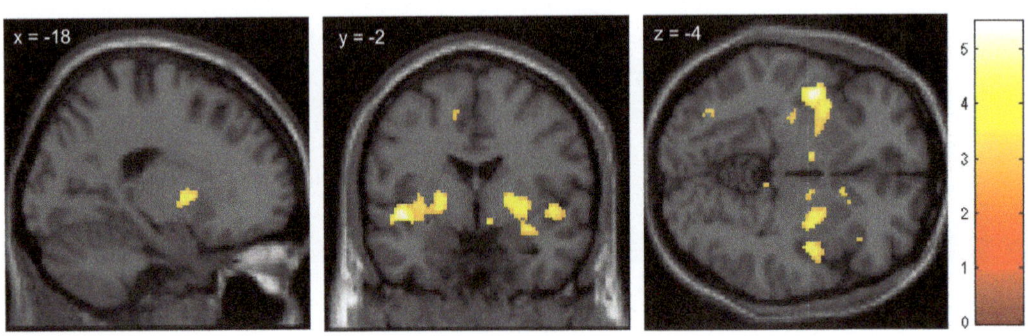

Figure 7. Reduced treatment response in the negative group is associated with increased activity of pain processing regions during the anticipation of pain. Images show BOLD activity (t-scores) during the anticipation phase (t-test: negative correlation of anticipatory activity [treated>untreated site] with the treatment response in the posterior insula for the negative group). For visualization purposes the images are thresholded at $p<0.005$. For details see Methods and Table 1 F1.

responses, independent of prior treatment experience. Furthermore, depression scores of our healthy volunteers were negatively correlated with the analgesic treatment response in the positive treatment history group indicating that depression may hamper the positive effects of prior treatment response. This observation highlights that the susceptibility to treatment history effects varies across individuals and indicates that patients with comorbid mood disorders may require particular attention.

Reframing (pharmaco-) therapy as a learning process that impacts therapeutic response over time and over therapy also yields important implications for the design and interpretation of clinical trials [40]. Prior treatment experiences or the participation in drug trials are currently neither systematically assessed nor accounted for in the statistical analysis of clinical trials. This neglect of the influence of treatment history on treatment efficacy might inadvertently contribute to the heterogeneity of responses in clinical trials and thereby reduce assay sensitivity (i.e. the sensitivity for drug placebo differences). Our data strongly suggest that the systematic assessment of the individual treatment history should be an essential part of any clinical trial.

While some implications of our study, such as the assessment of the patients' treatment history, can immediately be applied in the clinic, others require further investigation. In particular, we need to specify the critical time window during which prior effects can affect subsequent outcome, understand how the similarity of treatment approaches impacts the effect, and most importantly, how we can overcome negative and systematically use positive carry-over effects. In our study two locally applied "treatments" (i.e., a patch and an ointment) with presumably different pharmacological profiles were used. According to the conditioning literature carry-over effects are stronger the more similar the conditioned stimuli are in appearance. In support of this notion it has been shown that responses to two subsequent placebo treatments differ depending on treatment similarity [41]. If this holds true for learning effects in drug treatments these findings could motivate the use of different application forms (oral, intravenous, local etc.) after treatment failure in addition to pharmacodynamical considerations. Furthermore, psychological interventions could aid in overcoming the detrimental effects of negative treatment experiences. Additional studies are therefore needed to characterize the role of expectancy induced by the treatment experience.

Taken together, our study provides evidence that treatment history critically determines the response to a subsequent treatment at a behavioral and neurobiological level. Further, we show that the susceptibility for carry-over effects varies across individuals and is associated with trait anxiety and depression. Given the large number of patients with persisting health problems despite various treatment attempts, it seems reasonable to assume that negative treatment experiences and their detrimental effects for subsequent treatment approaches contribute substantially to increased health care costs and importantly, to prolonged suffering of our patients. Even though these experimental findings require replication in larger clinical populations, we feel that awareness of this effect is mandatory for every physician and concerted effort is required to avoid or overcome the negative effects of prior experience on treatment outcome.

Author Contributions

Conceived and designed the experiments: SK UB. Performed the experiments: SK. Analyzed the data: SK CR KF UB. Wrote the paper: SK KF CR KW MP UB.

References

1. Finniss DG, Kaptchuk TJ, Miller F, Benedetti F (2010) Biological, clinical, and ethical advances of placebo effects. Lancet 375: 686–695. Available: http://www.pubmedcentral.nih.gov/articlerender.fcgi?artid=2832199&tool=pmcentrez&rendertype=abstract. Accessed 2014 May 9.
2. Colloca L, Sigaudo M, Benedetti F (2008) The role of learning in nocebo and placebo effects. Pain 136: 211–218. Available: http://www.ncbi.nlm.nih.gov/pubmed/18372113. Accessed 2014 May 9.
3. Doering BK, Rief W (2012) Utilizing placebo mechanisms for dose reduction in pharmacotherapy. Trends Pharmacol Sci 33: 165–172. Available: http://www.ncbi.nlm.nih.gov/pubmed/22284159. Accessed 2014 May 9.
4. Voudouris NJ, Peck CL, Coleman G (1990) The role of conditioning and verbal expectancy in the placebo response. Pain 43: 121–128. Available: http://www.ncbi.nlm.nih.gov/pubmed/2277714. Accessed 2014 May 9.
5. Montgomery GH, Kirsch I (1997) Classical conditioning and the placebo effect. Pain 72: 107–113. Available: http://linkinghub.elsevier.com/retrieve/pii/S030439599700016X. Accessed 2014 May 7.
6. Wager TD, Rilling JK, Smith EE, Sokolik A, Casey KL, et al. (2004) Placebo-induced changes in FMRI in the anticipation and experience of pain. Science 303: 1162–1167. Available: http://www.ncbi.nlm.nih.gov/pubmed/14976306. Accessed 2014 May 7.
7. Colloca L, Benedetti F (2006) How prior experience shapes placebo analgesia. Pain 124: 126–133. Available: http://www.ncbi.nlm.nih.gov/pubmed/16701952. Accessed 2014 May 9.
8. Voudouris NJ, Peck CL, Coleman G (1985) Conditioned placebo responses. J Pers Soc Psychol 48: 47–53. Available: http://www.ncbi.nlm.nih.gov/pubmed/3981392. Accessed 2014 May 9.
9. Kessner S, Wiech K, Forkmann K, Ploner M, Bingel U (2013) The effect of treatment history on therapeutic outcome: an experimental approach. JAMA Intern Med 173: 1468–1469. Available: http://www.ncbi.nlm.nih.gov/pubmed/23780284. Accessed 2014 May 9.
10. Eippert F, Bingel U, Schoell ED, Yacubian J, Klinger R, et al. (2009) Activation of the opioidergic descending pain control system underlies placebo analgesia. Neuron 63: 533–543. Available: http://www.ncbi.nlm.nih.gov/pubmed/19709634. Accessed 2014 May 5.
11. Rolke R, Baron R, Maier C, Tölle TR, Treede RD, et al. (2006) Quantitative sensory testing in the German Research Network on Neuropathic Pain (DFNS): Standardized protocol and reference values. Pain 123: 231–243. doi:10.1016/j.pain.2006.01.041.
12. Laux L, Glanzmann P, Schaffner P, Spielberger CD (1981) State-Trait Anxiety Inventory (Spielberger, C.D., Gorsuch, R.L., Lushene, R.E., 1970) - Deutsche Version.
13. Spielberger CD, Gorsuch RL, Lushene PR, Vagg PR, Jacobs AG (1983) Manual for the State-Trait Anxiety Inventory (Form Y).
14. Radloff LS (1977) The CES-D Scale: A Self-Report Depression Scale for Research in the General Population. Appl Psychol Meas 1: 385–401. Available: http://apm.sagepub.com/content/1/3/385.abstract. Accessed 2014 April 29.
15. Hautzinger M, Bailer M (1993) ADS Allgemeine Depressionsskala. Weinheim: Beltz.
16. Levenson H (1972) Distinctions within the concept of internal-external control: Development of a new scale. Proc 80th Annu Conv Am Psychol Assoc 7: 259–260.
17. Levenson H (1973) Multidimensional locus of control in psychiatric patients. J Consult Clin Psychol 41: 397–404. doi:10.1037/h0035357.
18. Krampen G (1979) Differentiation of the construct "locus of control of reinforcement": German adaptation and application of the IPC-scales. Z Exp Angew Psychol 26: 573–595. Available: http://search.proquest.com/docview/616466088?accountid=10422.
19. Fruhstorfer H, Lindblom U, Schmidt WC (1976) Method for quantitative estimation of thermal thresholds in patients. J Neurol Neurosurg Psychiatry 39: 1071–1075. Available: http://jnnp.bmj.com/cgi/doi/10.1136/jnnp.39.11.1071. Accessed 2014 May 9.
20. Friston KJ, Ashburner J, Poline JB, Frith CD, Heather JD, et al. (1995) Spatial registration and normalisation of images. Hum Brain Mapp 2: 165–189.
21. Worsley KJ, Friston KJ (1995) Analysis of fMRI time-series revisited–again. Neuroimage 2: 173–181. Available: http://www.ncbi.nlm.nih.gov/pubmed/9343600. Accessed 2014 May 1.
22. Faymonville ME, Laureys S, Degueldre C, DelFiore G, Luxen A, et al. (2000) Neural mechanisms of antinociceptive effects of hypnosis. Anesthesiology 92: 1257–1267. Available: http://content.wkhealth.com/linkback/openurl?sid=WKPTLP:landingpage&an=00003643-200000002-00578. Accessed 2014 May 9.
23. Bingel U, Quante M, Knab R, Bromm B, Weiller C, et al. (2002) Subcortical structures involved in pain processing: Evidence from single-trial fMRI. Pain 99: 313–321. doi:10.1016/S0304-3959(02)00157-4.
24. Bingel U, Gläscher J, Weiller C, Büchel C (2004) Somatotopic representation of nociceptive information in the putamen: an event-related fMRI study. Cereb

Cortex 14: 1340–1345. Available: http://www.ncbi.nlm.nih.gov/pubmed/15217895. Accessed 2014 May 4.
25. Eickhoff SB, Amunts K, Mohlberg H, Zilles K (2006) The human parietal operculum. II. Stereotaxic maps and correlation with functional imaging results. Cereb Cortex 16: 268–279. Available: http://www.ncbi.nlm.nih.gov/pubmed/15888606. Accessed 2014 August 21.
26. Maldjian JA, Laurienti PJ, Kraft RA, Burdette JH (2003) An automated method for neuroanatomic and cytoarchitectonic atlas-based interrogation of fMRI data sets. Neuroimage 19: 1233–1239. doi:10.1016/S1053-8119(03)00169-1.
27. Lancaster JL, Woldorff MG, Parsons LM, Liotti M, Freitas CS, et al. (2000) Automated Talairach Atlas labels for functional brain mapping. Hum Brain Mapp 10: 120–131. doi:10.1002/1097-0193(200007)10:3<120::AID-HBM30>3.0.CO;2-8.
28. Apkarian AV, Bushnell MC, Treede R-D, Zubieta J-K (2005) Human brain mechanisms of pain perception and regulation in health and disease. Eur J Pain 9: 463–484. Available: http://www.sciencedirect.com/science/article/pii/S109038010400148X. Accessed 2014 April 29.
29. Petrides M, Pandya DN (1999) Dorsolateral prefrontal cortex: comparative cytoarchitectonic analysis in the human and the macaque brain and corticocortical connection patterns. Eur J Neurosci 11: 1011–1036. Available: http://www.ncbi.nlm.nih.gov/pubmed/10103094. Accessed 2014 September 1.
30. Bingel U, Tracey I (2008) Imaging CNS modulation of pain in humans. Physiology (Bethesda) 23: 371–380. Available: http://www.ncbi.nlm.nih.gov/pubmed/19074744. Accessed 2014 May 9.
31. Kong J, Gollub RL, Polich G, Kirsch I, Laviolette P, et al. (2008) A functional magnetic resonance imaging study on the neural mechanisms of hyperalgesic nocebo effect. J Neurosci 28: 13354–13362. Available: http://www.pubmedcentral.nih.gov/articlerender.fcgi?artid=2649754&tool=pmcentrez&rendertype=abstract. Accessed 2014 May 9.
32. Tracey I (2011) Can neuroimaging studies identify pain endophenotypes in humans? Nat Rev Neurol 7: 173–181. Available: http://www.ncbi.nlm.nih.gov/pubmed/21304481. Accessed 2014 May 2.
33. Wiech K, Ploner M, Tracey I (2008) Neurocognitive aspects of pain perception. Trends Cogn Sci 12: 306–313. Available: http://www.ncbi.nlm.nih.gov/pubmed/18606561. Accessed 2014 May 9.
34. Bingel U, Wanigasekera V, Wiech K, Ni Mhuircheartaigh R, Lee MC, et al. (2011) The effect of treatment expectation on drug efficacy: imaging the analgesic benefit of the opioid remifentanil. Sci Transl Med 3: 70ra14. Available: http://www.ncbi.nlm.nih.gov/pubmed/21325618. Accessed 2014 May 7.
35. Volkow ND, Wang G-J, Ma Y, Fowler JS, Zhu W, et al. (2003) Expectation enhances the regional brain metabolic and the reinforcing effects of stimulants in cocaine abusers. J Neurosci 23: 11461–11468. Available: http://www.ncbi.nlm.nih.gov/pubmed/14673011. Accessed 2014 May 9.
36. Suchman AL, Ader R (1992) Classic conditioning and placebo effects in crossover studies. Clin Pharmacol Ther 52: 372–377. Available: http://www.nature.com/doifinder/10.1038/clpt.1992.157. Accessed 2014 May 9.
37. Batterman RC, Lower WR (1968) Placebo responsiveness–influence of previous therapy. Curr Ther Res Clin Exp 10: 136–143. Available: http://www.ncbi.nlm.nih.gov/pubmed/4967001. Accessed 2014 May 9.
38. André-Obadia N, Magnin M, Garcia-Larrea L (2011) On the importance of placebo timing in rTMS studies for pain relief. Pain 152: 1233–1237. Available: http://www.ncbi.nlm.nih.gov/pubmed/21342747. Accessed 2014 May 9.
39. Organization WH (1986) Cancer pain relief. Cancer Pain Reli Geneva, Switzerland, World Heal Organ.
40. Colloca L (2011) Learned placebo analgesia in sequential trials: What are the Pros and Cons? Pain 152: 1215–1216. Available: http://www.ncbi.nlm.nih.gov/pubmed/21377800. Accessed 2014 May 9.
41. Whalley B, Hyland ME, Kirsch I (2008) Consistency of the placebo effect. J Psychosom Res 64: 537–541. Available: http://www.ncbi.nlm.nih.gov/pubmed/18440407. Accessed 2014 May 26.

Well-Loved Music Robustly Relieves Pain: A Randomized, Controlled Trial

Christine Hsieh[1]*, Jian Kong[1], Irving Kirsch[2,3], Robert R. Edwards[4], Karin B. Jensen[1,5], Ted J. Kaptchuk[2], Randy L. Gollub[1,5]

1 Department of Psychiatry, Massachusetts General Hospital and Harvard Medical School, Boston, Massachusetts, United States of America, **2** Program in Placebo Studies and the Therapeutic Encounter (PiPS), Harvard Medical School and Beth Israel Deaconess Medical Center, Boston, Massachusetts, United States of America, **3** Department of Psychology, Plymouth University, Plymouth, United Kingdom, **4** Department of Anesthesiology, Brigham and Women's Hospital, Boston, Massachusetts, United States of America, **5** Department of Radiology, Athinoula A. Martinos Center for Biomedical Imaging and Massachusetts General Hospital, Charlestown, Massachusetts, United States of America

Abstract

Music has pain-relieving effects, but its mechanisms remain unclear. We sought to verify previously studied analgesic components and further elucidate the underpinnings of music analgesia. Using a well-characterized conditioning-enhanced placebo model, we examined whether boosting expectations would enhance or interfere with analgesia from strongly preferred music. A two-session experiment was performed with 48 healthy, pain experiment-naïve participants. In a first cohort, 36 were randomized into 3 treatment groups, including music enhanced with positive expectancy, non-musical sound enhanced with positive expectancy, and no expectancy enhancement. A separate replication cohort of 12 participants received only expectancy-enhanced music following the main experiment to verify the results of expectancy-manipulation on music. Primary outcome measures included the change in subjective pain ratings to calibrated experimental noxious heat stimuli, as well as changes in treatment expectations. Without conditioning, expectations were strongly in favor of music compared to non-musical sound. While measured expectations were enhanced by conditioning, this failed to affect either music or sound analgesia significantly. Strongly preferred music on its own was as pain relieving as conditioning-enhanced strongly preferred music, and more analgesic than enhanced sound. Our results demonstrate the pain-relieving power of personal music even over enhanced expectations.

Trial Information: Clinicaltrials.gov NCT01835275.

Editor: Elvira Brattico, Cognitive Brain Research Unit, Finland

Funding: Funding was provided by the Harvard-MIT Health Sciences and Technology IDEA2 award (Hsieh) and NIH grant R01 AT 005280 (Gollub/Kaptchuk). The funders had no role in study design, data collection and analysis, decision to publish, or preparation of the manuscript.

Competing Interests: The authors have declared that no competing interests exist.

* Email: xtine.hsieh@gmail.com

Introduction

Music is a treatment that can affect pain perception through a complex set of past and present cues. Juslin and Vastfjall (2008), Salimpoor et al. (2011), and Koelsch (2009), among others, posited many ways through which music may activate regional brain networks mediating reward and anxiolytic effects that also overlap with regions involved in analgesia [1–9]. At the same time, music is an enactor of strong perceptual and behavioral responses, such as action tendency and emotional regulation [10], which may also contribute to modulation of pain perception. Scientific reports of pain relief date back to at least the time when Gardner (1960) used it to treat 1000 dental patients and found that using music and white noise, one quarter of the patients did not need additional analgesia during a dental procedure [11]. Amongst more recent music analgesia studies, positive emotions to music were seen to be a modulator of pain [12], but others did not find that music's cognitive and emotional effects were as influential on pain ratings as treatment expectancy [13]. Specific factors contributing to music analgesia have still not been established definitively [14].

No less complex than music are placebo responses, whose definition has evolved to emphasize psychosocial and contextual cues that generate objectively measurable psychobiological effects [15]. More specifically, beliefs, expectations, and previous treatment are all factors on the patient side that can influence the clinical outcome. Graded doses of increasing amounts of positive clinical contextual factors steadily produce more positive results [16]. Furthermore, research has begun to elucidate the underlying neurochemical and neuroanatomical substrates of placebo responses [3,17,18]. Expectancy in particular has emerged as one of the most well supported factors contributing to placebo analgesia [19,20]. Studies have shown that boosting expectations through conditioning leads to enhanced analgesia, as well as the opposite effect of hyperalgesia with induced negative expectations [21,22]. This linkage between expectancy, conditioning, and analgesia has been shown across a variety of conditioned stimuli,

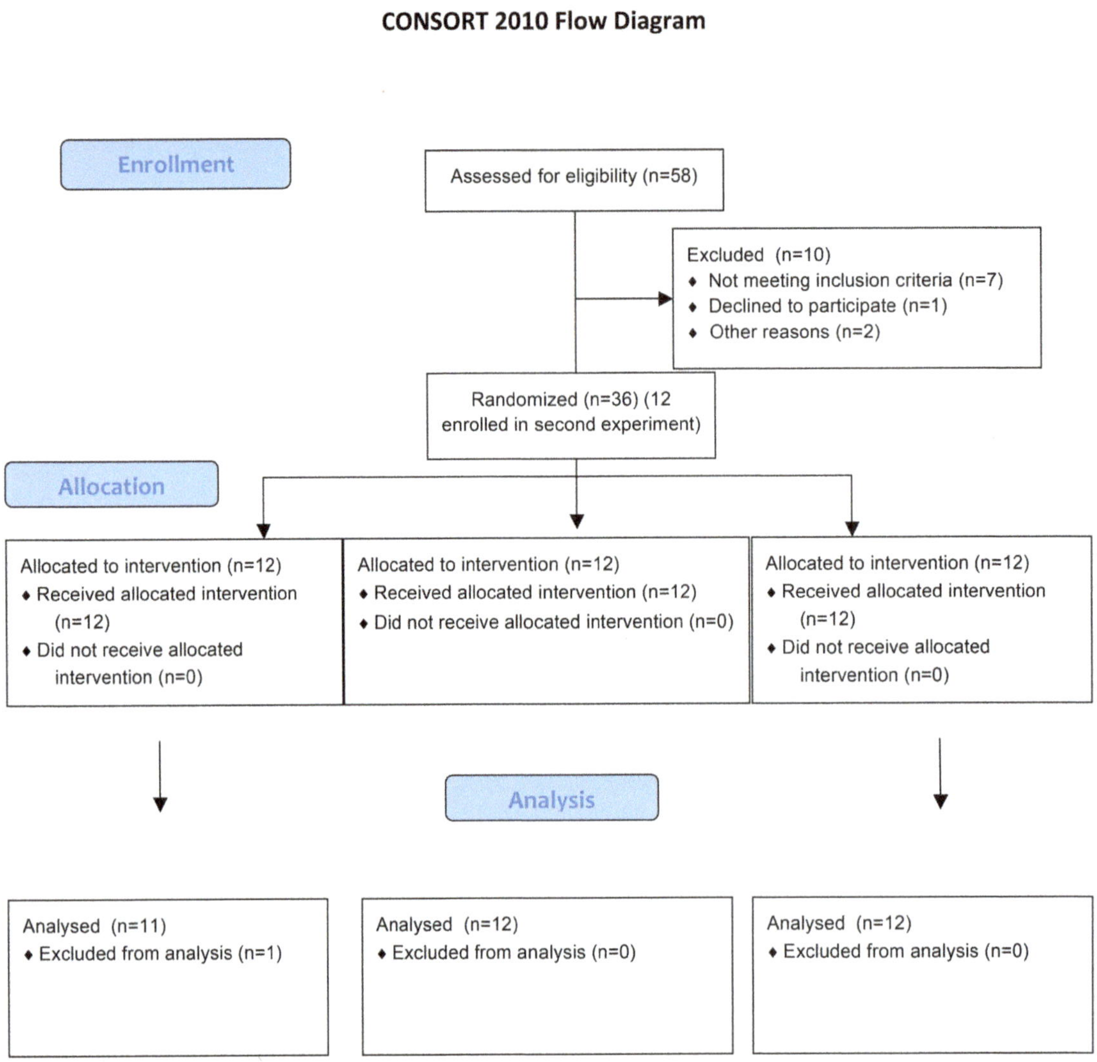

Figure 1. CONSORT Flowchart.

including acupuncture, creams, and visual cues [18,23,24]. Because of the countless ways we may modify subtle attitudes and actions in clinical circumstances, examining factors such as expectancy is of high interest for clinical translation of experimental analgesic outcomes.

To investigate whether the analgesic effect of an emotionally pleasurable stimulus, such as strongly preferred music, could be modified by the well studied conditioning paradigm used within placebo analgesia, we designed an experiment that juxtaposed music with conditioned-expectancy enhancement in two opposing ways - one in which conditioning aimed to enhance expectations of relief for music, and the second in which music would be put up against conditioned expectancy enhancement of a non-musical control sound. We used a well-validated conditioning procedure [19,25–28] of pairing lower heat pain stimuli with a target audio cue to achieve boosted analgesia. Our control group examined the analgesic effects of music and control sound alone. We were able to achieve the aim of shedding light on whether the analgesia of music would be enhanced or disrupted by expectancy-based placebo mechanisms.

Methods

Ethics Statement

All study procedures were carried out with Institutional Review Board approval from MIT COUHES (protocol #1206005109) and MGH (protocol #2012P000969), approved on June 27, 2012 and June 31, 2012 respectively. Data was collected at the Martinos Imaging Center in Charlestown, MA. All participants were taken through written informed consent prior to initiating any study procedures. The protocol for this trial and supporting CONSORT checklist are available as Checklist S1 and Protocol S1. This trial was registered under clinicaltrials.gov as trial #NCT01835275. Registration was completed after subject recruitment had begun due to a delay in assigning the appropriate Responsible Party to the record. The authors confirm that all ongoing and related trials for this intervention are registered.

Participants

Participants met the following criteria: ***Inclusion*** - healthy male and female adults aged 18–50, body mass index <30. ***Exclusion*** - current major medical, neurological, or psychiatric disease, pregnancy, advanced music training, instability of responses to experimental pain (see Study Procedures Section), non-fluent speaker of English, BDI-II (Beck Depression Inventory) [29,30] score greater than 13, previous experience in pain experiments, current or previous ear/nose/throat or hearing issues compromising ability to listen to audio stimuli. Volunteers were recruited by advertising via email, web, and bulletin board announcements. Recruitment took place from July 1, 2012 to January 23, 2013, and all study procedures were completed within the period from July 2012–January 2013.

Study Procedures

A two-session experiment was performed with 48 healthy, pain experiment-naïve participants. In a first cohort, 36 were randomized (via assignment to outcomes from a random number generator) into 3 treatment groups, including music conditioning, non-musical sound conditioning, and no-conditioning. The primary author completed the random sequence generation, enrollment, and participant assignments. Primary outcome measures included the change in subjective pain ratings to calibrated experimental noxious heat stimuli, as well as changes in treatment expectations on an Expectancy of Relief Scale (ERS). The ERS is a 0–10 scale (with 0 indicating "does not work at all" and 10 indicating "complete pain relief") used to measure the expectation of treatment pain relief [18]. We also acquired subjective responses to treatments assessed through semi-free form interviews and surveys. A separate replication cohort of 12 participants received only music conditioning following the main experiment. The flow of participants through the study can be found in Figure 1.

The two behavioral sessions were separated by a minimum of 2 days and a maximum of 10 days. Prior to coming to the experimental site, all participants were asked to acquire/choose a set of personal music that satisfied certain criteria for the study (see next section). During both sessions, participants received sets of calibrated noxious thermal stimuli using a Thermal Sensory Analyzer (TSA-II) or the Pathway CHEPS model (Contact Heat-Evoked Potential Stimulator) with a 3 cm×3 cm probe (Medoc Advanced Medical Systems, Rimat Yishai, Israel) running proprietary computerized visual analog scale software (COVAS). Each stimulus was 12 seconds long (2.5 second ramps with 7 second plateaus), and was delivered in blocks of 5 with a jittered average of 30 seconds between stimuli. After each stimulus, participants used 0–100 visual analog scales to rate the pain intensity and unpleasantness, with anchors of 0 = no pain and 100 = worst imaginable pain.

In the *first session*, participants underwent the consent process and screening questions, and we determined whether participants could report consistent, appropriate responses to the calibrated noxious thermal stimuli. Anchors for the pain ratings scales were explained verbally prior to administering the first set of stimuli. In the *second session* we repeated testing for appropriate responses to the thermal stimuli – only participants that performed consistently on the pain rating task (could reliably rate mild intensity pain stimuli as less painful than moderate intensity stimuli and have comparable ratings across sessions - within about 1 STD) would continue to further testing during the second session.

Participants who were eligible to continue first received identical baseline stimuli (calibrated individually during Session 1) on three spots of their right arms, in silence (Figure 2). Participants in conditioning groups then received a conditioning- expectancy manipulation procedure designed to enhance expectations of pain relief in response to their assigned treatment [26]. Participants in conditioning groups were first told that during the intended conditioned stimuli they could experience less pain: "Today we're testing a treatment for pain that is not yet in clinical use. The reason we're using ____ (this special frequency-filtered sound, your specially selected music) is because previous studies have shown it to have pain-relieving properties. This is what we're testing today, and we're just comparing it to ____ (the sound, the music), and silence." We then proceeded to pair the target conditioning stimuli with lowered pain levels, with the other audio (music or sound) paired with the baseline pain level. In the no-conditioning control group, we stated that *either* their music or the sound could have analgesic effects. Participants in this group then received two pain levels, with no audio paired. Finally, all groups underwent testing with stimuli identical to baseline, on the same three spots, within audio conditions of music, sound, and silence. All stimuli during the conditioning/variable pain block were applied to regions on the *left* arm, to avoid over-stimulation of regions on the right arm. We randomized order of low and high pain stimuli in the conditioning/variable block, and order of audio presentation during testing, across subjects. This resulted in equal numbers of subjects receiving each possible audio order within each group.

Expectancy was assessed with the ERS at time points including post-verbal suggestion, post-conditioning/variable pain, and post-testing (Figure 2). Expectancy ratings for both music and sound analgesia were requested in the no-conditioning group, as we treated music and sound equally within our verbal suggestion, and to provide baseline measures of ERS as compared to conditioned music and sound. Additionally, each subject rated their mood/valence, arousal, and perceived control using the three scales of the Self Assessment Manikin [31], and answered questions about their experience with the pain and audio after all baseline and testing blocks. At the end of the study all participants completed a final questionnaire assessing their belief in their specific treatment's efficacy, as well as providing further details on their experience with both their chosen sound and music samples. Questions were framed to neutrally assess opinion for both the effect of the sound and music samples.

In the music conditioning replication cohort that was enrolled after completion of the initial study, we added an explicit reminder that they would be receiving stimuli identical to that from baseline during the conditioning block to better ensure high expectations of music analgesia. The purpose of this group was to verify the effects of expectancy-enhancement on music analgesia in the first music conditioning group. The same ERS measures were taken as in the original cohort, and in addition we obtained one further ERS score at the end of Session 1 (orange arrow in Figure 2) *prior to* administration of the verbal suggestion for analgesia.

Music and sound sample criteria and choices

To determine individual song choices, we used a list of criteria designed to specify a particular controlled set of participants' personal music choices for analgesia. Prior to coming to the first study visit, all participants were asked to provide a set of songs (each at least 4 minutes long) that they love, had been familiar with for at least a few years, could listen to repeatedly, varied across a range from very relaxing to very energizing, did not evoke specific memories or chills, and that they had not seen the music video for. We excluded songs associated with specific visual memories including music videos in order to concentrate our study more on strong emotions associated with the music itself [4,32], and songs that consistently induced chills to ensure a more even set of strong emotional responses from all participants [1]. Participant songs were screened for these criteria during song rating and characterizing in Session 1. We created 4-min. song excerpts centered on the most favored part of each piece and of length appropriate for the pain trial blocks. To give further background

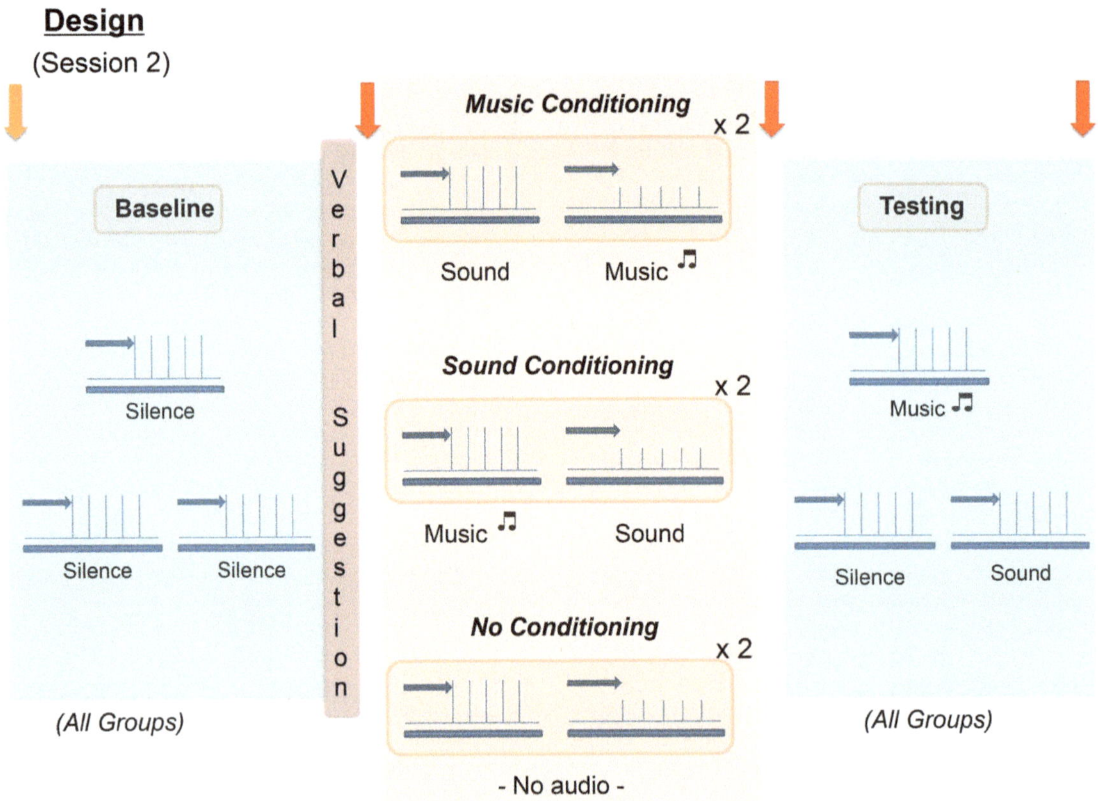

Figure 2. Schematic of Session 2. All subjects first receive identical baseline stimuli on three spots of their right arm. Conditioning groups were then given a verbal suggestion specific to their conditioned audio target, while the no-conditioning group was given a neutral suggestion. All groups then received four blocks of two stimulus intensities, with levels determined during Session 1 (target levels = 20–40 out of 100 and 55–70 out of 100 on the pain intensity VAS). Conditioning groups received lower heat levels when the conditioned audio stimulus was on, while the no-conditioning group received stimuli with silence. All groups were then tested with three audio conditions: music, sound, and silence, in randomized order across participants. Within each set of trials, lead-in arrows represent 1 minute of audio or silence that preceded the start of pain stimuli. In all groups ERS was assessed right after verbal suggestion, then following conditioning/variable pain, and after testing (red arrows). We added one more baseline ERS assessment within the music conditioning replication group at the end of session 1 (orange arrow).

on the participants' musical backgrounds, we excluded those with advanced music training (greater than 3 years of serious voice, instrument, or theory study), while including those with previous common music exposure limited to examples such as "music classes during grade school" or "a couple years of violin class when I was 12". Music preferences included a variety of genres, such as alternative, to country, to pop. On average, participants regarded music as "pretty important" to them.

The non-musical sound samples consisted of alternating, frequency-filtered noise clips that were chosen based on studies where participants perceived filtered noise to be less distressing than white noise [33,34]. During Session 2, all participants chose the song they wanted to listen to during the pain trials prior to their first exposure to audio. A list of these songs can be found as Music List S1.

Analysis

The primary outcomes were pre-post changes in pain intensity and unpleasantness. For the first cohort these data were analyzed using a 3×3 (conditioning by audio type) mixed model analysis of variance (ANOVA) with conditioning (music, sound, or none) as the between-subjects factor, and audio modality (music, sound or silence) as the within-subjects factor. We then compared pain intensity and unpleasantness in the replication cohort with the original music group using a 2×3 (group by audio) mixed model ANOVA. Bonferroni corrections were used for post hoc comparisons following significant main effects.

We examined expectancy in two ways. Participants in the no-conditioning group, where music and sound were presented equally, rated expected relief for both music and sound. These data were analyzed using a 3×2 (time by audio type) repeated measures ANOVA. Participants in the music and sound conditioning groups rated expected relief only for the audio type that was the focus of the verbal suggestion and conditioning. These data were analyzed using a 3×2 (time by conditioning) mixed model ANOVA. Statistical analyses were done using IBM SPSS Statistics version 20. Final sample sizes for sufficient power to detect outcomes were determined during an interim analyses conducted during data collection, based on previous work completed with the current study's methods by the laboratory. Finally, to analyze the semi-free form qualitative interview and survey data, we performed thematic analyses following the procedure and recommendations of Braun and Clark [35] to extract the themes most relevant to our research questions. All data was first coded, then iteratively collated and refined to maximize internal homogeneity and external heterogeneity of final themes. Extracts in the discussion were selected based on the strength of their congruency with the final themes.

Results

We enrolled 58 participants, from which 10 were dropped due to the following factors: the requirement of stable and reliable responses to pain stimuli necessary to perform the quantitative experiments, not wishing to continue, or not following study procedure guidelines. We studied 12 participants in each of four groups for a total of 48 participants (32 females), with average age 27±7. 36 of these comprised the initial cohort for which the main experiment was conducted. 12 participants served as a replication sample for the music conditioning group. All participants completing study procedures were included in the final analyses within originally assigned groups.

Pain Ratings

Examination of the distribution of changes in pain intensity and unpleasantness ratings revealed extreme positive kurtosis for intensity change scores for music (3.99). A box plot revealed one extreme outlier in the music conditioning group. With data from this participant removed, skewness and kurtosis for these six variables were all between +/−1. Hence, subsequent analyses were conducted with data where this one outlier was removed.

Table 1 displays baseline (pre) and test block (post) ratings of pain intensity and unpleasantness. Pre-post changes in these ratings are displayed in Figure 3. The 3×3 ANOVA on changes in pain intensity in the primary cohort revealed a significant main effect for audio type, $F(2,64) = 15.01$, $p<.001$, $eta^2 = .32$. Paired contrasts using a Bonferroni adjustment for multiple contrasts revealed that music decreased pain intensity significantly compared to both sound ($p = .026$) and silence ($p<.001$), whereas the difference between sound and silence failed to reach significance ($p = .059$). Neither the main effect for conditioning nor the conditioning by audio type interaction reached significance. It appears that the superiority of music over sound held regardless of conditioning. The 2×3 ANOVA comparing the original music conditioning group to the replication conditioning group showed a similar main effect for audio type, $F(2,42) = 7.38$, $p = .002$, $eta^2 = .26$, with music decreasing pain ($p = .051$) and silence increasing it ($p = .057$).

The 3×3 ANOVA on changes in pain unpleasantness in the primary cohort revealed a significant main effect for audio type, $F(2,64) = 15.43$, $p<.001$, $eta^2 = .33$. Paired contrasts using a Bonferroni adjustment for multiple contrasts revealed that music decreased pain unpleasantness significantly compared to both sound ($p = .015$) and silence ($p<.001$), and the difference between sound and silence just reached significance ($p = .05$). Neither the main effect for conditioning nor the conditioning by audio type interaction reached significance. For this aspect of the pain experience as well, it also appears that the superiority of music over sound, and of sound over silence at a statistical trend level, held regardless of conditioning. The 2×3 ANOVA comparing the original music conditioning group to the replication conditioning group showed a similar main effect for audio type, $F(2,42) = 8.44$, $p = .001$, $eta^2 = .29$, with music decreasing pain unpleasantness ($p = .013$) and no significant difference between sound and silence increasing it ($p = .174$).

Expectancy

The ANOVA in the no-conditioning group revealed a main effect for audio type, $F(1,11) = 43.70$, $p<.001$, $eta^2 = .80$). These participants expected much greater pain relief from music (Mean = 5.08; SD = 1.69) than from sound (Mean = 2.89; SD = 1.42), an effect that accounted for 80% of the variance. Neither the main effect for time nor the time by audio type interaction approached significance. The ANOVA in the two conditioning groups revealed a main effect for time, $F(2,42) = 6.05$, $p = .005$, $eta^2 = .22$. Polynomial contrast revealed a significant quadratic effect, $F(1,21) = 13.31$, $p = 002$, $eta^2 = .39$, in which expected relief increased following conditioning and then decreased after post-conditioning testing. The main effect for conditioning group did not approach significance. The group by time interaction was not significant ($p = .096$). Expectancy scores are shown in Figure 4. One participant in the music conditioning group failed to provide a pre-conditioning expectancy rating.

Table 1. Average Pain Ratings for all Groups.

Conditioning	Post Audio	Pain Intensity		Pain Unpleasantness	
		pre	*post*	*pre*	*post*
None	Music	55(13)	47(15)	46(20)	37(20)
	Sound	56(16)	56(15)	46(22)	47(20)
	Silence	58(15)	61(14)	48(23)	54(23)
Music	Music	59(19)	59(16)	50(19)	44(16)
	Sound	59(22)	63(16)	48(19)	51(15)
	Silence	57(16)	66(15)	49(16)	54(15)
Sound	Music	50(17)	47(17)	45(23)	42(24)
	Sound	49(14)	49(19)	44(21)	43(23)
	Silence	51(19)	55(20)	44(24)	51(25)
Music replication	Music	55(18)	48(15)	43(24)	35(19)
	Sound	55(15)	55(14)	43(21)	44(22)
	Silence	57(18)	61(14)	44(26)	49(23)

Mean (SD) ratings of pain intensity and unpleasantness for each audio type before and after the conditioning/variable pain phase for both cohorts. Note that all pre-pain stimuli occurred in silence (i.e. pre- ratings for music and sound are given for the corresponding skin spot of stimulation). One outlier subject has been removed from the original music conditioning group (as noted in text).

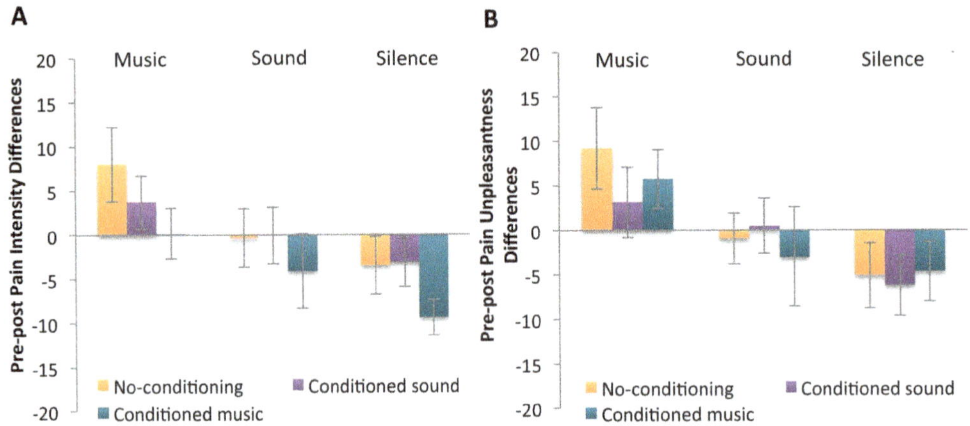

Figure 3. Average pain intensity and unpleasantness changes, all original groups. N = 35. Shown here are pre (baseline) minus post (testing) pain difference scores (mean ± SEM); positive values indicate analgesia. Panel A displays Pain Intensity, panel B displays Pain Unpleasantness.

Discussion

Without conditioned-expectancy enhancement, music had significantly higher measured positive expectancy and was most effective at decreasing pain, followed by sound over silence. Expected relief was boosted in the conditioning groups, however typical corresponding increases in analgesia [26,36–38] were not observed – the significant changes in expectancy did not link to pain relief. Music was the most pain relieving irrespective of conditioning, with enhanced music expectancy adding no further analgesia.

While some routes to analgesia, such as distraction and positive expectations of pain relief, have been seen to be additive [39], our experiment shows that preferred music and conditioning-enhanced expectancy do not appear to be, though our results are tempered by somewhat small group sizes. The powerful relationship individuals had with their music was displayed by the significantly higher expectancy for music in the no-conditioning group that explained 80% of the variance in expectancy ratings. Indeed, these high expectations could be indicative of overlapping mechanisms between music and expectancy-based placebo analgesia that may have precluded an analgesic boost from our conditioning procedure. We saw evidence that musical expectancy [8] and its associations with pleasure were in effect here, as our thematic analysis revealed that subjects regularly identified specific aspects of their songs that would "draw them in" and that they favored. The music selected for use in this experiment could have strongly activated dopaminergic pleasure centers and specifically the nucleus accumbens [5,9], implicated within analgesia as well [40]. These reward pathways could then have interacted at many levels with the opioidergic system to mediate analgesia [7,41,42]. In one preliminary study, results showed that an opiate receptor antagonist could potentially reduce the pleasurable chills response to music [43]; in a later PET study, music-induced chills activated the PAG region, an endogenous source of opiates [1]. Strong evidence exists that placebo analgesia expectations are also a form of reward expectancy [44–46] contributing to pain relief through representation of a more favorable homeostatic state. Thus, we would expect music and expectancy-based placebo analgesia to share at least some common pathways. This may explain in part why boosting expectancy did not necessarily enhance analgesia in our music conditioning group.

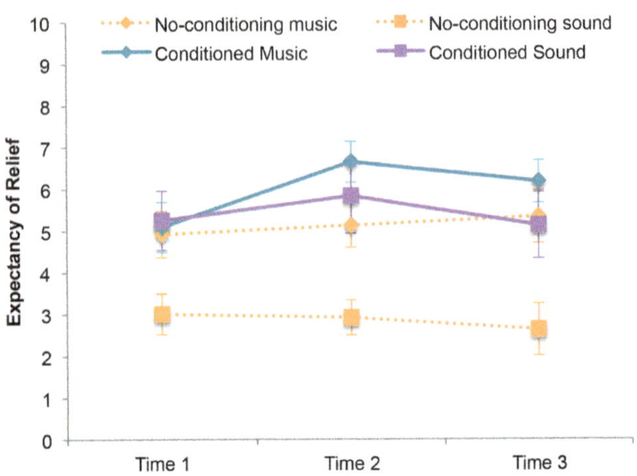

Figure 4. Average expectancy scores in all original groups, across all ERS assessment points. Means ± SEM are shown for N = 35. Time 1 occurs after verbal suggestion but prior to the conditioning phase in the conditioning groups, and prior to the matched variable pain phase in the no- conditioning group. Time 2 occurs immediately after the conditioning/variable pain phase, and Time 3 occurs after testing.

Additionally, the preferred personal music could have yielded maximal experimentally detectable endogenous analgesia in a ceiling effect. We believe that the strength of the analgesic effects were likely due to the latent conditioned relationships subjects had with their songs, leading to a more complex view of music as an analgesic agent. We suggest it can be viewed in the same framework that placebo responses are increasingly being seen in - that of a rich, nuanced set of contextual personal factors. An individual's song becomes connected over time to people, places, and circumstances such that there is a robust latent effect from the history and time spent with the music. Indeed, additional analyses of systematically gathered, qualitative participant experiences revealed themes consistent with those seen in the nascent field of neurobehavioral music research [14]: of *deep relationship with their music: "music has gotten me through a lot of hard times…it moves me regardless of mood, pain, emotion"; "I was really into my song. As in, I felt like I was in my song."*; of *music absorption*, where specific aspects of their music engaged them strongly, akin to Zatorre and Salimpoor's [8] concept of rewarding dynamics of musical expectancies. These "nodes" of pleasure could serve as "waypoints", as one subject described, during the pain experience. Further analyses of our data supported the existence of previously defined analgesic components of music, including perceived control and positive valence [12,13,47,48], and active music usage [49]. Subjects were able to consciously acknowledge bolstered feelings of control and positive valence: *"The specific music I chose makes me feel like I'm going somewhere, and can't be stopped. It makes me feel less vulnerable..."; "Music inherently makes me happy"; "music made me feel...energized and in control of myself"*. These statements were further confirmed by our qualitative review of perceived control and valence in the Self Assessment Manikin results. With respect to increased control, we saw a theme of *active coping and musical distraction* in that many participants reported purposely focusing on the music or that it was effective as a distraction from the pain: *"...chose this music because it was upbeat and energizing, which I knew would distract me"; "I focused on the song, listening to the lyrics and also knowing when the song, and my pain, was going to end"*. Strikingly, the heat pain was even felt to be the distractor rather than the center of attention for one subject: *"If anything it was more bothersome/unpleasant because it distracted me from the music"*. Consistent with previous efforts to define and isolate specific components of music analgesia, it is becoming clear that these factors are all distinct contributors.

We further propose that enhancing expectations for sound may not have boosted analgesia precisely because the conditioning phase, with lowered pain during sound samples, also included trials with powerfully rewarding music. If conditioning based expectancy modulation works through pathways common to music, then the presence of highly personal music during our attempted generation of increased sound expectancy would certainly interfere with that process. It would be akin to trying to show the glow of a lamp when the sun is shining brilliantly into the room. This cognitive conflict brings to mind the framing of belief and its effects on learning that Corlett et al (2010) put forth: "...sculpted connections...predict subsequent states of the internal and external world and respond adaptively; however, should that next state be surprising, novel or uncertain new learning is required." [50]. Most likely it was quite surprising for subjects in this group to feel greater pain to music than sound when their previous belief in their music undoubtedly would lead them to expect otherwise. Thus, this kind of prediction error could also have interfered with the manipulation process. Overall the findings indicate that social suggestion and first-hand experience of a phenomenon can be powerful enough to influence conscious expectation, but other factors from music and its long conditioned history with individuals may dominate endogenous mechanisms of pain relief. There appears to be much more behind music analgesia not captured by reports on expectancy scales. Our results show that two media (music and sound) of similarly boosted expectancy can still perform very differently for pain relief.

One caveat to mention is the somatotopic specificity that has been shown for placebo analgesia [28], which may have limited the conditioning effect possible in our paradigm to the left arm (where conditioning was carried out), versus the right testing arm. However, we believe it is unlikely that subjects' higher expectations post-conditioning would not transfer over to the right arm for the duration of the final three testing spots, as placebo analgesia is mainly mediated through the central nervous system and can thereby have effects in any part of the body. Still, future experiments may examine the conditioning effects when the test skin areas can be closer to the conditioning spots. An additional limitation of this experiment is that we do not know if non-musical sound can be conditioned when music is not present in the conditioning and testing phases; we note also that our small sample size may have precluded enough power for significance in some of our more specific comparisons. However, that sound expectancy was successfully boosted indicates that the procedure was not ineffective. With respect to the conditioning procedure, it is possible that the temperature difference must be even greater to enhance analgesia, though a difference too great can garner suspicion that a manipulation has taken place. Finally, though the interaction between time and group for the expectancy boost did not reach significance, we saw a trend towards a difference between music and sound conditioning. We speculate that with larger groups, future studies may see an additional boost to music analgesia from the conditioning procedure after all.

Conclusion

On the surface it seems that music should be amenable as a modulation target for the same reasons contextual placebo factors are being discussed for maximal clinical effect. Yet here, the combination of music with an expectancy-mediated conditioning procedure showed that music analgesia is not improved by these methods. On its own it performed just as well as it did following conditioning. Thus, despite the likely existence of many converging mechanisms of endogenous analgesia, music and expectancy-based placebo analgesia were not additive or synergistic in this study.

In her review, Tracey [7] put forth an intriguing consideration for the amelioration of pain: "...closely related to the subjective interpretation of a sensory stimulus is the concept of meaning...Even suffering can be rewarding if it has meaning to the sufferer." Music is indeed a medium filled with deep personal meaning, following closely alongside most of us as we wind our ways through life. With continued systematic study of healing components, we may still learn how to create whole new combinations of environments and contextual elements that lead to the alleviation of suffering.

Supporting Information

Checklist S1 CONSORT checklist for reporting randomized trials.
(DOC)

Music List S1 A list of the final song choices (with artist listed) that participants of each group chose to listen to during pain testing blocks in Session 2.
(DOCX)

Protocol S1 The full original detailed protocol submitted to the Partners Human Research Committee.
(DOC)

Acknowledgments

The authors would like to acknowledge the contributions of Rosa Spaeth, who assisted with data analysis and interpretation, and of Drs. Gregory Fricchione, M. Christian Brown, and Anne Blood, who assisted in the guidance of this work. We also acknowledge Amanda Cook, Alex Cheetham, and Sonya Freeman for their help in facilitating protocol approval and volunteer recruiting.

Author Contributions

Conceived and designed the experiments: CH JK IK RLG. Performed the experiments: CH. Analyzed the data: CH IK RRE RLG. Contributed reagents/materials/analysis tools: JK. Wrote the paper: CH IK KBJ TJK RLG.

References

1. Blood AJ, Zatorre RJ (2001) Intensely pleasurable responses to music correlate with activity in brain regions implicated in reward and emotion. Proc Natl Acad Sci U S A 98: 11818–11823.
2. Koelsch S, Fritz T, DY VC, Muller K, Friederici AD (2006) Investigating emotion with music: an fMRI study. Hum Brain Mapp 27: 239–250.
3. Benedetti F, Carlino E, Pollo A (2011) How placebos change the patient's brain. Neuropsychopharmacology 36: 339–354.
4. Juslin PN, Vastfjall D (2008) Emotional responses to music: the need to consider underlying mechanisms. Behav Brain Sci 31: 559–575; discussion 575–621.
5. Salimpoor VN, Benovoy M, Larcher K, Dagher A, Zatorre RJ (2011) Anatomically distinct dopamine release during anticipation and experience of peak emotion to music. Nat Neurosci 14: 257–262.
6. Koelsch S (2009) A neuroscientific perspective on music therapy. Ann N Y Acad Sci 1169: 374–384.
7. Leknes S, Tracey I (2008) A common neurobiology for pain and pleasure. Nat Rev Neurosci 9: 314–320.
8. Zatorre RJ, Salimpoor VN (2013) From perception to pleasure: Music and its neural substrates. Proc Natl Acad Sci U S A 110 Suppl 2: 10430–10437.
9. Salimpoor VN, van den Bosch I, Kovacevic N, McIntosh AR, Dagher A, et al. (2013) Interactions between the nucleus accumbens and auditory cortices predict music reward value. Science 340: 216–219.
10. Gabrielsson A (2001) Emotions in Strong Experiences with Music. In: Juslin PN, Sloboda JA, editors. Music and Emotion: Theory and Research. New York: Oxford University Press.
11. Gardner WJ, Licklider JC, Weisz AZ (1960) Suppression of pain by sound. Science 132: 32–33.
12. Roy M, Peretz I, Rainville P (2008) Emotional valence contributes to music-induced analgesia. Pain 134: 140–147.
13. Perlini AH, Viita KA (1996) Audioanalgesia in the Control of Experimental Pain. Canadian Journal of Behavioural Science 28: 292–301.
14. Bernatzky G, Presch M, Anderson M, Panksepp J (2011) Emotional foundations of music as a non-pharmacological pain management tool in modern medicine. Neurosci Biobehav Rev 35: 1989–1999.
15. Finniss DG, Kaptchuk TJ, Miller F, Benedetti F (2010) Biological, clinical, and ethical advances of placebo effects. Lancet 375: 686–695.
16. Kaptchuk TJ, Kelley JM, Conboy LA, Davis RB, Kerr CE, et al. (2008) Components of placebo effect: randomised controlled trial in patients with irritable bowel syndrome. BMJ 336: 999–1003.
17. Hall KT, Lembo AJ, Kirsch I, Ziogas DC, Douaiher J, et al. (2012) Catechol-O-methyltransferase val158met polymorphism predicts placebo effect in irritable bowel syndrome. PLoS One 7: e48135.
18. Kong J, Gollub RL, Rosman IS, Webb JM, Vangel MG, et al. (2006) Brain activity associated with expectancy-enhanced placebo analgesia as measured by functional magnetic resonance imaging. J Neurosci 26: 381–388.
19. Montgomery GH, Kirsch I (1997) Classical conditioning and the placebo effect. Pain 72: 107–113.
20. Kirsch I (2000) The response set theory of hypnosis. Am J Clin Hypn 42: 274–292.
21. Kong J, Gollub RL, Polich G, Kirsch I, Laviolette P, et al. (2008) A functional magnetic resonance imaging study on the neural mechanisms of hyperalgesic nocebo effect. J Neurosci 28: 13354–13362.
22. Bingel U, Wanigasekera V, Wiech K, Ni Mhuircheartaigh R, Lee MC, et al. (2011) The effect of treatment expectation on drug efficacy: imaging the analgesic benefit of the opioid remifentanil. Sci Transl Med 3: 70ra14.
23. Laverdure-Dupont D, Rainville P, Montplaisir J, Lavigne G (2009) Changes in rapid eye movement sleep associated with placebo-induced expectations and analgesia. J Neurosci 29: 11745–11752.
24. Kong J, Spaeth R, Cook A, Kirsch I, Claggett B, et al. (2013) Are all placebo effects equal? Placebo pills, sham acupuncture, cue conditioning and their association. PLoS One 8: e67485.
25. Voudouris NJ, Peck CL, Coleman G (1989) Conditioned response models of placebo phenomena: further support. Pain 38: 109–116.
26. Voudouris NJ, Peck CL, Coleman G (1990) The role of conditioning and verbal expectancy in the placebo response. Pain 43: 121–128.
27. Benedetti F, Pollo A, Lopiano L, Lanotte M, Vighetti S, et al. (2003) Conscious expectation and unconscious conditioning in analgesic, motor, and hormonal placebo/nocebo responses. J Neurosci 23: 4315–4323.
28. Price DD, Milling LS, Kirsch I, Duff A, Montgomery GH, et al. (1999) An analysis of factors that contribute to the magnitude of placebo analgesia in an experimental paradigm. Pain 83: 147–156.
29. Geisser ME, Roth RS, Robinson ME (1997) Assessing depression among persons with chronic pain using the Center for Epidemiological Studies-Depression Scale and the Beck Depression Inventory: a comparative analysis. Clin J Pain 13: 163–170.
30. Turner JA, Romano JM (1984) Self-report screening measures for depression in chronic pain patients. J Clin Psychol 40: 909–913.
31. Bradley MM, Lang PJ (1994) Measuring emotion: the Self-Assessment Manikin and the Semantic Differential. J Behav Ther Exp Psychiatry 25: 49–59.
32. Janata P (2009) The neural architecture of music-evoked autobiographical memories. Cereb Cortex 19: 2579–2594.
33. Villarreal EA, Brattico E, Vase L, Ostergaard L, Vuust P (2012) Superior analgesic effect of an active distraction versus pleasant unfamiliar sounds and music: the influence of emotion and cognitive style. PLoS One 7: e29397.
34. Roy M, Lebuis A, Hugueville L, Peretz I, Rainville P (2012) Spinal modulation of nociception by music. Eur J Pain 16: 870–877.
35. Braun V, Clarke V (2006) Using thematic analysis in psychology. Qualitative Research in Psychology 3: 77–101.
36. Kong J, Kaptchuk TJ, Polich G, Kirsch I, Vangel M, et al. (2009) Expectancy and treatment interactions: a dissociation between acupuncture analgesia and expectancy evoked placebo analgesia. Neuroimage 45: 940–949.
37. Amanzio M, Benedetti F (1999) Neuropharmacological dissection of placebo analgesia: expectation-activated opioid systems versus conditioning-activated specific subsystems. J Neurosci 19: 484–494.
38. Benedetti F, Arduino C, Amanzio M (1999) Somatotopic activation of opioid systems by target-directed expectations of analgesia. J Neurosci 19: 3639–3648.
39. Buhle JT, Stevens BL, Friedman JJ, Wager TD (2012) Distraction and placebo: two separate routes to pain control. Psychol Sci 23: 246–253.
40. Baliki MN, Geha PY, Fields HL, Apkarian AV (2010) Predicting value of pain and analgesia: nucleus accumbens response to noxious stimuli changes in the presence of chronic pain. Neuron 66: 149–160.
41. Scott DJ, Stohler CS, Egnatuk CM, Wang H, Koeppe RA, et al. (2007) Individual differences in reward responding explain placebo-induced expectations and effects. Neuron 55: 325–336.
42. Wager TD, Scott DJ, Zubieta JK (2007) Placebo effects on human mu-opioid activity during pain. Proc Natl Acad Sci U S A 104: 11056–11061.
43. Goldstein A (1980) Thrills in response to music and other stimuli. Physiological Psychology 8: 126–129.
44. de la Fuente-Fernandez R, Ruth TJ, Sossi V, Schulzer M, Calne DB, et al. (2001) Expectation and dopamine release: mechanism of the placebo effect in Parkinson's disease. Science 293: 1164–1166.
45. Lidstone SC, Schulzer M, Dinelle K, Mak E, Sossi V, et al. (2010) Effects of expectation on placebo-induced dopamine release in Parkinson disease. Arch Gen Psychiatry 67: 857–865.
46. Petrovic P, Dietrich T, Fransson P, Andersson J, Carlsson K, et al. (2005) Placebo in emotional processing–induced expectations of anxiety relief activate a generalized modulatory network. Neuron 46: 957–969.
47. Mitchell LA, MacDonald RA (2006) An experimental investigation of the effects of preferred and relaxing music listening on pain perception. J Music Ther 43: 295–316.
48. Mitchell LA, MacDonald RA, Brodie EE (2006) A comparison of the effects of preferred music, arithmetic and humour on cold pressor pain. Eur J Pain 10: 343–351.
49. Sloboda JA, O'neill SA (2001) Emotions in Everyday Listening to Music. In: Juslin PN, Sloboda JA, editors. Music and Emotion: Theory and Research. New York: Oxford University Press.
50. Corlett PR, Taylor JR, Wang XJ, Fletcher PC, Krystal JH (2010) Toward a neurobiology of delusions. Prog Neurobiol 92: 345–369.

Permissions

All chapters in this book were first published in PLOS ONE, by The Public Library of Science; hereby published with permission under the Creative Commons Attribution License or equivalent. Every chapter published in this book has been scrutinized by our experts. Their significance has been extensively debated. The topics covered herein carry significant findings which will fuel the growth of the discipline. They may even be implemented as practical applications or may be referred to as a beginning point for another development.

The contributors of this book come from diverse backgrounds, making this book a truly international effort. This book will bring forth new frontiers with its revolutionizing research information and detailed analysis of the nascent developments around the world.

We would like to thank all the contributing authors for lending their expertise to make the book truly unique. They have played a crucial role in the development of this book. Without their invaluable contributions this book wouldn't have been possible. They have made vital efforts to compile up to date information on the varied aspects of this subject to make this book a valuable addition to the collection of many professionals and students.

This book was conceptualized with the vision of imparting up-to-date information and advanced data in this field. To ensure the same, a matchless editorial board was set up. Every individual on the board went through rigorous rounds of assessment to prove their worth. After which they invested a large part of their time researching and compiling the most relevant data for our readers.

The editorial board has been involved in producing this book since its inception. They have spent rigorous hours researching and exploring the diverse topics which have resulted in the successful publishing of this book. They have passed on their knowledge of decades through this book. To expedite this challenging task, the publisher supported the team at every step. A small team of assistant editors was also appointed to further simplify the editing procedure and attain best results for the readers.

Apart from the editorial board, the designing team has also invested a significant amount of their time in understanding the subject and creating the most relevant covers. They scrutinized every image to scout for the most suitable representation of the subject and create an appropriate cover for the book.

The publishing team has been an ardent support to the editorial, designing and production team. Their endless efforts to recruit the best for this project, has resulted in the accomplishment of this book. They are a veteran in the field of academics and their pool of knowledge is as vast as their experience in printing. Their expertise and guidance has proved useful at every step. Their uncompromising quality standards have made this book an exceptional effort. Their encouragement from time to time has been an inspiration for everyone.

The publisher and the editorial board hope that this book will prove to be a valuable piece of knowledge for researchers, students, practitioners and scholars across the globe.

List of Contributors

Mei-Chi Chang and Ru-Hsiu Cheng
Biomedical Science Team, Chang Gung University of Science and Technology, Taoyuan,Taiwan

Hsiao-Hua Chang, Tong-Mei Wang, Jiiang-Huei Jeng and Chien-Yang Yeh
Laboratory of Pharmacology & Toxicology, Graduate Institute of Clinical Dentistry and Department of Dentistry, National Taiwan University Hospital and National Taiwan University Medical College, Taipei, Taiwan

Chiu-Po Chan and Sin-Yuet Yeung
Department of Dentistry, Chang Gung Memorial Hospital and Chang Gung University, Taipei, Taiwan

Bor-Ru Lin
Department of Diagnotherapeutics, National Taiwan University Hospital, Taipei, Taiwan

Bradley H. Lee, John Thomas Chan, Obhi Hazarika and Jeffrey W. Sall
Department of Anesthesia and Perioperative Care, University of California San Francisco, San Francisco, California, Unites States of America

Laszlo Vutskits
Department of Anesthesiology, Pharmacology and Intensive Care, University Hospital of Geneva, Geneva, Switzerland

Stephanie White
Department of Anesthesia, University of Iowa, Iowa City, Iowa, United States of America

Blanca Marquez de Prado
Department of Anesthesia, University of Iowa, Iowa City, Iowa, United States of America
Department of Molecular Physiology and Biophysics, University of Iowa, Iowa City, Iowa, United States of America

Andrew F. Russo
Department of Molecular Physiology and Biophysics, University of Iowa, Iowa City, Iowa, United States of America

Donna L. Hammond
Department of Anesthesia, University of Iowa, Iowa City, Iowa, United States of America
Department of Pharmacology, University of Iowa, Iowa City, Iowa, United States of America

Young Bin Joo, So-Young Bang and Tae-Hwan Kim
Department of Rheumatology, Hanyang University Hospital for Rheumatic Diseases, Seoul, Republic of Korea

Seung-Cheol Shim
Division of Rheumatology, Daejeon Rheumatoid & Degenerative Arthritis Center, Chungnam National University Hospital, Daejeon, Republic of Korea

Seunghun Lee and Kyung Bin Joo
Department of Radiology, Hanyang University Hospital for Rheumatic Diseases, Seoul, Republic of Korea

Jong Heon Kim
Department of Orthopedics, Hanyang University Hospital for Rheumatic Diseases, Seoul, Republic of Korea

Hye Joon Min
Department of anthropology, Cornell University, Ithaca, New York, United States of America

Proton Rahman
Department of Rheumatology, Memorial University, St. Clare's Mercy Hospital, St. John's, Newfoundland, Canada

Robert D. Inman
Division of Rheumatology, University of Toronto, Toronto Western Hospital, Toronto, Ontario, Canada

Milisa Blagojevic-Bucknall, Christian D. Mallen and Kate M. Dunn
Arthritis Research UK Primary Care Centre, Keele University, Keele, United Kingdom

Mujahed Shraim
Arthritis Research UK Primary Care Centre, Keele University, Keele, United Kingdom
Work Environment Department, University of Massachusetts Lowell, Lowell,
Massachusetts, United States of America
Center for Disability Research, Liberty Mutual Research Institute for Safety, Hopkinton, Massachusetts, United States of America

Michael R. Due, Aaron L. Randolph and Matthew S. Ripsch
Department of Anesthesia, Indiana University School of Medicine, Indianapolis, Indiana, United States of America

Fletcher A. White
Department of Anesthesia, Indiana University School of Medicine, Indianapolis, Indiana, United States of America
Department of Pharmacology and Toxicology, Indiana University School of Medicine, Indianapolis, Indiana, United States of America

Xiao-Fang Yang
Department of Pharmacology, College of Medicine, University of Arizona, Tucson, Arizona, United States of America

Yohance M. Allette and Erik T. Dustrude
Department of Cell Biology and Anatomy, Indiana University School of Medicine, Indianapolis, Indiana, United States of America

Sarah M. Wilson
Program in Medical Neurosciences, Paul and Carole Stark Neurosciences Research Institute, Indiana University School of Medicine, Indianapolis, Indiana, United States of America

Rajesh Khanna
Department of Pharmacology, College of Medicine, University of Arizona, Tucson, Arizona, United States of America
Department of Pharmacology and Toxicology, Indiana University School of Medicine, Indianapolis, Indiana, United States of America

Wei-Li Cao and Shi-Hai Xia
Postgraduate Training Base, Affiliated Hospital of Logistics University of the Chinese People's Armed Police Forces, Liaoning Medical University, Jinzhou, China,
Department of Hepatopancreatobiliary and Splenic Medicine, Affiliated Hospital of Logistics University of the Chinese People's Armed Police Forces, Tianjin, China

Wen-Shan Yan
Postgraduate Training Base, Affiliated Hospital of Logistics University of the Chinese People's Armed Police Forces, Liaoning Medical University, Jinzhou, China
Department of Endemic Area of Orthopedic Center Section III, Affiliated Hospital of Logistics University of the Chinese People's Armed Police Forces, Tianjin, China

Xiao-Hui Xiang and Kai Chen
Department of Hepatopancreatobiliary and Splenic Medicine, Affiliated Hospital of Logistics University of the Chinese People's Armed Police Forces, Tianjin, China

Eric W. de Heer
TopClinical Center for Body, Mind, and Health, GGz Breburg Tilburg, Tilburg, The Netherlands
Tilburg School of Behavioral and Social Sciences, Tranzo Department, University of Tilburg, Tilburg, The Netherlands

Marloes M. J. G. Gerrits and Brenda W. J. H. Penninx
Department of Psychiatry, EMGO Institute for Health and Care research, VU University Medical Centre, Amsterdam, The Netherlands

Aartjan T. F. Beekman
Department of Psychiatry, EMGO Institute for Health and Care research, VU University Medical Centre, Amsterdam, The Netherlands
GGZ inGeest, Mental Health Institute, Amsterdam, The Netherlands

Jack Dekker
Arkin, Mental Health Institute, Amsterdam, The Netherlands
Department of Clinical
Psychology, VU University, Amsterdam, The Netherlands

Harm W. J. van Marwijk
Department of General Practice, EMGO Institute for Health and Care Research, VU University Medical Centre, Amsterdam, The Netherlands

Margot W. M. de Waal
Department of Public Health and Primary Care, Leiden university Medical Centre, Leiden, The Netherlands

Philip Spinhoven
Institute of Psychology, Leiden University, Leiden, The Netherlands
Department of Psychiatry, Leiden University Medical Centre, Leiden, The Netherlands

Christina M. van der Feltz-Cornelis
TopClinical Center for Body, Mind, and Health, GGz Breburg Tilburg, Tilburg, The Netherlands
Tilburg School of Behavioral and Social Sciences, Tranzo Department, University of Tilburg, Tilburg, The Netherlands
Trimbos Institute, Utrecht, the Netherlands

Rogelio A. Coronado and Corey B. Simon
Department of Physical Therapy, University of Florida, Gainesville, Florida, United States of America

Carolina Valencia
Department of Applied Medicine and Rehabilitation, Indiana State University, Terra Haute, Indiana, Unites States of America

Jeffrey J. Parr
Department of Sports Medicine and Nutrition, University of Pittsburgh, Pittsburgh, Pennsylvania, United States of America

Paul A. Borsa
Department of Applied Physiology and Kinesiology, University of Florida, Gainesville, Florida, United States of America

Steven Z. George
Department of Physical Therapy, University of Florida, Gainesville, Florida, United States of America
Center for Pain Research and Behavioral Health, University of Florida, Gainesville, Florida, United States of America

Qian Sun, Yan Li
Department of gastroenterology, Shengjing Hospital Affiliated to China Medical University, Shenyang, Liaoning, China

Xavier Janssens and Filip De Keyser
Department of Rheumatology, Ghent University Hospital, Ghent, Belgium

Saskia Decuman
Department of Rheumatology, Ghent University Hospital, Ghent, Belgium
Department of Internal Medicine, Ghent University, Ghent, Belgium

Chongfei Yang, Lifeng Yu, Juliang Zhang, Qingsheng Zhu and Jinyu Zhu
Institute of Orthopaedic Surgery, Xijing Hospital, Fourth Military Medical University, Xi'an, China

Lingbo Kong and Dingjun Hao
Hong-Hui Hospital, Xi'an Jiaotong University College of Medicine,
Xi'an, China

Rui Ma
Department of Anesthesiology, Xijing Hospital, Fourth Military Medical University, Xi'an, China

Sarah McDavid, Mary Beth Bauer and Rebecca L. Brindley
Department of Anesthesiology, Vanderbilt University School of Medicine, Nashville, Tennessee, United States of America

Mark L. Jewell
Department of Pharmacology, Vanderbilt University School of Medicine, Nashville, Tennessee, United States of America

Kevin P. M. Currie
Department of Anesthesiology, Department of Pharmacology, and Vanderbilt Brain
Institute, Vanderbilt University School of Medicine, Nashville, Tennessee, United States of America

Shingo Matsuura, Kinuyo Ohara, Hiroki Komiya and Tetsuro Watase
Department of Endodontics, Nihon University School of Dentistry, Tokyo, Japan

Kohei Shimizu, Bunnai Ogiso and Keisuke Hatori
Department of Endodontics, Nihon University School of Dentistry, Tokyo, Japan
Divisions of Advanced Dental Treatment, Dental Research Center, Nihon University School of Dentistry, Tokyo, Japan

Kunihito Matsumoto
Department of Radiology, Nihon University School of Dentistry, Tokyo, Japan
Divisions of Advanced Dental Treatment, Dental Research Center, Nihon University School of Dentistry, Tokyo, Japan

Noboru Noma
Department of Oral Diagnosis, Nihon University School of Dentistry, Tokyo, Japan
Divisions of Clinical Research, Dental Research Center, Nihon University School of Dentistry, Tokyo, Japan

Yoshiyuki Tsuboi and Masamichi Shinoda
Department of Physiology, Nihon University School of Dentistry, Tokyo, Japan
Division of Functional Morphology, Dental Research Center, Nihon University School of Dentistry, Tokyo, Japan

Yuka Nakaya
Department of Oral Diagnosis, Nihon University School of Dentistry, Tokyo, Japan

Koichi Iwata
Department of Physiology, Nihon University School of Dentistry, Tokyo, Japan
Division of Functional Morphology, Dental Research Center, Nihon University School of Dentistry, Tokyo, Japan
Division of Applied System Neuroscience Advanced Medical Research Center, Nihon University Graduate School of Medical Science, Tokyo, Japan

Won-Mo Jung and Christian Wallraven
Department of Brain and Cognitive Engineering, Korea University, Seoul, Korea

Younbyoung Chae
Department of Brain and Cognitive Engineering, Korea University, Seoul, Korea
Acupuncture and Meridian Science Research Center, College of Korean Medicine,
Kyung Hee University, Seoul, Korea

In-Seon Lee, Hyejung Lee and Hi-Joon Park
Acupuncture and Meridian Science Research Center, College of Korean Medicine,
Kyung Hee University, Seoul, Korea

Dong-Seon Chang
Department of Human Perception, Cognition and Action, Max Planck Institute for Biological Cybernetics, Tu¨ bingen, Germany

Vitaly Napadow
Martinos Center for Biomedical Imaging, Massachusetts General Hospital, Harvard Medical School, Charlestown, Massachusetts, United States of America
Department of Biomedical Engineering, Kyunghee University, Yongin, Korea

Sulei Wang and Hui Yang
Department of Neurology, Nanjing Drum Tower Hospital Clinical College of Traditional Chinese and Western Medicine, Nanjing University of Chinese Medicine, Nanjing, P. R. China

Linjie Yu, Jiali Jin, Lai Qian and Hui Zhao
Department of Neurology, Affiliated Drum Tower Hospital of Nanjing University Medical School, Nanjing, P. R. China

Yun Xu and Xiaolei Zhu
Department of Neurology, Nanjing Drum Tower Hospital Clinical College of Traditional Chinese and Western Medicine, Nanjing University of Chinese Medicine, Nanjing, P. R. China
Department of Neurology, Affiliated Drum Tower Hospital of Nanjing University Medical School, Nanjing, P. R. China

Amanda Clarke and Derek Jones
School of Health, Community and Education Studies, Northumbria University, Newcastle, United Kingdom

Denis Martin
Health and Social Care Institute, Teesside University, Middlesbrough, United Kingdom

Patricia Schofield
School of Health and Social Care, University of Greenwich, London, United Kingdom,

Geraldine Anthony and Blair H. Smith
Medical Research Institute, University of Dundee, Dundee, United Kingdom

Paul McNamee and Denise Gray
chool of Medicine and Dentistry, University of Aberdeen, Aberdeen, United Kingdom

Divya Chander
Department of Anesthesiology, Perioperative and Pain Medicine, Stanford University School of Medicine, Stanford, California, United States of America

Paul S. García
Department of Anesthesiology, Atlanta VA Medical Center/Emory University, Atlanta, Georgia, United States of America

Jono N. MacColl, Sam Illing and Jamie W. Sleigh
Department of Anaesthesia, Waikato Clinical School, University of Auckland, Hamilton, New Zealand

Michihiro Osumi
Department of Neurorehabilitation, Graduate School of Health Science, Kio University, Nara, Japan
Neurocognitive Rehabilitation Center, Setsunan General Hospital, Osaka, Japan

Ryota Imai, Kozo Ueta, Satoshi Nobusako and Shu Morioka
Department of Neurorehabilitation, Graduate School of Health Science, Kio University, Nara, Japan

Anna H. Le, Luis A. Bonachea and Shelley L. Cargill
Department of Biological Sciences, San Jose´ State University, San Jose´ , California, United States of America

Jaime L. Watson, Tamara J. Hala, Rajarshi Putatunda, Daniel Sannie and Angelo C. Lepore
Department of Neuroscience, Farber Institute for Neurosciences, Sidney Kimmel Medical College at Thomas Jefferson University, Philadelphia, Pennsylvania, United States of America

Simon Kessner
Department of Neurology, University Medical Center Hamburg-Eppendorf, Hamburg, Germany

Katarina Forkmann
Department of Neurology, University Hospital Essen, University Duisburg-Essen, Essen, German

Christoph Ritter and Ulrike Bingel
Department of Neurology, University Medical Center Hamburg-Eppendorf, Hamburg, Germany
Department of Neurology, University Hospital Essen, University Duisburg-Essen, Essen, Germany

Katja Wiech
Nuffield Department of Clinical Neurosciences, John Radcliffe Hospital, University of Oxford, Oxford, United Kingdom, 4 Oxford Centre for Functional Magnetic Resonance Imaging of the Brain, Nuffield Department of Clinical Neurosciences, John Radcliffe Hospital, University of Oxford, Oxford, United Kingdom

Markus Ploner
Department of Neurology, Technische Universität München, Munich, Germany

Christine Hsieh and Jian Kong
Department of Psychiatry, Massachusetts General Hospital and Harvard Medical School, Boston, Massachusetts, United States of America

Karin B. Jensen and Randy L. Gollub
Department of Psychiatry, Massachusetts General Hospital and Harvard Medical School, Boston, Massachusetts, United States of America
Department of Radiology, Athinoula A. Martinos Center for Biomedical Imaging and Massachusetts General Hospital, Charlestown, Massachusetts, United States of America

Irving Kirsch
Program in Placebo Studies and the Therapeutic Encounter (PiPS), Harvard Medical School and Beth Israel Deaconess Medical Center, Boston, Massachusetts, United States of America
Department of Psychology, Plymouth University, Plymouth, United Kingdom

Robert R. Edwards
Department of Anesthesiology, Brigham and Women's Hospital, Boston, Massachusetts, United States of America

Ted J. Kaptchuk
Program in Placebo Studies and the Therapeutic Encounter (PiPS), Harvard Medical School and Beth Israel Deaconess Medical Center, Boston, Massachusetts, United States of America

Index